Advanced Therapeutics in Pain Medicine

T0239570

Advanced Therapeutics in Pain Medicine

Edited by
Sahar Swidan
Matthew Bennett

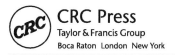

CRC Press
Taylor & Francis Group
Boca Raton London New York

CRC Press is an imprint of the
Taylor & Francis Group, an **informa** business

First edition published 2021
by CRC Press
6000 Broken Sound Parkway NW, Suite 300, Boca Raton, FL 33487-2742

and by CRC Press
2 Park Square, Milton Park, Abingdon, Oxon, OX14 4RN

© 2021 Taylor & Francis Group, LLC

CRC Press is an imprint of Taylor & Francis Group, LLC

Library of Congress Cataloging-in-Publication Data

Names: Swidan, Sahar, editor. | Bennett, Matthew (Matthew Thomas), editor.
Title: Advanced therapeutics in pain medicine / edited by Sahar Swidan, Matthew Bennett.
Description: First edition. | Boca Raton : CRC Press, 2021. | Includes bibliographical references and index. | Summary: "Chronic pain places a tremendous burden on both the patient and the healthcare system. The use of opioids to address pain has resulted in negative impacts. As practitioners work to undo the current opioid crisis, options to manage pain need a new approach. Advanced Therapeutics in Pain Medicine offers pioneering approaches to this intransigent problem providing a functional medicine approach toward treating pain. This book is dedicated to the advancement of non-opioid therapeutic options that offer real progress in reaching a future of better pain management. With an emphasis on pathophysiology, chapters review various types of pain and propose comprehensive treatment plans. These include manual therapies, novel pharmacologic and plant-based approaches, hormonal effects on pain pathways, as well as psychological and lifestyle interventions"-- Provided by publisher.
Identifiers: LCCN 2020044040 | ISBN 9781138585560 (hbk) | ISBN 9780367637989 (pbk) | ISBN 9780429504891 (ebk)
Subjects: MESH: Chronic Pain--therapy | Chronic Pain--physiopathology | Pain Management
Classification: LCC RB127 | NLM WL 704.6 | DDC 616/.0472--dc23
LC record available at https://lccn.loc.gov/2020044040

ISBN: 9781138585560 (hbk)
ISBN: 9780367637989 (pbk)
ISBN: 9780429504891 (ebk)

Typeset in Times
by Deanta Global Publishing Services, Chennai, India

Contents

Preface

Chronic pain is a crippling problem for society. According to the Centers for Disease Control and Prevention, more than one in five adults in the United States experiences chronic pain.[1] That is 50 million in the United States alone. Eight percent of the United States population has high-impact pain that is so severe it frequently limits life or work activities.[1] This places chronic pain as a leading medical condition and the main cause of disability worldwide. More patients suffer from chronic pain than diabetes, coronary heart disease, stroke, and cancer. Why are we doing so poorly in treating this condition?

We have done very well in treating acute pain. We have amazing pharmaceuticals that blunt acute pain exceptionally well, and treatment of acute pain has allowed for so many advancements in traditional western medicine—including surgical intervention, fracture care, and wound care. Our initial understanding of chronic pain was that it was acute pain that just did not subside. Understandably, we leaned heavily on the same pharmaceuticals for chronic pain as we used in acute pain—opioids.

Opioids work very well in the short term, but opioids seem to fail in the long run for a large number of people. Opioid dependency is a reliably expected outcome. Unfortunately, opioid misuse occurs in 21%–29% of users, and 8%–12% develop an overt opioid use disorder.[2] Between 1999 and 2018 nearly 450,000 people died from prescribed and illicit opioid overdose.[3] It is so tragic that so much pain and misery has been wrought from attempts to treat suffering.

There have been enormous regulatory pressures to stop using opioids. But what would come next for patients? Many providers and patients have relied on opioids as their only or most important tool for treating pain. Now this tool was being taken away. Should patients just live with chronic pain? There were many reports of patients being rapidly tapered from opioids with no real plan for next steps for pain treatment. Our personal clinical practices saw a large influx of these types of patients, some of whom had been outright abandoned.

There is a subset of patients with chronic pain who do very well with chronic opioid therapy. In our experience, this is more the exception than the rule. We agree with the Centers for Disease Control and Prevention that this subset of patients requires intense monitoring for harm reduction strategies. It is important to keep a clear eye on functional outcomes in this population as many patients see diminishing results over time.

Providers have traditionally been trained to treat the symptom of pain without necessarily understanding why the pain phenotype was there. So, where did it come from? Does all pain have the same cause? The same physiology? Our best understanding of the current studies on chronic pain explains that the immune, neurologic, and endocrine systems are interacting in a dysfunctional manner. So might there be a better way to manage pain instead of aiming all of our attention at the mu-opioid receptor?

If we start to think about pain from a systems biology or metabolic approach, it would require us to revisit our basic science years and remember some pain pathways. Those foundational training years were critical as we learned the interplay of all body systems and the physiological bases of health and disease. We must look at our patients from a unique perspective and take into account the entire ecosystem and how to best modulate it to treat chronic pain and not just band-aid the symptom. If we consider pain as a phenotypic expression of multiple complex systems, a one-size fits all approach probably will not suffice. We have seen this in clinical settings, and we believe this helps to explain our failure in treating chronic non-malignant pain. We will likely need to personalize the approach for each patient and address pain as "The N of 1 paradigm."

For a little under a decade, Dr. Sahar Swidan and I have discussed non-opioid treatment options for our chronic pain patients. We both have ample clinical experience in treating patients with chronic pain. As an orthopedic spine surgeon, I have taken a keen interest in the physiology of chronic pain, which was rooted in my fellowship training at the multi-disciplinary Texas Back

Institute where we embraced the use of neuromodulation and other modalities for chronic pain states. Sahar has spent many years working with medical teams weaning patients from ineffective high dose polypharmacy and opioids and will share many advanced modalities from her vast academic teachings around the world in this book. We both like to practice what we call logical and physiological medicine by looking at entire body systems and how the interactions of these systems drive pain and inflammation.

We put together a group of experts in their various fields to discuss innovative and functional medicine approaches to treating patients who suffer with chronic pain. These are important clinical topics to consider and address in this difficult patient population. Our goal in this book is to give the clinician additional tools to use in treating this complex and multi-system dysfunction that we see in our patients. We must look at the connection between Neuro–Endocrine–Immune dysfunction that we see in our chronic pain patients and personalize treatment. Our one-size approach to most disease states is no longer sustainable as we see the skyrocketing numbers of chronic disease and the level of inflammation that our patients have.

This leads us to another consideration. How do we perform trials and studies to evaluate the utility of these interventions? In theory, one would design a study with a population of like patients and intervene on some but not others. But if chronic pain is only the phenotype, how do we gather a group of individuals with a similar pain phenotype under our current diagnostic capabilities? Might some of these patients' normal findings be in the tails of a normal distribution? How do we adequately, accurately, and safely evaluate a N of 1 paradigm? With this is mind, let me be the first to say that not all of the approaches in this book have been subjected to intense clinical study. The reader will find that some chapters are more of philosophy on how to approach the patient with chronic pain. Do these approaches need study? Certainly. But we must keep in mind that the traditional/historical standard approach to the patient with chronic pain has not been subjected to study either. We hope that you find these particular chapters useful as you work with patients to discover what physiologic processes have gone awry. Other chapters describe techniques that may not be as amenable to our traditional "gold-standard" randomized double blinded studies as they are to more individualized treatment by their very nature. So what are we left with? We believe this work provides a springboard to reimagine the way we think about and treat our patients with chronic pain as we learn to look at the patient as a person who is subjected to complex physiologic interactions. Some of these interactions have become perturbed and result in problematic downstream outcomes—namely the phenotype of pain. We definitely need more robust and thoughtful studies in this patient population—but we need to stop chasing the symptom and start understanding and correcting the metabolic disturbances.

Every medical specialty will have patients that will complain of some sort of pain, and it is critical that we try to find the root cause of the pain and not just band-aid the pain with opioids and other pharmaceuticals. This work will be useful to help you start to recognize and treat the root cause problems rather than concentrating on the symptom of pain.

REFERENCES

1. Dahlhamer J, Lucas J, Zelaya, C, et al. Prevalence of Chronic Pain and High-Impact Chronic Pain Among Adults — United States, 2016. *MMWR Morb Mortal Wkly Rep* 2018;67:1001–1006.
2. Vowles KE, McEntee ML, Julnes PS, Frohe T, Ney JP, van der Goes DN. Rates of opioid misuse, abuse, and addiction in chronic pain: a systematic review and data synthesis. *Pain.* 2015;156(4):569-576.
3. Wide-ranging online data for epidemiologic research (WONDER). Atlanta, GA: CDC, National Center for Health Statistics; 2020. Available at http://wonder.cdc.gov.

Editors

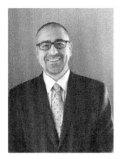

Dr. Matthew Bennett is a fellow of the American Academy of Orthopedic Surgeons. He received his medical doctorate at Upstate Medical University in Syracuse, New York, where he was invited to complete a surgical internship and orthopedic residency program. He continued his training in operative and non-operative spine care at the multidisciplinary Texas Back Institute in Plano, Texas.

He has been a physician leader and educator teaching traditional surgical skills in cooperation with industry partners. Recognizing the opportunity to look beyond our current paradigms, he became board certified and an advanced fellow in anti-aging and regenerative medicine. He currently serves as medical director of Spine Care and Pain Management in a busy clinical practice at United Health Services Medical Group in Binghamton, New York.

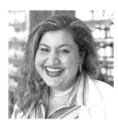

Dr. Sahar Swidan is President and CEO of Pharmacy Solutions in Ann Arbor, Michigan. She is also Adjunct Associate Professor of Clinical Research and Leadership at George Washington University School of Medicine and Health Sciences and Adjunct Clinical Associate Professor of Pharmacy at Wayne State University.

Dr. Swidan received her Doctor of Pharmacy degree and completed a 3-year research fellowship in Bio-Pharmaceutics and Gastroenterology at the University of Michigan. Following her fellowship, she became Director of Pharmacy at Chelsea Community Hospital and the clinical pharmacist for the in-patient head and chronic pain service.

Dr. Swidan is board certified and an advanced fellow in anti-aging and regenerative medicine. She is an internationally renowned speaker in the areas of pain management, headaches, and HRT. She has authored several book chapters, articles, and patient education material in head and general pain management and personalized medicine.

Most recently, Dr. Swidan has contributed to authoring *Metabolic Therapies in Orthopedics, Second Edition*, which provides continued knowledge on how optimizing metabolic pathways can improve the success of regenerative therapies through emerging technologies, integrative approaches, clinical research, and compelling evidence from over 30 experts. Dr. Swidan provides key insight in the areas of drug-related muscular pain and sarcopenia and the effects of hormones on the musculoskeletal system.

Contributors

Ellen Antoine, DO, FACEP, ABOIM, IFMCP
Medical Director
The Center for Fully Functional Health
Carmel, Indiana

Scott Antoine, DO, FACEP, ABOIM, FMNFM, IFMCP
Medical Director
The Center for Fully Functional Health
Carmel, Indiana

Matthew Bennett, MD, FABOS, ABAARM, FAARFM
Medical Director
Spine Care and Pain Management
United Health Services
Johnson City, New York

David Bilstrom, MD
Medical Director
International Autoimmune Institute
Bingham Center for Functional Medicine
Bingham Healthcare
Blackfoot, Idaho

Hal S. Blatman, MD
Medical Director
Blatman Health and Wellness Center
Affiliate Faculty Bastyr University
Cincinnati, Ohio

Jeffrey S. Block, MD
Founder, Nurturing Nature Group Consultants
Adjunct Professor, Department of
  Anesthesiology
University of Miami Miller School of Medicine
Miami, Florida

Hyla Cass, MD
Diplomat of the American Board of Psychiatry
  and Neurology (ABPN)
Diplomat of the American Board of Integrative
  Holistic Medicine (ABIHM)
Associate Editor of *Total Health* magazine
Marina del Ray, California

Randy A. Fink, MD, FACOG
Medical Director
Miami Center of Excellence and Florida
  Keys Obstetrics & Gynecology
Miami, Florida

Bradley D. Fullerton, MD, FAAPMR
Texas A&M University College of Medicine,
  Round Rock Campus
Medical Director-ProloAustin
Austin, Texas

Raphael Gonzales, PhD
Senior Vice President of Research &
  Development
RESTEM LLC
Corona, California

Kai-Uwe Kern, MD
Institute for Pain Medicine
Pain Practice
Wiesbaden, Germany

Ellen Klepack, PharmD
Principal Consultant
San Diego, California

Jennifer Kljajic, LCSW
Director of Health Coaching and Therapy
  Lucid Lane
Los Altos, California

Sarah Martin, PhD
David Geffen School of Medicine at UCLA
Los Angeles, California

Sharon McQuillan, MD
New You Medical-CEO and Founder
Great Healthworks-Chief Science Officer
A4M/MMI -Director of the Stem Cell
  Fellowship
Fort Lauderdale, Florida

Richard F. Mestayer, III, MD
Medical Director of NAD+ Research Inc.
President, Medical Director
Springfield Wellness Center
Springfield, Louisiana

Vy Phan, BS
National Institutes of Health
Rehabilitation Medicine Department,
    Clinical Center
Bethesda, Maryland

Samantha Rafie, PhD
University of California
San Diego/VA San Diego Healthcare System
San Diego, California

Sarah Rispinto, PhD
Department of Psychiatry/Psychology
Center for Comprehensive Pain Recovery
    Neurological Institute
Cleveland Clinic
Cleveland, Ohio

Todd D Rozen, MD, FAAN
Mayo Clinic Florida
Department of Neurology
Jacksonville, Florida

Mara Rubin, PharmD
Clinical Pharmacist-Pediatrics
Department of Pharmacy
Nationwide Children's Hospital
Columbus, Ohio

Charles E. Schultz, MD
University of Michigan
Department of Neurology
Ann Arbor, Michigan

Jay P. Shah, MD
National Institutes of Health
Rehabilitation Medicine Department
    Clinical Center
Bethesda, Maryland

Pamela W. Smith, MD, MPH, MS
Co-Director, Master's Program in
    Metabolic Medicine
Morsani College of Medicine
University of South Florida
Tampa, Florida

Brian Spitsbergen, PhD, LPC, CAADC
Division Director-Substance Use Disorder and
    Recovery Support Services
Wellspring Lutheran Services
Oak Park, Michigan

Pamela Stratton, MD
National Institutes of Health
Office of the Clinical Director
National Institute of Neurological Disorders
    and Stroke
Bethesda, Maryland

**Sahar Swidan, PharmD, ABAAHP,
FAARFM, FACA**
Adjunct Associate Professor of Clinical
    Research and Leadership at George
    Washington University School of Medicine
    and Health Sciences
Adjunct Clinical Associate Professor of
    Pharmacy at Wayne State University
Pharmacy Solutions-President and CEO
Ann Arbor, Michigan

Dr. Ahmed Zaafran, MD
Chief Medical Officer, Lucid Lane
Assistant Professor of Anesthesiology (Affiliated)
Stanford University School of Medicine
Palo Alto, California

1 Physiology of the Pain System

Matthew Bennett and Sahar Swidan

CONTENTS

In order to better understand the treatment options for patients in chronic pain, it is incumbent upon us to review our understanding of the pain system. By better understanding the pain system, we hope to show how our current pain treatment paradigms have fallen short; in doing so, we hope to encourage better pain management.

Nociception exists at the intersection of the nervous system, the immune system, and the endocrine system. There exists a significant cross-talk between these, previously considered independent, pathways. Shared receptors allow ligands to have effects across systems and create a coordinated pain system. The pain experience is even more complex as it includes psychological and social variables.

Acute pain typically develops a well-coordinated and predictable signal from the periphery to the central nervous system where it is processed and ultimately observed. The nociceptive signal is generally a useful signal that alerts the organism to injury. On the other hand, chronic pain has been considered to be akin to a disease state. Patients with chronic pain syndromes are not typically experiencing an unending supply of acute pain. Rather, these patients have had their pain systems fundamentally altered. As we attempt to understand the pain system in these patients with chronic pain, it is critical to understand that the pain signal is frequently being modulated on its journey from creation to observation. From the initial activation of peripheral nociceptors, to spinal cord signaling, to synthesis of a pain perception and emotional processing in the brain, there are many opportunities to either enhance or suppress the pain experience. Modulation occurs within and because of the nervous system, the immune system, and the endocrine system.

First, we will consider the acute pain system and overview how it operates in its natural unaltered state. Notably missing from this overview is the endocannabinoid system which will be fully covered in its own dedicated chapter.

PERIPHERAL SYSTEM

We will begin our review of the pain system by starting peripherally. Information from the outside world enters the organism through various different receptors. Non-nociceptive or innocuous information is collected by Pacinian corpuscles detecting vibration and pressure, Meissner's corpuscles detecting light touch, Merkel nerve endings detecting mechanical pressure and position, and Ruffini corpuscles detecting stretch. Innocuous sensory information meant to describe touch, pressure, and proprioception is received from the skin, muscle, and joints.

Painful information is conveyed by nociceptors which detect a wide range of thermal, chemical, or mechanical perturbations through a variety of mechanisms, including bare nerve endings which either react to specific noxious stimuli or are polymodal and respond to a variety of noxious stimuli. Painful information is relayed from the skin, muscles, joints, viscera, and various neural structures. Specific transducer channels are present on the nerve ending, allowing specific chemicals to activate the receptor. For instance, the transient receptor potential vanilloid-1 (TRPV1) receptor is activated by temperatures >43°C as well as capsaicin from the chili pepper plant. In addition, then endocannabinoid anandamide may also act as an endogenous ligand.[1] Transient receptor potential M member 8 (TRPM8) is activated by temperatures <25–28°C as well as menthol. The frequency at which the afferent fires is dependent upon the intensity of the stimulus.[2] Importantly, the frequency of afferent firing is also dependent upon the resting potential of the axon—which can be modified.

AXONS

Sensory information is relayed via sensory neurons. Primary sensory neurons can be divided into two main categories: those which relay innocuous non-painful information (Aβ-fibers) and those that relay painful nociceptive information (Aδ and C-fibers). Innocuous information is communicated through the peripheral nerve on low-threshold Aβ-fibers which are large in diameter, highly myelinated, and allow for quick action potentials.

Nociception is carried on primary afferent fibers by Aδ fibers or C fibers. Aδ-fibers are smaller in diameter and thinly myelinated, making them slower conducting (4–30 m/sec) than Aβ-fibers but much quicker than C-fibers.[2] Aδ fibers are mechanoreceptors or thermoreceptors that respond to either low- or high-threshold stimuli. Aδ fibers are small, myelinated, and fast conducting. Myelinated axons usually contain specialized terminals that are sensitive to mechanical distortion.[1] C-fibers are the smallest fibers and non-myelinated, making them the slowest conducting fiber type (2.5 m/sec).[3] These free nerve endings are activated by high-intensity stimuli. C-fibers are polymodal—meaning they respond to mechanical stimuli, thermal stimuli, chemical stimuli, or a combination. Some C-fibers respond only to thermal stimuli. Almost all C-fibers respond to chemical stimuli—specifically capsaicin.[4]

The velocity differential between fiber types leads to the experience of first pain and second pain. Aδ-fibers convey the initial quick shallow pain. It is the C-fibers that convey the slower but deeper, more spread out, and more intense pain. Furthermore, C-fibers are more numerous in peripheral nerves than myelinated fibers, further explaining the pain experience.[2] Specific variability in the proportions of each fiber sub-type is just one example of how certain bodily locations can create a "signature" pain experience. For example, pain from visceral organs is typically poorly localized, deep, and dull.[5]

At rest, the primary afferent shows very little baseline activity. Once activated by either physical or chemical stimuli, the primary afferent activates voltage-sensitive sodium (Na_v) channels, allowing the inflow of sodium and resulting depolarization of the axon. It is these Na_v channels that allow for the utility of local anesthetics. Na_v channels are broadly blocked with lidocaine. Interestingly, analgesia produced by the blockade of Na_v 1.7 in the mouse is reversible by naloxone, suggesting a connection to the endogenous opioid system.

Alterations in Na_v channels explain some of the variability in the pain experience. Three sodium channels have been associated with peripheral neurons—Na_v 1.7, Na_v 1.8, and Na_v 1.9 play a key role in neurotransmitter release. By altering these channels, different neurotransmitter outputs are noted at the spinal cord synapse. The human gene SCN9A encodes for the Na_v 1.7 channel. Mutations in this gene can result in chronically painful conditions (such as inherited primary erythromelalgia, paroxysmal extreme pain disorder, painful small fiber neuropathy/episodic pain syndrome) or painless conditions (such as channelopathy-associated insensitivity to pain).[6] In the absence of Na_v 1.7, substance P release no longer occurred from mouse sensory neurons.[7] Na_v channel alterations can be seen in other pathological states such as nerve injury. Loss of Na_v 1.7 is linked to transcriptional upregulation of *Penk*—the precursor of met-enkephalin. Combined, this suggests that these Na_v channels are more complex than mere on/off switches that allow or disallow conduction along the axon. They can direct gene expression back at the dorsal root ganglia (DRG). It is interesting to consider that congenital anomalies in the Na_v channels, resulting in congenital insensitivity to pain, might be in part dependent on increased endogenous opioid activity—but somehow without any development of tolerance (which is markedly different than what is observed with exogenous opioid delivery).[8]

CENTRAL SYSTEM

The primary afferent summarizes nociceptive information from the periphery and feeds this information centrally into the spinal cord. But first, it passes through the cell body of the axon—the DRG. The DRG is the bulbous portion of the nerve seen in the neuroforamen of the spine. It is a pseudo-unipolar type neuron, meaning there is an axon on either side of the cell body that together act as a single axon. Small glial cells surround and support these cells. Nutrients are supplied via gap junctions. The DRG is the control center for the neuron, housing the genetic code for the nerve, and, as such, synthesizes neuropeptides. It follows that the DRG is a powerful modulatory location—more on this in future chapters.

SPINAL CORD

The primary afferent continues through the dorsal root to the dorsal column where the first synapse occurs. Here innocuous and noxious information diverges. First, a final brief note on innocuous information. The large myelinated primary afferent non-nociceptive fibers traverse the top of the dorsal horn through Lissauer's tract and then ascend the spinal cord through the white matter of the dorsal column or decussate to the contralateral ventral spinothalamic tract.[2]

Nociceptive information enters Lissauer's tract and then innervates the gray matter of the dorsal horn where primary afferents finally synapse in the dorsal horn of the spinal cord. In the dorsal horn of the spinal cord, neurotransmission occurs via two mechanisms. Glutamate released from the primary afferent and mediated by the α-amino-3-hydroxy-5-methyl-4-isoxazolepropionate (AMPA)-type glutamate receptor produces a robust but short-lasting depolarization of the second-order neuron.[2] The second mechanism consists of peptides that produce a delayed and longer-lasting discharge as compared to the AMPA receptors. These peptidergic neurons contain peptide neurotransmitters such as CGRP, substance P, and growth factors such as brain-derived neurotropic factor. Peptides can enhance nociception, thus playing a role in central sensitization.[2]

DORSAL HORN EXCITABILITY

It is the dorsal horn synapse which allows for significant modulation of the pain signal. Inhibitory modulation pathways are both supraspinal as well as local. We will look at local modulation first. While all neurons synapse at least once before continuing their ascent to the brain, some neurons experience multiple synapses where interneurons can affect transmission. Most of the nociceptive neurons synapse in the superficial portion of the dorsal horn within the anatomic locations of Rexed laminae I and II. Laminae II contains interneurons that modulate the signal with either excitatory or inhibitory neurotransmitters. Glutamate is the excitatory neurotransmitter while γ-aminobutyricacid (GABA) is the inhibitory neurotransmitter. GABA and glycine are major inhibitory neurotransmitters which are active both pre-synaptic as well as post-synaptic. GABA serves as a ligand for both $GABA_A$ and $GABA_B$ receptors. Both $GABA_A$ and glycine receptors increase Cl^- conductance.

GABA$_B$ functions as a G protein-coupled receptor. GABA and glycine have more of an impact on the larger Aβ fibers than the smaller fiber types. The modulation is not that simple and other modulatory substances are also found in the dorsal horn including adenosine, choline acetyltransferase, CCK, corticotropin-releasing factor, dynorphin, enkephalin, galanin, glycine, neurotensin, neuropeptide Y, somatostatin, substance P, and thyrotropin-releasing hormone. Each of these substances modulates the signal in various ways.

Lamina V contains wide dynamic range (WDR) neurons responding to both painful and non-painful stimuli. Aβ fibers typically project into lamina III and deeper. High-threshold C fibers project into the more superficial lamina I and II. Following peripheral nerve injury, it has been noted that A fibers can sprout into the more superficial lamina I and II, resulting in low-threshold mechanoreceptor activation being interpreted as deep pain.[2]

SUPRASPINAL MODULATION

In addition to local signal modulation, there are supraspinal pathways that impact the dorsal horn. The supraspinal pathway (or descending pathway) originates from the brain and travels to the dorsal horn of the spinal cord, creating a top-down component utilizing serotonin and norepinephrine. Midbrain periaqueductal gray (PAG), dorsolateral pons, and rostroventral medulla all play important roles in this descending pain pathway. The descending pathways were originally considered as a pain inhibition pathway only. However, it is now known that these descending pathways can be both facilitatory as well as inhibitory.

The midbrain's PAG plays a central role in the descending pain pathway. The hypothalamus has topographic projections onto the PAG. Forebrain projections from the limbic system are also noted. Together, these regions affect the PAG to project to the rostroventral medulla (RVM) and the pons, utilizing substance P, glutamate, and cholinergic neurons to impact the pain processing system. Opiate receptors are noted in the PAG (as well as the amygdala and midline medulla). Opiates inhibit the inhibitory (GABA) output to the medulla. As a result, the bulbospinal pathway is activated via noradrenergic and serotoninergic pathways.

In the pons, the locus coeruleus projects norepinephrine toward the spinal cord as well as into the thalamus and forebrain. The forebrain projections appear to alter affective components of behavior, while the spinal projections inhibit pain transmission in the dorsal horn via α$_2$ receptors on the dorsal horn. α$_2$ receptor binding is both pre-synaptic on the C fibers and post-synaptic on the dorsal horn neurons. Opiates inhibit the activity of the cells of the locus coeruleus. During withdrawal from opiates, the increased activity of these cells becomes symptomatic. Clonidine has been used as an antagonist to blunt the withdrawal effect.

The nucleus raphe magnus in the caudal pons/rostral medulla projects serotoninergic neurons spinally toward the dorsal horn of the spinal cord as well as the limbic forebrain. Here, serotonin may actually excite pain processing. This pathway may play an important role in pain chronification. This pathway may also hold insight as to how higher centers can impact the nocebo effect.[9] This may occur via neurotopins. Specifically, BDNF from the PAG binds to TrkB in the RVM. This process is mediated by NMDA receptors.[9] In addition, neuron-glial interactions play a role when nerve injury is present by the CCL2 chemokine binding to astrocytes in the RVM.[10] The prefrontal, anterior cingulate cortex (ACC) and amygdala coordinate this inhibitory and excitatory balance.[11–13] It appears as though the analgesic properties of antidepressants may be mediated more by their impact on norepinephrine than on serotonin.

Projections from the rostral ventromedial medulla (RVM) directly synapse with the dorsal horn of the spinal cord. These cells are both serotonergic and non-serotonergic. In addition, there are cells from the RVM that project back to the dorsolateral pons, utilizing enkephalin as inhibitory and SP as excitatory neurotransmitters.

Diffuse noxious inhibitory controls (DNICs) are a spinal-medullary-spinal mechanism where harmless but noxious stimuli may inhibit the responsiveness of WDR neurons in the spinal cord.[9]

This pathway is not dependent on the PAG or RVM. Rather, it is dependent on a supraspinal loop through the dorsal reticular nucleus.[2]

In addition to sustained C fiber input activating wide dynamic range neurons, there is direct communication with the medullary raphe nuclei that results in the excitation of bulbo-serotonin pathways that activate 5-hydroxytyptamine (5-HT$_3$) receptors on lamina V neurons. The use of 5-HT$_3$ inhibitors can reduce this state.[14]

SPINOTHALAMIC TRACT

From the dorsal horn neurons, spinothalamic tract (STT) cells carry the information ventral and decussate via the anterior white commissure to the white matter in the lateral and ventrolateral funiculi, which makes up the spinothalamic tract and ascend the spinal cord. STT cells may be sensitive to "high-threshold" input or respond to a variety of thermal, mechanical, and nociceptive input—known as "wide dynamic range" neurons. The axons of the STT cells terminate in a lateral or medial pain pathway. The lateral axons terminate in the posterior ventrobasal thalamic complex (VPL), while the medial axons terminate in the medial and intralaminar thalamus. The lateral pain pathway is responsible for transmitting discriminative information about the location and quality of the pain to the thalamus, primary, and secondary somatosensory cortices. On the other hand, the medial pathway transmits information to the midline brainstem, hypothalamus, amygdala, medial, and intralaminar thalamus which impact the limbic structures to activate the emotional and autonomic responses to pain.[2]

STT axons also terminate in spinoreticular pathways which impact descending pain pathways, autonomic responsiveness, alerting responses, and limbic responses. The descending pathway can help to balance between facilitation and inhibition of the pain pathway. The subnucleus reticularis dorsalis (SRD) of the dorsal medullary reticular formation plays an important role in this process.

BRAIN CONSIDERATIONS

The brain does not merely witness the nociceptive signal. It actively participates in constructing the nociceptive signal. The spinothalamic tract ultimately communicates with higher nociception processing centers within the brain. The lateral thalamic nuclei, SI, and SII somatosensory cortices play a sensory discriminative role. The medial thalamic nuclei, and anterior and medial cingulate cortices interpret the emotional significance of the stimuli via the limbic system. The insula, cerebellum, and prefrontal cortex contribute to memory and fear avoidance behaviors. The lentiform nucleus, and cerebellum are involved in reflexive motor responsiveness.[2]

The limbic system is a set of brain structures on either side of the thalamus that directs emotion, behavior, motivation, long-term memory, and olfaction. The mesolimbic pathway is part of the reward circuit. Dopaminergic neurons in the ventral tegmental area (VTA) of the midbrain project to the forebrain nucleus accumbens (NAc). Burst firing of dopaminergic neurons into the NAc serves as a reward signal and is inhibited by tonic GABA input.[15] Opioids inhibit GABAergic tone on these neurons, while pain relief directly engages dopamine circuitry.[15] The mesolimbic pathway has been implicated in depression, anxiety, pain sensation, anticipation of analgesia or placebo-induced analgesia, and chronic pain.[16] Different types of pain can impact different aspects of the VTA and result in either activation or inhibition. In this way, dopamine release is variable based on various pain signals.[16] These dopaminergic pathways are variably altered with stress as well as opioids. Dynorphin and the kappa opioid receptor can play a role in impairing dopamine release in the Na.[16]

Some are questioning the specificity of particular regions. Some regions may respond preferentially to painful stimulus, but not specifically (or only) to a pain stimulus where actual or potential tissue damage is occurring.[17] There are several examples of regions that initially appeared to be specific for nociception, but on further study respond to more generalized input. In one instance, facial pain elicited the activation of a neuron close to SII, but so did a novel or threatening object approaching the visually receptive field.[18] In another example, noxious heat produced a response in several neurons in the ACC, but these same neurons were also activated when subjects watched the experimenter receive painful stimuli.[19] Care needs to be taken in assigning nociceptive causation to these brain regions. Nevertheless, if neuroimaging is able to identify target brain regions (or more likely patterns of regions) that show increased activity correlated with increased pain intensity, then this neuroimaging may potentially allow us to predict which interventions might be most impactful to specific groups of people.[17]

Much of the cortical responses to pain can be modulated with opioid analgesics. In women, more opioid receptors are available in the presence of high estrogen levels.[20] Dopamine may also play a role in the pain response. High D2/D3 receptor availability in the striatum is associated with higher pain intensity.[21]

Cognitive attention to and distraction from stimuli also appear to play a role in the nociceptive processing of pain. During distraction there is an interaction between the anterior cingulate cortex and the frontal cortex. This results in modulation of the PAG and thalamus and decreases activity in the cortical sensory regions, which ultimately results in the decreased perception of pain.[22,23]

Anticipation of pain also impacts the pain experience. The expectation of pain intensity is necessary for maximal activation of the afferent pain circuitry and maximal perceived pain intensity.[24,25] It has been suggested that the descending pain pathways are modulated by cognitive suggestions and may impact the system at the dorsal horn of the spinal cord.

The placebo effect has been associated with changes in endogenous opioid release in the prefrontal cortex, anterior cingulate cortex, insula, nucleus accumbens, and ventral striatum.[26] The descending pain pathway via the PAG appears to play a role in pain modulation. Not surprisingly, naloxone can block placebo analgesia.[27] In a knee arthritis trial, placebo response was noted to correlate with fMRI activity in the right midfrontal gyrus but not in those responsive to duloxetine. Interestingly, in some subjects the duloxetine was able to further activate the placebo response, while in other patients the drug interfered with the placebo response.[28]

OTHER CONSIDERATIONS

The orexin system appears to play a role in nociception. The orexin (hypocretin) system is composed of two G-protein coupled receptors (Ox_1 and Ox_2) and two neuropeptides (orexin-A and orexin-B). The neuropeptides are produced in the hypothalamus and their receptors are widely dispersed throughout the CNS. Orexin-A activates both Ox_1 and Ox_2. Orexin-B activates only Ox_2.[29] The orexin system is involved in a variety of processes including arousal, reward-seeking behavior, energy homeostasis, sensory modulation, stress processing, or locomotion, cognition, endocrine functions, visceral functions, and pain modulation.[30] Orexin-A has shown antinociceptive effects in the brain and spinal cord while orexin-B has shown little antinociceptive effect.[31] In the brain, orexin-A may be mediated by Ox_1 in the RVM and PAG. Orexin-A may also activate H1 or H2 receptors that release histamine at supraspinal levels, blocking the antinociceptive effect of orexin-A. Blocking the H1 and H2 receptors may induce more antinociception.[29] In the spinal cord, orexin-A may act on the DRG by elevating Ca^{2+} concentration in certain neurons.[29] In stressful situations, orexin expression is increased in the hypothalamus, activating the Ox_1 receptor in the PAG to produce analgesia through 2-arachidonoylglycerol (2-AG) and the endocannabinoid system.[32] Nociceptin—also known as orphanin FQ (N/OFQ)— is a neuropeptide implicated in a number of physiologic responses. N/OFQ has been shown to make contact with orexin cells both pre- and post-synaptic and inhibit their activity and thus block stress-induced analgesia.[33]

In a rheumatoid arthritis model, daily administration of intravenous orexin-A induced a significant pain reduction and serum nerve growth factors.[34] Acupuncture analgesia is likely at least in part obtained through the orexin system. Electroacupuncture was shown to increase lower than normal levels of orexin-A in the hypothalamus, PAG, and spinal cord. Naloxone could not inhibit orexin-A-induced analgesia.[35]

In summary, the nociceptive system is not just a bottom-up system of connections that relays painful information to consciousness. Ascending and descending pathways exist to modulate the pain experience in real-time. There is a top-down component that allows for cognitive and emotional control over nociception. Importantly, the brain itself plays an active role in pain pathways and sculpting the pain experience. In this chapter, we reviewed the basics of the pain pathway. We have yet to discuss pain modulation which occurs both peripherally and centrally and is of critical importance when considering the chronic pain patient. Any effective strategy to treat patients with chronic pain must take these multiple variables into account.

REFERENCES

1. D'Mello, R., & Dickenson, A.H. (2008). Spinal cord mechanisms of pain. *Br J Anaesth, 101*(1), 8–16. doi:10.1093/bja/aen088
2. Benzon, H.T. (2014). *Practical Management of Pain* (5th ed.). Philadelphia, PA: Elsevier/Mosby.
3. Gasser, H.S. (1950). Unmedullated fibers originating in dorsal root ganglia. *J Gen Physiol, 33*(6), 651–690.
4. Julius, D., & Basbaum, A.I. (2001). Molecular mechanisms of nociception. *Nature, 413*(6852), 203–210. doi:10.1038/35093019
5. Gebhart, G.F. (1996). Visceral polymodal receptors. *Prog Brain Res, 113*, 101–112.
6. Sexton, J.E., Cox, J.J., Zhao, J., & Wood, J.N. (2018). The genetics of pain: implications for therapeutics. *Annu Rev Pharmacol Toxicol, 58*, 123–142. doi:10.1146/annurev-pharmtox-010617-052554
7. Minett, M.S., Nassar, M.A., Clark, A.K., Passmore, G., Dickenson, A.H., Wang, F., ... Wood, J.N. (2012). Distinct Nav1.7-dependent pain sensations require different sets of sensory and sympathetic neurons. *Nat Commun, 3*, 791. doi:10.1038/ncomms1795
8. Emery, E.C., Luiz, A.P., & Wood, J.N. (2016). Nav1.7 and other voltage-gated sodium channels as drug targets for pain relief. *Expert Opin Ther Targets, 20*(8), 975–983. doi:10.1517/14728222.2016.1162295
9. Chapman, C.R., & Vierck, C.J. (2017). The transition of acute postoperative pain to chronic pain: an integrative overview of research on mechanisms. *J Pain, 18*(4), 359.e1–359.e38. doi:10.1016/j.jpain.2016.11.004
10. Brink, T.S., Pacharinsak, C., Khasabov, S.G., Beitz, A.J., & Simone, D.A. (2012). Differential modulation of neurons in the rostral ventromedial medulla by neurokinin-1 receptors. *J Neurophysiol, 107*(4), 1210–1221. doi:10.1152/jn.00678.2011
11. Kobayashi, S. (2012). Organization of neural systems for aversive information processing: pain, error, and punishment. *Front Neurosci, 6*, 136. doi:10.3389/fnins.2012.00136
12. Mobbs, D., Marchant, J.L., Hassabis, D., Seymour, B., Tan, G., Gray, M., ... Frith, C.D. (2009). From threat to fear: the neural organization of defensive fear systems in humans. *J Neurosci, 29*(39), 12236–12243. doi:10.1523/JNEUROSCI.2378-09.2009
13. Ossipov, M.H., Morimura, K., & Porreca, F. (2014). Descending pain modulation and chronification of pain. *Curr Opin Support Palliat Care, 8*(2), 143–151. doi:10.1097/SPC.0000000000000055
14. McCleane, G.J., Suzuki, R., & Dickenson, A.H. (2003). Does a single intravenous injection of the 5HT3 receptor antagonist ondansetron have an analgesic effect in neuropathic pain? A double-blinded, placebo-controlled cross-over study. *Anesth Analg, 97*(5), 1474–1478.
15. Cahill, C.M., & Taylor, A.M. (2017). Neuroinflammation-a co-occurring phenomenon linking chronic pain and opioid dependence. *Curr Opin Behav Sci, 13*, 171–177. doi:10.1016/j.cobeha.2016.12.003
16. Massaly, N., Moron, J.A., & Al-Hasani, R. (2016). A trigger for opioid misuse: chronic pain and stress dysregulate the mesolimbic pathway and kappa opioid system. *Front Neurosci, 10*, 480. doi:10.3389/fnins.2016.00480
17. Mouraux, A., & Iannetti, G.D. (2018). The search for pain biomarkers in the human brain. *Brain, 141*(12), 3290–3307. doi:10.1093/brain/awy281
18. Dong, W.K., Chudler, E.H., Sugiyama, K., Roberts, V.J., & Hayashi, T. (1994). Somatosensory, multisensory, and task-related neurons in cortical area 7b (PF) of unanesthetized monkeys. *J Neurophysiol, 72*(2), 542–564. doi:10.1152/jn.1994.72.2.542
19. Hutchison, W.D., Davis, K.D., Lozano, A.M., Tasker, R.R., & Dostrovsky, J.O. (1999). Pain-related neurons in the human cingulate cortex. *Nat Neurosci, 2*(5), 403–405. doi:10.1038/8065

20. Zubieta, J.K., Smith, Y.R., Bueller, J.A., Xu, Y., Kilbourn, M.R., Jewett, D.M., … Stohler, C.S. (2002). Mu-opioid receptor-mediated antinociceptive responses differ in men and women. *J Neurosci*, *22*(12), 5100–5107.

21. Martikainen, I.K., Hagelberg, N., Jääskeläinen , S.K., Hietala, J., & Pertovaara, A. (2018). Dopaminergic and serotonergic mechanisms in the modulation of pain: in vivo studies in human brain. *Eur J Pharmacol*, *834*, 337–345. doi:10.1016/j.ejphar.2018.07.038

22. Tracey, I., Ploghaus, A., Gati, J.S., Clare, S., Smith, S., Menon, R.S., & Matthews, P.M. (2002). Imaging attentional modulation of pain in the periaqueductal gray in humans. *J Neurosci*, *22*(7), 2748–2752. https://www.ncbi.nlm.nih.gov/pubmed/11923440

23. Valet, M., Sprenger, T., Boecker, H., Willoch, F., Rummeny, E., Conrad, B., … Tolle, T.R. (2004). Distraction modulates connectivity of the cingulo-frontal cortex and the midbrain during pain–an fMRI analysis. *Pain*, *109*(3), 399–408. doi:10.1016/j.pain.2004.02.033

24. Keltner, J.R., Furst, A., Fan, C., Redfern, R., Inglis, B., & Fields, H.L. (2006). Isolating the modulatory effect of expectation on pain transmission: a functional magnetic resonance imaging study. *J Neurosci*, *26*(16), 4437–4443. doi:10.1523/JNEUROSCI.4463-05.2006

25. Kong, J., Gollub, R.L., Rosman, I.S., Webb, J.M., Vangel, M.G., Kirsch, I., & Kaptchuk, T.J. (2006). Brain activity associated with expectancy-enhanced placebo analgesia as measured by functional magnetic resonance imaging. *J Neurosci*, *26*(2), 381–388. doi:10.1523/JNEUROSCI.3556-05.2006

26. Zubieta, J.K., Bueller, J.A., Jackson, L.R., Scott, D.J., Xu, Y., Koeppe, R.A., … Stohler, C.S. (2005). Placebo effects mediated by endogenous opioid activity on mu-opioid receptors. *J Neurosci*, *25*(34), 7754–7762. doi:10.1523/JNEUROSCI.0439-05.2005

27. Levine, J.D., Gordon, N.C., & Fields, H.L. (1978). The mechanism of placebo analgesia. *Lancet*, *2*(8091), 654–657.

28. Tétreault, P., Mansour, A., Vachon-Presseau, E., Schnitzer, T.J., Apkarian, A.V., & Baliki, M.N. (2016). Brain connectivity predicts placebo response across chronic pain clinical trials. *PLOS Biol*, *14*(10), e1002570. doi:10.1371/journal.pbio.1002570

29. Razavi, B.M., & Hosseinzadeh, H. (2017). A review of the role of orexin system in pain modulation. *Biomed Pharmacother*, *90*, 187–193. doi:10.1016/j.biopha.2017.03.053

30. Chiou, L.C., Lee, H.J., Ho, Y.C., Chen, S.P., Liao, Y.Y., Ma, C.H., … Wang, S.J. (2010). Orexins/hypocretins: pain regulation and cellular actions. *Curr Pharm Des*, *16*(28), 3089–3100.

31. Cady, R.J., Denson, J.E., Sullivan, L.Q., & Durham, P.L. (2014). Dual orexin receptor antagonist 12 inhibits expression of proteins in neurons and glia implicated in peripheral and central sensitization. *Neuroscience*, *269*, 79–92. doi:10.1016/j.neuroscience.2014.03.043

32. Ho, Y.C., Lee, H.J., Tung, L.W., Liao, Y.Y., Fu, S.Y., Teng, S.F., … Chiou, L.C. (2011). Activation of orexin 1 receptors in the periaqueductal gray of male rats leads to antinociception via retrograde endocannabinoid (2-arachidonoylglycerol)-induced disinhibition. *J Neurosci*, *31*(41), 14600–14610. doi:10.1523/JNEUROSCI.2671-11.2011

33. Xie, X., Wisor, J.P., Hara, J., Crowder, T.L., LeWinter, R., Khroyan, T.V., … Kilduff, T.S. (2008). Hypocretin/orexin and nociceptin/orphanin FQ coordinately regulate analgesia in a mouse model of stress-induced analgesia. *J Clin Invest*, *118*(7), 2471–2481. doi:10.1172/JCI35115

34. Mohamed, A.R., & El-Hadidy, W.F. (2014). Effect of orexin-A (hypocretin-1) on hyperalgesic and cachectic manifestations of experimentally induced rheumatoid arthritis in rats. *Can J Physiol Pharmacol*, *92*(10), 813–820. doi:10.1139/cjpp-2014-0258

35. Feng, X.M., Mi, W.L., Xia, F., Mao-Ying, Q.L., Jiang, J.W., Xiao, S., … Wu, G.C. (2012). Involvement of spinal orexin A in the electroacupuncture analgesia in a rat model of post-laparotomy pain. *BMC Complement Altern Med*, *12*, 225. doi:10.1186/1472-6882-12-225

2 Neuro–Endocrine–Immune Dysfunction in the Chronic Pain Patient

Matthew Bennett

CONTENTS

Acute pain typically presents a well-orchestrated experience providing useful information about tissue damage. However, in the chronic pain patient, this communication mechanism gets disrupted. Many steps in the pathway can become perturbed. Aberrations in the neurological system, endocrine system, and immune system impact the pain experience in patients with chronic pain. Neuro–endocrine–immune dysfunction in chronic pain patients helps to explain some of our clinical failures in this arena. Many of the strategies that are effective and compassionate for patients in acute pain have been relatively ineffective and perhaps even counterproductive in treating the growing chronic pain epidemic.

We have previously considered the normal functioning pain system. In review, ascending pathways move from the periphery from primary receptors through primary afferent axons through the pseudo-unipolar dorsal root ganglia (DRG) to the first synapse at the dorsal horn of the spinal cord. Once in the central nervous system, the signal is modulated by both local and descending pathways. Descending pathways from the forebrain and hypothalamus project onto the limbic system and periaqueductal gray in the midbrain to the rostroventral medulla and finally join the multiple synapses in the dorsal horn of the spinal cord. Once the signal is molded by local and descending controls it decussates to the contralateral spinal cord where it ascends via the spinothalamic tract to the ventral posterior nucleus of the thalamus. With the signal in the brain, third-order neurons project to the somatosensory cortex and other brain regions.

We will start by considering neurologic alterations in the system—peripheral, central, auto-nomic, and even cellular energetics. The immune system interactions will be discussed. Finally, endocrine alterations will be explored.

PERIPHERAL SENSITIZATION

The primary afferent pathway can change into a more sensitive state, becoming more efficient at relaying nociceptive information to central pathways—known as primary or peripheral sensitiza-tion. Several systems are known to impact peripheral sensitization. In peripheral sensitization the afferent itself, the immune system, the endocrine system, and other non-neuronal cells all contribute to the increased activity and sensitization of the primary afferent nociceptor. Tissue injury acti-vates several pathways. In addition to nociception, injury also results in tissue damage and immune activation—both local and global. The result of this tissue damage is a peripheral "inflammatory soup"—peptides (bradykinin), neurotransmitters (serotonin), prostaglandins, and neurotrophins (nerve growth factor) are released which sensitize the nociceptors. The C fiber afferent terminals themselves contribute to this peripheral sensitization by releasing substance P and calcitonin gene-related peptide (CGRP) which induce non-neuronal cells to induce a progressive inflammatory response including local vasodilation, plasma extravasation, and the degranulation of mast cells.

Immune cells become activated which further serves to feed forward this primary or peripheral sensitization. Histamine is released by mast cells, basophils, and platelets. Serotonin is released by mast cells and platelets. These amines result in reddening and swelling in the skin and radiation of pain.

MAST CELLS

Mast cells may play a particularly important role in this regard by secreting pre-stored mediators. Bradykinin, substance P, TNF-α, nerve growth factor, prostaglandins, tryptase, and histamine are released by mast cells and impact nearby nerves. Inappropriate mast cell activation can occur by specific mutation sets. Unregulated mediator release can result in recruitment of normal local and distant mast cells that sets off a cascade of mast cell activation.[1] In addition, mast cells recruit eosinophils, neutrophils, macrophages, and T-cells which further release their own set of inflamma-tory mediators, further sensitizing the nociceptive pathways.

This peripheral nociceptive sensitization results in central upregulation of pain pathways. Furthermore, mast cells also impact the central pain processing pathways. (We will consider the process of central sensitization separately.) Mast cells reside on the brain side of the blood–brain barrier of the infundibulum, pituitary, hypothalamus, and thalamus and communicate with neu-rons, glia, and vascular endothelial cells.[1,2] Mast cell function can rapidly alter brain function by the widespread addition of histamine. These central effects can ultimately stimulate more mast cell activation and create a positive feedback loop.[1]

Mast cell activation can result in increased pain symptoms in the chest, stomach, upper abdomen, lower abdomen, bones, joints, muscles, and nerves or connective tissue.[3] Opioids and non-steroidal anti-inflammatory drugs can trigger mast cell activation.[1] There are no official guidelines for the treatment of mast cell activation disease.[1]

PERIPHERAL SENSITIZATION

With peripheral sensitization, other non-neuronal substances become activated as well. Non-kallikrein, trypsin, and physical trauma activate Factor XII. Bradykinin is synthesized from Factor XII via the kinin-kallikrein system which results in vasodilation, increased vascular permeability, and also sensitizes the primary afferent terminals. Resident mast cells sensitize nociceptors possibly via bradykinin release.[4]

As tissue is injured, phospholipases become activated. Phospholipases free arachidonic acid. Cyclooxygenase converts arachidonic acid into eicosanoids such as prostaglandin E_2, thromboxane A_2, and prostacyclin. These pro-inflammatory eicosanoids can result in increased excitability of C fibers. There are modifiable lifestyle inputs that alter the balance of pro-inflammatory to anti-inflammatory eicosanoids which may ultimately have the ability to impact the overall inflammatory levels. More on this in a later chapter.

Inflammatory cytokines such as tumor necrosis factor alpha and interleukin-1β are released by macrophages. These cytokines bind directly to C fibers. These inflammatory cytokines are also noted as important upregulators in neuroma sensitization. Thrombin and trypsin are released which activates specific receptors.

Up-activation of the immune system may play an important role in maintaining chronic pain states. Multiple mechanisms exist to control the magnitude of inflammation. The endocrine and autonomic nervous systems play a role in controlling inflammation. As we have seen, the magnitude of inflammation has a direct bearing on nociception. The hypothalamic–pituitary–adrenal axis (HPA), the sympatho-adrenal axes, nociceptive neurons, and the sympatho-neural system are all contributing factors. The autonomic nervous system regulates physiological systems by integrating afferent inputs from internal and external environments with the neuronal system, endocrine system, and cell modulated responses.

ENDOCRINE AND INFLAMMATION

The HPA is involved in nociception and serves as an intermediary between the neuro and endocrine and immune systems. These systems normally communicate to maintain physiologic homeostasis. There has been a relative history of skepticism surrounding the relevance of this system to the pain experience; but the current literature suggests a mechanistic pathway of communication.[5] Various immune cells including lymphocytes and monocytes have receptors for corticosteroids, insulin, prolactin, growth hormone, somatostatins, estrogens, testosterone, leptin, ghrelin, opioids, corticosteroids, neuropeptide Y, and vasoactive intestinal polypeptide. Neuronal cells and endocrine organs express receptors for immune-derived cytokines and growth factors. There is a true bi-directional communication between these systems.

AUTONOMIC NERVOUS SYSTEM AND INFLAMMATION

The autonomic nervous system is made up of the sympathetic nervous system, the parasympathetic nervous system, and the enteric nervous system (ENS). The enteric nervous system directly controls the gastrointestinal (GI) tract.[6] A key role of the autonomic system is the regulation of acute inflammatory responses at local and systemic levels.[7] The sympathetic nervous system secretes catecholamines such as epinephrine and norepinephrine which induces changes in bone marrow, thymus, spleen, and lymph nodes. Catecholamines can regulate immune proliferation, cytolytic activity, cytokine release, antibody release, and chemotaxis by binding to adrenoreceptors on lymphoid organs and immune cells. Norepinephrine and epinephrine increase lymphocyte proliferation and inhibit cytotoxic activity. Dopamine inhibits both proliferation and cytotoxic activity.[8] In addition, peripheral vasoconstriction occurs which can result in chronic muscular ischemia.

The sympathetic nervous system is also involved in the inflammatory milieu in joint spaces by regulating plasma extravasation in the synovium by the activity of sympathetic post-ganglionic fibers but not by the release of norepinephrine onto terminal receptors. Rather, there may be a sympathetic-sensory neuron coupling that sustains this chronic inflammatory state.[7] Central control also plays a role. The HPA axis appears to control inflammatory changes as well. Systemic corticosterone induces remote cells such as leukocytes or endothelial cells to produce annexin-1 which impacts the sympathetic terminals in the synovium, decreasing the local inflammatory environment.[7]

The parasympathetic nervous system is controlled by the vagus nerve. Vagus nerve activation releases norepinephrine from splenic neurons which bind to β2 adrenergic receptors on splenic T-cells which favors choline acetyltransferase stimulation. The result is acetylcholine production.[9] Acetylcholine binds to the α7 subunit of the nicotinic acetylcholine receptor on macrophages in the spleen, resulting in decreased NF-κB activity. The result is decreased cytokine synthesis.[8] Patients with autoimmune disease and non-resolving inflammation display impaired vagus nerve signaling.[10] Vagus nerve stimulation can limit leukocyte migration into the joints of these patients.[11] Fish oil has been shown to enhance vagus nerve activity.[12]

Vagal afferents project through the celiac branches of the abdominal vagus nerve and may be associated with the gut-associated lymphoid tissue (GALT). Here in the gut is a location for major interaction between the autonomic nervous system and the immune system. The gut also has significant interactions with the central nervous system. The gastrointestinal tract may play a central role in communication—hence the growing interest in the brain–gut axis communication.

The ENS can communicate with the CNS via the sensory pathways of the vagus nerve in the parasympathetic nervous system. Likewise, the efferent motor pathways of the prevertebral ganglion can provide communication via the sympathetic nervous system.[13] The microbiome of the gut can also impact the CNS either by direct effect on the vagus nerve or via microbial metabolic products that can have either a direct impact on the enteric cells or a direct impact on the brain by crossing the blood–brain barrier.[13,14] One example of this is serotonin. Only approximately 3% of the body's serotonin is found in the CNS. The vast majority is found in the intestine.[15] Various bacteria and bacterial products—such as short-chain fatty acids—modulate serotonin production.[13,16,17]

Microbiome alterations can clinically impact the pain experience. A recent poster presentation comparing the microbiome of twins with and without chronic widespread pain (CWP) has shown that Firmicutes of families Ruminococcaceae and Lachnospiraceae were decreased in patients with CWP, with an increase in different Firmicutes families, Bacteroidetes, and proteobacteria. Alpha diversity was also decreased in CWP. These findings held true even while controlling for BMI.[18] Likewise, a case report showed that fecal microbiota transplantation was able to relieve painful diabetic neuropathy.[19] Not only are there mechanistic reasons to believe that gut modifications may impact the pain experience, but clinical models are becoming apparent.

The gut may also influence the blood–brain barrier (BBB). The endothelium of the cerebral microvasculature protects neural function by preventing the passage of many circulating molecules—such as neurotransmitters and bacteria—from entering the brain.[20] Inflammation may disrupt the BBB and allow inflammatory substances such as lipopolysaccharide to enter the brain, allowing the ratcheting up of neuroinflammation by exciting microglia cells.[21] The gut microbiome may be correlated to the development of hyperpermeable gut which may directly or indirectly impact the BBB.[21,22] These issues are in the early stages of being worked out, but this remains an area where our understanding may continue to evolve.

Another pathway used by the central nervous system to communicate with the immune system is via a neuropeptidergic pathway. When nociceptors are activated, the axons themselves release neuropeptides that have been noted to further impact the activity of the neurons. Substances such as CGRP, SP, adrenomedullin, neurokinin A and BV, vasoactive intestinal peptide (VIP), neuropeptide Y (NPY), and gastrin-releasing peptide (GRP) are examples of these type of neuropeptides. These neuropeptides also modulate innate and adaptive immune cells. Mast cell degranulation increases. Neutrophil activation and chemotaxis increase. T-cell activation and proliferation increase. Macrophage activation and phagocytosis capability increase.[8]

The cytokine pathway is another means to allow cross-talk between the immune system and the central nervous system. It is not only immune cells that display cytokine receptors—neurons do as well. IL-1, TNF-α, IL-6, IL-2, and IFN-γ contribute to increased chemotaxis, activation, and proliferation of immune cells. These cytokines can also bind to CNS in regions where the BBB is deficient, by carrier-mediated transport mechanisms, or by altering the BBB permeability, allowing neutrophil and leukocyte infiltration into brain tissue.[8] Glia cells have been shown to secrete cytokines.[23,24] Cytokines may act in the periphery, binding to peripheral sensory neurons or to the autonomic vagus nerve.[25] Cytokines may impact the hypothalamus and affect the HPA.[26,27]

Mechanistically, it follows that chronic inflammatory pressure from chronic smoldering infections, oxidative stress, or environmental stress/toxins may be important obstacles in treating the patient with chronic pain.

MORE ON PERIPHERAL SENSITIZATION

Neurotrophic factors also play an important role in peripheral sensitization. After peripheral nerve injury, the physiology of the nerve itself can become altered. Nerve injury can stimulate nerve growth factor (NGF) expression. NGF promotes the growth and repair of nerves. Satellite glial cells in the DRG synthesize more NGF when needed. Mast cells and fibroblasts release NGF as well. NGF binds to tyrosine kinase (TrkA) on $A\delta$ and C fibers which activates these primary afferent terminals by upregulating Na_v channels.[4]

In peripherally injured nerves, increased densities of Na_v channels can be noted which can result in increased spontaneous discharges of the nerve. Independent pacemakers have been noted in surgically damaged nerves. Increased expressions of receptors along an injured axon have also been noted which can result in increased sensitivity.[4] Peripheral nerve transection results in the formation of neuromas. These neuromas are sensitized by immune activation by cytokines such as TNF (as previously described). Both A and C fibers show ectopic activity. The autonomic nervous system impacts the damaged nerve as well. Postganglionic sympathetic efferents sprout into the nerve injury site as well, further sensitizing the nerve in response to catecholamine release. The postganglionic terminals are influenced by nerve growth factor released from local Schwann cells to release catecholamines which excite the injured nerve and the nerve's dorsal root ganglia (DRG). Prostanoids also enhance the opening of TTX-insensitive sodium channels on the afferent terminals.[28]

Injured tissue is noted to have a lower pH and higher K+ concentration compared to non-injured tissue. Channels present on C fibers are activated by higher H+ concentrations. TRPV1/acid-sensing ion channels (ASICs) are just one example.[28]

The primary afferents themselves are also noted to play a role in the local inflammatory milieu. CGRP and SP are released from the peripheral terminals of the C fibers. CGRP and SP result in vasodilation, plasma extravasation, and degranulation of mast cells. This leads to the previously mentioned reddening and swelling.

During primary sensitization, intracellular signaling pathways such as the activation of protein kinase A (PKA)[29] and protein kinase C (PKC)[30] result in the phosphorylation and resultant activation of receptors such as TRPV1. The action of prostaglandin is also noted to upregulate PKA which also activates Na_v 1.8 and 1.9 channels.[31] Both of these intracellular alterations result in increased afferent activation. Extracellular pathways can also become activated. Phosphatidylinositol-3 kinase (PI3K), activated via an extracellular signal-regulated kinase (ERK)-dependent manner, can also sensitize TRPV1.[32,33]

It is important to note that while primary sensitization occurs peripherally, central mechanisms via the endocrine system can play an important role. Stressors can activate the hypothalamus to direct the pituitary to secrete adrenocorticotropic hormone (ACTH), macrophage migration inhibitory factor (MIF), and pituitary adenylate cyclase-activating polypeptide (PACAP). ACTH stimulates the release of cortisol and norepinephrine from the adrenal glands which act on and modulate the immune system (lymphocytes, granulocytes, and macrophages). The immune cells secrete cytokines, chemokines that modulate inflammatory responses in the skin. Skin inflammation has a reciprocal effect on the immune cells via cytokines, chemokines, prostaglandins, leukotrienes, nitric oxide, and melanocyte-stimulating hormone impacting the production of inflammatory mediators such as cytokines.[34]

DRG

The primary afferent summarizes the nociceptive information from the periphery and feeds this information centrally toward the spine where the signal passes through the primary afferent cell body—the dorsal root ganglia (DRG). The DRG is yet another location where nociceptive information can be modulated. The DRG is impacted by repetitive stimulation and adjusts gene transcription. The DRG synthesizes modulatory neuropeptides that are rapidly transported antegrade and retrograde, impacting the sensitivity of the nociceptor.[28] Within the DRG, multiple cell bodies are encased in a small region. These cell bodies can pathologically cross-talk. This short circuit process is known as ephaptic-transmission and results in increased excitation[32] and pain outside of the originally injured location. Ephaptic-transmission can also occur in the periphery in the case of peripheral neuromas. A large low-threshold fiber such as an Aβ fiber can create activation in a high-threshold fiber such as an Aδ fiber—essentially turning innocuous information into nociception.

The cell bodies of the DRG are surrounded by small glial cells (SGCs) that support and supply nutrients to these cell bodies via gap junctions. In the presence of induced inflammation, there is increased gap junction coupling and boosting of neuronal excitability. This can further drive the pain sensation beyond the field of injury. Pro- and anti-inflammatory cytokines create a milieu that influences the interaction. In cases of chronic pain, these interactions can fail to resolve themselves.[4]

CENTRAL SENSITIZATION

The pain pathway can be modulated from within the central nervous system as well by a phenomenon called central sensitization. The dorsal horn itself can modulate its own excitability. Repetitive activation of nociceptive input can alter the ascending pain pathway. Persistent C fiber activation of lamina I and lamina V occurs with tissue injury and inflammation. Lamina V's WDR neurons enhance the dorsal horn's response to further nociceptive input. WDR neurons are unique in that the intensity of the response increases with increased frequency of stimulation even though the strength of the stimulation stays constant. This can result in over-excitation of the nociceptive signal. In addition, the receptive field of activated neurons enlarges so that dermatomal areas not previously activated are now responsive. This effect has been called "wind-up."[35] Chronic neuropathic pain has been linked to WDR neurons. WDR neurons are also activated by sympathetic pathways and can be temporarily blocked by sympathetic blockade.[36]

Bliss and Lomo described long-term potentiation (LTP) in the hippocampus where brief high-frequency coincident input resulted in a persistent increase in synaptic efficacy.[37] This phenomenon was later recorded in the spinal cord as part of the central sensitization process.[38,39] This synaptic plasticity shares striking similarities with the process of memory.[40] With LTP, the facilitation manifested after the stimulus—that is to say that for some time, only a low level of nociception was required to sustain the stimulation. Nociceptive inputs that are normally sub-threshold create excitation. This is distinct from wind-up where the facilitation occurs with continued stable but high-frequency stimulation.[41] Long-term depression (LTD) is an opponent process to LTP. LTD occurs in response to weak or low-frequency stimulation.[4]

The N-methyl-D-aspartate (NMDA) receptor has been well-implicated in the development of wind-up. The NMDA receptor is an ionotropic glutamate receptor (glutamate receptor and an ion channel). At normal resting potential, the ionophore channel is blocked by Mg^{2+}. With the Mg^{2+} block in place, glutamate will not be able to open the channel. However, with repetitive stimulation by AMPA and SP, the Mg^{2+} block is removed. If secondary glycine or D-serine sites are also occupied, activation of the NMDA receptor by glutamate can then allow entry of Ca^{2+} and Na^+ into the cell, and K^+ out of the cell. So not only is the cell depolarized, but there are increased intracellular stores of Ca^{2+} as well. Wind-up has been prevented by the administration of NMDA receptor antagonists.[42-44]

The increased intracellular concentration of Ca^{2+} promotes the externalization of phospholipases to the cell membrane which then cleave arachidonic acid and is acted upon by cyclooxygenase to produce prostanoids. Prostaglandins act pre- and post-synaptically. The pre-synaptic effect enhances the opening of voltage gated calcium channels. Post-synaptically, glycine receptors are inhibited. Glycine typically acts as an inhibitory neurotransmitter on the second-order neuron.

Increased intracellular concentration of Ca^{2+} also results in increased levels of nitric oxide synthase which in the presence of arginine allows for the release of nitric oxide. Nitric oxide impacts the pre-synaptic neuron to enhance the release of excitatory glutamate neurotransmitter.

Increased intracellular concentration of Ca^{2+} also activated multiple protein kinases. Protein kinases result in multiple changes. Amino acid sites on NMDA and AMPA receptors are phosphorylated, lowering the activation threshold. Phospholipase-A_2 is phosphorylated which activates transcription factors such as nuclear factor-KB, which increased the synthesis of inflammatory proteins, channels, receptors, and transcription factors.[28]

With nerve injury, there is an upregulation several types of sodium channels (especially the $\alpha_2\delta$ subunit) and downregulation of potassium channels. This is noted at the superficial dorsal horn in the substantia gelatinosa and in the DRG. Hence, the anti-nociceptive actions of gabapentin or intrathecal ziconotide.

Central sensitization can also occur from non-neuronal cells resident in the central nervous system. In addition to neurons, the central nervous system contains supportive glia cells such as astrocytes, microglia, and oligodendrocytes. Astrocytes envelop the synapse and secrete and absorb neurotransmitters. Microglia are essentially resident macrophages in the CNS. These glia cells are considered to be an important contributor to the synapse—so much so that the synapse has been referred to as tripartite. Microglia typically exist in a resting state. With appropriate stimulation, glia cells can shift into an activated, reactive, pro-inflammatory response profile—creating neuronal excitability and removing the "brake" on excitability. Sensory afferents can increase glutamate release. Upregulation in the number and conductance of calcium-permeable AMPA and NMDA receptors is noted. Inhibitory GABA receptors are down regulated. Glial glutamate transporters are downregulated. Astrocytes typically regulate extracellular glutamate concentration by utilizing an active uptake system. However, during certain situations, these stores can be dumped out, resulting in significant increases in glutamate concentration. Astrocytes may become "activated" after microglial activation and communicate on a broader network basis via gap junctions which may result in the reversal of glutamate transporters. Once microglia become activated, they do not return to a normal resting state but remain "primed."

Neurotransmitters such as glutamate, SP, and ATP can be taken up by glia cells to activate them. Second-order neurons can secrete fractalkine which activate the microglia. Circulating cytokines may activate glia cells. Astrocytes may themselves communicate with the microglia via S-100 protein or cytokines. Peripheral nerve injury can elicit endogenous danger signals or "alarmins" which activate the glia by binding to innate immune pattern recognition receptors such as toll-like receptors. Examples include degradation products of the extracellular matrix, components of circulating blood not normally having access to the extracellular space—such as fibrinogen—or substances released from damaged or dying cells (nuclear protein HMBG1, HSP, or DNA). The activation of toll-like receptors (TLRs) activates glia cells. TLR4 agonists have been shown in DRG cells to increase intracellular Ca^{2+} and lead to the release of neurotransmitters.[45,46] In the presence of bone cancer, there is significant activation of glia.

DORSAL HORN MODULATION

Local inhibitory pathways are interesting in that, over time, an inhibitory pathway can become excitatory and create a positive feedback loop. At baseline, there is a normal Cl^- gradient with Cl^- concentrations higher outside of the neuron than inside the neuron. This is established by the action of an active Cl^- transporter pushing Cl^- out of the cell. Typically, $GABA_A$ and glycine receptors are inhibitory secondary to their function as a Cl^- ionophore and allow the influx of Cl^- into the cell according to its gradient—diminishing the chance of a successful action potential. There are two receptor sites on GABA receptors. The active site binds GABA, muscimol, gaboxadol, and bicu-culine, while drugs such as benzodiazepines, alcohol, and barbiturates bind to different allosteric binding sites. After nerve injury, the Cl^- transporter activity becomes diminished. As a result, the Cl^- concentration becomes reversed with higher concentrations of Cl^- inside of the neuron. Now, these ionophore receptors result in membrane depolarization—improving the likelihood of a successful action potential.

GABA interneurons are at risk with repetitive excitatory dorsal horn stimulation. As NMDA receptor activation increases, there is an increase in intracellular Ca^{2+} concentrations. At some point, the Ca^{2+} buffering capacity of the mitochondria in these cells is overrun and apoptosis ensues. As a result, pain inhibition is even further degraded.[47]

Opioids play a role in modulating pain throughout the CNS. While opiates are presumed analogues to endogenous opioids such as enkephalin, dynorphin, and β-endorphin, there is little evidence showing the role played by these endogenous opioids in the pain system. Opioids bind to the μ-opioid receptor primarily on the C fiber afferents (located in the superficial dorsal horn and cell bodies of the deeper dorsal horn neurons) inhibiting neuronal discharge. Aβ fibers are also present here but are not typically affected by opioids. The pre-synaptic opioid effect works primarily by preventing the opening of Ca^{2+} channels which limits peptide neurotransmitter release (such as SP). Post-synaptic neurons experience K^+ channel activation which results in hyperpolarization.[28]

BRAIN

As discussed in the last chapter, the brain does not merely function as a receiver of the pain signal. Instead, it actively manipulates and sculpts the signal. Spontaneous pain is an interesting scenario. fMRI evidence suggests that some patients with chronic lower back pain may have different brain regions directing the pain experience. High sustained pain in patients with chronic back pain was primarily noted in the medial prefrontal cortex—a region typically associated with emotional assessment in relation to self, not typically associated with pain processing. This activity was correlated with the intensity of the perceived pain. However, when these same patients experienced an increasing phase of pain, the activated brain regions were similar to control subjects—such as the insula. When thermal stimulation was applied, the intensity of activation of the medial prefrontal cortex was correlated to the intensity of spontaneous pain, while the activation of the insula correlated to the intensity of thermal stimulation.[48] Another meta-analysis has shown that in chronic pain patients, the prefrontal cortex shows stronger activation, while other cortical areas and the thalamus show a weaker response.[49] It appears as though the baseline pain perception in chronic pain patients may be originating from the altered and different brain circuits; but this is not to say that the more traditional pain circuits are not functioning. In fact, they appear to activate when challenged with a nociceptive input.

Brain pathways may be altered in patients with chronic neuropathic pain. Magnetic resonance spectroscopy (MRS) is a non-invasive measure of the in vivo concentration of metabolites in the brain. An MRS study on spinal cord injury patients showed significant decreased concentrations of N-acetyl aspartate (NAA) and a trend toward an increased concentration of myo-inositol in paraplegic patients with chronic neuropathic pain. Decreases in NAA concentrations are considered reflections of degenerative neuronal disease in processes such as brain tumors, epilepsy, amyotrophic lateral sclerosis, Parkinson's, and Huntington's diseases. Myo-inositol is felt to be a glial marker. It was hypothesized that deafferentation of the thalamus was responsible.[50] Furthermore, SPECT studies have shown increases in blood flow to the thalamus in a similar population during times of increased pain.[51] Thalamic activity was also noted to be diminished in patients with CRPS and post-herpetic neuralgia.[52,53]

In patients with chronic low back pain, MRS studies have also shown decreased NAA and glucose in the dorsolateral prefrontal cortex, cingulate, and sensorimotor cortex.[54] In addition, reductions in total gray matter volume in the dorsolateral prefrontal cortex are correlated to the duration of chronic pain.[55] Patients with chronic low back pain also show decreases in gray matter density in bilateral striatum (primarily in the nucleus accumbens and extending into the caudate and putamen) and insula, and in the left sensorimotor cortex.[56] A strengthened nucleus accumbens medial prefrontal cortex connection predicts a transition to chronic pain.[56] Sensorimotor and mesolimbic changes appear to play an important role in the chronification of pain.

Patients with centralized pain show a diminished opioid receptor binding capacity in portions of the posterior midbrain, medial thalamus, and the insular, temporal, and prefrontal cortices contralateral to the painful side, whereas patients with peripheral neuropathic pain do not show any decreased opioid receptor binding. This was shown in a study using positron emission tomography (PET) and [11C] diprenorphine to compare the in vivo distribution abnormalities of brain opioid receptors.[57]

Limbic system dysfunction in patients with chronic pain may precipitate depression and mood disorders.[58–60] Although the mechanism has not been fully elucidated, elevated levels of NAc brain-derived neurotrophic factor (BDNF), neuroinflammation in the basal ganglia, and other limbic structures may play an important role.[59] The prevalence of depression ranges from 30 to 80%, and suicide is more common in patients with chronic pain than any other medical disorder except for bipolar disease.[59]

ENDOCRINE SYSTEM

Multiple mechanisms exist to control the magnitude of inflammation. As we have seen, the magnitude of inflammation has a direct bearing on nociception. The hypothalamic–pituitary–adrenal axis (HPA), the sympatho-adrenal axes, nociceptive neurons, and the sympatho-neural system are all contributing factors. The autonomic nervous system regulates physiological systems by integrating afferent inputs from internal and external environments with the neuronal system, endocrine system, and cell modulated responses.

The HPA is involved in nociception and serves as an intermediary between the neuro and endocrine and immune systems. These systems normally communicate to maintain physiologic homeostasis. There has been a relative history of skepticism surrounding the relevance of this system to the pain experience; but the current literature suggests a mechanistic pathway of communication.[5] Various immune cells, including lymphocytes and monocytes, have receptors for corticosteroids, insulin, prolactin, growth hormone, somatostatins, estrogens, testosterone, leptin, ghrelin, opioids, corticosteroids, neuropeptide Y, and vasoactive intestinal polypeptide. Neuronal cells and endocrine organs express receptors for immune-derived cytokines and growth factors. There is a true bi-directional communication between these systems.

Pain has profound effects on the HPA system. Pain activates the hypothalamus to release corticotropin-releasing hormone (CRH), gonadal-releasing hormone (GRH), and thyroid-releasing hormone (TRH). These activate the pituitary and then end organs to release hormones that ultimately play a role in pain control—cortisol, pregnenolone, DHEA, testosterone, progesterone, estrogen, triiodothyronine (T_3), and thyroxine (T_4).[61] If pain levels become severe enough, these levels may be seen to elevate.[62,63] Over time, with sustained severe pain, the HPA may not be able to provide sufficient hormone levels, and serum levels may drop.[63–65] Hypercortisolemia may result in calcium resorption (osteoporosis, joint degeneration, tooth decay, nephrolithiasis, vertebral compression fractures), hypertension, hyperlipidemia, obesity, and mental deterioration.[61] Hypocortisolism produces weight loss, muscle wasting, mental apathy, hypotension, brown pigmentation on the skin, or even sudden death.[61]

The hypothalamic–pituitary–gonadal axis (HPG) plays a role in nociception. These initial observations occurred by noting variations in several painful conditions in relation to the menstrual cycle. Temporomandibular joint dysfunction, fibromyalgia syndrome, irritable bowel syndrome (IBS), interstitial cystitis (IC), and migraine can show cyclical variations.[66] These findings suggest that rapidly falling estrogen plays a role in pain. Stabilizing hormone levels (with oral contraceptives) or abolishing hormone levels with GnRH antagonists or menopause can improve IBS and IC but worsen migraine (unless an additional low-dose estrogen is given).[67] Pregnancy analgesia can also improve pain conditions such as migraine and pelvic pain.[68] Androgens also play a role in pain. Rheumatoid arthritis patients have lower androgen levels than sex-based controls and improve with exogenous androgen administration.[69] Interestingly in a 2007 study on transgender patients, one out of three of male to female transitions developed chronic pain, and those who did not develop chronic pain appeared to develop increased sensitivity to pain. On the other hand, one out of every two female to male transition patients who had chronic pain before transition appeared to improve with the administration of androgens.[70] Testosterone and progesterone function as analgesics in the brain. Testosterone modulates endogenous opioids in the brain and modulates dorsal horn response to neuropathic pain. Progesterone mediates spinal cord hypersensitivity after nerve root damage. Estrogen increases μ-opioid receptor availability in the brain and modulates dorsal horn response to pain. Estrogen alters T- and B-cell proliferation and phenotype as well as changing the cytokine and immunoglobulin balance. Progesterone has an anti-inflammatory impact on the immune system. Testosterone decreases cellular immune response.[67]

Pituitary hormones impact nociception. Growth hormone (GH) production and the resulting insulin-like growth factor-1 (IGF-1) production mediate immune cell proliferation or the survival of immune cells such as T-lymphocytes and inhibit the dexamethasone-induced inhibition of T-cell proliferation.[71] Prolactin sustains antibody response and cell-mediated immunity.[72] The immune system also influences the endocrine system. Inflammatory cytokines have also been shown to result in hormone resistance—such as insulin, glucocorticoids, GH, and IGF-1.[5]

Stress has a large impact on the nociceptive system. Stress activates the HPA and the sympathetic nervous system. On one hand, the HPA can create stress-induced analgesia. Hormonal or neural signals of injury can lead to the activation of the hypothalamic periventricular nucleus which induces the release of pro-opiomelanocortin (POMC). POMC is cleaved into various peptides including beta-endorphin which binds to μ-opioid receptors to dampen neuronal excitability by inhibiting voltage-gated Ca^{2+} channels and/or opening K^+ channels in the periphery, DRG, PAG, and RVM.[4] On the other hand, chronic stress or fear can activate the HPA and sympathetic nervous system, creating multiple downstream effects. The activation of the HPA axis results in an increased production of glucocorticoids.

MITOCHONDRIA

Mitochondria likely play a role in chronic pain. Universally known as being the power production center of the cell, the mitochondria do more than merely supply ATP. They are also involved in the creation of reactive oxygen species, mitochondrial permeability transition pore—which may lead to mitochondrial death in reperfusion injury[73]—apoptotic pathways, and intracellular calcium mobilization.[74] Each of these may play a role in neuropathic pain.[75] Mitochondrial division appears to play an important role in the creation and sustaining of some types of neuropathic pain. By inhibiting mitochondrial division in sensory neurons, mechanical hyperalgesia, normally brought on by anti-HIV drug 2,3-dideoxycytidine or the cancer drug oxaliplatin, was decreased. There was less hypersensitivity created by reactive oxygen species. In addition, inhibiting mitochondrial division also showed a treatment effect by reversing mechanical hyperalgesia secondary to the inflammatory mediators TNF-α, glial-derived neurotrophic factor, and the nitric oxide donor NOR-3.[76]

While the inhibition of mitochondrial division appears to play an important role in the treatment and protection of neuropathic pain, the loss of mitochondrial function in Schwann cells can also lead to the development of progressive neuropathy. By creating mitochondrial dysfunction in peripheral nerve Schwann cells (by deleting mitochondrial transcription factor-A gene), it was shown that a progressive peripheral neuropathy developed with age. These were associated with nerve conduction abnormalities as well as muscle denervation.[77] Clinically, Schwann cell mitochondrial abnormalities have been identified in some neuropathies.[78,79]

Calcium modulation and the creation of reactive oxygen species are other important mitochondrial elements in the chronic pain state. We know that, during central sensitization, NMDA receptors lead to increased Ca^{2+} concentrations in the dorsal horn. By blocking mitochondrial uptake of Ca^{2+}, NMDA receptor activation did not lead to central sensitization.[80] Mitochondrial oxidative phosphorylation is a major source of superoxide ions found in excited neurons and is typically controlled by superoxide dismutase.[81] Scavenging superoxide significantly reduces mechanical hyperalgesia.[82] This provides a strong mechanistic explanation for the role of the mitochondria in central sensitization.

LEPTIN AND GHRELIN

Leptin is typically considered to play a role in metabolism, being produced by adipocytes in a fed state. However, leptin levels have been noted to increase during acute infection, and acute and chronic inflammatory processes. Leptin also appears to be a potent immunomodulatory hormone and may play a role in several autoimmune pathways.[83] Leptin increases phagocytic activity and cytokine secretion. It can stimulate neutrophil chemotaxis and oxidative burst. It can increase the activity of natural killer cells.[8] Leptin promotes the switch toward Th1 activity.[84] Leptin promotes pro-inflammatory cytokine secretion and may play a role in enhancing autoimmune disorders.[85] It is interesting to note that women show increased serum leptin levels compared to age- and BMI-matched men.[86]

On the other hand, ghrelin is produced primarily in the stomach during non-fed states and serves not only as an orexigen controlling energy expenditure, but also as a GH secretagogue receptor. Ghrelin and GH secretagogue receptor are also found on immune cells such as lymphocytes, monocytes, and dendritic cells. Ghrelin has anti-inflammatory effects on the immune system.[5]

CONCLUSION

In the chronic pain patient, there are multiple pathways that are disrupted or altered. A more comprehensive approach to unwinding this situation is likely to be more effective than our current strategies. Chronic opioid therapy falls short in many respects. The following chapter will discuss this further.

REFERENCES

1. Wirz, S., & Molderings, G.J. (2017). A practical guide for treatment of pain in patients with systemic mast cell activation disease. *Pain Phys*, 20(6), E849–E861.
2. Afrin, L.B., Pöhlau, D., Raithel, M., Haenisch, B., Dumoulin, F.L., Homann, J., … Molderings, G.J. (2015). Mast cell activation disease: an underappreciated cause of neurologic and psychiatric symptoms and diseases. *Brain Behav Immun*, 50, 314–321. doi:10.1016/j.bbi.2015.07.002
3. Jennings, S., Russell, N., Jennings, B., Slee, V., Sterling, L., Castells, M., … Akin, C. (2014). The mastocytosis society survey on mast cell disorders: patient experiences and perceptions. *J Allergy Clin Immunol Pract*, 2(1), 70–76. doi:10.1016/j.jaip.2013.09.004
4. Chapman, C.R., & Vierck, C.J. (2017). The transition of acute postoperative pain to chronic pain: an integrative overview of research on mechanisms. *J Pain*, 18(4), 359.e1–359.e38. doi:10.1016/j.jpain.2016.11.004
5. Taub, D.D. (2008). Neuroendocrine interactions in the immune system. *Cell Immunol*, 252(1–2), 1–6. doi:10.1016/j.cellimm.2008.05.006
6. Costa, M., Brookes, S.J., & Hennig, G.W. (2000). Anatomy and physiology of the enteric nervous system. *Gut*, 47(Suppl. 4), iv15–19; discussion iv26. doi:10.1136/gut.47.suppl_4.iv15
7. Jänig, W., & Green, P.G. (2014). Acute inflammation in the joint: its control by the sympathetic nervous system and by neuroendocrine systems. *Auton Neurosci*, 182, 42–54. doi:10.1016/j.autneu.2014.01.001
8. Procaccini, C., Pucino, V., De Rosa, V., Marone, G., & Matarese, G. (2014). Neuro-endocrine networks controlling immune system in health and disease. *Front Immunol*, 5, 143. doi:10.3389/fimmu.2014.00143

9. Rosas-Ballina, M., Olofsson, P.S., Ochani, M., Valdés-Ferrer, S.I., Levine, Y.A., Reardon, C., … Tracey, K.J. (2011). Acetylcholine-synthesizing T cells relay neural signals in a vagus nerve circuit. *Science*, 334(6052), 98–101. doi:10.1126/science.1209985

10. Tracey, K.J. (2007). Physiology and immunology of the cholinergic antiinflammatory pathway. *J Clin Invest*, 117(2), 289–296. doi:10.1172/JCI30555

11. Saeed, R.W., Varma, S., Peng-Nemeroff, T., Sherry, B., Balakhaneh, D., Huston, J., … Metz, C.N. (2005). Cholinergic stimulation blocks endothelial cell activation and leukocyte recruitment during inflammation. *J Exp Med*, 201(7), 1113–1123. doi:10.1084/jem.20040463

12. Holguin, F., Téllez-Rojo, M.M., Lazo, M., Mannino, D., Schwartz, J., Hernández, M., & Romieu, I. (2005). Cardiac autonomic changes associated with fish oil vs soy oil supplementation in the elderly. *Chest*, 127(4), 1102–1107. doi:10.1378/chest.127.4.1102

13. Khlevner, J., Park, Y., & Margolis, K.G. (2018). Brain-gut axis: clinical implications. *Gastroenterol Clin North Am*, 47(4), 727–739. doi:10.1016/j.gtc.2018.07.002

14. Smith, P.A. (2015). The tantalizing links between gut microbes and the brain. *Nature*, 526(7573), 312–314. doi:10.1038/526312a

15. Gershon, M.D. (2013). 5-Hydroxytryptamine (serotonin) in the gastrointestinal tract. *Curr Opin Endocrinol Diabetes Obes*, 20(1), 14–21. doi:10.1097/MED.0b013e32835bc703

16. Reigstad, C.S., Salmonson, C.E., Rainey, J.F., 3rd, Szurszewski, J.H., Linden, D.R., Sonnenburg, J.L., … Kashyap, P.C. (2015). Gut microbes promote colonic serotonin production through an effect of short-chain fatty acids on enterochromaffin cells. *FASEB J*, 29(4), 1395–1403. doi:10.1096/fj.14-259598

17. Yano, J.M., Yu, K., Donaldson, G.P., Shastri, G.G., Ann, P., Ma, L., … Hsiao, E.Y. (2015). Indigenous bacteria from the gut microbiota regulate host serotonin biosynthesis. *Cell*, 161(2), 264–276. doi:10.1016/j.cell.2015.02.047

18. Stalteri, M.F., Lachance, G., Baleanu, A., Bowyer, R., Jackson, M., & Williams, F. (2018). Association studies of chronic widespread pain and the gut microbiome. Paper presented at the World Congress on Pain, Boston, MA.

19. Cai, T.T., Ye, X.L., Yong, H.J., Song, B., Zheng, X.L., Cui, B.T., … Ding, D.F. (2018). Fecal microbiota transplantation relieve painful diabetic neuropathy: a case report. *Med (Baltim)*, 97(50), e13543. doi:10.1097/MD.0000000000013543

20. Abbott, N.J. (2002). Astrocyte-endothelial interactions and blood-brain barrier permeability. *J Anat*, 200(6), 629–638. doi:10.1046/j.1469-7580.2002.00064.x

21. Obrenovich, M.E.M. (2018). Leaky gut, leaky brain? *Microorganisms*, 6(4). doi:10.3390/microorganisms6040107

22. Lanza, G., Bella, R., Cantone, M., Pennisi, G., Ferri, R., & Pennisi, M. (2018). Cognitive impairment and celiac disease: is transcranial magnetic stimulation a trait d'union between gut and brain? *Int J Mol Sci*, 19(8). doi:10.3390/ijms19082243

23. Fontana, A., & Grob, P.J. (1984). Astrocyte-derived interleukin-1-like factors. *Lymphokine Res*, 3(1), 11–16.

24. Giulian, D., Baker, T.J., Shih, L.C., & Lachman, L.B. (1986). Interleukin 1 of the central nervous system is produced by ameboid microglia. *J Exp Med*, 164(2), 594–604.

25. Marvel, F.A., Chen, C.C., Badr, N., Gaykema, R.P., & Goehler, L.E. (2004). Reversible inactivation of the dorsal vagal complex blocks lipopolysaccharide-induced social withdrawal and c-Fos expression in central autonomic nuclei. *Brain Behav Immun*, 18(2), 123–134. doi:10.1016/j.bbi.2003.09.004

26. Berkenbosch, F., van Oers, J., del Rey, A., Tilders, F., & Besedovsky, H. (1987). Corticotropin-releasing factor-producing neurons in the rat activated by interleukin-1. *Science*, 238(4826), 524–526.

27. Sapolsky, R., Rivier, C., Yamamoto, G., Plotsky, P., & Vale, W. (1987). Interleukin-1 stimulates the secretion of hypothalamic corticotropin-releasing factor. *Science*, 238(4826), 522–524.

28. Benzon, H.T. (2014). *Practical Management of Pain* (5th ed.). Philadelphia, PA: Elsevier/Mosby.

29. Bhave, G., Zhu, W., Wang, H., Brasier, D.J., Oxford, G.S., & Gereau, R.W.t. (2002). cAMP-dependent protein kinase regulates desensitization of the capsaicin receptor (VR1) by direct phosphorylation. *Neuron*, 35(4), 721–731.

30. Bhave, G., Hu, H.J., Glauner, K.S., Zhu, W., Wang, H., Brasier, D.J., … Gereau, R.W. (2003). Protein kinase C phosphorylation sensitizes but does not activate the capsaicin receptor transient receptor potential vanilloid 1 (TRPV1). *Proc Natl Acad Sci U S A*, 100(21), 12480–12485. doi:10.1073/pnas.2032100100

31. Julius, D., & Basbaum, A.I. (2001). Molecular mechanisms of nociception. *Nature*, 413(6852), 203–210. doi:10.1038/35093019

32. D'Mello, R., & Dickenson, A.H. (2008). Spinal cord mechanisms of pain. *Br J Anaesth*, 101(1), 8–16. doi:10.1093/bja/aen088

33. Zhuang, Z.Y., Xu, H., Clapham, D.E., & Ji, R.R. (2004). Phosphatidylinositol 3-kinase activates ERK in primary sensory neurons and mediates inflammatory heat hyperalgesia through TRPV1 sensitization. *J Neurosci*, 24(38), 8300–8309. doi:10.1523/JNEUROSCI.2893-04.2004

34. Roosterman, D., Goerge, T., Schneider, S.W., Bunnett, N.W., & Steinhoff, M. (2006). Neuronal control of skin function: the skin as a neuroimmunoendocrine organ. *Physiol Rev*, 86(4), 1309–1379. doi:10.1152/physrev.00026.2005

35. Mendell, L.M., & Wall, P.D. (1965). Responses of single dorsal cord cells to peripheral cutaneous unmyelinated fibres. *Nature*, 206, 97–99.

36. Roberts, W.J., & Foglesong, M.E. (1988). Spinal recordings suggest that wide-dynamic-range neurons mediate sympathetically maintained pain. *Pain*, 34(3), 289–304.

37. Bliss, T.V., & Lomo, T. (1973). Long-lasting potentiation of synaptic transmission in the dentate area of the anaesthetized rabbit following stimulation of the perforant path. *J Physiol*, 232(2), 331–356.

38. Ikeda, H., Heinke, B., Ruscheweyh, R., & Sandkuhler, J. (2003). Synaptic plasticity in spinal lamina I projection neurons that mediate hyperalgesia. *Science*, 299(5610), 1237–1240. doi:10.1126/science.1080659

39. Ikeda, H., Stark, J., Fischer, H., Wagner, M., Drdla, R., Jäger, T., & Sandkühler, J. (2006). Synaptic amplifier of inflammatory pain in the spinal dorsal horn. *Science*, 312(5780), 1659–1662. doi:10.1126/science.1127233

40. Ji, R.R., Kohno, T., Moore, K.A., & Woolf, C.J. (2003). Central sensitization and LTP: do pain and memory share similar mechanisms? *Trends Neurosci*, 26(12), 696–705. doi:10.1016/j.tins.2003.09.017

41. Woolf, C.J. (2011). Central sensitization: implications for the diagnosis and treatment of pain. *Pain*, 152(3 Suppl.), S2–15. doi:10.1016/j.pain.2010.09.030

42. Kristensen, J.D., Hartvig, P., Karlsten, R., Gordh, T., & Halldin, M. (1995). CSF and plasma pharmacokinetics of the NMDA receptor antagonist CPP after intrathecal, extradural and i.v. administration in anaesthetized pigs. *Br J Anaesth*, 74(2), 193–200.

43. Kristensen, J.D., Karlsten, R., Gordh, T., & Berge, O.G. (1994). The NMDA antagonist 3-(2-carboxypiperazin-4-yl)propyl-1-phosphonic acid (CPP) has antinociceptive effect after intrathecal injection in the rat. *Pain*, 56(1), 59–67.

44. Kristensen, J.D., Svensson, B., & Gordh, T. Jr. (1992). The NMDA-receptor antagonist CPP abolishes neurogenic 'wind-up pain' after intrathecal administration in humans. *Pain*, 51(2), 249–253.

45. Hutchinson, M.R., Bland, S.T., Johnson, K.W., Rice, K.C., Maier, S.F., & Watkins, L.R. (2007). Opioid-induced glial activation: mechanisms of activation and implications for opioid analgesia, dependence, and reward. *Sci World J*, 7, 98–111. doi:10.1100/tsw.2007.230

46. Watkins, L.R., Hutchinson, M.R., Rice, K.C., & Maier, S.F. (2009). The 'toll' of opioid-induced glial activation: improving the clinical efficacy of opioids by targeting glia. *Trends Pharmacol Sci*, 30(11), 581–591. doi:10.1016/j.tips.2009.08.002

47. Whiteside, G.T., & Munglani, R. (2001). Cell death in the superficial dorsal horn in a model of neuropathic pain. *J Neurosci Res*, 64(2), 168–173. doi:10.1002/jnr.1062

48. Baliki, M.N., Chialvo, D.R., Geha, P.Y., Levy, R.M., Harden, R.N., Parrish, T.B., & Apkarian, A.V. (2006). Chronic pain and the emotional brain: specific brain activity associated with spontaneous fluctuations of intensity of chronic back pain. *J Neurosci*, 26(47), 12165–12173. doi:10.1523/JNEUROSCI.3576-06.2006

49. Apkarian, A.V., Bushnell, M.C., Treede, R.D., & Zubieta, J.K. (2005). Human brain mechanisms of pain perception and regulation in health and disease. *Eur J Pain*, 9(4), 463–484. doi:10.1016/j.ejpain.2004.11.001

50. Pattany, P.M., Yezierski, R.P., Widerström-Noga, E.G., Bowen, B.C., Martinez-Arizala, A., Garcia, B.R., & Quencer, R.M. (2002). Proton magnetic resonance spectroscopy of the thalamus in patients with chronic neuropathic pain after spinal cord injury. *AJNR Am J Neuroradiol*, 23(6), 901–905.

51. Ness, T.J., San Pedro, E.C., Richards, J.S., Kezar, L., Liu, H.G., & Mountz, J.M. (1998). A case of spinal cord injury-related pain with baseline rCBF brain SPECT imaging and beneficial response to gabapentin. *Pain*, 78(2), 139–143.

52. Fukui, S., Matsuno, M., Inubushi, T., & Nosaka, S. (2006). N-acetylaspartate concentrations in the thalami of neuropathic pain patients and healthy comparison subjects measured with (1).H-MRS. *Magn Reson Imaging*, 24(1), 75–79. doi:10.1016/j.mri.2005.10.021

53. Fukumoto, M., Ushida, T., Zinchuk, V.S., Yamamoto, H., & Yoshida, S. (1999). Contralateral thalamic perfusion in patients with reflex sympathetic dystrophy syndrome. *Lancet*, 354(9192), 1790–1791. doi:10.1016/S0140-6736(99)03746-0

54. Grachev, I.D., Fredrickson, B.E., & Apkarian, A.V. (2000). Abnormal brain chemistry in chronic back pain: an in vivo proton magnetic resonance spectroscopy study. *Pain*, 89(1), 7–18.

55. Apkarian, A.V. (2004). Cortical pathophysiology of chronic pain. *Novartis Found Symp*, 261, 239–245; discussion 245–261.

56. Baliki, M.N., Petre, B., Torbey, S., Herrmann, K.M., Huang, L., Schnitzer, T.J., … Apkarian, A.V. (2012). Corticostriatal functional connectivity predicts transition to chronic back pain. *Nat Neurosci*, 15(8), 1117–1119. doi:10.1038/nn.3153

57. Maarrawi, J., Peyron, R., Mertens, P., Costes, N., Magnin, M., Sindou, M., … Garcia-Larrea, L. (2007). Differential brain opioid receptor availability in central and peripheral neuropathic pain. *Pain*, 127(1–2), 183–194. doi:10.1016/j.pain.2006.10.013

58. Cahill, C.M., Cook, C., & Pickens, S. (2014). Migraine and reward system-or is it aversive? *Curr Pain Headache Rep*, 18(5), 410. doi:10.1007/s11916-014-0410-y

59. Cahill, C.M., & Taylor, A.M. (2017). Neuroinflammation-a co-occurring phenomenon linking chronic pain and opioid dependence. *Curr Opin Behav Sci*, 13, 171–177. doi:10.1016/j.cobeha.2016.12.003

60. Cahill, C.M., Taylor, A.M., Cook, C., Ong, E., Moron, J.A., & Evans, C.J. (2014). Does the kappa opioid receptor system contribute to pain aversion? *Front Pharmacol*, 5, 253. doi:10.3389/fphar.2014.00253

61. Tennant, F. (2013). The physiologic effects of pain on the endocrine system. *Pain Ther*, 2(2), 75–86. doi:10.1007/s40122-013-0015-x

62. Khoromi, S., Muniyappa, R., Nackers, L., Gray, N., Baldwin, H., Wong, K.A., … Blackman, M.R. (2006). Effects of chronic osteoarthritis pain on neuroendocrine function in men. *J Clin Endocrinol Metab*, 91(11), 4313–4318. doi:10.1210/jc.2006-1122

63. Tennant, F., & Hermann, L. (2002). Normalization of serum cortisol concentration with opioid treatment of severe chronic pain. *Pain Med*, 3(2), 132–134. doi:10.1046/j.1526-4637.2002.02019.x

64. Tennant, F. (2000). Intractable pain is a severe stress state associated with hypercortisolemia and reduced adrenal reserve. *Drug Alcohol Depend*, 60(Suppl. 1), 220–221.

65. Tennant, F. (2012). How to use adrenocorticotropin as a biomarker in pain management. *Pract Pain Manag*, 12, 62–66.

66. LeResche, L. (2000). *Epidemiologic Perspectives on Sex Differences in Pain* (R.B. Fillingim, Ed.). Seattle, WA: IASP Press.

67. Vincent, K., & Tracey, I. (2008). Hormones and their interaction with the pain experience. *Rev Pain*, 2(2), 20–24. doi:10.1177/204946370800200206

68. Carvalho, B., Angst, M.S., Fuller, A.J., Lin, E., Mathusamy, A.D., & Riley, E.T. (2006). Experimental heat pain for detecting pregnancy-induced analgesia in humans. *Anesth Analg*, 103(5), 1283–1287. doi:10.1213/01.ane.0000239224.48719.28

69. Aloisi, A.M., & Bonifazi, M. (2006). Sex hormones, central nervous system and pain. *Horm Behav*, 50(1), 1–7. doi:10.1016/j.yhbeh.2005.12.002

70. Aloisi, A.M., Bachiocco, V., Costantino, A., Stefani, R., Ceccarelli, I., Bertaccini, A., & Meriggiola, M.C. (2007). Cross-sex hormone administration changes pain in transsexual women and men. *Pain*, 132(Suppl. 1), S60–S67. doi:10.1016/j.pain.2007.02.006

71. Dorshkind, K., & Horseman, N.D. (2000). The roles of prolactin, growth hormone, insulin-like growth factor-I, and thyroid hormones in lymphocyte development and function: insights from genetic models of hormone and hormone receptor deficiency. *Endocr Rev*, 21(3), 292–312. doi:10.1210/edrv.21.3.0397

72. Esquifino, A.I., Arce, A., Alvarez, M.P., Chacon, F., Brown-Borg, H., & Bartke, A. (2004). Differential effects of light/dark recombinant human prolactin administration on the submaxillary lymph nodes and spleen activity of adult male mice. *Neuroimmunomodulation*, 11(2), 119–126. doi:10.1159/000075321

73. Halestrap, A.P. (2009). What is the mitochondrial permeability transition pore? *J Mol Cell Cardiol*, 46(6), 821–831. doi:10.1016/j.yjmcc.2009.02.021

74. Sui, B.D., Xu, T.Q., Liu, J.W., Wei, W., Zheng, C.X., Guo, B.L., … Yang, Y.L. (2013). Understanding the role of mitochondria in the pathogenesis of chronic pain. *Postgrad Med J*, 89(1058), 709–714. doi:10.1136/postgradmedj-2012-131068

75. Reichling, D.B., & Levine, J.D. (2011). Pain and death: neurodegenerative disease mechanisms in the nociceptor. *Ann Neurol*, 69(1), 13–21. doi:10.1002/ana.22351

76. Ferrari, L.F., Chum, A., Bogen, O., Reichling, D.B., & Levine, J.D. (2011). Role of Drp1, a key mitochondrial fission protein, in neuropathic pain. *J Neurosci*, 31(31), 11404–11410. doi:10.1523/JNEUROSCI.2223-11.2011

77. Viader, A., Golden, J.P., Baloh, R.H., Schmidt, R.E., Hunter, D.A., & Milbrandt, J. (2011). Schwann cell mitochondrial metabolism supports long-term axonal survival and peripheral nerve function. *J Neurosci*, 31(28), 10128–10140. doi:10.1523/JNEUROSCI.0884-11.2011

78. Kalichman, M.W., Powell, H.C., & Mizisin, A.P. (1998). Reactive, degenerative, and proliferative Schwann cell responses in experimental galactose and human diabetic neuropathy. *Acta Neuropathol*, 95(1), 47–56.
79. Schröder, J.M. (1993). Neuropathy associated with mitochondrial disorders. *Brain Pathol*, 3(2), 177–190.
80. Kim, H.Y., Lee, K.Y., Lu, Y., Wang, J., Cui, L., Kim, S.J., … Chung, K. (2011). Mitochondrial Ca(2+) uptake is essential for synaptic plasticity in pain. *J Neurosci*, 31(36), 12982–12991. doi:10.1523/JNEUROSCI.3093-11.2011
81. Schwartz, E.S., Kim, H.Y., Wang, J., Lee, I., Klann, E., Chung, J.M., & Chung, K. (2009). Persistent pain is dependent on spinal mitochondrial antioxidant levels. *J Neurosci*, 29(1), 159–168. doi:10.1523/JNEUROSCI.3792-08.2009
82. Kim, H.K., Park, S.K., Zhou, J.L., Taglialatela, G., Chung, K., Coggeshall, R.E., & Chung, J.M. (2004). Reactive oxygen species (ROS) play an important role in a rat model of neuropathic pain. *Pain*, 111(1–2), 116–124. doi:10.1016/j.pain.2004.06.008
83. Lago, R., Gómez, R., Lago, F., Gómez-Reino, J., & Gualillo, O. (2008). Leptin beyond body weight regulation–current concepts concerning its role in immune function and inflammation. *Cell Immunol*, 252(1–2), 139–145. doi:10.1016/j.cellimm.2007.09.004
84. Procaccini, C., Jirillo, E., & Matarese, G. (2012). Leptin as an immunomodulator. *Mol Aspects Med*, 33(1), 35–45. doi:10.1016/j.mam.2011.10.012
85. Fraser, D.A., Thoen, J., Reseland, J.E., Førre, O., & Kjeldsen-Kragh, J. (1999). Decreased CD4+ lymphocyte activation and increased interleukin-4 production in peripheral blood of rheumatoid arthritis patients after acute starvation. *Clin Rheumatol*, 18(5), 394–401.
86. Garcia-Gonzalez, A., González-Lopez, L., Valera-Gonzalez, I.C., Cardona-Muñoz, E.G., Salazar-Paramo, M., Gonzalez-Ortiz, M., … Gamez-Nava, J.I. (2002). Serum leptin levels in women with systemic lupus erythematosus. *Rheumatol Int*, 22(4), 138–141. doi:10.1007/s00296-002-0216-9

3 The Opioid Epidemic

Matthew Bennett

CONTENTS

Despite the intention of the modern medical community, opioids have not lived up to the inherent promise of providing safe antinociceptive treatment for those in chronic pain. The reasons for this are complex and include physiologic shortcomings, safety issues, psychological confounders, societal implications, and regulatory and oversight concerns. This chapter will concentrate on the physiologic shortcomings. This work will not discuss the inherent risks of opioid diversion, abuse, misuse, or accidental overdose and death. These are important issues, but outside of the scope of our discussion. In addition, the context of this discussion is in the consideration of chronic non-malignant pain. The argument being presented is that opioids often do not function well for chronic non-malignant pain. However, they continue to serve important functions in acute pain, cancer pain, and palliative care.

OPIOID OVERVIEW

Opioids are natural or synthetic substances that bind to opiate receptors. An opiate is a drug derived from opium—from the poppy plant *Papaver somniferum*. Morphine, codeine, thebaine, and papaverine are examples of opiates. Semi-synthetic opioids include drugs such as hydrocodone, oxycodone, oxymorphone, hydromorphone, and heroin. Synthetic opioids include methadone, fentanyl, and tramadol.

Opiates bind to various opioid receptors scattered throughout the body in the central nervous system, peripheral nervous system, gastrointestinal tract, and blood cells. There are multiple sub-types of opioid receptors, but the most clinically important are mu (μ), kappa (κ), and delta receptors (δ). μ-opiate receptors (MOP) have a high affinity for endogenous enkephalins and beta-endorphin and a low affinity for dynorphin. Morphine is the prototypical MOP agonist. κ-opiate receptors (KOP) have a high affinity for endogenous dynorphin. KOP act as a natural anti-reward system. δ-opiate receptors (DOP) have an affinity for enkephalin. The role of DOP in the pain system is not fully elucidated. Although not a true opioid receptor, the opioid-receptor-like receptor 1 (ORL1) shares a high sequence identity with true opioid receptors. Nociceptin/orphanin FQ (N/OFQ) binds the ORL1 and plays a role in analgesia and opioid tolerance.

Opioid receptors are G protein-coupled receptors (GPCR) with seven transmembrane helical loops—three intracellular loops and three extracellular loops. The extracellular loops contain the pocket in which the signaling molecules bind. Acute stimulation of the receptor results in activation of the G-protein and a blocking of the voltage-gated dependent calcium channel which prevents the flow of calcium into the neurons. A potassium channel is also activated—pumping K^+ ions out of the neuron. The result is hyperpolarization, activation of components of the mitogen-activated proteins (MAP) kinase cascade, and a decrease in neurotransmitter release such as glutamate and substance P.[1] Ultimately analgesia results.

Opioids typically result in profound analgesia when given acutely. Neuroadaptation interferes with the ability of opioids to provide long-term analgesia, especially when given continuously, and may actually produce opposite effects such as increasing existent pain or facilitating the development of chronic pain by activating endogenous counter-regulatory systems.[1,2] Neuroadaptation occurs within the nociception system activated by the opioid—giving rise to tolerance by altering MOP. Opioids can also paradoxically result in the development of pain hypersensitivity by activating pro-nociceptive systems.

OPIOID FAILURE

Worsening pain routinely occurs during the treatment of chronic pain states with opioid analgesics. Tolerance describes a pharmacologic experience where the same dose of medication results in a diminished physiologic response—this can be in regard to analgesia or in the experience of side effects. Tolerance commonly occurs and, while frustrating, can be overcome by dose escalation. On the other hand, hyperalgesia describes decreased pain thresholds and increased pain intensity. Hyperalgesia is a form of central or secondary sensitization (which includes a necessary initial component of tolerance). When the hyperalgesia results from opioid administration, this worsened pain situation cannot be overcome with dose escalation—rather, this exacerbates the phenomenon.

MOP and δ-opioid receptor (DOP) activation lead to a cascade of events that desensitizes signaling. Disruption of the capacity of the receptor to interact with G-proteins or a sequestration of the receptor away from the cell surface have been described.[3] Changes in the phosphorylation state of the receptors at serine, threonine, or tyrosine residues can provide binding sites for adaptor or uncoupling molecules such as arrestins.[4]

NMDA PATHWAY

Activated N-methyl-D-aspartate (NMDA) receptors play a central role in the development of hyperalgesia. The excitatory neurotransmitter glutamine blinds to α-amino-3-hydroxy-5-methyl-4-isoxazoleopropionic acid (AMPA), kainite, and NMDA receptors. NMDAR are ionotropic glutamate receptors that, once bound by glutamate and glycine (or D-serine), open and allow cations (Ca^{2+}) to enter the neuron. The ion channel can be blocked by Mg^{2+} or Zn^{2+}. The influx of calcium activates protein kinase C (PKC)—which among other phosphorylation events lowers the threshold to release the Mg^{2+} block on the NMDAR.[5] NMDA receptors (NMDAR) are typically considered to control plasticity and memory. Opioids may play a role in creating spinal pain memory. Hyperalgesia has been attributed to the pre-synaptic N-methyl-D-aspartate (NMDA) receptor.[6]

Repeated intrathecal administration of morphine results in tolerance and hyperalgesia through both NMDA and non-NMDA receptor activation. A single administration of ultra-short-acting remifentanil produces long-term potentiation at the C fiber synapses in the dorsal horn of the spinal cord by activating spinal NMDA receptors.[7] Opioids potentiate the impact of glutamate on the NMDA receptor, probably through a protein kinase C (PKC) pathway. This likely results in an increased open probability, reduction of the Mg^{2+} block, and recruitment of more NMDA receptors to the membrane surface.[8] Chronic opioid treatment also decreases the availability of glutamate transporters—thus more glutamate is available to affect the NMDA receptors.[8] Both chronic opioid availability and increased NMDA receptor activation lead to an increase in PKC expression in the dorsal horn of the spinal cord, which leads to a positive feedback loop.[9] NMDA receptor activation also leads to apoptosis of spinal dorsal horn neurons that express glutamic acid decarboxylase for the synthesis of the inhibitory neurotransmitter GABA.[10] The result is less normal inhibition of the pronociceptive signal. Blocking of the NMDA receptor may be a very helpful treatment option and diminish the impact of opioid-induced hyperalgesia.[9,11,12] As a NMDAR antagonist, ketamine has been anecdotally used as a treatment for central sensitization. Only recently have consensus guidelines been published.[13]

NON-NMDR PATHWAYS

Other non-NMDAR pathways exist. Chronic morphine exposure induces increases in the phosphorylation of MAPK including p38, extracellular signal-regulated protein kinase (ERK), and c-Jun N-terminal kinase (JNK). MAP kinase activation is noted in the sciatic nerve and spinal cord after morphine administration.[14] MAPK phosphorylates phospholipase A_2 which results in the activation of NF-κB and the synthesis and overexpression of cyclooxygenase (COX) and transient receptor potential vanilloid 1 (TRPV1).[5]

The non-opioid orexin pathway also plays a role in the development of opioid tolerance. Blocking orexin pathways prior to initiating opioid exposure can prolong the onset of opioid tolerance. The orexin receptor-rich locus coeruleus may play an important role in this phenomenon.[15]

The descending pain pathways project from the midbrain periaqueductal grey (PAG) to the noradrenergic cells of the pons to the rostral ventromedial medulla (RVM) and dorsal horn of the spinal cord. These pathways provide for both facilitatory and inhibitory pain modulation.

Tonic activation of descending bulbospinal (medulla to spinal cord) pain facilitatory loops from the rostral ventromedial medulla (RVM) to the spinal cord play a role in opioid-induced hyperalgesia. Opioid exposure in the RVM can lead to an increased descending facilitation of pain.[16] Upregulation of spinal dynorphin has been implicated.[1] An increase in dynorphin enhances primary afferent neurotransmitter release.[1] Dynorphin has also been shown to potentiate NMDA receptors.[17] Upregulated spinal dynorphin is pronociceptive and is required for the maintenance of persistent neuropathic pain.[18] Lesioning the dorsolateral funiculus prevents the increase of dynorphin and the presence of the excitatory neuropeptide calcitonin gene-related protein (CGRP).[19] In the same vein, treatment with a selective k-opioid receptor antagonist also reduced established opioid-induced hyperalgesia.[20]

GENETIC IMPLICATIONS

Morphine also impacts epigenetic mechanisms that result in hyperalgesia and tolerance by changes in long-term gene expression in the pain system. Histone acetylation and deacetylation help to control gene expression. Histone acetyltransferase (HAT) enzymes transfer an acetyl group onto histones. The result is a more relaxed chromatin structure (euchromatin) and greater gene transcription. This relaxed structure can be "undone" by histone deacetylase (HDAC) transforming to a more condensed form (heterochromatin). Increasing morphine dose enhances the expression of acetylated histone H3 lysine9 (aceH3K9) in the dorsal spinal cord, which regulates the expression of dynorphin and brain-derived neurotrophic factor (BDNF).[21] HAT inhibitors prior to morphine exposure (such as curcumin) have reduced the development of opioid-induced hyperalgesia.[1,22] Conversely, HDAC inhibitor injections after morphine exposure prolong the morphine hyperalgesia and tolerance.[22] Preventing the acetylation of histones or blocking BDNF or dynorphin may reduce hyperalgesia.

After intrathecal administration of morphine, mammalian target of rapamycin (mTOR) (now known as "mechanistic" TOR) expression in the dorsal horn of the spinal cord increases. The presence of mTOR, which governs most protein translation, leads to tolerance and hyperalgesia via activation of the phosphoinositide 3-kinase/Akt pathway (PI3K). Inhibition of mTOR by intrathecal rapamycin blocked the induction and maintenance of morphine tolerance and hyperalgesia.[23] mTOR also regulates microglia and astrocytes.[24]

GLIAL CELLS

Glial cells play an important role in creating a neuroinflammatory state. As non-neuronal cells inhabiting the central nervous system and peripheral nervous system, glial cells play a supportive role in maintenance and regulation. Glial cells include oligodendrocytes, astrocytes, ependymal cells, and microglia in the central nervous system. Schwann cells and satellite cells support the peripheral nervous system. Microglia cells are particularly important and serve as resident macrophages in the brain and spinal cord, and as such are active against damaged neurons and infectious agents. At rest, microglia do not typically contribute to the synaptic milieu of neurotransmitters. This is in contrast to astrocytes which play an active function in taking up and releasing neurotransmitters.

Spinal microglia are activated in many animal models of pain enhancement, including pain arising from trauma-, inflammation-, or chemotherapy-induced peripheral nerve damage, bone cancer, spinal cord injury, spinal nerve injury, multiple sclerosis, migraine, radiculopathy, and others.[2] Under certain circumstances microglia and astrocytes can shift from their quiescent state to an activated pro-inflammatory state. In this activated state, glia release pro-inflammatory cytokines (IL-1, TNF, IL-6), chemokines, arachidonic acid and prostaglandins, ATP, excitatory amino acids and D-serine, nerve growth factor, reactive oxygen species, nitric oxide, and enkephalins.[2] The result is increased neuronal excitability by upregulating AMPA and NMDA receptors, downregulating GABA receptors, and downregulating glial glutamate transporters.[2]

Glial cells play a role in tolerance and hyperalgesia by contributing to a pro-inflammatory state and secreting chemokines and cytokines. Morphine administration results in the activation of matrix metalloproteinase-9 (MMP9) in the satellite cells of the DRG which results in the increased release of IL-1β.[25] The blockade of IL-1β receptor in the spinal cord results in decreasing tolerance and hyperalgesia.[26]

Chemokine and cytokine secretion from microglia and lymphocytes contributes to analgesic tolerance. After chronic morphine exposure, the chemokine fractalkine (CX3CL1) can be cleaved from the neuron cell membrane changing from the inactive form into the active form. This cleavage occurs secondary to glutamate signaling, presumably from opioid-induced NMDA receptor activation. CX3CL1 can bind to its CX3CR1 receptor on microglia. CX3CL1 induces the release of IL-1 from the spinal cord which opposes morphine analgesia. Co-administration of morphine with a neutralizing antibody against CX3CL1 potentiated acute morphine analgesia and attenuated the development of tolerance, hyperalgesia, and allodynia.[26] The same occurs in the periaqueductal grey (PAG).[27]

HYPERALGESIA

Morphine-induced hyperalgesia appears to have a distinct pathway from tolerance. Hyperalgesia requires microglia. Specifically, morphine-induced hyperalgesia requires the expression of P2X4 receptor in the microglia. Chronic exposure to morphine causes an increase in P2X4 receptor expression by a μ-receptor-dependent mechanism. P2X4 receptor stimulation results in the release of brain-derived neurotrophic factor (BDNF). BDNF through TrkB downregulates a K^+-Cl^- cotransporter (KCC2) expression in lamina I neurons causing an impairment in Cl^- extrusion through a μ-receptor-independent mechanism. So, a μ-receptor-dependent mechanism is required to activate the microglia, but a μ-receptor-independent mechanism is responsible for the microglia-neuron signaling. Toll-like receptor 4 (TLR4) was not involved in the μ-receptor independent mechanism.[28]

TLR4 does play a role in the antinociceptive and hyperalgesic effect of morphine. TLR4 is predominantly expressed by microglia and is typically considered the receptor that senses endotoxin (lipopolysaccharide [LPS]). It is also the receptor responsible for the establishment of and maintenance of ongoing neuropathic pain by the release of substances released from neuron damage.[29] Activation of TLR4 activates the ceramide pathway in glial cells which results in the activation of PI3k/Akt, NF-κB, and MAP kinase (MAPK).[2] Inflammatory cytokine overexpression and pain hypersensitivity occur. Morphine-3-glucoronide (M3G), an otherwise inactive morphine metabolite, activates TLR4 and results in opposing acute and chronic opioid analgesia, contributing to opioid-induced hyperalgesia, dependence, and reward.[2,30] This has been shown in both the spinal cord and the PAG.[31] Interference with the TLR4 receptor via multiple mechanisms potentiates the magnitude and duration of morphine analgesia.[32]

In animal models, opioid exposure has been shown to result in increased latent pain sensitization. A single opioid exposure activates NMDA-dependent pronociceptive systems, leading to long-term pain vulnerability after analgesia.[33] In animal models, 7 days after an inflammatory event, a second inflammatory event creates a hyperalgesic response. This hyperalgesic response is exaggerated by exposure to fentanyl during the first inflammatory event. NMDA receptor blockade prevents this central sensitization event.[34] Another animal model showed that a small dose of heroin was ineffective at producing hyperalgesia, but when given several days after opioid exposure hyperalgesia ensued. Hyperalgesia was prevented by NMDA receptor blockade.[35] The inflammatory system is also impacted by MOP priming. After repeat MOP activation, prostaglandin E_2 (PGE_2) administration results in markedly prolonged hyperalgesia. These findings were still present after 1 month.[36] Similarly, 5-day opioid exposure 10 days after nerve injury prolonged injury-induced pain hypersensitivity for months after the cessation of morphine.[37] The morphine-induced spinal NOD-like receptor protein 3 (NLRP3) inflammasomes and associated release of IL-1β from microglia were responsible. A "two-hit hypothesis" from the microglia—the first from the nerve injury and the second from the opioid exposure—is likely responsible for this prolonged pain response.[37]

Non-nociceptive environmental stress may also play a role in the priming of the microglia cells. Non-nociceptive environmental stress typically leads to the release of endogenous opioids. However, repetitive non-nociceptive environmental stress prolonged hyperalgesia after opioid pretreatment for up to 4 months.[33]

ENDOCRINE DISRUPTION

Opioid administration—particularly sustained or intrathecal exposure—impacts the hypothalamic–pituitary–adrenal axis (HPA). HPA dysfunction creates common endocrine abnormalities such as changes in energy and libido. However, more importantly, HPA dysfunction can contribute to the chronic pain phenotype and worsen pain outcomes.

Testosterone is the most commonly considered affected hormone. In both humans and animals, chronic opioid administration decreases gonadotropin-releasing hormone (GnRH) from the hypothalamus—perhaps by inhibiting biosynthesis.[38] Luteinizing hormone (LH) secretion from the pituitary decreases. Opioids directly inhibit LH release from the pituitary as well. FSH impact is limited. Testosterone, estradiol, and progesterone secretion are inhibited. This can lead to menstrual irregularities in women.[39] Hypogonadism was noted in 86% of men receiving intrathecal opiates while the rate for sustained release oral opioids was 89%.[40,41] Interestingly, this was not seen in those treated with buprenorphine.[42]

Symptoms associated with lower sex hormone levels are frequently seen in the chronic pain population. Sex hormones play an important role in analgesia.[43] In a large population study, independent of age, body mass index, health and lifestyle factors, and osteoarthritis, women with androstenedione or estradiol levels in the lowest tertile had more chronic pain. In men with chronic pain, estradiol levels were also lower. The lowest tertile of 17-hydroxyprogesterone in women was associated with 38% more new onset pain.[44] Under stressful states, salivary testosterone levels fall (while salivary cortisol levels increase), pain ratings increase, and pain thresholds decrease.[45]

It is not surprising that the osteoporotic compression fracture rate is 1.5–6 times higher with opioid use.[46] This further complicates the questions regarding the correlation between epidural steroid injections and osteoporotic compression fractures.[47] Sexual dysfunction is noted in multiple studies.[39] Decreased sexual behavior may be due to the direct action of opioids on μ and δ receptors in the hypothalamus.[38]

DHEA levels are correlated with the pain experience. Higher DHEA-S is correlated with elevated pain thresholds and higher pain tolerances in post-menopausal woman.[48] There seems to be an influence of decreased levels of DHEA-S and increased pain sensitivity in post-menopausal women with fibromyalgia syndrome.[48] DHEA levels have been shown to be depressed in opioid users in a dose-dependent fashion, while adrenocorticotropic hormone (ACTH) levels remained normal.[49]

Changes in glucocorticoid activity are noted in the chronic pain state and have been noted in several chronic conditions—such as fibromyalgia, chronic fatigue, chronic pelvic pain, and temporomandibular joint disorder.[50] Morning cortisol levels should register the highest of the day. Blunted awakening cortisol response is predictive of pain and fatigue.[51] Patients with lumbar disc herniations with lower morning cortisol levels had lower physical function, perceived lower possibility of influencing their pain, and were more prone to catastrophize.[52] Not all painful states decrease morning cortisol. To the contrary, in women with chronic widespread pain, morning cortisol was elevated.[53]

Nerve injury increases spinal glucocorticoid receptors.[54] There is evidence that increased corticosterone combined with nerve injury may worsen allodynia. Transient dorsal horn microglia activation is noted with corticosterone. More importantly, increased activation of dorsal horn extracellular signal-regulated kinase phosphorylation (pERK) likely influences NMDA receptors to create allodynia through central sensitization.[54]

Unfortunately, chronic opioid exposure may decrease glucocorticoid response to ACTH, but lead to chronically elevated glucocorticoid levels.[39] It is interesting to note that opioids impact the circadian rhythm of the HPA axis. Constant plasma levels of β-endorphin, ACTH, and cortisol were seen throughout the day rather than typical circadian variations.[55] An opioid-induced elevation of glucocorticoid levels further exacerbates a dysfunctional glucocorticoid system.

The impact of opioids on thyroid function does not appear to be significant. Opioids can stimulate thyroid-stimulating hormone (TSH) via the hypothalamus—primarily through κ-receptors.[39] In a hypothyroid patient, there may be implications.[38]

Acute opioid administration results in an increase in growth hormone (GH) secretion.[39] The chronic administration of intrathecal opioids is more complex. Chronic intrathecal administration of opioids has been associated with GH deficiency in a small number of patients (15%).[40]

AUTONOMIC NERVOUS SYSTEM

The upregulation of norepinephrine (NE) receptors on the terminals of nociceptive afferents has been implicated in hyperalgesia and allodynia in nerve injury and complex regional pain syndrome (CRPS).[56] Sympathetic/sensory coupling has been implicated in the DRG. Chronic opioid exposure has been shown to increase catecholamine secretion via the brainstem. Hypertension may be a complicating issue.[57]

Chronic opioid treatment for non-malignant pain has not provided overwhelmingly positive outcomes for patients despite a decade of fairly aggressive prescribing. Chronic opioid use may be complicated by tolerance, hyperalgesia, and neuroimmune and endocrine dysfunction which may worsen the clinical picture. When opioids are chosen for chronic pain, these limitations should be taken into account.

REFERENCES

1. Rivat, C., & Ballantyne, J. (2016). The dark side of opioids in pain management: basic science explains clinical observation. *Pain Rep*, 1(2), e570. doi:10.1097/PR9.0000000000000570
2. Watkins, L.R., Hutchinson, M.R., Rice, K.C., & Maier, S.F. (2009). The 'toll' of opioid-induced glial activation: improving the clinical efficacy of opioids by targeting glia. *Trends Pharmacol Sci*, 30(11), 581–591. doi:10.1016/j.tips.2009.08.002

3. Johnson, E.E., Christie, M.J., & Connor, M. (2005). The role of opioid receptor phosphorylation and trafficking in adaptations to persistent opioid treatment. *Neurosignals*, 14(6), 290–302. doi:10.1159/000093044

4. Ferguson, S.S. (2001). Evolving concepts in G protein-coupled receptor endocytosis: the role in receptor desensitization and signaling. *Pharmacol Rev*, 53(1), 1–24.

5. Benzon, H.T. (2014). *Practical Management of Pain* (5th ed.). Philadelphia, PA: Elsevier/Mosby.

6. Zhao, Y.L., Chen, S.R., Chen, H., & Pan, H.L. (2012). Chronic opioid potentiates presynaptic but impairs postsynaptic N-methyl-D-aspartic acid receptor activity in spinal cords: implications for opioid hyperalgesia and tolerance. *J Biol Chem*, 287(30), 25073–25085. doi:10.1074/jbc.M112.378737

7. Drdla, R., Gassner, M., Gingl, E., & Sandkühler, J. (2009). Induction of synaptic long-term potentiation after opioid withdrawal. *Science*, 325(5937), 207–210. doi:10.1126/science.1171759

8. Ruscheweyh, R., & Sandkühler, J. (2005). Opioids and central sensitisation: II. Induction and reversal of hyperalgesia. *Eur J Pain*, 9(2), 149–152. doi:10.1016/j.ejpain.2004.05.011

9. Mao, J., Price, D.D., & Mayer, D.J. (1994). Thermal hyperalgesia in association with the development of morphine tolerance in rats: roles of excitatory amino acid receptors and protein kinase C. *J Neurosci*, 14(4), 2301–2312.

10. Mao, J., Sung, B., Ji, R.R., & Lim, G. (2002). Neuronal apoptosis associated with morphine tolerance: evidence for an opioid-induced neurotoxic mechanism. *J Neurosci*, 22(17), 7650–7661.

11. Marek, P., Ben-Eliyahu, S., Gold, M., & Liebeskind, J.C. (1991). Excitatory amino acid antagonists (kynurenic acid and MK-801) attenuate the development of morphine tolerance in the rat. *Brain Res*, 547(1), 77–81.

12. Trujillo, K.A., & Akil, H. (1991). Inhibition of morphine tolerance and dependence by the NMDA receptor antagonist MK-801. *Science*, 251(4989), 85–87.

13. Cohen, S.P., Bhatia, A., Buvanendran, A., Schwenk, E.S., Wasan, A.D., Hurley, R.W., … Hooten, W.M. (2018). Consensus guidelines on the use of intravenous ketamine infusions for chronic pain from the American society of regional anesthesia and pain medicine, the American academy of pain medicine, and the American society of anesthesiologists. *Reg Anesth Pain Med*, 43(5), 521–546. doi:10.1097/AAP.0000000000000808

14. Chen, Y., Geis, C., & Sommer, C. (2008). Activation of TRPV1 contributes to morphine tolerance: involvement of the mitogen-activated protein kinase signaling pathway. *J Neurosci*, 28(22), 5836–5845. doi:10.1523/JNEUROSCI.4170-07.2008

15. Razavi, B.M., & Hosseinzadeh, H. (2017). A review of the role of orexin system in pain modulation. *Biomed Pharmacother*, 90, 187–193. doi:10.1016/j.biopha.2017.03.053

16. Vanderah, T.W., Suenaga, N.M., Ossipov, M.H., Malan, T.P., Jr., Lai, J., & Porreca, F. (2001). Tonic descending facilitation from the rostral ventromedial medulla mediates opioid-induced abnormal pain and antinociceptive tolerance. *J Neurosci*, 21(1), 279–286.

17. Lai, J., Ossipov, M.H., Vanderah, T.W., Malan, T.P., Jr., & Porreca, F. (2001). Neuropathic pain: the paradox of dynorphin. *Mol Interv*, 1(3), 160–167.

18. Wang, Z., Gardell, L.R., Ossipov, M.H., Vanderah, T.W., Brennan, M.B., Hochgeschwender, U., … Porreca, F. (2001). Pronociceptive actions of dynorphin maintain chronic neuropathic pain. *J Neurosci*, 21(5), 1779–1786.

19. Gardell, L.R., Wang, R., Burgess, S.E., Ossipov, M.H., Vanderah, T.W., Malan, T.P., Jr., … Porreca, F. (2002). Sustained morphine exposure induces a spinal dynorphin-dependent enhancement of excitatory transmitter release from primary afferent fibers. *J Neurosci*, 22(15), 6747–6755.

20. Liang, D.Y., Sun, Y., Shi, X.Y., Sahbaie, P., & Clark, J.D. (2014). Epigenetic regulation of spinal cord gene expression controls opioid-induced hyperalgesia. *Mol Pain*, 10, 59. doi:10.1186/1744-8069-10-59

21. Sahbaie, P., Liang, D.Y., Shi, X.Y., Sun, Y., & Clark, J.D. (2016). Epigenetic regulation of spinal cord gene expression contributes to enhanced postoperative pain and analgesic tolerance subsequent to continuous opioid exposure. *Mol Pain*, 12. doi:10.1177/1744806916641950

22. Liang, D.Y., Li, X., & Clark, J.D. (2013). Epigenetic regulation of opioid-induced hyperalgesia, dependence, and tolerance in mice. *J Pain*, 14(1), 36–47. doi:10.1016/j.jpain.2012.10.005

23. Xu, J.T., Zhao, J.Y., Zhao, X., Ligons, D., Tiwari, V., Atianjoh, F.E., … Tao, Y.X. (2014). Opioid receptor-triggered spinal mTORC1 activation contributes to morphine tolerance and hyperalgesia. *J Clin Invest*, 124(2), 592–603. doi:10.1172/JCI70236

24. Lisi, L., Aceto, P., Navarra, P., & Dello Russo, C. (2015). mTOR kinase: a possible pharmacological target in the management of chronic pain. *BioMed Res Int*, 2015, 394257. doi:10.1155/2015/394257

25. Nakamoto, K., Kawasaki, S., Kobori, T., Fujita-Hamabe, W., Mizoguchi, H., Yamada, K., … Tokuyama, S. (2012). Involvement of matrix metalloproteinase-9 in the development of morphine tolerance. *Eur J Pharmacol*, 683(1–3), 86–92. doi:10.1016/j.ejphar.2012.03.006

26. Johnston, I.N., Milligan, E.D., Wieseler-Frank, J., Frank, M.G., Zapata, V., Campisi, J., ... Watkins, L.R. (2004). A role for proinflammatory cytokines and fractalkine in analgesia, tolerance, and subsequent pain facilitation induced by chronic intrathecal morphine. *J Neurosci*, 24(33), 7353–7365. doi:10.1523/JNEUROSCI.1850-04.2004

27. Chen, X., Geller, E.B., Rogers, T.J., & Adler, M.W. (2007). The chemokine CX3CL1/fractalkine interferes with the antinociceptive effect induced by opioid agonists in the periaqueductal grey of rats. *Brain Res*, 1153, 52–57. doi:10.1016/j.brainres.2007.03.066

28. Ferrini, F., Trang, T., Mattioli, T.A., Laffray, S., Del'Guidice, T., Lorenzo, L.E., ... De Koninck, Y. (2013). Morphine hyperalgesia gated through microglia-mediated disruption of neuronal Cl⁻ homeostasis. *Nat Neurosci*, 16(2), 183–192. doi:10.1038/nn.3295

29. Hutchinson, M.R., Zhang, Y., Brown, K., Coats, B.D., Shridhar, M., Sholar, P.W., ... Watkins, L.R. (2008). Non-stereoselective reversal of neuropathic pain by naloxone and naltrexone: involvement of toll-like receptor 4 (TLR4). *Eur J Neurosci*, 28(1), 20–29. doi:10.1111/j.1460-9568.2008.06321.x

30. Hutchinson, M.R., Northcutt, A.L., Hiranita, T., Wang, X., Lewis, S.S., Thomas, J., ... Watkins, L.R. (2012). Opioid activation of toll-like receptor 4 contributes to drug reinforcement. *J Neurosci*, 32(33), 11187–11200. doi:10.1523/JNEUROSCI.0684-12.2012

31. Eidson, L.N., & Murphy, A.Z. (2013). Blockade of toll-like receptor 4 attenuates morphine tolerance and facilitates the pain relieving properties of morphine. *J Neurosci*, 33(40), 15952–15963. doi:10.1523/JNEUROSCI.1609-13.2013

32. Hutchinson, M.R., Zhang, Y., Shridhar, M., Evans, J.H., Buchanan, M.M., Zhao, T.X., ... Watkins, L.R. (2010). Evidence that opioids may have toll-like receptor 4 and MD-2 effects. *Brain Behav Immun*, 24(1), 83–95. doi:10.1016/j.bbi.2009.08.004

33. Rivat, C., Laboureyras, E., Laulin, J.P., Le Roy, C., Richebé, P., & Simonnet, G. (2007). Non-nociceptive environmental stress induces hyperalgesia, not analgesia, in pain and opioid-experienced rats. *Neuropsychopharmacology*, 32(10), 2217–2228. doi:10.1038/sj.npp.1301340

34. Rivat, C., Laulin, J.P., Corcuff, J.B., Célèrier, E., Pain, L., & Simonnet, G. (2002). Fentanyl enhancement of carrageenan-induced long-lasting hyperalgesia in rats: prevention by the N-methyl-D-aspartate receptor antagonist ketamine. *Anesthesiology*, 96(2), 381–391.

35. Célèrier, E., Laulin, J.P., Corcuff, J.B., Le Moal, M., & Simonnet, G. (2001). Progressive enhancement of delayed hyperalgesia induced by repeated heroin administration: a sensitization process. *J Neurosci*, 21(11), 4074–4080.

36. Araldi, D., Ferrari, L.F., & Levine, J.D. (2015). Repeated mu-opioid exposure induces a novel form of the hyperalgesic priming model for transition to chronic pain. *J Neurosci*, 35(36), 12502–12517. doi:10.1523/JNEUROSCI.1673-15.2015

37. Grace, P.M., Strand, K.A., Galer, E.L., Urban, D.J., Wang, X., Baratta, M.V., ... Watkins, L.R. (2016). Morphine paradoxically prolongs neuropathic pain in rats by amplifying spinal NLRP3 inflammasome activation. *Proc Natl Acad Sci U S A*, 113(24), E3441–E3450. doi:10.1073/pnas.1602070113

38. Seyfried, O., & Hester, J. (2012). Opioids and endocrine dysfunction. *Br J Pain*, 6(1), 17–24. doi:10.1177/2049463712438299

39. Vuong, C., Van Uum, S.H., O'Dell, L.E., Lutfy, K., & Friedman, T.C. (2010). The effects of opioids and opioid analogs on animal and human endocrine systems. *Endocr Rev*, 31(1), 98–132. doi:10.1210/er.2009-0009

40. Abs, R., Verhelst, J., Maeyaert, J., Van Buyten, J.P., Opsomer, F., Adriaensen, H., ... Van Acker, K. (2000). Endocrine consequences of long-term intrathecal administration of opioids. *J Clin Endocrinol Metab*, 85(6), 2215–2222. doi:10.1210/jcem.85.6.6615

41. Daniell, H.W. (2002). Hypogonadism in men consuming sustained-action oral opioids. *J Pain*, 3(5), 377–384.

42. Bliesener, N., Albrecht, S., Schwager, A., Weckbecker, K., Lichtermann, D., & Klingmüller, D. (2005). Plasma testosterone and sexual function in men receiving buprenorphine maintenance for opioid dependence. *J Clin Endocrinol Metab*, 90(1), 203–206. doi:10.1210/jc.2004-0929

43. Tennant, F. (2013). The physiologic effects of pain on the endocrine system. *Pain Ther*, 2(2), 75–86. doi:10.1007/s40122-013-0015-x

44. de Kruijf, M., Stolk, L., Zillikens, M.C., de Rijke, Y.B., Bierma-Zeinstra, S.M., Hofman, A., ... van Meurs, J.B. (2016). Lower sex hormone levels are associated with more chronic musculoskeletal pain in community-dwelling elderly women. *Pain*, 157(7), 1425–1431.

45. Choi, J.C., Chung, M.I., & Lee, Y.D. (2012). Modulation of pain sensation by stress-related testosterone and cortisol. *Anaesthesia*, 67(10), 1146–1151. doi:10.1111/j.1365-2044.2012.07267.x

46. Vestergaard, P., Rejnmark, L., & Mosekilde, L. (2006). Fracture risk associated with the use of morphine and opiates. *J Intern Med*, 260(1), 76–87. doi:10.1111/j.1365-2796.2006.01667.x

47. Mandel, S., Schilling, J., Peterson, E., Rao, D.S., & Sanders, W. (2013). A retrospective analysis of vertebral body fractures following epidural steroid injections. *J Bone Joint Surg Am*, 95(11), 961–964. doi:10.2106/JBJS.L.00844

48. Freitas, R.P., Lemos, T.M., Spyrides, M.H., & Sousa, M.B. (2012). Influence of cortisol and DHEA-S on pain and other symptoms in post menopausal women with fibromyalgia. *J Back Musculoskelet Rehabil*, 25(4), 245–252. doi:10.3233/BMR-2012-0331

49. Daniell, H.W. (2006). DHEAS deficiency during consumption of sustained-action prescribed opioids: evidence for opioid-induced inhibition of adrenal androgen production. *J Pain*, 7(12), 901–907. doi:10.1016/j.jpain.2006.04.011

50. Hannibal, K.E., & Bishop, M.D. (2014). Chronic stress, cortisol dysfunction, and pain: a psychoneuroendocrine rationale for stress management in pain rehabilitation. *Phys Ther*, 94(12), 1816–1825. doi:10.2522/ptj.20130597

51. Tak, L.M., & Rosmalen, J.G. (2010). Dysfunction of stress responsive systems as a risk factor for functional somatic syndromes. *J Psychosom Res*, 68(5), 461–468. doi:10.1016/j.jpsychores.2009.12.004

52. Johansson, A.C., Gunnarsson, L.G., Linton, S.J., Bergkvist, L., Stridsberg, M., Nilsson, O., & Cornefjord, M. (2008). Pain, disability and coping reflected in the diurnal cortisol variability in patients scheduled for lumbar disc surgery. *Eur J Pain*, 12(5), 633–640. doi:10.1016/j.ejpain.2007.10.009

53. Stehlik, R., Ulfberg, J., Zou, D., Hedner, J., & Grote, L. (2018). Morning cortisol and fasting glucose are elevated in women with chronic widespread pain independent of comorbid restless legs syndrome. *Scand J Pain*, 18(2), 187–194. doi:10.1515/sjpain-2018-0026

54. Alexander, J.K., DeVries, A.C., Kigerl, K.A., Dahlman, J.M., & Popovich, P.G. (2009). Stress exacerbates neuropathic pain via glucocorticoid and NMDA receptor activation. *Brain Behav Immun*, 23(6), 851–860. doi:10.1016/j.bbi.2009.04.001

55. Facchinetti, F., Grasso, A., Petraglia, F., Parrini, D., Volpe, A., & Genazzani, A.R. (1984). Impaired circadian rhythmicity of beta-lipotrophin, beta-endorphin and ACTH in heroin addicts. *Acta Endocrinol Copenh*, 105(2), 149–155.

56. Harden, R.N., Rudin, N.J., Bruehl, S., Kee, W., Parikh, D.K., Kooch, J., … Gracely, R.H. (2004). Increased systemic catecholamines in complex regional pain syndrome and relationship to psychological factors: a pilot study. *Anesth Analg*, 99(5), 1478–1485. table of contents. doi:10.1213/01.ANE.0000132549.25154.ED

57. Thosani, S., & Jimenez, C. (2011). Opioid-induced biochemical alterations of the neuroendocrine axis. *Expert Rev Endocrinol Metab*, 6(5), 705–713. doi:10.1586/eem.11.55

4 Endogenous Cannabinoid Receptors and Medical Cannabis

Jeffrey S. Block

CONTENTS

HISTORICAL CONSIDERATIONS AND CLINICAL PRECEDENT

"Primum non nocere" (first do no harm) is a guiding maxim for clinicians, and concern for balancing risk with benefit is central to treatment decisions in patient care. Most responsible clinicians will not advise their patients to pursue a particular treatment regimen without conclusive clinical evidence and peer review confirmation regarding the relative safety and efficacy of a given treatment.

Yet the compassionate physician will also be mindful of the ethical obligation to ease suffering with whatever tools might be available, and wherever possible. In this context, the medicinal use of cannabis currently presents a conundrum in need of bioethical rationale.

This chapter considers clinical aspects of cannabis when used for the treatment of pain (Figure 4.1). It includes how cannabinoid medicines may augment or substitute for the use of opioids, the history and development of their therapeutic use, and the importance of a unique receptor system through which plant-derived cannabinoids exert their effects. An appreciation of this receptor system's biologic context will assist the clinician's understanding and evaluation of limited human trials, including the emergence of cannabidiol (CBD) used as a medicine. Taken together, they inform the discussion of clinical applications to which the chapter turns, such as dosing guidance, routes of administration, and risks and contraindications, as well as public health concerns from contaminants to dependence.

A physician's skillful art of observing the non-medical use of a substance can contribute to the development of unique medical applications; this has notable parallels to the development of contemporary uses of cannabis. Despite some of the horrors associated with 19th-century experimental medicine, one of the sentinel events leading to modern healthcare was the first documented use of ether as an anesthetic, when American physician Crawford Long administered it for a surgical procedure on March 30, 1842, a date later commemorated as national "Doctor's Day" in recognition of physicians' noble efforts to alleviate pain and suffering. The properties of ether that lend to its use providing anesthesia were first identified by a young Dr. Long through observing the effects on individuals who used the drug recreationally, a practice popularly known in its day as "ether frolics" (Figure 4.2).*

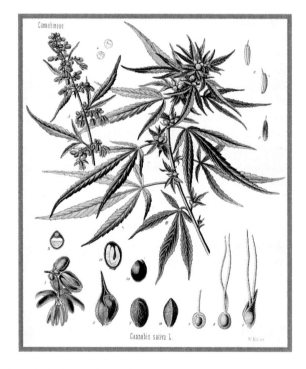

FIGURE 4.1   Classic botanical print depicting *Cannabis sativa* (Kohler; 1887).

---

* Nitrous oxide was similarly popular in that era, with public exhibitions devoted to its recreational use as "laughing gas."
  Long's insight on the application to patient care made him a hero in his home state of Georgia, which later dedicated one
  of its two citizen statues in the U.S. Capitol Rotunda to him for his contributions to alleviating surgical pain.

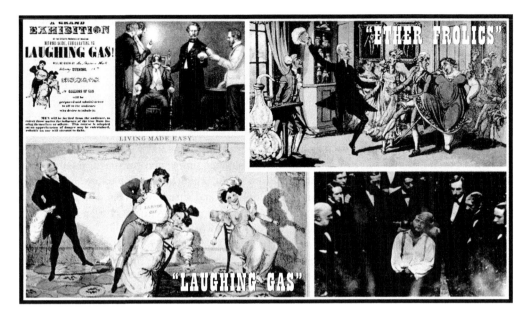

FIGURE 4.2 Eighteenth-century social recreation featuring diethyl ether referred to as "ether frolics," and nitrous oxide popularly known as "laughing gas" (Jeffrey S. Block, MD).

A similar observational initiative is evolving for clinicians to incorporate cannabinoid-based medicines within their armamentarium. Most major medical schools currently offer only limited training on pain management and cannabinoids, and this has raised bioethical objections. However, it is less an indictment of any lack of interest in emerging treatments than a reflection of the pragmatic training that is necessarily focused on preparing future licensed practitioners to achieve certain minimum education standards as confirmed through the current examination and licensure process. Until physician education includes the knowledge required to answer questions about how and why endogenous cannabinoid signaling might be therapeutically exploited using plant-derived cannabinoid medicines, the burden currently falls on individual clinicians of good conscience to educate themselves about this promising area. For the time being, individuals who do so are to be commended.

As much as a new scientific understanding of the therapeutic applications of cannabis is recent and emerging, its medicinal use has an extraordinarily long history, with its oldest documentation appearing in Chinese medicine dated to circa 2700 BC. Cannabis reached Western medicine's physicians in the mid-19th century through the French who observed its use in Egypt, and by the British in colonialized India, who chronicled Ayurvedic medicine. Between 1840 and 1900, upwards of 100 articles about the medical use of cannabis were published in Western medical journals, primarily touting its utility as an analgesic and antispasmodic. Cannabis was added to the United States Pharmacopoeia in 1852, where it would remain for 90 years until federal laws made the production of cannabis medicines prohibitively expensive. During that era, most major pharmaceutical companies provided multiple cannabis formulations, often combined with other substances. As that was also the era of bunk remedies and medical quackery, skepticism about the therapeutic utility of cannabis would have been warranted, but concern about unfounded claims was not the basis for restricting it. The first federal law aimed at criminalizing "marihuana" was enacted in 1937 with little debate or acknowledgement of its potential therapeutic properties. The sole exception was the testimony of Dr. William C. Woodward, the legislative counsel of the American Medical Association, who warned that prohibiting it "loses sight of the fact that future investigation may show that there are substantial medical uses for cannabis."* He announced his

---

* U.S. Congress, House of Representatives, Committee on Ways and Means, *Taxation of Marihuana, Hearing before the Committee on Ways and Means*, 75th Cong., 1st sess., May 4, 1937.

opposition to the bill and sought to dispel any impression that either the AMA or enlightened medical opinions sponsored this legislation.

Indeed, the tax act and the subsequent Controlled Substances Act of 1970 classifying "marijuana" as a Schedule 1 substance continue to stymie research in the United States. Today, cannabis remains uniquely challenging to study, subject to not only extra review constraints, but also tightly controlled limitations on the supply of research materials. Despite those barriers, cannabinoid researchers elsewhere in the world have shared substantial successes investigating both the endogenous system and the action of cannabis plant-derived molecules on it.

During the 19th century, water-soluble alkaloids extracted from plants were isolated and became the source of such medicines as aspirin, atropine, morphine, quinine, and cocaine. Cannabis is fundamentally different because its active molecules are lipids, which are insoluble in water and more difficult to chemically isolate. Furthermore, the complexity and variability of cannabis are inherent within the plant's rich repertoire of bioactive chemical components. While Victorian chemists had considerable success identifying alkaloids because they form crystalline solids when combined with acids, cannabinoids would need to wait until new techniques were developed in the following century. There is a long history of human use of cannabis for treating a variety of maladies; however, only a limited number of modern clinical trials that meet current standards for evidence-based medicine exist. Additionally, because little is known about effective dosing and about the long-term effects of chronic downregulating of this newly discovered receptor system, longitudinal studies are needed that are consistent with how these plant-based cannabinoids are used by patients. Clinical trials and preclinical anecdotal findings include not just the plant preparations commonly recognized as "medical marijuana" but other plant-based pharmaceutical medicines such as nabiximols (Sativex®) and cannabidiol (Epidiolex®), as well as synthetic cannabinoids such as dronabinol (Marinol®) and nabilone (Cesamet). Taken collectively, these all are considered to be "cannabinoid medicines" in that they interact with our endogenous receptors. Cannabinoid medicines represent a class of drugs, not a single substance, so research findings or patient experience with any given cannabinoid product cannot be generalized to others in the class. As will be discussed later in this chapter, many factors influence the effects and efficacy of cannabinoid medicines.

Today, as a result of social media and other informal information sharing, many patients hear anecdotal reports suggesting cannabis may help or even cure a remarkably diverse range of conditions. Hyperbole is rampant in these accounts, particularly regarding curative potential, and even knowledgeable patients often hold mistaken beliefs about medical cannabis.[1] The dearth of clinical research has led to a reliance on anecdotal reports, but the plural of anecdote is not data, and most of these reports lack the scientific method's meaningful evidence. Nonetheless, preclinical studies provide the basis for robust clinical investigations, and reviews by reputable professional bodies such as the Institutes of Medicine and the National Academies of Sciences, Engineering, and Medicine have identified sound clinical studies supporting the anecdotal and preclinical indications for medicinal cannabis use. Perhaps nowhere has this been more evident than for treating pain, which has been far and away the subject of the greatest number of clinical trials.

Before turning to a discussion of those trials, a consideration of the robust research on the role and function of the endogenous cannabinoid receptor system will help illuminate the implications of those clinical studies and the potential of future developments.

MAINTAINING PHYSIOLOGIC BALANCES

THE ROLES OF RECEPTORS AND THEIR LIGANDS

The second half of the 20th century can be regarded as the golden age of scientific discovery for how and why human receptor systems function. Exploration continues, with an eye to better understandings of how a receptor's functions can be targeted not just with medicines that operate directly on the receptors, but also with treatments that enhance, inhibit, or block the metabolism of natural substances that interact with these unique receptors. While receptors and the natural ligands that attach to them are often described as locks and keys, molecules of other substances that are capable of activating those receptors need not resemble the molecular structure of natural ligands. The lock-and-key metaphor for describing an endocannabinoid receptor's activation can seem misleading when exogenous ligand molecules produce differing degrees of receptor engagement (Figure 4.3).

The "orthosteric" receptor site is where the primary interaction occurs between that receptor and either its natural ligand, or a drug that produces direct agonism or antagonism of that receptor. Agonists, which activate the receptor, and antagonists, which can counter-balance the receptor's action, operate at these specific sites. For some receptors, equally important are their "allosteric" receptor sites: alternative areas to which therapeutic molecules can bind in order to modulate selective innate effects of the receptor's activation. Allosteric modulators offer significant therapeutic promise for leveraging endogenous receptor function, without otherwise causing the consequences of unnatural receptor activation.

A MASTER REGULATORY SYSTEM'S MECHANISM OF ACTION

Among the receptor systems identified in the last century, several have important implications for treatment, such as the dopamine and serotonin systems. But none hold quite the significance of the endogenous cannabinoid system (ECS),[2] as it plays a regulatory role with other bodily systems that maintains the physiological balances of *homeostasis*.

Cannabinoid receptors are part of the Class A family of G protein-coupled receptors (GPCR), which are implicated in nearly all physiological functions of the peripheral and central nervous systems, and in various peripheral organs. The ECS fulfills an essential regulatory role in the body's

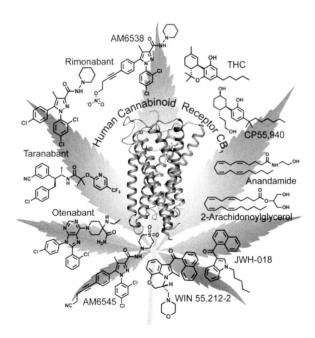

FIGURE 4.3 A model of the CB_1 receptor shows the structure of the receptor in green, along with the stabilizing molecule AM6538 in the central binding pocket. The researchers used this model to examine how different cannabinoid molecules bind to and activate the receptor. Credit: Yekaterina Kadyshevskaya, Stevens Laboratory, USC https://phys.org/news/2016-10-marijuana-receptor.html#jCp CB_1 receptor's central binding site and stabilizing research molecule shown in green, surrounded by other test molecules, natural ligands Anandamide & 2-AG, and cannabis plant-derived Δ-9 tetrahydrocannabinol (THC) (Yekaterina Kadyshevskaya, Stevens Laboratory, USC).

biochemistry and physiology, operating to maintain physiological system balances by keeping their functions within tenable parameters. Many different types of receptors can influence the activity of one another by enhancing or inhibiting their effects, but the ECS operates as a constant fine-tuning master system that attenuates the action of all other receptor systems, including those of the endorphin receptor system central to stress and pain responses.[3] Cannabinoid receptors are so ubiquitous and important, a recent NIH review concluded that "modulating ECS activity may have therapeutic potential in almost all diseases affecting humans."[4] In summary, the ECS is the central regulatory system for maintaining a physiological balance sometimes referred to as *homeostasis*, not only in mammals, but also in all animals.[5,6] The components of the ECS are expressed in nearly all parts of the human body throughout every stage of life, and they exert influence on nearly all other receptor systems' neurotransmitters, including dopamine, serotonin, melatonin, and acetylcholine.[7–9]

THE UBIQUITOUS ENDOCANNABINOID SYSTEM

All physiological systems' functions are subordinate to endocannabinoid receptors' effects, and the abundance of cannabinoid receptors in the human body is most remarkable, being roughly 4 times more than dopamine D2 receptors and 12 times more than mu-opiate receptors. The ECS differs from other receptor systems not just by being the only lipid-based neurotransmitter system; it is also unique in that it has not one, but two ligands that exert their collective effects on two types of lipophilic cannabinoid receptors designated as CB_1 and CB_2. By comparison, the dopaminergic system has a single ligand neurotransmitter, dopamine, that is capable of acting on 5 different receptors, while the endorphins are known to act on at least 20 different receptors.[10] The ECS also employs a unique retrograde feedback loop to affect pre-synaptic signaling (Figure 4.4). Both of the endogenous cannabinoids, N-arachidonylethanolamine (AEA) also known as anandamide—dubbed "anandamide" from the Sanskrit word for "bliss"—and 2-arachidonylglycerol (2-AG), are found in the post-synaptic neuron membrane within a lipid ring encircling synapses that keep the endocannabinoids and their receptors sequestered from their aqueous surroundings. They are produced on-site and on-demand. These cannabinoids then travel retrograde, backwards to the

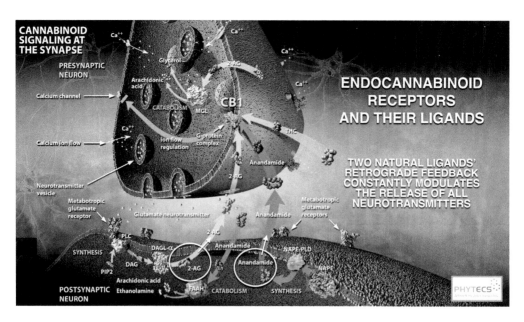

FIGURE 4.4 Post-synaptic retrograde cannabinoid signaling serves as a feedback loop at the neuron's synapse (Phytecs, Inc.; artwork by John Karapelou, Text by Phytecs).

pre-synaptic cannabinoid receptor associated with that transmitting neuron to modulate the release of all neurotransmitters, including glutamate.

Concentrations of localized CB_2 receptors appear in the brain in connection with its injury, as well as neurodegenerative conditions such as Parkinsonism. After a head injury or stroke that may frequently produce cell death, endocannabinoids produced at that site of brain injury mitigate the increase of glutamate signaling. The expression of CB_2 receptors in response to inflammation or injury is not limited to the brain. Glutamate manipulation may hold significance for pain management because overproduction of this stimulatory chemical is also implicated in neuropathic pain associated with conditions such as diabetes, multiple sclerosis, HIV/AIDS, and cancer.[8]

Considerably more work is needed to fully describe the pharmacology of the orthosteric and allosteric modulators operating on the ECS, but much is already known. The endocannabinoid anandamide is a partial agonist, operating as a modulator more in the periphery, outside the CNS. Anandamide functions as a partial receptor agonist affecting the neurons that regulate pain signaling by controlling the chemical gates through which pain signals access the CNS. By contrast, the endocannabinoid 2-AG is a total agonist, fully activating the cannabinoid receptors. 2-AG has been referred to as the workhorse of the ECS, serving as a point-to-point retrograde messenger to provide fundamental brain and spinal cord functions. Major endocannabinoids are rapidly deactivated by reuptake mechanisms and degrading enzymes.[11,12] Cannabinoid receptor activity is also selectively modified by the binding of ligands at allosteric sites on receptors.

ECS signaling is generally linked to cell proliferation, cell differentiation, cell movement, and cell death.[13] Cannabinoid receptors are most abundant on the cell surface's plasma membranes, as well as on the endoplasmic reticulum and around the cell nucleus. Cannabinoid receptors may also be present on other organelles within the cell, including mitochondria.[14] The locations and activities of CB_1 receptors are highly dynamic, allowing significant effects derived from receptor signaling. CB_1 receptors are ubiquitous in the CNS, peripheral nerve terminals, and within some extra-neuronal sites, with concentrations in areas that agree with what is known about cannabinoid effects on neurophysiology.[11,15]

PLANT-DERIVED MOLECULES ENGAGE ENDOGENOUS RECEPTORS

THE EFFECTS OF BIOACTIVE CANNABIS PLANT CHEMICALS LEAD TO THE DISCOVERY OF RECEPTORS AND ENDOCANNABINOIDS

While the endogenous *cannabinoid* system (ECS) carries the plant's name because study of cannabis effects led to the system's discovery, the bodily regulatory system is in fact exponentially older than the plant. All animals, vertebrates and even invertebrates, have an ECS, the oldest identified being the sea squirt, a creature that developed nearly 600 million years ago.[5] By comparison, cannabis developed as a distinct botanical genus no earlier than 34 million years ago during the Oligocene epoch, and its closest genetic relative, hops, did not appear as a species in the fossil record until only around 6 million years ago.[16] The appearance of a botanical compound that interacts with a much older animal receptor system may support a teleological or ethnobotanical contention that there is a coevolutionary relationship in which plants have developed highly sophisticated chemistries to cooperatively appeal to creatures, unwittingly assisting with those plants' reproduction and dissemination, as well as to repel insect and animal herbivore threats. An understanding of the plant's survival rationale also helps to explain why its bitter-tasting defensive chemical alkaloids when used as medicines often are taken along with a proverbial "spoonful of sugar" to make their ingestion more palatable.

Molecular similarities attest to the core of biochemical evolutionary links between plants and animals. This becomes apparent when comparing the critical energy molecules of plants and animals. Light energy processing is possible through chlorophyll that allows photosynthesis, while animals'

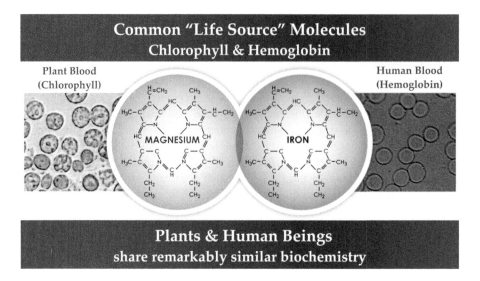

FIGURE 4.5 Other than their respective 2^+ cations (magnesium in chlorophyll, and iron in hemoglobin), these Kingdom of Life-defining molecules share remarkably similar biochemistries.

hemoglobin molecule is responsible for O_2 exchange to derive energy. The mere substitution of magnesium (a 2^+ cation) at the core of chlorophyll with iron (another 2^+ cation) dramatically changes that molecule into serving as hemoglobin. This similarity of molecular structure is most remarkable when one considers the resulting essential consequence of each molecule's unique bioactive purpose (Figure 4.5).

The discovery process of identifying active plant compounds and then searching for the bodily system with which they interact has proven fruitful in many instances, although compiling the supporting evidence can often be time- and cost-consuming. Aspirin's analgesic properties were commercially known for nearly a century before the discovery of prostaglandins and, of course, opium's analgesic effects were known for thousands of years before endorphins and enkephalins were identified. In 1974 endorphins were discovered through plant-based phyto-opioids derived from the opium poppy and morphine. In 1992 endocannabinoids were discovered through phyto-cannabinoids produced by the cannabis plant, and in 1997 endovanilloids were discovered through phyto-vanilloids including the chili pepper and capsaicin (Figure 4.6).

Ethnobotanical observations of how plants affect pain have helped to identify these three distinct endogenous receptor systems, each of which has been revealed through their plants' unique chemical contributions. These three receptor systems have complementary pathways that collectively may help treat pain more safely and effectively when used in a balanced therapeutic manner. Several decades before the discovery of any of these receptors particularly important to pain perception, major pharmaceutical companies had already attempted to mitigate side effects by combining only small amounts of all three plant substances for use as an elixir.

Some components of the cannabis plant, such as cannabidiol and cannabinol, were described by chemists in the 1940s, but it would take until 1964 before the definitive structure and biosynthesis of cannabis' best-known bioactive molecule, Δ-9 tetrahydrocannabinol (THC), were determined.*

Complementing what is known about the molecular structure of THC and CBD, elucidating these cannabinoids' biosynthesis and breakdown revealed a single parent chemical—geranyl-pyrophosphate—that derives not only other cannabinoids, but also the plant's terpenes, chemical molecules

---

* Israeli biochemist Rafael Mechoulam's lab is credited with not only the discovery of THC's structure and biosynthesis, but also of the CB receptors' natural ligands. The importance of his life's work validates his being regarded as the "Father of Cannabinoid Medicine."

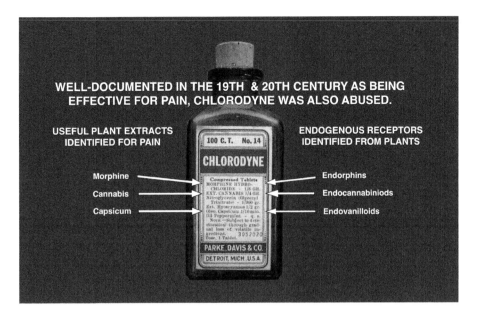

FIGURE 4.6 Pre-dating their respective receptors' discoveries, pharmaceutical products containing combinations of plant-sourced chemicals were common in formulary.

that animals perceive as smells. Plant cannabinoids exist naturally in a non-psychoactive acid form, and each has its own unique bioactivity. Only upon exposure to air and heating does the loss of CO_2 by decarboxylation change the living plant's precursor acid form known as THCA into THC, cannabis' only psychoactive molecule. The consumption and digestion of THC allowing subsequent liver metabolism results in 11 hydroxy THC, a more potent psychoactive cannabinoid known to also have a considerably longer effective half-life than does its precursor molecule, THC (Figure 4.7).

The identification of the cannabis plant's primary psychotropic phytocannabinoid enabled a search for the receptor system within which it interacts. It took nearly 30 years until THC was revealed to engage CB receptors as a unique stereo-specific isomer, fitting a natural receptor's "lock-and-key" analogy, and giving its plant family name to this newly discovered "endocannabinoid" receptor system. This led to a far more essential discovery: the endogenous receptor-activating ligand that THC mimics. Not simply one, but two different endogenous ligands were discovered in 1994. Each of these endogenous cannabinoids, N-arachidonylethanolamine (AEA) and 2-arachidonylglycerol (2-AG), can attach to either of the CB receptors. Since then, many other minor lipid metabolites having molecular structures similar to anandamide and 2-AG have been identified that also may exert effects on the two cannabinoid receptors.

Endocannabinoid receptors:

- CB_1
- CB_2

Endogenous ligands:

- 2-arachidonylglycerol (2-AG)
- N-arachidonylethanolamine (AEA or anandamide)

For all of the importance of plant–human interactions in identifying endogenous mechanisms and targets for analgesia, future therapeutic applications will have less to do with the plant's chemicals, and more to do with other pharmacological ways to manipulate the ECS. This integrating system

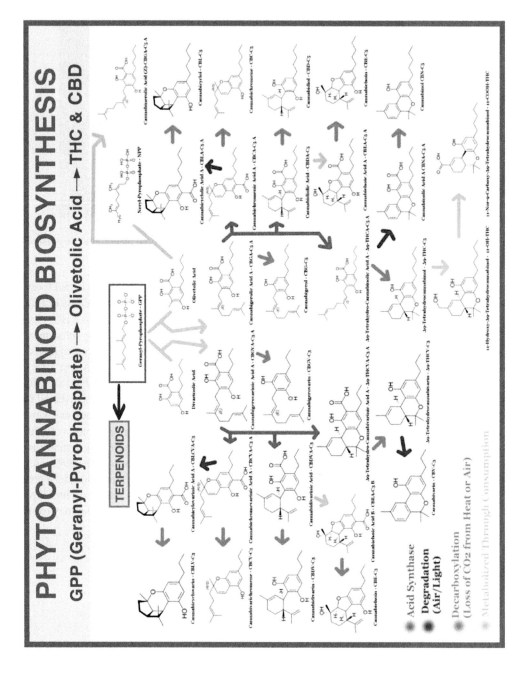

FIGURE 4.7   Several natural and physiologic conditions influence the primary phytocannabinoids' biosynthetic pathways (Smokereports.com).

appears to be the body's key regulatory mechanism, particularly in the brain, where it is known to affect memory, pain perception, and mood among other things.

CANNABIS MODULATES OPIATES AS ENDOCANNABINOIDS MODULATE ENDORPHINS

Opioid medications are important tools in the treatment of pain, but their well-known central nervous system (CNS) and gastrointestinal side effects are often poorly tolerated. As opioid overdosing frequency has become epidemic in the United States, their use has come under intense scrutiny. Among the proposed alternatives to opioid and other pharmaceutical pain treatments is medical cannabis (marijuana). The emerging evidence indicates that cannabinoids can exert opioid-sparing effects seen at both pharmacological and behavioral levels,[17–22] although a recent Australian 4-year cohort study failed to confirm changes in opioid effectiveness.[23] While the scarcity of clinical evidence for the medicinal use of cannabis poses a challenge for treatment decision-making, the expansive scope of chronic pain and frequency of opioid abuse suggest conventional treatments are insufficient.

Clinical decisions are based on our knowledge of the risks and benefits of available treatments, including those that have yet to receive full acceptance. For all of the limitations on clinical research utilizing plant-derived cannabinoids, a wealth of insight derives from understanding the supporting basic science. Appreciating the mechanism of action can inform decisions about where future benefits may lie for patient care. The evidence for the efficacy of cannabis as an analgesic includes a wealth of anecdotal patient reports, human clinical trials, experimental animal studies, and laboratory research. The preclinical findings on comparative safety and potential efficacy have thus far found limited confirmation in clinical trials for chronic pain. Studies indicating the efficacy of cannabis in the treatment of pain have been well-summarized in the consensus conclusions of expert reviews conducted by the Institutes of Medicine (IOM) in 1999 and again in 2017 by the National Academies of Sciences, Engineering and Medicine (NASEM).[24,25] These meta-analyses of randomized clinical trials and other research studies found "substantial evidence" that cannabinoid medicines are effective in the treatment of pain. Importantly, the NASEM report also finds evidence of opioid substitution with cannabinoid use consistent with initial survey data of medical cannabis users and statistical analyses of opioid prescription reductions in states where medical cannabis is available.[26–28]

Before considering those findings and clinical recommendations, an understanding of what has been established about how endogenous receptors and their natural ligands function helps to illuminate why several plant-derived or "phyto-"cannabinoids—key active components in the cannabis plant—hold such promise for treating a startlingly broad range of conditions, including pain. As the 1999 IOM report notes, "basic biology indicates a role for cannabinoids in pain and control of movement, which is consistent with a possible therapeutic role in these areas."

The experience of pain is a complex phenomenon involving the interaction of a number of biological systems having psychological and social aspects. Of course, *pain* in and of itself is not a "diagnosis" per se, but a symptom of many diseases and injuries. Because pain is a subjective state for which there are no reliable objective measures, caution is required in assessing the validity and reliability of data. Researching its amelioration presents a significant challenge, particularly in assessing a substance such as cannabis, which generally produces obvious psychoactive effects that make assessing a placebo difficult.

Physiologically, pain processing is mediated through the central, autonomic, and peripheral nervous systems, all of which are potential targets for cannabinoids. Cannabinoids act on pain through mechanisms that are distinct from opioids, and it appears that these overlapping pathways may explain their synergistic and opioid-sparing effects. Cannabinoid receptors have been identified in peripheral, spinal, and supra-spinal sites and play a clear role in CNS pain signaling. Brain sites involved in cannabinoid analgesia reflect the role of descending pathways of neural connections from the brain to the spinal cord. Research indicates that both CB_1 and CB_2 receptors play independent roles in controlling peripheral pain.

Pain is also one of the oldest documented reasons for which people have traditionally used cannabis therapeutically—from the role of cannabis in traditional Chinese medicine and Ayurvedic practices, to its introduction in Western medicine in the 1840s. Chronic pain has the most robust scientific evidence for the effectiveness of cannabinoids in its treatment and is the qualifying condition for the vast majority of patients enrolled in state medical marijuana programs that recognize pain and the condition(s) with which it may be associated, constituting in some states more than 90% of registrants.[1]

CHEMICAL COMPLEXITY OF THE CANNABIS PLANT

Δ-9 TETRAHYDROCANNABINOL (THC) AND CANNABIDIOL (CBD)

Δ-9 tetrahydrocannabinol (THC) has been the focus of considerable inquiry that has produced indications of its efficacy for managing nausea, appetite loss, and, of particular interest, pain. Like anandamide, THC is a partial agonist of cannabinoid receptors. The collective effect of several cannabinoids, terpenes, and other chemicals in the whole cannabis plant has been consistently shown to produce superior perceived effects when compared with cannabinoid isolates such as THC or synthetic cannabinoids, both in terms of maximizing efficacy and minimizing side effects. This is often referred to as an "entourage effect," but that term can be a bit misleading in that it implies that THC is the star or leader and the other chemicals contributing are "hangers on." A more accurate way to refer to this chemical synergy might be as an "ensemble effect," as the whole plant's constituents work in concert, often without THC itself coordinating the full balanced orchestration. This presents significant clinical difficulty in that the total components of this ensemble have yet to be uniformly researched, and the FDA requires drug makers to follow good manufacturing practices to deliver a reliably consistent, known dose of bioactive chemicals. Whole-plant "botanical" cannabis products that contain many chemicals are exponentially more challenging to study than medicines that contain known amounts of only one or two cannabinoids.

Cannabidiol (CBD) has received considerable recent attention as a potential therapeutic agent for a host of conditions. Since CBD is not intoxicating, it may offer a more favorable side-effect profile than medicines containing THC. A recent Critical Review of CBD by the World Health Organization's Expert Committee on Drug Dependence (ECDD) concluded that CBD poses no risk of abuse or dependence and recommended that pure CBD extracts not be subject to scheduling. The WHO's expert determination on CBD mirrors that of the FDA experts who evaluated the CBD medication Epidiolex® and concluded that its safety profile and lack of abuse potential indicate that it should not be scheduled as a strictly controlled substance.

CBD is a negative allosteric modulator of CB_1 receptors, meaning that it modifies some, but not all of a cannabinoid receptor's normal functions.[29] For instance, even though CBD does not activate CB_1 receptors directly, it can slow the rapid degradation of the endocannabinoid anandamide to prolong and enhance its natural effects on CB_1 receptors. As an allosteric modulator, CBD is capable of attenuating some of the dysphoric side effects from Δ-9 tetrahydrocannabinol (THC), such as paranoia.

Another allosteric modulator, the endogenous hormone pregnenolone also produces an allosteric inhibitory action on CB_1 receptors that reduces the psychotropic effects unique to THC. Pregnenolone synthesis increases in response to THC administration, and exogenous administration has been proposed as a method of mitigating THC's central side effects.[30] Similarly, CBD modulates the effects of the partial agonist THC on CB_1 receptors, inhibiting some of the intoxicating effects of THC by adjusting anandamide levels and modifying adenosine uptake. CBD also appears to inhibit the digestive metabolism of THC edibles that through liver metabolism produce its considerably longer lasting and more potent psychotropic metabolite, 11-hydroxy-THC. At CB_2 receptors,

CBD can function as a partial agonist, not fully activating the receptors but attenuating them, much as THC does at CB_1 receptors.[31]

Phytocannabinoids such as CBD have many targets other than CB_1 and CB_2, and CBD may be considered as the epitome of polypharmacy. It can interface with a host of other enzymes, transporters, ion channels, ligand-gated ion channels, GPCRs, and nuclear hormone receptors. CBD can stimulate adenosine receptors and provide indirect pain relief by modulating other receptors indirectly. Perhaps most significant among these for CBD and pain may be the Transient Receptor Potential (TRP) channels, particularly those designated as Transient Receptor Potential Vanilloid One (TRPV1) channels, which appear to contribute to the control of inflammation, pain, and temperature sensation. Both CBD and anandamide can stimulate TRPV1 channel activity. The extent to which CBD appears to activate, and over time may desensitize TRPV1 through receptor downregulation, helps to explain CBD's analgesic and anti-inflammatory effects. Other minor phytocannabinoids (not THC) also appear active on TRPV1.[32]

CBD seems to function in diverse ways, stimulating receptors, enzymes, and other proteins as an agonist, antagonist, and allosteric modulator. CBD also acts indirectly by inhibiting the degradation of ECS components such as anandamide and other neurotransmitters. When administered alone, CBD may be acutely ineffective at low doses of less than 200 mg/day, while CBD administered in larger doses (i.e., 200–800 mg per day) can produce many discernible therapeutic effects. Those effects can be observed at significantly lower doses when administered in combination with THC. Lower doses of CBD and THC in a 1:1 ratio can produce comparable effects to high doses of CBD in isolation, as noted in relation to seizure control.

CBD modulates the effects of THC through direct and indirect mechanisms. In addition to augmenting anandamide levels and modifying adenosine uptake, and without causing sedation, CBD can counteract paranoia and anxieties that can result from THC exposure, particularly in "cannabisnaïve" users, by activating complementary receptor functions that have anxiolytic effects. CBD also potentiates the amino acid tryptophan found in turkey and other foods that is known to be associated with elevated mood and relaxation. All of these can be positive effects in patients with pain, who often suffer associated anxiety and dysphoria.

Rodent studies, anecdotal reports, and data collected by cannabis product manufacturers provide evidence that CBD may be effective in both topical and systemic treatments for certain localized pain, particularly arthritis.[8] Research has shown that the joints of rheumatoid arthritis sufferers have a high concentration of responding CB_2 receptors, consistent with their on-site, on-demand protective role in fighting inflammation and injury.[33] Some arthritis sufferers report that disease progression slows or ceases, even with topical cannabinoid medicine use.

FDA APPROVAL OF CBD AS A MEDICINE

Most prominent among the potential applications of CBD has been its use for seizure control. Plant extracts producing CBD have been shown in clinical trials and numerous anecdotal reports to mitigate seizures associated with several disorders, even among refractory patients.[34,35] The U.S. Food and Drug Administration (FDA) approved Epidiolex® in 2018 as a standardized, dose-control CBD medication manufactured from cannabis plants. It was approved only for Dravet syndrome and Lennox–Gastaut syndrome (LGS), two rare pediatric seizure disorders, following clinical trials that were facilitated by an "orphan drug" designation that provides incentives for the development of drugs to treat rare diseases affecting only small populations.[36] Subsequent to the approval of Epidiolex®, the DEA issued a scheduling order in September 2018 placing only "FDA-approved drugs that contain CBD derived from cannabis and no more than 0.3% tetrahydrocannabinol" in Schedule V, the least restrictive controlled substance category.[37] In April 2020, the FDA removed Epidiolex® from drug scheduling entirely, meaning it is no longer a controlled substance. Currently that designation exclusively applies to Epidiolex and does not impact the Schedule I status of any other CBD product. It is nonetheless a significant milestone in cannabinoid medicine development and opens the door to similar plant-derived CBD-isolate drugs or products.

The approval and scheduling of Epidiolex® have contributed to confusion over the legality of other CBD products. Many companies are aggressively marketing CBD products as legal to ship to all 50 states, which they are not as of the time of this publication. Some claim that because the Controlled Substances Act of 1970 (CSA) identifies THC by name as a Schedule I substance but makes no mention of CBD, CBD is not scheduled. Others claim that because the CSA distinguishes between Schedule I marijuana and hemp (a varietal of the cannabis plant containing less than 0.3% THC), any CBD derived from hemp is legal. In 2016, the DEA rejected these arguments in published guidance, noting that phytocannabinoid extracts will remain covered by the CSA and that any plant material from which more than negligible amounts of cannabinoids can be extracted is by definition marijuana, and not hemp.[38] In fact, the testing of products marketed as "hemp-derived CBD extracts" has revealed that most of them contain little to no CBD.[39] The Farm Bill of 2018 may facilitate access to CBD derived from hemp, as it contains language to exclude hemp extracts from the Controlled Substances Act, but the FDA has not released rules for hemp-derived CBD as of the time of this publication.*

ADDITIONAL BIOACTIVE CHEMICAL COMPONENTS IN CANNABIS

The total cannabinoid content of a product offers only a crude index of therapeutic effect, since much of the end-user experience is dictated by other chemicals acting in concert, including the 100-plus cannabinoids in plant material and abundant terpenes. While the ratio of cannabinoids, particularly between THC and CBD, may help predict many effects, terpenes figure more prominently than was realized until very recently. Of interest in relation to the clinical trials conducted in the development of the standardized, dose-controlled plant extract medicine nabiximols, is that the approximate 1:1 THC:CBD ratio was demonstrated to be most effective for analgesia. That balanced ratio is characteristic of some historical landrace strains of cannabis cultivated over thousands of years, but as the illicit "recreational" market developed, that ratio would tip dramatically to the intoxicating THC, as the intoxicant-modulating CBD and certain terpenes were recessively bred out of commercial cannabis. The development or reclamation of CBD-rich hybrids of cannabis has been a renewed interest for contemporary medical cannabis cultivators.

Medical cannabis dispensaries and product manufacturers still mistakenly label their products based on a perceived distinction between different species types of cannabis plants, with indica or sativa respectively identified as being either sedative or energizing. While there is an historical basis to the evolutionary development of plant phenotypes (indica cannabis varietals developed in northern latitudes, while sativa types came from equatorial regions), recent genomic analyses of cannabis plants reveal that contemporary plants should essentially be regarded as hybrids of the two, with little chemical distinction in terms of their cannabinoid profiles. Where pronounced differences appear is in the plant's terpenes. Terpenes are the bioactive chemicals that give all plants their smells. These and other chemicals can influence receptor activity, including analgesia. An example is the reported sedative effects of some CBD-dominant cannabis hybrids. While CBD has demonstrated anxiolytic effects that may contribute to relaxation, hypnotic sedation is typically associated with the terpene known as myrcene, which is often abundant in CBD-dominant varietals having both sedative and analgesic properties. Myrcene is the likely source of what is a colloquial term called "couch lock"—a perceived inability to engage in physical movement or activities that appears to result from myrcene's hypnotic effect. Other terpenes and cannabinoid profiles can produce a range of distinguishable effects.† This explains why patients often tend to prefer particular

---

* CBD can also be found in some varieties of hops, the closest genetic relative to cannabis. A California company claims to have derived CBD oil extracts from *Humulus kriya*, an Asian hops variety cross-bred with Indian hemp, and a Canadian company is developing hemp-based beer that they say will include CBD.

† Considerable amounts of myrcene can also be found in hops, cannabis' closest genetic relative. In eastern Europe it is still possible to find pillows stuffed with hops that are used as a sleep aid.

varieties, types of products, or methods of delivery, and why availability of a wide diversity of products can be helpful.

RESEARCH: EVIDENCED-BASED DATA VS. ANECDOTAL EXPERIENCES

The evidence in support of cannabinoids as a treatment for acute, inflammatory, and neuropathic pain includes preclinical laboratory and animal studies, as well as experimental and clinical trials with humans. Though research has been limited by the constraints of drug scheduling and other administrative barriers, there is considerably more evidence for the efficacy of cannabinoids in the treatment of pain than for any other application. That evidence has been well-summarized by a pair of commissioned federal reviews, first in the 1999 report of the Institutes of Medicine (IOM) and then in the 2017 report of the National Academies of Sciences, Engineering, and Medicine (NASEM).[*]

INSTITUTES OF MEDICINE (1999)

Only 7 years after the discovery of the ECS, the IOM report noted that "cannabinoids likely have a natural role in pain modulation"—a conclusion that has been further developed and supported by basic research—and that cannabinoid drugs hold particular therapeutic promise for pain relief. The authors acknowledge that pain is the most common symptom for which patients seek treatment, and research findings on the analgesic properties of cannabinoids are consistent with anecdotal reports on how cannabis appears to modulate pain. Animal models of acute, inflammatory, and neuropathic pain have all responded positively to CB receptor Δ-9 THC agonists. The patient groups the report identifies as most likely to benefit from cannabinoid medicines are cancer patients being treated with chemotherapy; postoperative pain patients, particularly those experiencing nausea or vomiting from opioids; patients with spinal-cord injury, peripheral neuropathic pain, or central post-stroke pain; chronic pain patients with insomnia; and AIDS patients with cachexia, neuropathy, and other significant pain syndromes. This suggests that cannabinoids may be useful and indicated for a variety of reasons including:

- Synergism with other analgesics
- For patients who have developed a critical tolerance or intolerance to opioids
- Conditions for which cannabinoids may be safer than other medications
- Situations in which certain side effects may have clinical usefulness
- Efficacy for a remarkably broad spectrum of illnesses

Pain management experts consider neuropathic pain to be among the most challenging of pain syndromes to treat. The IOM report points to the treatment of neuropathic pain with cannabinoids as particularly promising based on experiments treating rodent models of neuropathic pain with cannabinoids capable of helping treat two problematic types of increased pain sensitivity—allodynia and hyperalgesia—associated with neural changes resulting from chronic pain. Cannabinoids showed potency and efficacy comparable to opioids in those experiments. The IOM also notes the efficacy of THC shown in three studies of treating severe cancer pain resistant to opioid treatment.[24] Those conclusions are borne out by subsequent clinical research addressed in a 2017 comprehensive report from the National Academies of Sciences, Engineering, and Medicine.

NATIONAL ACADEMIES OF SCIENCES, ENGINEERING, AND MEDICINE (2017)

The National Academies of Sciences, Engineering, and Medicine (NASEM) report reflects a consensus conclusion of a graded critical meta-analysis of the 24,000 relevant scientific publications on

---

[*] What was formerly known as the Institutes of Medicine is now a part of the National Academies.

cannabinoids since the time of the IOM report in 1999. Of all those publications, 100 studies were selected as meeting the clinical criteria. Evaluation of these study results produced a consensus conclusion that "there is substantial evidence that cannabis is an effective treatment for chronic pain in adults" (NASEM 2017, 90). Their report focused on five systematic reviews of clinical studies using cannabinoid medicines. For chronic pain, they relied primarily on one extensive review that included 28 randomized clinical trials on pain involving 2,454 participants that compared cannabinoid treatment to placebo, and another that compared cannabinoid medicine to amitriptyline for neuropathy.[40] Plant-derived cannabinoids of various types were used in 22 trials, while a synthetic analog of THC, nabilone, was used in five. Neuropathy was the focus in 17 of those trials. Other pain studies included cancer and chemotherapy-induced pain, multiple sclerosis, rheumatoid arthritis, and musculoskeletal pain. Plant-based treatments were approximately 40% more likely than controls to produce significant analgesia across all pain conditions. Inhalation was the route of administration in just one of the studies included in the review, but the NASEM authors note that its results were both comparable with other routes, and consistent with a different review of five other trials of inhaled cannabis in the treatment of neuropathic pain.[25]

As previously emphasized, the results of these and other controlled human trials are consistent with more voluminous anecdotal patient reports, experimental animal studies, and laboratory research, all of which point to the utility of cannabinoid medicines as analgesics. Systematic reviews of clinical studies of treating animals with cannabinoids—whether whole-plant products, isolate extracts, or synthetic analogs—found that study conclusions were largely consistent in showing that cannabinoids demonstrate a modest effect on pain, regardless of type of cannabinoid or type of pain, including arthritis, spinal cord injury, and neuropathy. The distress associated with neuropathic pain is a particularly challenging condition to treat. Another systematic review coordinated by the U.S. Department of Veterans Affairs concluded that limited evidence suggests that cannabis may alleviate neuropathic pain in some patients, but insufficient evidence exists for other types of chronic pain.[41]

Multiple sclerosis (MS) is another often painful condition for which the NASEM found "substantial evidence" of cannabinoid medicines being efficacious. Most randomized clinical trials of cannabinoid medicines in the treatment of MS have evaluated the effects on muscle spasticity, a condition that impairs function in 90% of these patients at some point during their illness. A more recent review of randomized MS trials also found that cannabinoids, including smoked cannabis, are superior to placebo in relief of pain and spasticity.[42] Both subjective patient reports and objective clinical measures of spasticity indicate some efficacy, but subjective reports of effect are consistently greater than objective measures. This disparity has led some to suggest that the clinical measures are flawed by limitations in design, and others to speculate that the euphoric side effects of cannabinoids are distracting patients from painful spasticity sufficiently to produce reports of improvement without significant change in muscle tone. MS patients may experience other symptom improvements with cannabinoid medicines, such as reductions in anxiety and depression, that may contribute to the differences between subjective reporting and objective clinical assessments.

For the estimated 100 million persons with chronic pain in the United States, second only to lower back pain is severe headache and/or neck pain.[43] The NASEM report does not address cannabinoid treatment for migraine and other headaches, as clinical trials are lacking, but many migraine sufferers report relief using cannabis, often prophylactically in low doses.[44] Growing understanding of the neurological and vascular mechanism of migraines indicates involvement of the ECS affecting the serotonin and endorphin receptors on which it operates, suggesting that exogenous cannabinoids may not just have a role in treatment but provide an "ideal" medication.[45] A recent review of preclinical studies and clinical trials identifies historical reports from the 19th and early 20th century that cannabis preparations were effective in both aborting and preventing headaches, as well as several modern case reports and patient surveys that found the same, but the lack of clinical trials means evidence for cannabinoid treatment of migraines and other headaches is inconclusive.[46] Migraine headache's disease-targeted therapy suggests that cannabis breeding for cultivar-specific synergistic ratios of cannabinoids, terpenes, and other phytochemicals may result in predictable user effects to improve symptoms (Figure 4.8).

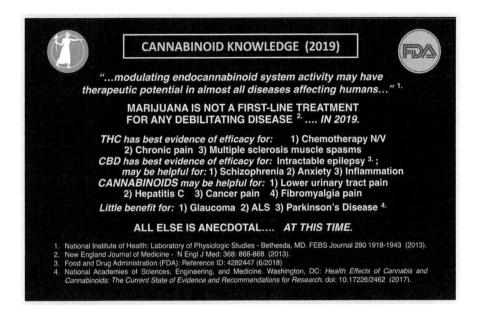

FIGURE 4.8 The significant promise of endocannabinoid science's research development is currently constrained by limited evidence-based data (Jeffrey S. Block, MD).

The multiple effects of cannabinoid medicines are not available à la carte. For many patients, the inseparable broad-spectrum effects can be a benefit because one medication may provide multiple mechanisms of therapeutic actions. For many pain conditions, anti-inflammatory and analgesic effects are both helpful. For chronic pain, psychosocial symptoms such as depression and anxiety often also require concurrent interventions, such that the euphoric side effects of cannabinoid medicines may be effective in treating those symptoms as well.

EDUCATION: CLINICAL RATIONALE TO CANNABINOIDS USED AS MEDICINE

A CONCEPT MODEL DESCRIBING THE ROLES OF ENDOCANNABINOIDS

The components of the ECS are expressed in nearly all parts of the human body throughout every stage of life. Upon conception and continuing until death, the actions of messages that are produced by endocannabinoids, alone or in combination with other mediators, support all basic life-sustaining functions. From the perspective that all animals' genetic ability to evolve relies on maintaining an effective balance with life's continuous stressors, a healthy animal's naturalized response requires an effective endocannabinoid system's nurturing to ensure its ultimate survival.[2]

As an educational concept, the endocannabinoid receptors' clinical role can be regarded as constantly integrating the balance of five general functions that are collectively essential to sustaining life. This receptor system's general purpose is in supporting the ability to eat, sleep, relax, forget, and to protect from the consequences of disease as age advances. Growth and development's dependence on balanced eating and sleeping is obvious and is a critical role of CB_1 receptor function. Understanding ECS wide function even explains the holistic and scientifically elusive so-called "brain–gut connection" (Figure 4.9).

The ability to recover from life's relentless physical and psychological stress is directed through endocannabinoids. This recovery requires not only time to physically relax and recover, but also the ability to forget. Effective processing of new memories occurs in the brain's hippocampus, which is replete with CB_1 receptors. The filtering of memories through effective CB_1 receptor function is a genetically hard-wired protective mechanism, essential for behavioral health.

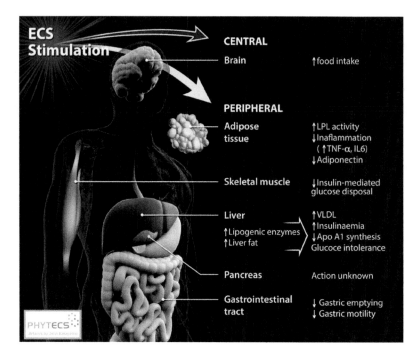

FIGURE 4.9   Stimulation of the endocannabinoid system (ECS) connects the brain's central influences with peripheral organ system metabolism (Phytecs, Inc.; artwork by John Karapelou).

Intolerably painful physical, psychological, or spiritual experiences are selectively filtered through this part of the brain, and pathologic inabilities to forget intolerable situations can lead to pain sensitivity and avoidance behaviors such as are seen in patients suffering from post-traumatic stress disorders (PTSD). Conversely, the astute clinician may also observe that a patient's inability to forget a pleasurable experience leads to their inability to control seeking that circumstance; then such pleasure-seeking behavior may cause the patient to suffer from the consequences of an addiction's dependency.

As life's experiences accrue, the endocannabinoid system's effect on selectively filtering painful and pleasurable experiences may be a critical determinant in the development of one's behavioral personality. Because so little is known about the biochemical basis of personality, it is intriguing to consider that the endocannabinoid system's contributions to functional health might be central to the understanding of this elusive human characteristic.

In contrast, CB_2 receptor functions play a particularly important protective role by mitigating the physiologic consequences of disease. CB_2 receptors are generally thought of as being plentiful in the abdomen in proximity to where the majority of cells of immune lineage are known to exist but are cellularly ubiquitous in that they have been identified not only in vascular cells, but also in adipocytes, B-lymphocytes, and macrophages. CB_2 receptors are primarily associated with cells of innate immune lineage derived from the bone marrow. In the CNS, CB_2 receptor expression is associated with responses to injury by modulating inflammation. CB_2 receptors help maintain pivotal balances and are able to respond when and where an organism is threatened by the effects of disease or injury. In a clinical sense, corrective physiologic changes modulated through CB_2 receptors may be those which allow a disease to become chronic, when an inability to respond to the progression of disease would otherwise result in death. This possibility emphasizes the clinical importance of future innovations that exploit this receptor system's subtle, yet essential health function (Figure 4.10).

One of the few places where cannabinoid receptors are *not* found is within the portion of the brain stem's medulla and pons devoted to respiration. This neuroanatomical advantage helps explain cannabis' lethal dose safety profile; even with its abuse, no respiratory depression fatal overdoses attributed only to cannabis have ever been documented. Experimental safety challenges in reliable

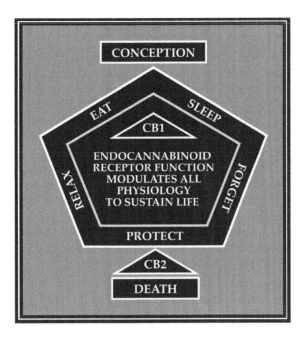

FIGURE 4.10 An applied clinical model consistent with CB_1 and CB_2 receptor functions and endocannabinoids' life-sustaining health rationale (Jeffrey S. Block, MD).

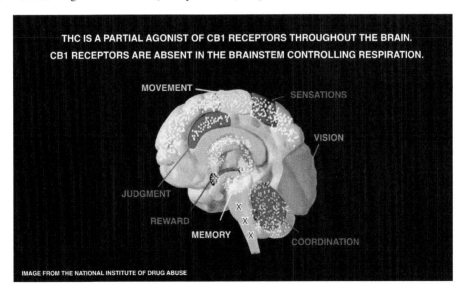

FIGURE 4.11 The distribution of CB_1 receptors in the brain explains THC's known effects on functions including memory, judgment, and coordination (image by NIDA www.drugabuse.gov/publications/drugfacts/marijuana).

animal models include studies in which monkeys and dogs were administered extraordinarily large doses of THC, equivalent to a human being consuming 63,000 times a standard 10 mg dose, without lethal injury from central respiratory depression (Figure 4.11).[47]

Complicating this picture of cannabinoid receptor modulation, activation, and deactivation are compounds recently described as "super agonists"—synthetic compounds that bind to cannabinoid receptors much more intensely and overdrive their response. Super-agonist chemicals with street names such as "K2" and "Spice" are misleadingly referred to as synthetic "marijuana" but were originally developed as experimental laboratory molecules never intended for human use. These synthetic cannabinoid analog products are not infrequently abused by school-age youth, and can pose substantial dangers, including death.[48]

Excessive doses of cannabis, typically in the form of edible products whose potency is often discovered too late, can cause acute discomfort manifested as paranoia and dysphoria in individuals that may lead to emergency room visits after ingestion, but physical or psychological injury does not result. In contrast, the use of synthetic super agonists such as K2 and Spice may result in serious injury or death, because sometimes these drugs are manufactured in combination with potentiating chemicals thought to prolong the intoxicating effects, such as anticoagulants including warfarin, as found in rat poison. These synthetic drugs are not chemically similar to THC or other phytocannabinoids but can strongly bind to cannabinoid receptors, exerting up to 100 times more effect.[49]

Cannabinoids, both endogenous ligands and exogenous molecules (plant-derived or synthetic), produce a wide range of receptor activity, consistent with their role as modulators of bodily functions. A crucial difference between endogenous and exogenous cannabinoids is the locations they affect and their duration of action. While endocannabinoids are produced on-site and on-demand and are created and degraded very rapidly, exogenous plant-based and synthetic cannabinoids typically produce system-wide effects that persist far longer.

CLINICAL CONSIDERATIONS OF CANNABINOID MEDICINES

Behavioral research has established that most patients have already experimented with using cannabis therapeutically before asking their physicians about it—if they ask at all.[1] The concern patients have for how their doctor perceives them, coupled with a fear of being stigmatized as a marijuana user, indicates that patients using cannabis medicinally often fail to disclose that use to their doctors.[50] The robust market in cannabis makes independent experimental use possible in ways that are not seen using conventional medications. As a result, it behooves clinicians to not just be prepared for such questions, but to be assertive about broaching it with patients for whom cannabis may be a legitimate treatment option.

While some individuals may hide their therapeutic use of a stigmatized drug, others may ask physicians for medications outside the bounds of accepted treatment. Research indicates that 20% of individuals who present themselves in emergency room visits as having acute pain are seeking opioid medication for questionable or non-therapeutic reasons.[51] Clinical guidelines for managing addiction liability include continuity of care and use of signed treatment agreements to describe and minimize risks, an approach that has been recommended for medical cannabis.[52]

DOSING GUIDANCE

Clinicians are rightfully concerned with providing accurate medication dosing directions for their patients. Though plants have been the source of treatments throughout most of human history, botanical medicines pose a challenge for accurate dosing because of the difficulty in obtaining reliably standardized products. The complexity and variability of botanical medicines contributed to the 20th century's turn away from plant remedies to pharmaceuticals based on isolated active ingredients that can be synthetically manufactured with consistency.

This complexity and variability are particularly true of medicinal cannabis products and of the plant itself, all of which are highly variable in their chemical components. Even carefully cultivated cannabis plants of the same varietals, including clones from the same parent plant, may result in end-product variability with differing cannabinoid and terpene profiles. This is multifactorial and can depend on a given plant flower's chemical variability, how and where it was grown, when it was harvested, and how it was dried and cured. Additionally, non-standardized chemical testing reports can vary significantly in assessing products, further complicating the matter (Figure 4.12).

As with most medications, "start low and go slow" is a sound strategy for cannabinoid medicine therapies in most conditions. The variability of commonly available cannabis products is

Generic Name and Delivery Route	Brand Name	Doses and/or Components	Dosages Used in Selected Trials	DEA (USA) Schedule
CANNABINOID FORMULARY DOSING AND SCHEDULING (2019)				
Cannabis species plant (Multiple routes)	Marijuana hybrids Sativa / Indica	THC 4% - >28%? CBD 0% - >15%?	1% - 8% THC self-titrated	Schedule I (1970)
Cannabis species plant (capsule extract)	*Cannador* (Germany)	THC 2.5% CBD 1.25%	Max 1.25 mg/kg/d Max 25.0 mg/kg/d	Schedule I (1970)
Nabilone (capsule)	*Cesamet*	1.0 mg synthetic cannabinoid	1.0 mg BID 0.5 -1.0 mg hs	Schedule II (2006)
Dronabinol (liquid)	*Syndros*	5.0 mg synthetic THC analog	2.1 mg/BID 4.2 mg/m2	Schedule II (2010)
Dronabinol (tablets)	*Marinol*	2.5 mg synthetic THC analog	1.25 mg/BID 10.00 mg/BID	Schedule III (1998)
Nabiximols (oral spray extract)	*Sativex* (England)	THC 2.7 mg CBD 2.5 mg	Max THC 65/d Max CBD 120/d	Under FDA evaluation
Cannabidiol (oral oil extract)	*Epidiolex* (England)	(98% CBD)	2 - 25 mg/kg/d	Schedule V (2018)

FIGURE 4.12 Summary of current cannabinoid medicines with their available component doses, research trial dose ranges, and Drug Enforcement Administration schedule (Jeffrey S. Block, MD).

compounded and confounded by considerable variance in patient experiences based on inconsistent product types and routes of administration, use timing and routines, and physiologic set points. What counts as a sub-optimal dose in one individual may be a robust effective treatment in another, and this often changes with individuals over time. Some of those differences may be associated with developed tolerance via receptor downregulation, but changes in sensitivity can affect some long-time users such that they report decreasing their dosing over time with comparable results. What serves as a low or high dose will vary between individuals based on that person's experience with cannabis use, their physiology, and the route of administration. Many state regulatory agencies have set dosing standards or "serving sizes" at 10 mg THC, but doses as low as the clinical threshold of 2.5 mg THC or 2.5 mg of balanced ratio THC:CBD products are commonly manufactured and used effectively by cannabis-naïve patients. CBD dosing should be carefully integrated as part of a patient's overall pharmaceutical management because it can induce some cytochrome p450 enzymes, suggesting that it has clinical relevance concerning the breakdown of other medications, including blood-thinners and other anxiolytics.

PARADOXICAL DOSE-DEPENDENT EFFECTS ON PAIN

For pain patients, care with dosing is especially important, as THC and whole-plant preparations have been shown to exhibit dose-dependent effects that are paradoxically biphasic. Relatively low doses typically produce effective mild to moderate analgesia, but high doses can actually intensify pain sensations. This dose-dependent characteristic features a narrow window of effective dosing (ED) that may explain early clinical studies of cannabinoid analgesia that produced inconclusive results. The doses of THC vary between clinical trials, and the studies included in the NASEM report produced some indication of dose-dependent effects. The importance of dose was also seen in studies of vaporized cannabis involving acute pain,[53,54] but a similar study found analgesic effects to not be dose-dependent.[55] Anecdotal reports of pain intensification typically entailed relatively large doses. Escalation in dosing can occur when a patient believes the amount taken was insufficient, and subsequently takes more. That can happen when the time to onset of effect is underestimated, as is more common with edible cannabis product's slower GI absorption. Failure to achieve the desired level of analgesia can also contribute to a cannabis user surpassing the effective dose range as more and more is taken in hopes of achieving more relief.

Increasing cannabinoid dosing may cause increasing side effects, hence diminishing its overall therapeutic value. This is most profound with synthetic cannabinoids. When comparing synthetic cannabinoid medications such as dronabinol and nabilone, many patients prefer the whole plant's balanced chemicals, critically describing the THC isolates as having "all of the side effects without all of the benefits." At high doses, the effects of THC alone may be not just hyperalgesia but acute anxiety and dysphoria. As mentioned earlier, CBD modulates these concerning effects of THC through direct and indirect mechanisms.

ROUTES OF ADMINISTRATION

In addition to varietal differences, the effects of cannabinoid medicines can be dramatically altered by their route of administration, including inhalation, mucosal absorption, oral ingestion, and topical application. Smoking is the method most commonly employed by cannabis users, not only because of tradition and ease of use, but also because inhalation's speed of onset allows for quick symptom relief and effective titration management. It only takes a few seconds before the cannabis user perceives an initial effect, and up to a few minutes until its peak effects are realized. The byproducts of smoke inhalation nonetheless make it an undesirable method. However, by heating plant material to a temperature below combustion, but sufficient to aerosolize the volatile cannabinoid and terpene oils, vaporizing provides the benefits of inhalation's speed of onset without smoking's byproducts. Lessons learned from tobacco smoking's combustion release of cancer-causing benzene and polycyclic aromatic hydrocarbons remain a concern, although epidemiological studies have failed to find an association between cannabis smoking and the health risks associated with tobacco smoking, such as lung cancer, emphysema, or chronic obstructive pulmonary disease.[56–58]

Inhalation is well-known to accelerate nicotine's central and systemic blood levels, but deference to the lungs' critical function of gas exchange has largely limited their use to deliver local therapeutic bronchodilators and anti-inflammatory medications. Nevertheless, when compared to combustion, vaporization's lower temperatures minimally adulterate the cannabis plant's bioactive component chemicals.

While many vaporizers of cannabis oils and flowers are commercially available, devices that allow precise, consistent temperature control are ideal, as different temperatures will release varying combinations of cannabinoids and terpenes. Some experienced cannabis users may report reduced effectiveness because vaporizing lacks cues associated with smoking that may produce an independent placebo effect, but vaporizing appears to deliver cannabinoids at least as well as smoking and better preserves a given varietal's terpene profile. Multiple clinical trials have shown vaporization to be an effective delivery method for pain management, and a crossover trial of vaporization and smoking found vaporized delivery produced higher blood THC levels and more acute effects at both low and moderate doses.[59]

Oral-mucosal delivery methods are utilized for Sativex and Epidiolex, and other sprays and hard candies provide absorption through the mucous membranes of the mouth, with some content known to advance to absorption from digestion. Mucosal absorption offers superior speed of onset when compared with edible products, as well as a more systemic bodily effect than inhalation, that delivers cannabinoids far more rapidly to the brain. Cannabis suppositories are also available and may be preferred by patients with persistent nausea, as well as those using higher dosages that would not be well-tolerated through edibles.

Edible cannabis products come in many varieties, from infused chocolate and candies, to cookies and sodas. Cannabis tinctures suspended in alcohol or glycerin, similar to those of the last century, are widely available and can be added to food products or taken directly. Edible ingestion results in not only the longest time to onset, but also the longest duration of effect. The prolonged time to onset means naïve users may mistakenly believe that they have already experienced a full effect long before they actually do, and so they may then ingest even more cannabis. This is the most common way to an acutely uncomfortable experience that may induce intense paranoia that not infrequently brings an intoxicated dysphoric patient to the emergency room. The consequences are compounded by the more intense psychoactivity of 11-hydroxy-THC, the Δ-9THC metabolite produced by liver metabolism during digestion. The duration of effect from edibles lends itself to their use for overnight treatments, when extended relief and sleep assistance are primary goals. Many pain patients who are cannabis-savvy also report using low-dose edibles to maintain a baseline of analgesia, with inhalation for breakthrough pain.

Topical cannabis products are often combined with other therapeutic or aromatic creams and oils for treating arthritis or muscle pain. The evidence in support of topical application is limited to anecdotal reports, although some cannabis product manufacturers have been collecting data through individual and crowd sourcing in a more systemic fashion. As with all subjective reporting in the absence of objective clinical measures, caution is required in assessing the validity and reliability of these data. Of extra concern in the case of cannabinoid medicines are the potentially confounding effects of euphoria and memory impairment, which may individually or in tandem influence both the immediate experience and its recall.

RISKS AND CONTRAINDICATIONS

The important role of clinicians in educating their adult patients about the potential risks involved in cannabis use needs to be emphasized when making it available for therapeutic purposes. Cannabis dependence and impairment are significant public health issues, but complications from cannabis use are poorly documented. Multiple animal studies of extreme cannabinoid exposure indicate at worst mild risks from its use. In humans, three primary relative contraindications for cannabis use are pre-existing or genetic predispositions to mental health disorders, heart problems, and pregnancy.

Individuals with a variety of mental health disorders appear to gravitate to cannabis use because of a subjective perception of improved symptoms. Particularly in the naïve user, higher doses (e.g., greater than 15–20 mg of THC) can induce feelings of panic and anxiety that can be problematic. Side effects of chronic cannabis intoxication, including performance declines, are more often seen in recreational consumers. Limited clinical research suggests cannabinoids may be effective in treating schizophrenia.[60,61] The NASEM report notes substantial evidence of a statistical association between cannabis use and development of schizophrenia and other psychoses, and an increased rate of cannabis use is associated with a genetic predisposition to schizophrenia.[62]

Cannabis use consistently produces tachycardia and vascular dilation, which rarely may elevate the risk of a myocardial infarction in individuals with pre-existing heart problems.[63] Those individuals with heart disease are more likely to develop chest pain after acutely consuming cannabis. While cannabis use can increase heart rate and systolic blood pressure, a decrease in peripheral vascular resistance can also result in orthostatic hypotension.[64]

Pregnancy contraindicates many medications, though, as with all individuals, physicians and patients should weigh the risks and benefits to arrive at clinical decisions. Lower birth weight is the most serious reported association with maternal cannabis use, but that may be explained by the prevalence of smoking as a delivery method and the concomitant CO and CO_2 exposure that can create hypoxia in the fetus and limit growth. A study of neonates and infants in a population of heavy cannabis users found no developmental or other problems.[65,66] Ethnobotanical use of cannabis by some Caribbean cultures has traditionally treated first-trimester hyperemesis by drinking cannabis teas to remedy the nutritional risks and restore the systemic fluid needs associated with this malady.[67,68] Due to the ethical challenges associated with studying women during pregnancy, any potential consequences from cannabis use on fetal stem cells causing long-term effects are poorly understood.

The antiemetic and appetite-stimulating properties of cannabis have been reported to benefit women afflicted with severe morning sickness with fewer side effects than other medications, but should women suffering from morning sickness during pregnancy use marijuana to control their nausea? In states with medical cannabis programs, health experts, regulatory officials, and most patient advocates have consistently answered "no" in the form of public service announcements and warning labels on cannabis packaging. Nevertheless, a statewide cross-sectional study in Colorado found that nearly 70% of dispensary workers endorsed using cannabis for first-trimester morning sickness, and fewer than a third spontaneously recommended consulting a healthcare professional about it.[69]

In contrast to morning sickness in gravid women, cannabis hyperemesis syndrome is a rare but serious adverse event associated with chronic cannabis use. This is a paradoxical condition in which an individual with consistent long-term exposure to cannabis may suddenly develop uncontrollable vomiting following cannabis use.[70–72] This effect is striking given the well-documented and far more common *anti*emetic effects of cannabis use. Symptoms are reportedly often relieved by a hot shower or bath. While the etiology of the cannabis hyperemesis syndrome remains unclear, cannabinoids are known to inhibit calcium channels, and calcium channel blocking is associated with nausea.[73] Furthermore, calcium channels are temperature-sensitive, and heat increases channel firing that mitigates nausea, which may explain why afflicted patients often report that a hot shower or bath relieves their hyperemesis. The paradoxical nature of the syndrome and its rarity even among populations of heavy chronic users suggest factors other than plant constituents including that an autoimmune phenomenon may be responsible. Another explanation posited by some knowledgeable with cannabis cultivation practices is chronic exposure to azadirachtin, the active chemical compound in the biopesticide neem oil, which is commonly used in organic farming.

CONTAMINANTS AND TESTING

Pesticides of all types are a concern with cannabis cultivation, and inadequate regulation and testing in some U.S. state markets have resulted in cultivators using chemical insecticides and fungicides on their cannabis crops. A random testing of cannabis commercially available in California and Washington legal markets detected residual pesticide contaminants with known potential for serious health effects in a majority of analyzed samples.[74] Health Canada requires testing for pesticides in the medical cannabis distributed through their program and conducts its own random testing of products. In 2018, two Canadian suppliers were required to recall their pesticide-contaminated products.[75]

In recent years many U.S. states have adopted regulations for what can be used safely in cannabis products intended for human consumption and require testing of products. Due to federal prohibition, universal guidelines have not been developed, and organic certification standards are unavailable for cannabis cultivation. The absence of a United States Pharmacopeia disposition on cannabis standards led the American Herbal Pharmacopeia (AHP) to issue a monograph on cannabis purity and identity standards in 2014. The American Herbal Products Association (AHPA) has similarly produced guidelines for regulators on cannabis products, including cultivation, storage, manufacturing, and dispensing. Both groups acted in collaboration with subject matter experts and patient advocates, and their standards have subsequently been widely adopted by certifying standards organizations and state agencies in the United States. Global standards organizations such as ASTM International, formerly known as the American Society for Testing and Materials, are also working to establish uniform protocols for analytic testing and other aspects of cannabis production.

Life-threatening pulmonary complications subsequent to the increased use of vaporizing devices have been recently reported. While infectious diseases do not appear to be responsible, other contaminants including tocopheryl (vitamin E) acetate remain suspect and have been investigated as a source of chemical burns progressing to reactive airway pneumonitis. Consistent state guidelines directing the enforcement of production standards have not been established while cannabis remains under federal prohibition. The Centers for Disease Control urged doctors to report suspected cases to their state health agencies, and the Food and Drug Administration is collecting information about illnesses related to e-cigarettes and vaping.[76]

The broad range of ECS effects requires caution in pharmacological applications. The effects of long-term chronic use of exogenous cannabinoids on the system's function is unknown; however, limited studies of medical cannabis users enrolled for more than 30 years in the federal government's

Investigational New Drug program have found no adverse health consequences.[77] Possible down-regulation of endogenous cannabinoid receptors such as is seen in other receptor systems requires longitudinal studies to determine significance, but this may be a neuroadaptive factor of cannabis dependence. A 2012 investigation by the National Institute of Drug Abuse addressed the ECS's receptor's plasticity as measured by its ability to regenerate after chronic heavy exposure. Cannabis users sequestered without access to the drug had a near total recovery of their brain's full complement of CB_1 receptors after only four weeks of monitored abstinence.[78]

Where significant patient outcome problems have been seen is with drugs that block cannabinoid receptor activity. The role of endocannabinoids in metabolism and appetite has made the ECS a target for the development of drugs to treat metabolic syndrome. Rimonabant (Acomplia® or SR141716) is one such drug that works as an inverse agonist at CB_1 to reduce hunger and weight gain, but at considerable cost to overall endocannabinoid tone. Although weight loss was documented with rimonabant, serious adverse side effects included nausea, seizures, depression, and suicidality, leading to withdrawal of the drug after two years on the foreign market.[79] In this case, drug development failed to appreciate the full extent of the CB_1 endocannabinoid receptor's broad range of non-specific central effects.

CONTEMPORARY CANNABIS AND ITS MEDICALIZATION

LEGAL STATUS AND ACCREDITABLE PRACTICE STANDARDS

Cannabis is undergoing a social process of "medicalization" similar to what has been described with how contested illnesses come to be recognized as legitimate and within the domain of medicine.[1] That process differentiates medicinal cannabis use from drug abuse and is reflected in the various medical access laws and institutional initiatives such as professional organization endorsements. Physician-led initiatives directed through the American Society of Cannabinoid Medicine (ASCM) provide responsible legislative guidance and leadership to advance high-quality education and clinical research. Physician-focused organizations including the American Academy of Cannabinoid Medicine and the Society of Cannabis Clinicians provide a basis through which contemporary practice standards are being established. Such standards of care are essential to assess and correct for negative patient outcomes. Accreditable goals will be essential to this emerging healthcare sector's ultimate success. Enforcing these practices through licensing dependent on accreditation will ensure continuous quality improvement benefits, similar to the metrics used elsewhere in healthcare. The medicalization of cannabis is currently incomplete, but it is slowly being incorporated into physician education and practice, and gradually becoming less controversial.

Until then, as a Schedule I substance, cannabis cannot be legally "prescribed" anywhere in the United States. Federal courts have ruled that First Amendment protections of free speech cover doctor–patient communications, including the written "recommendations" required to participate in state medical cannabis programs. Doctors who recommend cannabis to their patients may experience heightened scrutiny from their peers, including state medical boards. These boards in states with medical cannabis programs have begun to develop limited practice standards for recommending cannabis. Those typically entail a physical exam and preservation of patient records, but minimal follow-up requirements to assess patient outcome. Careful re-evaluation is important to determine underlying conditions producing pain or other symptoms that may necessitate additional therapeutic or curative interventions. Cannabis can be considered as a *complementary* palliative medicine; however, at this time its recommendation should not be intended as an *alternative* medicine if that implies it to be a substitute for the evidence-based data essential to Western medicine's diagnostic and therapeutic advances.

Guidelines vary between countries such as Israel and Canada that allow access via a physician's prescription. Health Canada has developed medical cannabis access regulations, and the Canadian Medical Association, the Canadian Medical Protective Association, and the College of Family Physicians of Canada have published practice guidelines for responsibly treating chronic pain and other debilitating illnesses.[80–84]

FUTURE DEVELOPMENTS

At this time, whole-plant preparations of cannabinoids and terpenoids produce multiple effects that are inseparable from one another. Future phytocannabinoid medicines may be developed which can exert their effects in isolated areas, including operating in the periphery on pain and other conditions without crossing the blood–brain barrier to include central effects. Developing methods of selectively inhibiting the psychoactive side effects of THC, such as increased synthesis of pregnenolone, may also enhance the versatility and tolerability of cannabinoid medicines.

E-cigarette technology developed for nicotine delivery has recently extended to the systemic absorption of vaporized cannabis plant flower oils by utilizing so-called vape pens. While many vaporizers of cannabis are commercially available, devices that allow precise, consistent temperature control are ideal, as different temperatures will release varying combinations of these cannabinoid and terpene chemicals. Nevertheless, the black market operating within a largely unregulated vaporizing device industry currently appears to be responsible for increasing pulmonary deaths. These lethal complications associated with inhaled super-heated carrier chemicals or contaminants will renew clinical interest in the dermal absorption of therapeutic lipids.

Topical application and transdermal methods of delivery using nanoscale molecules such as liposomes improve the local site-specific and systemic delivery of the lipophilic cannabinoids and terpenoids produced by the cannabis plant. Nanotechnology can facilitate the transportation of these drugs across epithelial and endothelial barriers, as well as extending their bioactivity and retention in the body to allow a more effective duration of treatment.[85]

Drug development may profitably focus on enhancing natural ECS activity, but basic lifestyle adjustments are also likely to contribute to a healthier ECS response to stressors. That may be as simple as advising patients not only on the importance of exercise and sleep, which are both tied to ECS function, but also on what to eat. Because the endogenous ligand anandamide and other important, related lipids are synthesized in humans from omega-3 fatty acids (such as fish oil), dietary adjustments or supplements may also serve to improve ECS function.

The biosynthesis and degradation of enzymes such as fatty acid amide hydrolase (FAAH) and monoglyceride lipase (MGL) that break down endocannabinoids are prime targets for new drug development. Manipulating these enzymes may harness innate processes that counteract disease states, and plant-derived molecules such as cannabidiol (CBD) hold significant promise for this. Allosteric modulators of endocannabinoid receptors other than CBD are a target of future drug development, as their effects on the receptors' activity can potentially enhance endogenous cannabinoid function.

The 2019 case report of a woman who did not manifest anxiety or perceive pain as a noxious stimulus discovered that she had a pseudogene microdeletion compromising FAAH's breakdown of anandamide.[86] Not unexpectedly, this individual's extraordinary phenotype also appears to cause other central nervous system side effects, including memory impairment. Future work will help to understand if targeting this link using viral short hairpin RNA or gene-editing techniques could be effective as an analgesic or anxiolytic drug development strategy.

THE CONTEMPORARY CLINICIAN'S RESPONSIBLE ROLE

Clinicians will recognize that pain can pose special challenges and, when intolerable, can drive patients to desperate measures. Seeking relief from the physical, psychological, or spiritual symptoms of disease is a natural instinct that contributes to therapeutic uses of many substances, including cannabis. Beyond the pragmatics of dealing honestly and directly with patient choice, the remarkable safety profile of cannabinoids can give clinicians an added measure of confidence in recommending them for patients who are not achieving adequate analgesia with more conventional treatments, particularly those who suffer from neuropathies or other intractable conditions. The complexity of the evolving legal landscape for cannabinoid medicines will continue to require

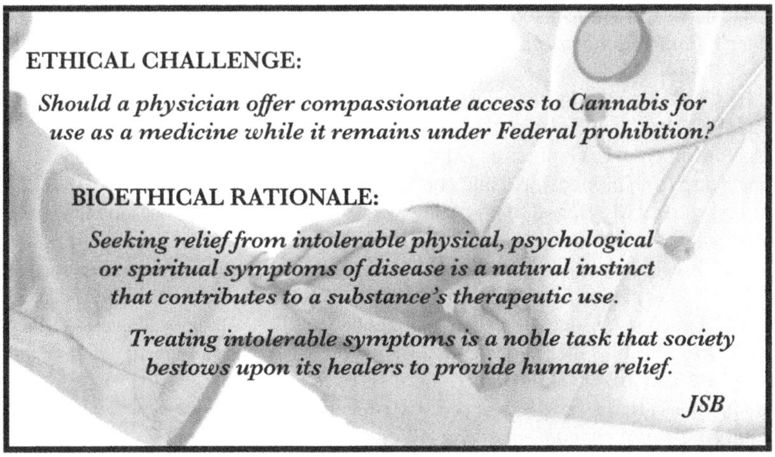

ETHICAL CHALLENGE:

Should a physician offer compassionate access to Cannabis for use as a medicine while it remains under Federal prohibition?

BIOETHICAL RATIONALE:

Seeking relief from intolerable physical, psychological or spiritual symptoms of disease is a natural instinct that contributes to a substance's therapeutic use.

Treating intolerable symptoms is a noble task that society bestows upon its healers to provide humane relief.

JSB

FIGURE 4.13 Bioethics can offer rational solutions to public health's most challenging problems (Jeffrey S. Block, MD).

attention, and physicians should act accordingly by first acknowledging that the treatment of intolerable symptoms to provide humane relief is a noble task that society bestows upon its healers (Figure 4.13).

This imperative is perhaps seen and felt most acutely in the treatment of children. The suffering of children with seizure disorders has inspired parents, physicians, and policymakers to act on their behalf. The successful clinical trials of the first plant-based cannabinoid pharmaceutical medicine (cannabidiol) and its recent Schedule V designation have completed the initial steps toward making a more complete armamentarium available to physicians. Several other companies are following suit, and cannabinoids are likely to be featured in many pharmaceutical formularies of the future.

The clinician faced with a patient in intolerable pain has an obligation to not just feel compassion, but to do what is possible to alleviate that suffering without causing harm. As the limitations of opioid options become more evident, the search for safe and effective solutions has rightfully included cannabinoid medicines. Despite barriers to research, randomized clinical trials provide substantial evidence of the analgesic potential of cannabinoids, confirming animal experiments, laboratory science, and what is known about the purpose of the endocannabinoid receptor system. As clinicians consider how to apply these discoveries, they may do well to heed the ethical standards which physicians have historically promised to uphold, whether the Hippocratic oath to "apply for the benefit of the sick all measures that are required," or that of Maimonides to seek the strength, time, and opportunity to correct acquired beliefs and extend the domain of knowledge.

REFERENCES

1. Newhart M., Dolphin W. *The Medicalization of Marijuana: Legitimacy, Stigma, and the Patient Experience*. New York, NY: Routledge; 2019.
2. Di Marzo V.D., Melck D., Bisogno T., Petrocellis L.D. Endocannabinoids: endogenous cannabinoid receptor ligands with neuromodulatory action. *Trends Neurosci* 1998;21(12):521–528.
3. Befort K. Interactions of the opioid and cannabinoid systems in reward: insights from knockout studies. *Front Pharmacol* 2015;6(6).
4. Pacher P., Kunos G. Modulating the endocannabinoid system in human health and disease–Successes and failures. *FEBS J* 2013;280(9):1918–1943.
5. Elphick M.R. The evolution and comparative neurobiology of endocannabinoid signalling. *Philos Trans R Soc Lond B Biol Sci* 2012;367(1607):3201–3215.
6. Vaughn L., Denning G., Stuhr K., de Wit H., Hill M., Hillard C. Endocannabinoid signalling: has it got rhythm? *Br J Pharmacol* 2010;160(3):530–543.

7. Russo E.B. The role of cannabis and cannabinoids in pain management. In: B.E. Cole, M.V. Boswell, eds. *Weiner's Pain Management: A Practical Guide for Clinicians*. Boca Raton, FL: CRC Press; 2006:823–844.
8. Russo E.B. Cannabinoids in the management of difficult to treat pain. *Ther Clin Risk Manag* 2008;4(1):245–259.
9. Gifford A.N., Bruneus M., Gatley S.J., Volkow N.D. Cannabinoid receptor-mediated inhibition of acetylcholine release from hippocampal and cortical synaptosomes. *Br J Pharmacol* 2000;131(3):645–650.
10. Dalayeun J.F., Norès J.M., Bergal S. Physiology of beta-endorphins: a close-up view and a review of the literature. *Biomed Pharmacother* 1993;47(8):311–320.
11. Pertwee R.G. Targeting the endocannabinoid system with cannabinoid receptor agonists: pharmacological strategies and therapeutic possibilities. *Philos Trans R Soc Lond B Biol Sci* 2012;367(1607):3353–3363.
12. Piomelli D. The molecular logic of endocannabinoid signalling. *Nat Rev Neurosci* 2003;4(11):873–884.
13. Prenderville J.A., Kelly Á.M., Downer E.J. The role of cannabinoids in adult neurogenesis. *Br J Pharmacol* 2015;172(16):3950–3963.
14. Busquets-Garcia A., Bains J., Marsicano G. CB1 receptor signaling in the brain: extracting specificity from ubiquity. *Neuropsychopharmacology* 2017;43(1):4.
15. Console-Bram L., Marcu J., Abood M.E. Cannabinoid receptors: nomenclature and pharmacological principles. *Prog Neuropsychopharmacol Biol Psychiatry* 2012;38(1):4–15.
16. McPartland J.M. Cannabis systematics at the levels of family, genus, and species. *Cannabis Cannabinoid Res* 2018;3(1):203–212.
17. Boehnke K.F., Litinas E., Clauw D.J. Medical cannabis use is associated with decreased opiate medication use in a retrospective cross-sectional survey of patients with chronic pain. *J Pain* 2016;17(6):739–744.
18. Reiman A., Welty M., Solomon P. Cannabis as a substitute for opioid-based pain medication: patient self-report. *Cannabis Cannabinoid Res* 2017;2(1):160–166.
19. Nielsen S., Sabioni P., Trigo J.M., et al. Opioid-sparing effect of cannabinoids: a systematic review and meta-analysis. *Neuropsychopharmacology* 2017;42(9):1752–1765.
20. Lucas P., Walsh Z. Medical cannabis access, use, and substitution for prescription opioids and other substances: a survey of authorized medical cannabis patients. *Int J Drug Policy* 2017;42:30–35.
21. Cichewicz D.L., Martin Z.L., Smith F.L., Welch S.P. Enhancement of μ opioid antinociception by oral delta9-tetrahydrocannabinol: dose-response analysis and receptor identification. *J Pharmacol Exp Ther* 1999;289(2):859–867.
22. Cichewicz D.L. Synergistic interactions between cannabinoid and opioid analgesics. *Life Sci* 2004;74(11):1317–1324.
23. Campbell G., Hall W.D., Peacock A., et al. Effect of cannabis use in people with chronic non-cancer pain prescribed opioids: findings from a 4-year prospective cohort study. *Lancet Public Health* 2018;3(7):e341–e350.
24. IOM. *Marijuana and Medicine: Assessing the Science Base*. Washington, DC: The National Academies Press; 1999.
25. NASEM NAoS, Engineering and Medicine. *The Health Effects of Cannabis and Cannabinoids: The Current State of Evidence and Recommendations for Research*. Washington, DC: The National Academies Press; 2017.
26. Bradford A.C., Bradford W.D., Abraham A., Bagwell Adams G. Association between US state medical cannabis laws and opioid prescribing in the medicare part D population. *JAMA Intern Med* 2018;178(5):667–672.
27. Liang D., Bao Y., Wallace M., Grant I., Shi Y. Medical cannabis legalization and opioid prescriptions: evidence on US medicaid enrollees during 1993–2014. *Addiction* 2018;113(11):2060–2070.
28. Lucas P., Walsh Z., Crosby K., et al. Substituting cannabis for prescription drugs, alcohol and other substances among medical cannabis patients: the impact of contextual factors. *Drug Alcohol Rev* 2016;35(3):326–333.
29. Ibeas Bih C., Chen T., Nunn A.V., Bazelot M., Dallas M., Whalley B.J. Molecular targets of cannabidiol in neurological disorders. *Neurotherapeutics* 2015;12(4):699–730.
30. Vallée M., Vitiello S., Bellocchio L., et al. Pregnenolone can protect the brain from cannabis intoxication. *Science* 2014;343(6166):94–98.
31. Morales P., Reggio P., Jagerovic N. An overview on medicinal chemistry of synthetic and natural derivatives of cannabidiol. *Front Pharmacol* 2017;8:422.
32. De Petrocellis L., Ligresti A., Moriello A.S., et al. Effects of cannabinoids and cannabinoid-enriched cannabis extracts on TRP channels and endocannabinoid metabolic enzymes. *Br J Pharmacol* 2011;163(7):1479–1494.

33. Gui H., Liu X., Wang Z.-W., He D.-Y., Su D.-F., Dai S.-M. Expression of cannabinoid receptor 2 and its inhibitory effects on synovial fibroblasts in rheumatoid arthritis. *Rheumatology* 2014;53(5):802–809.

34. Devinsky O., Cross J.H., Laux L., et al. Trial of cannabidiol for drug-resistant seizures in the dravet syndrome. *N Engl J Med* 2017;376(21):2011–2020.

35. Pamplona F.A., da Silva L.R., Coan A.C. Potential clinical benefits of CBD-rich cannabis extracts over purified CBD in treatment-resistant epilepsy: observational data meta-analysis. *Front Neurol* 2018;9:759.

36. FDA approves first drug comprised of an active ingredient derived from marijuana to treat rare, severe forms of epilepsy [press release]. June 25, 2018.

37. DEA. Schedules of controlled substances: placement in schedule V of certain FDA-approved drugs containing cannabidiol; corresponding change to permit requirements. Final order. *Fed Regist* 2018;83(189): 48950–48953.

38. DEA. Clarification of the new drug code (7350) for Marijuana extract. https://www.deadiversion.usdoj .gov/schedules/marijuana/m_extract_7350.html2017

39. Bonn-Miller M.O., Loflin M.J.E., Thomas B.F., Marcu J.P., Hyke T., Vandrey R. Labeling accuracy of cannabidiol extracts sold online. *JAMA* 2017;318(17):1708–1709.

40. Whiting P.F., Wolff R.F., Deshpande S., et al. Cannabinoids for medical use: a systematic review and meta-analysis. *JAMA* 2015;313(24):2456–2473.

41. Nugent S., Morasco B., O'Neil M., et al. The effects of cannabis among adults with chronic pain and an overview of general harms: a systematic review. *Ann Intern Med* 2017;167(5):319–331.

42. Torres-Moreno M., Papaseit E., Torrens M., Farré M. Assessment of efficacy and tolerability of medicinal cannabinoids in patients with multiple sclerosis: a systematic review and meta-analysis. *JAMA Network Open* 2018;1(6):e183485.

43. Institute of Medicine Committee on Advancing Pain Research Care, and Education. *Relieving Pain in America: A Blueprint for Transforming Prevention, Care, Education, and Research.* Washington, DC: National Academies Press; 2011.

44. Krashin D., Murinova N., Mannava A., Schorn N., Murin M. *Marijuana Use in Headache.* Boston, MA: World Congress on Pain; 2018.

45. Russo E.B. Hemp for headache: an in-depth historical and scientific review of cannabis in migraine treatment. *J Cannabis Ther* 2001;2:21–92.

46. Lochte B.C., Beletsky A., Samuel N.K., Grant I. The use of cannabis for headache disorders. *Cannabis Cannabinoid Res* 2017;2(1):61–71.

47. Thompson G.R., Rosenkrantz H., Schaeppi U.H., Braude M.C. Comparison of acute oral toxicity of cannabinoids in rats, dogs and monkeys. *Toxicol Appl Pharmacol* 1973;25(3):363–372.

48. Seely K., Lapoint J., Moran J., Fattore L. Spice drugs are more than harmless herbal blends: a review of the pharmacology and toxicology of synthetic cannabinoids. *Prog Neuropsychopharmacol Biol Psychiatry* 2012;39(2):234–243.

49. Tai S., Fantegrossi W.E. Synthetic cannabinoids: pharmacology, behavioral effects, and abuse potential. *Curr Addict Rep* 2014;1(2):129–136.

50. Kondrad E.C., Reed A.J., Simpson M.J., Nease D.E. Lack of communication about medical marijuana use between doctors and their patients. *J Am Board Fam Med* 2018;31(5):805–808.

51. Grover C.A., Elder J.W., Close R.J., Curry S.M. How frequently are 'classic' drug-seeking behaviors used by drug-seeking patients in the emergency department? *West J Emerg Med* 2012;13(5):416–421.

52. Wilsey B., Atkinson J.H., Marcotte T.D., Grant I. The medicinal cannabis treatment agreement: providing information to chronic pain patients through a written document. *Clin J Pain* 2015;31(12):1087–1096.

53. Wilsey B.L., Marcotte T.D., Deutsch R., Zhao H., Prasad H., Phan A. An exploratory human laboratory experiment evaluating vaporized cannabis in the treatment of neuropathic pain from spinal cord injury and disease. *J Pain* 2016;17(9):982–1000.

54. Wallace M., Schulteis G., Atkinson J.H., et al. Dose-dependent effects of smoked cannabis on capsaicin-induced pain and hyperalgesia in healthy volunteers. *Anesthesiology* 2007;107(5):785–796.

55. Wilsey B., Deutsch R., Samara E., et al. A preliminary evaluation of the relationship of cannabinoid blood concentrations with the analgesic response to vaporized cannabis. *J Pain Res* 2016;9:587–598.

56. Hashibe M., Morgenstern H., Cui Y., et al. Marijuana use and the risk of lung and upper aerodigestive tract cancers: results of a population-based case-control study. *Cancer Epidemiol Biomarkers Prev* 2006;15(10):1829–1834.

57. Huang Y.H., Zhang Z.F., Tashkin D.P., Feng B., Straif K., Hashibe M. An epidemiologic review of marijuana and cancer: an update. *Cancer Epidemiol Biomarkers Prev* 2015;24(1):15–31.

58. Tashkin D.P. Effects of marijuana smoking on the lung. *Ann Am Thorac Soc* 2013;10(3):239–247.

59. Spindle T.R., Cone E.J., Schlienz N.J., et al. Acute effects of smoked and vaporized cannabis in healthy adults who infrequently use cannabis: a crossover trial. *JAMA Network Open* 2018;1(7):e184841.

60. Osborne A.L., Solowij N., Weston-Green K. A systematic review of the effect of cannabidiol on cognitive function: Relevance to schizophrenia. *Neurosci Biobehav Rev* 2017;72:310–324.

61. Manseau M., Goff D. Cannabinoids and schizophrenia: risks and therapeutic potential. *Neurotherapeutics* 2015;12(4):816–824.

62. Power R.A., Verweij K.J., Zuhair M., et al. Genetic predisposition to schizophrenia associated with increased use of cannabis. *Mol Psychiatry* 2014;19(11):1201–1204.

63. Desai R., Patel U., Sharma S., et al. Recreational marijuana use and acute myocardial infarction: insights from nationwide inpatient sample in the United States. *Cureus* 2017;9(11):e1816.

64. Goyal H., Awad H.H., Ghali J.K. Role of cannabis in cardiovascular disorders. *J Thorac Dis* 2017;9(7):2079–2092.

65. Hayes J.S., Dreher M.C., Nugent J.K. Newborn outcomes with maternal marihuana use in Jamaican women. *Pediatr Nurs* 1988;14(2):107–110.

66. Hayes J.S., Lampart R., Dreher M.C., Morgan L. Five-year follow-up of rural Jamaican children whose mothers used marijuana during pregnancy. *West Indian Med J* 1991;40(3):120–123.

67. Dreher M.C., Nugent K., Hudgins R. Prenatal marijuana exposure and neonatal outcomes in Jamaica: an ethnographic study. *Pediatrics* 1994;93(2):254–260.

68. Dreher M. Crack heads and roots daughters: the therapeutic use of cannabis in Jamaica. *J Cannabis Therap* 2002;2(3–4):121–133.

69. Dickson B., Mansfield C., Guiahi M., et al. Recommendations from cannabis dispensaries about first-trimester cannabis use. *Obstet Gynecol* 2018;131(6):1031–1038.

70. Khattar N., Routsolias J.C. Emergency department treatment of cannabinoid hyperemesis syndrome: a review. *Am J Ther* 2018;25(3):e357–e361.

71. Simonetto D.A., Oxentenko A.S., Herman M.L., Szostek J.H. Cannabinoid hyperemesis: a case series of 98 patients. *Mayo Clin Proc* 2012;87(2):114–119.

72. Galli J.A., Sawaya R.A., Friedenberg F.K. Cannabinoid hyperemesis syndrome. *Curr Drug Abuse Rev* 2011;4(4):241–249.

73. Twitchell W., Brown S., Mackie K. Cannabinoids inhibit N- and P/Q-type calcium channels in cultured rat hippocampal neurons. *J Neurophysiol* 1997;78(1):43–50.

74. Russo E. Current therapeutic cannabis controversies and clinical trial design issues. *Front Pharmacol* 2016;7:309.

75. Health Canada. Health Canada testing of cannabis for medical purposes for unauthorized pest control products. *Gov Can Publ* 2018. Accessed January 7, 2019.

76. CDC, Centers for Disease Control. CDC urges clinicians to report possible cases of unexplained vaping-associated pulmonary illness to their state/local health department. In: Clinician Outreach and Communication Activity. 2019. Published August 14, 2019.

77. Russo E., Mathre M.L., Byrne A., et al. Chronic cannabis use in the compassionate investigational new drug program. *J Cannabis Ther* 2002;2(1):3–57.

78. Hirvonen J., Goodwin R.S., Li C.T., et al. Reversible and regionally selective downregulation of brain cannabinoid CB1 receptors in chronic daily cannabis smokers. *Mol Psychiatry* 2012;17(6):642–649.

79. Moreira F.A., Crippa J.A. The psychiatric side-effects of rimonabant. *Rev Bras Psiquiatr* 2009;31(2):145–153.

80. CMPA. Medical marijuana: guidance for Canadian doctors. https://www.ccmpa -acpm.ca/en/advice-p ublications/browse-articles/2014/medical-marijuana-new-regulations-new-college-guidance-for-can adian-doctors. Published 2018. Accessed January 7, 2019.

81. Allan G., Ramji J., Perry D., et al. Simplified guideline for prescribing medical cannabinoids in primary care. *Can Fam Phys* 2018;64(2):111–120.

82. Fischer B., Russell C., Sabioni P., et al. Lower-risk cannabis use guidelines: a comprehensive update of evidence and recommendations. *Am J Public Health* 2017;107(8):e1–e12.

83. CFPC, College of Family Physcicians of Canada. *Authorizing Dried Cannabis for Chronic Pain or Anxiety: Preliminary Guidance from the College of Family Physicians of Canada.* Mississauga, ON, 2014.

84. CMA. CMA statement: authorizing marijuana for medical purposes. https://www.cma.ca/Assets/asse ts-library/document/en/advocacy/CMA_Policy_Authorizing_Marijuana_for_Medical_Purposes_ Update_2015_PD15-04-e.pdf. Published 2015. Accessed January 7, 2019.

85. AZoNano. *Nanotechnology for Drug Delivery Applications.* Published November 1, 2017.

86. Habib A.M., Okorokov A.L., Hill M.N., et al. Microdeletion in a FAAH pseudogene identified in a patient with high anandamide concentrations and pain insensitivity. *Br J Anaesth* 2019;123(2):e249–e253.

5 Sex Hormones and Pain Control

Pamela W. Smith

CONTENTS

INTRODUCTION

Severe pain has major effects on the endocrine system. As science progresses, the role that sex hormones play in pain control is being further examined. In addition, hormone abnormalities may result if the individual experiences chronic pain. These abnormalities serve as biomarkers for the presence of intense pain and the need to replace hormones to achieve pain control. Initially severe pain causes a hyperarousal of the hypothalamic–pituitary–adrenal (HPA) system which results in elevated serum hormone levels such as adrenocorticotropin, cortisol, and pregnenolone. If the pain does not resolve, the HPA system cannot maintain its normal hormone production and balance. Consequently, levels of some hormones may decline. Conversely, several hormones are so critical for pain control that a deficiency may further enhance the pain.[1]

SEX HORMONES IN WOMEN

This chapter will begin by examining the major sex hormone in a woman's body which is estrogen, produced mainly by the ovaries. Women have estrogen receptor sites throughout their system including the brain, muscles, bone, bladder, gut, uterus, ovaries, vagina, breasts, eyes, heart, lungs, and blood vessels, to name a few. Estrogen has 400 critical functions, some of which are the following:[2–14]

- Stimulates the production of choline acetyltransferase, an enzyme which prevents Alzheimer's disease
- Increases metabolic rate
- Improves insulin sensitivity
- Regulates body temperature
- Helps prevent muscle damage
- Helps maintain muscle
- Improves sleep
- Reduces risk of cataracts

- Helps maintain the elasticity of arteries
- Dilates small arteries
- Increases blood flow
- Inhibits platelet stickiness
- Decreases the accumulation of plaque on arteries
- Enhances magnesium uptake and utilization
- Maintains the amount of collagen in the skin
- Decreases blood pressure
- Decreases LDL and prevents its oxidation
- Helps maintain memory
- Increases reasoning and new ideas
- Helps with fine motor skills
- Increases the water content of skin and is responsible for its thickness and softness
- Enhances the production of nerve-growth factor
- Increases HDL by 10 to 15%
- Reduces the overall risk of heart disease by 40 to 50%
- Decreases lipoprotein(a)
- Acts as a natural calcium channel blocker to keep arteries open
- Enhances energy
- Improves mood
- Increases concentration
- Maintains bone density
- Helps prevent glaucoma
- Increases sexual interest
- Reduces homocysteine
- Decreases wrinkles
- Protects against macular degeneration
- Decreases the risk of colon cancer
- Helps prevent tooth loss
- Aids in the formation of neurotransmitters in the brain such as serotonin which decreases depression, irritability, anxiety, and pain sensitivity
- Increases glucose and oxygen transport to the neurons
- Maintains the blood–brain barrier
- Protects neurons
- Increases the production of choline acetyltransferase, which is needed for the production of acetylcholine, the main neurotransmitter of memory

Progesterone is another sex hormone synthesized by the ovaries that has many functions in a woman's body, including the following:[2,15–20]

- Balances estrogen
- Has a positive effect on her sleeping pattern
- Helps build bone
- Helps prevent anxiety, irritability, and mood swings
- Helps bladder function
- Regulates the smooth muscle in the gut so that the body can break down food into nutrients that are absorbed to be used elsewhere in the body

Testosterone falls into a class of hormones called androgens which are commonly referred to as "male" hormones but which are present in women as well. Testosterone is made in the ovaries, and a small amount is also made in the adrenal glands. It has numerous functions, which include:[21–26]

- Decreases bone deterioration
- Decreases excess body fat
- Aids with pain control
- Elevates norepinephrine in the brain consequently having an antidepressant effect
- Helps maintain memory
- Increases muscle mass and strength
- Increases muscle tone
- Increases sense of emotional well-being, self-confidence, and motivation
- Increases sexual interest

It is paramount that women maintain hormonal balance of all of their steroid hormones throughout their lifetime to help maintain optimal function as well as to aid in pain control.

SEX HORMONES IN MALES

Testosterone is the main sex hormone produced by the male. It is produced by the Leydig cells in the testes, and a small amount is also produced in the adrenal glands. Men have hormone receptors in several locations in their body. Testosterone has many functions, including the following:[27–41]

- Important for sexual interest
- Involved in the making of protein and muscle formation
- Helps manufacture bone
- Improves oxygen uptake throughout the body
- Helps control blood sugar
- Needed for normal sperm development
- Regulates acute HPA responses under dominance challenge
- Helps regulate cholesterol
- Helps maintain a powerful immune system
- Aids in mental concentration
- Improves mood
- Helps protect the brain against Alzheimer's disease
- Regulates the population of thromboxane A2 receptors on megakaryocytes and platelets and consequently platelet aggregation
- Aids in pain control

Progesterone also has the following functions in a male's body:[42]

- Influences spermiogenesis
- Sperm capacitation/acrosome reaction
- Testosterone biosynthesis in the Leydig cells
- Blocking of gonadotropin secretion
- Sleep improvement
- Regulates immune system
- Positive cardiovascular effects
- Regulates kidney function
- Affects adipose tissue
- Regulates behavior
- Affects the respiratory system

Androgens aromatize into estrogens via the enzyme aromatase. Estrogens, at low levels, are important for a male to help maintain memory and bone structure.[43]

PREGNENOLONE IN WOMEN AND MEN

Pregnenolone makes estrogen, progesterone, testosterone, DHEA, and cortisol in both men and women. It also has the following functions:[44–48]

- Regulates the balance between excitation and inhibition in the nervous system
- Increases resistance to stress
- Improves energy both physically and mentally
- Enhances nerve transmission
- Reduces pain and inflammation
- Blocks the production of acid-forming compounds
- Modulates the neurotransmitter GABA
- Helps to repair nerve damage
- Promotes mood elevation
- Modules NMDA receptors
- Regulates pain control, learning, memory, and alertness

ADRENAL HORMONES IN WOMEN AND MEN

Dehydroepiandrosterone (DHEA), which is made in adrenal glands and a small amount in the brain and the skin, has many wonderful functions in both women and men, including the following:[49–54]

- Breaks down into estrogen and testosterone
- Decreases cholesterol
- Decreases formation of fatty deposits
- Prevents blood clots
- Increases bone growth
- Promotes weight loss
- Increases brain function
- Increases lean body mass
- Increases sense of well-being
- Helps one deal with stress
- Supports the immune system
- Helps the body repair and maintain tissues
- Decreases allergic reactions
- Lowers triglycerides

Cortisol, which is likewise made in the adrenal glands, is one of the most valuable hormones in the body. It is essential for life. If the body stops manufacturing it, the individual will shortly expire. Therefore, it is preferentially made from pregnenolone over the remainder of the steroidogenic pathway due to its overwhelming importance in the body. Cortisol has the following functions:[55–71]

- Balances blood sugar
- Controls weight
- Regulates immune system response
- Modulates the stress reaction
- Regulates sleep
- Involved in protein synthesis
- Controls mood and thoughts
- Influences testosterone/estrogen ratio
- Influences DHEA/insulin ratio

- Affects pituitary/thyroid/adrenal system
- Regulates bone turnover rate
- Participates with aldosterone in sodium reabsorption
- Is an anti-inflammatory
- Regulates pain control

THE EFFECTS OF PAIN ON SEX HORMONES

Severe pain has significant effects on the endocrine system.[1,72–78] Intense pain activates the hypot halamic–pituitary–adrenal–thyroid–gonadal (HPATG) system, which is the major stress-control mechanism of the body.[79–82] The purpose of this system is to produce additional hormones in the thyroid, adrenals, and gonads, and secrete them into the system, as they are required by the body for many pain-control functions, including the protection and regeneration of injured tissue, immuno-logic activity, and metabolic controls.[81–84]

HORMONES AND PAIN CONTROL

The critical pain-control hormones that are produced in glands outside the CNS are cortisol, preg-nenolone, dehydroepiandrosterone (DHEA), progesterone, testosterone, estrogen, and thyroid.[47,85–98] Tennant, in his landmark article, examines the major pain-control mechanisms of each sex hor-mones in the steroidogenic pathway.[1] Adequate pain control may not be achieved without hormonal homeostasis. Among the primary pain-control functions of these hormones are immune and anti-inflammatory actions, cellular protection, tissue regeneration, glucose control; and modulation of CNS receptors, the blood–brain barrier, and nerve conduction.[47,97–105]

One of the best investigated of these hormones is estrogen. Studies have shown that there are many estrogenic influences on pain processing in women.[106] Estrogen has both pronociceptive and antinociceptive actions.[107–109] In addition, an animal study revealed that estrogen replacement sig-nificantly increased anti-inflammatory IL-10 levels peripherally and centrally, as well as decreasing pro-inflammatory tumor necrosis factor alpha (TNF-alpha) and IL-1B levels.[110]

Likewise, studies have shown that patients in pain with low serum testosterone levels need replacement for not only the traditional reasons, but also for testosterone's neuroprotective, neuro-genic, and analgesic properties.[87,92,111–114] Testosterone has mostly antinociceptive action in both men and women.[107, 108] Furthermore, White et al. revealed that low or deficient testosterone serum levels are linked to a high risk for an inflamed nociceptive nervous system and resultant chronic pain states. The study showed that testosterone applied transdermally to individuals with fibromyalgia was an effective therapy for chronic pain control.[115]

Consequently, if hormone levels are low or even suboptimal, hormone replacement therapy should be considered before prescribing opioids, which put the patient at risk for opioid-induced suppression of the endocrine system.[116–120] Replacement of pregnenolone, DHEA, estrogen, proges-terone, and/or testosterone is rightfully emerging as a new therapy for pain management.[121,122]

In addition, some patients with severe and chronic pain fail to obtain adequate pain relief with standard drug therapies, including low to moderate dosages of opioids. A study was done to help characterize these individuals and develop treatment strategies for them. In the trial, a serum hor-mone profile consisting of adrenocorticotropin, cortisol, pregnenolone, progesterone, dehydroepian-drosterone, and testosterone was obtained on over 60 people with chronic pain who failed standard treatments. The study revealed that hormone abnormalities were biomarkers of severe, uncontrolled pain. In addition, in patients who were unsuccessful in achieving pain relief with traditional thera-pies, hormone replacement may be indicated. [123]

Interestingly, patients who have mild pain or pain that is intermittent tend to have normal serum sex hormone levels.[124] Many of these patients, however, may have elevated cortisol levels. These indi-viduals are not appropriate candidates for opioid medications or other more intense interventions.

Yet, with the demands of severe pain, the tissues in the hypothalamus, pituitary, adrenals, gonads, or thyroid may not sustain serum concentrations of some hormones and levels may drop below normal. Consider replacing these hormones before starting narcotic pain control medications including therapies for cortisol dysfunction.[125,126]

In fact, chronic cortisol abnormalities, when levels are elevated or depressed, are the major hormonal problem in chronic pain patients, although the prevalence of cortisol abnormalities in chronic pain patients is unknown.[125,127] The stress response results in cortisol levels that are initially elevated, and then if the pain is chronic, cortisol levels over time become depressed. Cortisol is a potent anti-inflammatory hormone, and its dysfunction is prone to result in extensive inflammation due to the activation of a proinflammatory stress response that is acute. Likewise with chronic stress, cortisol dysfunction results in unregulated inflammation following reactivation of the stress response, which may contribute to a cycle of pain, inflammation, and depression. Furthermore, pain itself is a stressor that may reactivate a proinflammatory stress response which is now changed due to abnormal cortisol levels.[128] In addition, studies have shown associations among inflammatory cytokines, stress-related chronic pain, and low salivary cortisol levels.[129,130] Furthermore, dwindling cortisol levels have been observed in patients with different stress-related disorders such as chronic fatigue syndrome, fibromyalgia, and post-traumatic stress disorder. Data suggest that these disorders are characterized by a symptom triad of enhanced stress sensitivity, pain, and fatigue.[131]

There are also numerous mechanisms by which widespread inflammation may contribute to pain since pain is a major component of the inflammatory response. The reactivation of a stress response that has not been balanced releases proinflammatory sympathetic catecholamines. Likewise, the impaired anti-inflammatory function of cortisol may intensify and prolong the inflammatory response.[132] Similarly, physical injury during a state of stress-induced hypocortisolism may result in a persistent inflammatory response that impairs healing instead of beginning the healing process. Additionally, the prolonged elevation of inflammatory cytokines sensitizes nociceptors which increases the patient's sensitivity to pain. Furthermore, chronic reactivation of the stress response by inflammatory mediators that are not controlled and emotional responsiveness that is increased may add to the inflammatory response, reinforce an abnormal stress response, and intensify the cycle of stress, inflammation, and pain.[131,133] Likewise, following chronic reactivation of the HPA axis, cortisol dysfunction and inflammation may directly facilitate pain transmission via impaired modulation or repeated nociceptor activation by inflammatory mediators.[128]

For all of the reasons above, the benefits of hormone replacement and balancing of the cortisol response are paramount prior to the initiation of pain control medications, particularly long-acting opioids. [134]

OPIOID SUPPRESSION OF HORMONES

Opioids, particularly those that are long-acting or delivered by the intrathecal route, may suppress some hormone production,[117,118,135–137] although the exact dosages that may produce suppression have not been determined.[100,120] It is the consistency of sustained-action opioids that produces a brain concentration that does not allow the HPATG system to produce its normal output of hormones.[118,119,138] Suppressed levels of testosterone are the most common issue with opioid administration, but cortisol, pregnenolone, and DHEA may also be suppressed.[120,137] Lower levels of testosterone are believed to be due to the tendency of opioids to preferentially suppress gonadotropin-releasing hormone.[136] Consequently, testosterone suppression with long-acting and intrathecal opioids occurs in the majority of these patients.[120,136] In fact, a study revealed that testosterone is suppressed in men with regular opioid use regardless of opioid type.[139] Suppression may begin within 90 days of the opioid being prescribed, and testosterone levels may remain low as long as the opioids are given. Consequently, patients who are prescribed long-term opioids should be screened for hormonal dysfunction and also be re-evaluated every 6 months. If the levels are low, individuals should be prescribed hormone replacement since, as discussed previously in this chapter, low levels of sex hormones are commonly associated with poor pain control. Hormone replacement has been reported to relieve allodynia and hyperalgesia in some patients.[126] In clinical practice, hormone replacement may have to be given for appropriate candidates without knowing precisely which mechanism is primarily responsible for the hormone deficiency.[121] Furthermore, given the CNS effects of certain hormones, analgesics such as anti-depressants, neuropathic agents, and opioids may not achieve maximal analgesic responses without hormonal balance.[1,2,84,90,92,94,95,126]

CONCLUSION

The basic physiologic effect of pain on the endocrine system is one of severe stress. Pain initially stimulates the HPATG system to produce and secrete higher levels of hormones from the adrenals, gonads, and thyroid, which travel to target tissues including injured nerves and the CNS. These hormones provide anti-inflammatory, immunologic, and regenerative properties which protect and heal the cells. In the stimulation phase of severe pain, hormone levels are elevated. If pain persists unrestrained for too long, the hormonal system is commonly unable to tolerate the stress of the pain itself, and hormone production may be reduced, causing hormone levels to become suboptimal. The most serious hormone complication of severe chronic pain is the negative impact that occurs upon cortisol. In fact, hormone levels serve as biomarkers for uncontrolled pain. Before considering therapy with long-acting opioids and other pain treatment modalities that carry risks, a hormone assessment should be made to determine whether a chronic pain patient has normal serum or salivary levels of cortisol, pregnenolone, DHEA, estrogen, progesterone, and testosterone and replace if the patient is an appropriate candidate. With this new approach, the use of opioids and other pain medications can be minimized if hormone balance is achieved prior to introduction of these agents and even after the use of these medications to help lower dosages and possible side effects.

REFERENCES

1. Tennant, F., "The physiologic effects of pain on the endocrine system," *Pain Ther* 2013; 2(2):75–86.
2. Smith, P., *What You Must Know About Women's Hormones*, Garden City Park, NY: Square One Publishers, 2010.
3. Fink, G., et al., "Estrogen control of central neurotransmission: effect on mood, mental state, and memory," *Cell Mol Neurobiol* 1996; 16(3):325–44.
4. Felson, D., et al., "Aromatase inhibitors and the syndrome of arthralgias with estrogen deprivation," *Arthritis Rheum* 2005; 52(9):2594–98.
5. Di Paolo, T., et al., "Modulation of brain dopamine transmission by sex steroids," *Rev Neurosci* 1994; 5(1):27–41.
6. Miller, V., et al., "Vascular effects of estrogen and progesterone," in *Estrogens and Progestogens in Clinical Practice*, Fraser, J., Ed., New York: Harcourt Publishers, 2000.
7. Miller, V., et al., "Vascular actions of estrogens: functional implications," *Pharmacol Rev* 2008; 60(2):210–41.
8. Stirone, C., et al., "Estrogen increases mitochondrial efficiency and reduces oxidative stress in cerebral blood vessels," *Mol Pharmacol* 2005; 68(4):959–65.
9. Duckles, S., et al., "Estrogen and mitochondria: a new paradigm for vascular protection?" *Mol Interv* 2006; 6(1):26–35.
10. Niki, E., et al., "Estrogens as antioxidants," *Methods Enzymol* 1990; 186:330.
11. Puder, J., et al., "Estrogen modulates the hypothalamic-pituitary-adrenal and inflammatory cytokine responses to endotoxin in women," *J Clin Endocrinol Metab* 2001; 86(6):2403–08.
12. Xu, H., et al., "Estrogen reduces neuronal generation of Alzheimer's β-amyloid peptides," *Nat Med* 1998; 4(4):447–51.
13. Weiland, N., "Estradiol selectively regulates agonist binding sites on the N-methyl-d-aspartate receptor complex in the CA1 region of the hippocampus," *Endocrinology* 1992; 131(2):662–68.
14. Wise, P., et al., "Minireview: neuroprotective effects of estrogen—New insights in mechanisms of action," *Endocrinology* 2001; 142(3):969–73.

15. Carmody, B., et al., "Progesterone inhibits human infragenicular arterial smooth muscle cell proliferation induced by high glucose and insulin concentrations," *J Vasc Surg* 2002; 36(4):833–38.
16. Rosano, G., et al., "Natural progesterone, but not medroxyprogesterone acetate, enhances the beneficial effect of estrogen on exercise-induced myocardial ischemia in postmenopausal women," *J Am Coll Cardiol* 2000; 36(7):2154–59.
17. Prior, J., "Progesterone as a bone-tropic hormone," *Endocr Rev* 1990; 11(2):386–98.
18. Taylor, D., "Perimenstrual symptoms and syndromes: guidelines for symptom management and self-care," *Obstet Gynecol* 2005; 595:228–41.
19. Solomon, C., et al., "Long or highly irregular menstrual cycle as a marker for the risk of type 2 diabetes mellitus," *JAMA* 2001; 286(19):2421–26.
20. Stein, D., "The case for progesterone," *Ann N Y Acad Sci* 2005; 1052:152–69.
21. Almeida, O., "Sex playing with the mind. Effects of oestrogen and testosterone on mood and cognition," *Arq Neuropsiquiatr* 1999; 57(3A):701–06.
22. Ehrenreich, H., et al., "Psychoendocrine sequelae of chronic testosterone deficiency," *J Psychiatr Res* 1999; 33(5):379–87.
23. Davis, S., et al., "Testosterone influences libido and well-being in women," *Curr Opin Obstet Gynecol* 1997; 9(3):177–80.
24. Brincat, M., et al., "Sex hormones and skin collagen content in postmenopausal women," *Br Med J* 1983; 287(6402):1337–38.
25. Rohr, U., "The impact of testosterone imbalance on depression and women's health," *Maturitas* 2002; 41(Suppl 1):S25–S46.
26. Monjo, M., et al., "Direct effects of testosterone, 17 beta-estradiol, and progesterone on adrenergic regulation in cultured brown adipocytes: potential mechanism for gender-dependent thermogenesis," *Endocrinology* 2003; 144(11):4923–30.
27. van den Beld, A.W., et al., "Measures of bioavailable serum testosterone and estradiol and their relationships with muscle strength, bone density, and body composition in elderly men," *J Clin Endocrinol Metab* 2000; 85(9):3276–82.
28. Swerdloff, R., et al., "Androgen deficiency and aging in men," *West J Med* 1993; 159(5):579–85.
29. Vermeulen, A., "Androgens in the aging male," *J Clin Endocrinol Metab* 1991; 73(2):221–4.
30. Mehta, P., et al., "The social endocrinology of dominance: basal testosterone predicts cortisol changes and behavior following victory and defeat," *J Pers Soc Psychol* 2008; 94(6):1078–93.
31. Ajayi, A., et al., "Testosterone increases human platelet thromboxane A2 receptor density and aggregation responses," *Circulation* 1995; 91(11):2742–47.
32. Webb, C., et al., "Effects of testosterone on coronary vasomotor regulation in men with coronary heart disease," *Circulation* 1999; 100(16):1690–96.
33. Channer, K., et al., "Cardiovascular effects of testosterone: implications of the 'male menopause?' *Heart* 2003; 89(2):121–22.
34. Yaffe, K., et al., "Sex hormones and cognitive function in older men," *J Am Geriatr Soc* 2002; 50(4):707–12.
35. Thilers, P., et al., "The association between endogenous free testosterone and cognitive performance: a population-based study in 35 to 90 year-old men and women," *Psychoneuroendocrinology* 2006; 31(5):565–76.
36. Güder, G., et al., "Low circulating androgens and mortality risk in heart failure," *Heart* 2010; 96(7):504–09.
37. Torkler, S., et al., "Inverse association between total testosterone concentrations, incident hypertension and blood pressure," *Aging Male* 2011; 14(3):176–82.
38. Hyde, Z., et al., "Low free testosterone predicts mortality from CVD but not other causes: the health in men study," *J Clin Endocriol Metab* 2012; 97(1):179–89.
39. Rizza, R., "Androgen effect on insulin action and glucose metabolism," *Mayo Clin Proc* 2000; 75(Suppl):S61–4.
40. Stellato, R., et al., "Testosterone, sex hormone-binding globulin, and the development of type 2 diabetes in middle-aged men: prospective results from the Massachusetts male aging study," *Diabetes Care* 2000; 23(4):490–94.
41. Ma, R., et al., "Erectile dysfunction predicts coronary heart disease in type 2 diabetes," *J Am Coll Cardiol* 2008; 51(21):2045–50.
42. Oettel, M., et al., "Progesterone: the forgotten hormone in men? *Aging Male* 2004; 7(3):236–57.
43. Gibbs, R., et al., "Estrogen and cognition: applying preclinical findings to clinical perspectives," *J Neurosci Res* 2003; 74(5):637–43.

44. Akwa, Y., et al., "Neurosteroids: biosynthesis, metabolism, and function of pregnenolone and dehydro-epiandrosterone in the brain," *J Steroid Biochem Mol Biol* 1991; 40(1–3):71–81.

45. Havlíková, H., et al., "Sex- and age-related changes in epitestosterone in relation to pregnenolone sulfate and testosterone in normal subjects," *J Clin Endocrinol Metab* 2002; 87(5):2225–31.

46. Labrie, F., et al., "Marked decline in serum concentrations of adrenal C19 sex steroid precursors and conjugated androgen metabolites during aging," *J Clin Endocrinol Metab* 1997; 82(8):2396–402.

47. Mayo, W., et al., "Pregnenolone sulfate and aging of cognitive functions: behavioral, neurochemical, and morphological investigations," *Horm Behav* 2001; 40(2):215–17.

48. Vallée, M., et al., "Role of pregnenolone, dehydroepiandrosterone and their sulfate esters on learning and memory in cognitive aging," *Brain Res Rev* 2001; 37(1–3):301–12.

49. De Bruin, V., et al., "Cortisol and dehydroepiandrosterone sulfate plasma levels and their relationship to gaining, cognitive function, and dementia," *Brain Cogn* 2002; 50(2):316–23.

50. Buffington, C., et al., "Case report: amelioration of insulin resistance in diabetes with dehydroepian-drosterone," *Am J Med Sci* 1993; 306(5):320–24.

51. Villareal, D., et al., "Effect of DHEA on abdominal fat and insulin action in elderly women and men: a randomized controlled trial," *JAMA* 2004; 292(18):2243–48.

52. Watson, R., et al., "Dehydroepiandrosterone and diseases of aging," *Drugs Aging* 1996; 9(4):274–91.

53. Yamaguchi, Y., et al., "Reduced serum dehydroepiandrosterone levels in diabetic patients with hyperin-sulinaemia," *Clin Endocrinol (Oxf)* 1998; 49(3):377–83.

54. Barrett-Conner, E., et al., "A prospective study of dehydroepiandrosterone sulfate, mortality, and cardiovascular disease," *N Engl J Med* 1986; 315(24):1519–24.

55. Carlson, L., et al., "Relationships among cortisol (CRT), dehydroepiandrosterone-sulfate (DHEAS), and memory in a longitudinal study of healthy elderly men and women," *Neurobiol Aging* 1999; 20(3):315–24.

56. Whitworth, J., et al., "Cardiovascular consequences of cortisol excess," *Vasc Health Risk Manag* 2005; 1(4):291–99.

57. Kelly, J., et al., "Cortisol and hypertension," *Clin Exp Pharmacol Physiol* 1998; 25(S1):S51–6.

58. Hamer, M., et al., Cortisol responses to mental stress and incident hypertension in healthy men and women," *J Clin Endocrinol Metab* 2012; 97(1):E29–E34.

59. Hamer, M., et al., "Cortisol responses to mental stress and the progression of coronary artery calcification in healthy men and women," *PLOS ONE* 2012; 7(2):e31356.

60. Hewagalamulage, S., et al., "Stress, cortisol, and obesity: a role for cortisol responsiveness in identifying individuals prone to obesity," *Domest Anim Endocrinol* 2016; 56(Suppl):S112–20.

61. Rosmond, R., et al., "The hypothalamic-pituitary-adrenal axis activity as a predictor of cardiovascular disease, type 2 diabetes and stroke," *J Inter Med* 2000; 247(2):188–97.

62. Krajnak, K., "Potential contribution of work-related psychosocial stress to the development of cardiovascular disease and type II diabetes: a brief review," *Environ Health Insights* 2014; 8(Suppl 1):41–5.

63. Nijm, J., et al., "Inflammation and cortisol response in coronary artery disease," *Ann Med* 2009; 41(3):224–33.

64. Jonasson, L., et al., "Stress-induced release of the S100A8/A9 alarmin is elevated in coronary artery disease patients with impaired cortisol response,". *Sci Rep* 2017; 7(1):17545.

65. Fantidis, P., et al., "Morning cortisol production in coronary heart disease patients," *Eur J Clin Invest* 2002; 32(5):304–08.

66. Ronaldson, A., et al., "Diurnal cortisol rhythm is associated with adverse cardiac events and mortality in coronary artery bypass patients," *J Clin Endocrinol Metab* 2015; 100(10):3676–82.

67. Elenkov, I., "Systemic stress-induced Th2 shift and its clinical implications," *Int Rev Neurobiol* 2002; 52:163–86.

68. Cohen, S., "Psychological stress and susceptibility to upper respiratory infections," *Am J Respir Crit Care Med* 1995; 152(4 Pt.2):S53–8.

69. Kunz-Ebrecht, S., et al., "Cortisol responses to mild psychological stress are inversely associated with proinflammatory cytokines," *Brain Behav Immun* 2003; 17(5):373–83.

70. Ohlin, B., et al., "Chronic psychosocial stress predicts long-term cardiovascular morbidity and mortality in middle-aged men," *Eur Heart J* 2004; 25(10):867–73.

71. Yehuda, R., et al., "Circadian rhythm of salivary cortisol in holocaust survivors with and without PTSD," *Am J Psychiatr* 2005; 162(5):998–1000.

72. Glynn, C., et al., "Biochemical changes associated with intractable pain," *Br Med J* 1978; 1(6108):280–81.

73. Moore, R., et al., "Increased cortisol excretion in chronic pain," *Anaesthesia* 1983; 38(8):788–91.

74. Nakagawa, H., et al., "Study of the stress response to acute pain in the awake human," *Pain Clin* 1994; 7:317–24.

75. Shenkin, H., "The effect of pain on the diurnal pattern of plasma corticoid levels," *Neurology* 1964; 14:1112–17.

76. Straub, R., et al., "Involvement of the hypothalamic–pituitary–adrenal/gonadal axis and the peripheral nervous system in rheumatoid arthritis: viewpoint based on a systemic pathogenetic role," *Arthritis Rheum* 2001; 44(3):493–507.

77. Tennant, F., "Intractable pain is a severe stress state associated with hypercortisolemia and reduced adrenal reserve," *Drug Alcohol Depend* 2000; 60(Suppl 1):220–21.

78. Griep, E., et al., "Function of the hypothalamic–pituitary–adrenal axis in patients with fibromyalgia and low back pain," *J Rheumatol* 1998; 25(7):1374–81.

79. Ibid., Tennant, 2000.

80. Cutolo, M., et al., "Hypothalamic–pituitary–adrenocortical axis function in premenopausal women with rheumatoid arthritis not treated with glucocorticoids," *J Rheumatol* 1999; 26:282–88.

81. Chrousos, G., "The hypothalamic–pituitary–adrenal axis and immune-mediated inflammation," *N Engl J Med* 1995; 332(20):1351–62.

82. Bateman, A., et al., "The immune–hypothalamic–pituitary-adrenal axis," *Endocr Rev* 1989; 10(1):92–112.

83. McEwen, B., et al., "The role of adrenocorticoids as modulators of immune function in health and disease: neural, endocrine and immune interactions," *Brain Res Rev* 1997; 23(1–2):79–133.

84. McEwen, B., et al., "Adrenal steroid receptors and actions in the nervous system," *Physiol Rev* 1986; 66(4):1121–88.

85. Fischer, L., et al., "The protective role of testosterone in the development of temporomandibular joint pain," *J Pain* 2007; 8(5):437–42.

86. Guth, L., et al., "Key role for pregnenolone in combination therapy that promotes recovery after spinal cord injury," *Proc Natl Acad Sci U S A* 1994; 91(25):12308–12.

87. Harbuz, M., et al., "A protective role for testosterone in adjuvant-induced arthritis," *Br J Rheumatol* 1995; 34(12):1117–22.

88. Ørstavil, K., et al., "Pain and small-fiber neuropathy in patients with hypothyroidism," *Neurology* 2006; 67(5):786–91.

89. Ren, K., et al., "Progesterone attenuates persistent inflammatory hyperalgesia in female rats: involvement of spinal NMDA receptor mechanisms," *Brain Res* 2000; 865(2):272–77.

90. Stafford, E., et al., "Gonadal hormone modulation of mu, kappa, and, delta opioid antinociception in male and female rats," *J Pain* 2006; 6:261–74.

91. Leonelli, E., et al., "Progesterone and its derivatives are neuroprotective agents in experimental diabetic neuropathy: a multimodal analysis," *Neuroscience* 2007; 144(4):1293–304.

92. Mensah-Nyagan, A., et al., "Evidence for a key role of steroids in the modulation of pain," *Psychoneuroendocrinology* 2009; 34(Suppl 1):S169–77.

93. Aloisi, A., et al., "Testosterone affects pain-related responses differently in male and female rats," *Neurosci Lett* 2004; 361(1–3):262–64.

94. Aloisi, A., et al., "Sex hormones, central nervous system and pain," *Horm Behav* 2006; 50(1):1–7.

95. Dawson-Basoa, M., et al., "Estrogen and progesterone activate spinal kappa-opiate receptor analgesic mechanisms," *Pain* 1996; 64(3):608–15.

96. Ceccon, M., et al., "Distinct effect of pregnenolone sulfate on NMDA receptor subtypes," *Neuropharmacology* 2001; 40(4):491–500.

97. Jones, K., "Gonadal steroids and neuronal regeneration: a therapeutic role," *Adv Neurol* 1993; 59:227–40.

98. Kimonides, V., et al., "Dehydroepiandrosterone (DHEA) and DHEA-sulfate (DHEAS) protect hippocampal neurons against excitatory amino acid-induced neurotoxicity," *Proc Natl Acad Sci USA* 1998; 95(4):1852–57.

99. McMahon, M., et al., "Effects of glucocorticoids on carbohydrate metabolism," *Diabetes Metab Rev* 1988; 4(1):17–30.

100. Munck, A., et al., "Physiological functions of glucocorticoids in stress and their relation to pharmacological actions," *Endocr Rev* 1984; 5(1):25–44.

101. Schlechte, J., et al., "Decreased glucocorticoid receptor binding in adrenal insufficiency," *J Clin Endocrinol Metab* 1982; 54(1):145–49.

102. Wiegers, G., et al., "Induction of cytokine receptors by glucocorticoids: functional and pathological significance," *Trends Pharmacol Sci* 1998; 19(8):317–21.

103. Barnes, P., "Anti-inflammatory actions of glucocorticoids: molecular mechanisms," *Clin Sci (Lond)* 1998; 94(6):557–72.

104. Horner, H., et al., "Glucocorticoids inhibit glucose transport in cultured hippocampal neurons and glia," *Neuroendocrinology* 1990; 52(1):57–63.

105. Penza, P., et al., "Painful neuropathy in subclinical hypothyroidism: clinical and neuropathological recovery after hormone replacement therapy," *Neurol Sci* 2009; 30(2):149–51.

106. Amandusson, A., A. Blomqvist, "Estrogenic influences in pain processing," *Front Neuroendocrinol* 2013; 34(4):329–49.

107. Gupta, A., et al., "Sex-based differences in brain alterations across chronic pain conditions," *J Neurosci Res* 2017; 95(1–2):604–16.

108. Craft, R., "Modulation of pain by estrogens," *Pain* 2007; 132(Suppl 1):S3–S12.

109. Vincent, K., I. Tracey, "Sex hormones and pain: the evidence from functional imaging," *Curr Pain Headache Rep* 2010; 14(5):396–403.

110. Shivers, K., et al., "Estrogen alters baseline and inflammatory-induced cytokine levels independent from hypothalamic-pituitary-adrenal axis activity," *Cytokine* 2015; 72(2):121–29.

111. Hau, M., et al., "Testosterone reduces responsiveness to nociceptive stimuli in a wild bird.," *Horm Behav* 2004; 46(2):165–70.

112. Pednekar, J., et al., " Role of testosterone on pain threshold in rats," *Indian J Physiol Pharmacol* 1995; 39(4):423–24.

113. Stoffel, E., et al., "Gonadal hormone modulation of mu, kappa, and delta opioid antinociception in male and female rats," *J Pain* 2005; 6(4):261–74.

114. Tennant, F., et al., "Testosterone replacement in chronic pain patients," *Prac Pain Manag* 2010; 10(6):12–5.

115. White, H., et al., "A novel use for testosterone to treat central sensitization of chronic pain in fibromyalgia patients," *Int Immunopharmacol* 2015; 27(2):244–48.

116. Aloisi, A., et al., "Chronic pain therapy and hypothalamic-pituitary-adrenal axis impairment," *Psychoneuroendocrinology* 2011; 36(7):1032–39.

117. Abs, R., et al., "Endocrine consequences of long-term intrathecal administration of opioids," *J Clin Endocrinol Metab* 2000; 85(6):2215–22.

118. Daniell, H., "Hypogonadism in men consuming sustained-action oral opioids," *J Pain* 2002; 3(5):377–84.

119. Daniell, H., "Opioid endocrinopathy in women consuming prescribed sustained-action opioids for control of nonmalignant pain," *J Pain* 2008; 9(1):28–36.

120. Vuong, C., et al., "The effects of opioids and opioid analogs on animal and human endocrine systems," *Endocr Rev* 2010; 31(1):98–132.

121. Tennant, F., "Hormone therapies: newest advance in pain care,"*Pract Pain Manag* 2011; 11:98–105.

122. Tennant, F., "Complications of uncontrolled, persistent pain," *Pract Pain Manag* 2004; 4(1):11–4.

123. Tennant, F., "Hormone abnormalities in patients with severe and chronic pain who fail standard treatments," *Postgrad Med* 2015; 127(1):1–4.

124. Khorami, S., et al., "Effect of chronic osteoarthritis pain on neuroendocrine function in men," J *Clin Endocrinol Metab* 2006; 91(11):4313–18.

125. Tennant, F., et al., "Normalization of serum cortisol concentration with opioid treatment of severe chronic pain," *Pain Med* 2002; 3(2):132–34.

126. Tennant, F., "How to use adrenocorticotropin as a biomarker in pain management," *Pract Pain Manag* 2012; 12:62–6.

127. Ibid., Tennant, 2000.

128. Hannibal, K., et al., "Chronic stress, cortisol dysfunction, and pain: a psychoneuroendocrine rationale for stress management in pain rehabilitation," *Phys Ther* 2014; 94(12):1816–25.

129. Brydon, L., et al., "Synergistic effects of psychological and immune stressors on inflammatory cytokine and sickness responses in humans," *Brain Behav Immun* 2009; 23(2):217–24.

130. Colloca, L., et al., "Nocebo hyperalgesia: how anxiety is turned into pain," *Curr Opin Anaesthesiol* 2007; 20(5):435–39.

131. Fries, E., et al., "A new view on hypocortisolism," *Psychoneuroendocrinology* 2005; 30(10):1010–16.

132. Jankord, R., et al., "Limbic regulation of hypothalamo-pituitary-adrenocortical function during acute and chronic stress," *Ann NY Acad Sci* 2008; 1148:64–73.

133. Tsigos, C., et al., "Hypothalamic-pituitary-adrenal axis, neuroendocrine factors and stress," *J Psychosom Res* 2002; 53(4):865–71.

134. Nieman, L., et al., "The diagnosis of cushing syndrome: an endocrine society clinical practice guideline," *J Clin Endocrinol Metab* 2008; 93(5):1526–40.

135. Roberts, L., et al., "Sex hormone suppression by intrathecal opioids: a prospective study," *Clin J Pain* 2002; 18(3):144–48.
136. Finch, P., et al., "Hypogonadism in patients treated with intrathecal morphine," *Clin J Pain* 2000; 16(3):251–54.
137. Daniell, H., "DHEA deficiency during consumption of sustained-action prescribed opioids: evidence for opioid-induced inhibition of adrenal androgen production," *J Pain* 2006; 7(12):901–07.
138. Arnaldi, G., et al., "Diagnosis and complications of cushing syndrome: a consensus statement," *J Clin Endocrinol Metab* 2003; 88(12):5593–602.
139. Bawor, M., et al., "Testosterone suppression in opioid users: a systematic review and meta-analysis," *Drug Alcohol Depend* 2015; 149:1–9.

6 Managing Pain in the Presence of Autoimmune Disease

David Bilstrom

CONTENTS

One of the leading causes of death in female children and women in all age groups up to 65 years of age is autoimmune disease (AD).[1] $100 billion per year is spent in the U.S. for AD-related care compared with $50 billion for all cancer care.[1] Only $591 million is spent by the NIH on AD research compared to $6.1 billion spent on cancer research.[1] The number-one most popular health topic requested by callers to the National Women's Health Information Center is AD.[1]

ADs have classically been considered as multiple different disease states. However, AD could also be considered as one disease that can affect different body parts in different people. The term "polyautoimmunity" has been put forward to better describe this idea. This also helps to describe why, once a person is diagnosed with one AD, they are much more likely to be diagnosed with another AD or multiple ADs.

AD can present with many symptoms when the autoimmune process becomes active. Pain is a symptom that is extremely common in people with an AD and has a huge impact on quality of life. The medications that are typically used to combat AD and the associated pain may potentially contribute to worsening within the very organ systems contributing to the AD in the first place.[2-5]

Joint pain can be a primary symptom in many ADs such as rheumatoid arthritis and sacroiliitis. Because of the specificity in the body part attacked, antibodies can also attack voltage-gated potassium channels (VGKC).[6] The attack on VGKC can cause a broad spectrum of neuronal hypersensitivity disorders. Pain may present in isolation or in association with other neurologic signs such as muscle cramps and twitching which can be regional or diffuse or even seizures.[6]

In Hashimoto's thyroiditis, thyroid dysfunction can present with multiple signs and/or symptoms. As such, it has been referred to as "The Great Mimicker."

Moreover, the biochemical and physiologic changes in the body that cause AD are the same changes that can lead to pain conditions that are not specifically AD pain. Fibromyalgia (FM) is not an AD, but a large percentage of people with an AD also have FM.[7] Whereas 1–2% of the U.S. overall has FM, 20% of people with rheumatoid arthritis have FM.[7] These changes in the body causing the AD also cause the FM-related pain.

In order to optimally treat the pain in someone with an AD, a better understanding of why the body starts to attack itself is required.

ETIOLOGY OF AD AND IMMUNE SYSTEM DYSREGULATION

GENETICS AND TERRAIN PLUS ENVIRONMENTAL TRIGGERS

So how does a person develop an AD and the pain that goes with it? There appears to be some very specific circumstances that must occur in order to start the autoimmune process (Figure 6.1).

Genetics: We used to think that genes were hard wired and destined to be expressed. However, we have a much better understanding now of epigenetics and the effect of environment on genes being turned on or off. The Human Genome Project sought to sequence our genes, and with this information it was thought that all disease could be reversed or prevented by simply altering "bad genes." However, after 10 years and nearly $3 billion, results thus far have found a few very rare genetic diseases (involving 50 to 100 people in the world) that could be totally reversed using this information.[8] More important in the reversal of chronic disease is optimizing gene expression: turning on "good" genes and off "bad" genes. Seven to 8% of the human genome is consistent with viral DNA.[9,10] Pieces of viral DNA have slowly but surely been incorporated into the human genome over time. The bulk of these were integrated during primate evolution. Subsequent mutations in these sequences have rendered older insertions nonfunctional, but some of the younger and more intact sequences have been linked to disease.[11] These genes need to be shut down, as otherwise proteins will be produced that would make us sick. Many bad genes that need to be turned off are on the "X" chromosome.[12] Because women have two copies and men only have one, this appears to be one of the reasons why women acquire more ADs than men.[12] A close genetic relationship appears to exist among AD, explaining the clustering in individuals and families as well as a common pathway of disease.[1]

Terrain: The "terrain" in our bodies includes things like how we are eating, sleeping, exercising, and managing stress. How are our vitamin levels and mineral levels? How healthy is our gastrointestinal tract? Do we have chronic infections? Are we carrying a lot of environmental toxins or

Genetics + Terrain ➔ Environmental Triggers

FIGURE 6.1 Environmental triggers.

internally generated toxic byproducts of metabolism because we can't clear them effectively? How is the overall hormone balance?

I like to think of terrain like a backyard swimming pool and, ideally, a backyard swimming pool should have crystal clear water. On the other hand, that same backyard swimming pool could be covered in thick algae.

Environmental triggers: Once genetics come into play and the terrain is altered, the immune system has the potential to become dysfunctional enough to create an AD. All that now needs to occur to begin the AD is an environmental trigger. It is very challenging to be a human being as something always seems to be happening that is trying to derail us. We may not have slept well the night before. We caught the flu. A woman gives birth to her third child after a difficult pregnancy or delivery. You were in a car accident. You have just had a surgery. Someone you loved has just died. You got very sick on a trip out of the country. A lot of stress was happening at work or at home over a prolonged period of time. At times, people can tell you exactly what started the whole process that eventually led to a diagnosis of an AD. "I have never felt well since _____." The blank can be filled by "the birth of my third child," "that car accident," "the death of my mother," "since I got travelers' diarrhea on that trip," "since all that stress surrounding my divorce," etc.

LOSING THE IMMUNE SYSTEM SET POINT

The immune system. Not upregulated. Not downregulated. But both at the same time.

So how does the immune system become so disrupted that a person develops an AD? The immune system is a great example of how the body loves balance. In most areas, you don't want to be too high or too low. There is a "sweet spot" or "set point" right in the middle (Figure 6.2).[13] Having a low iron level is bad just as having too much iron is bad also. Having two little estradiol is bad but so is too much estradiol. When a person loses the immune system "set point," their system starts to become both upregulated and downregulated at the same time. Upregulated immune system issues include allergies, asthma, and all the ADs. Downregulated immune system issues include colds, flus, infections, recurrent infections, and cancer.[13] As time marches on, they develop new immune system issues on top of the old ones. This is why, when a person develops one AD, they are more likely to get a second, third, fourth, or fifth.[14]

Oftentimes, when someone is diagnosed with AD, they are offered medications that try to suppress the overactive or upregulated aspect of the immune system dysregulation. They try and push the immune system down. Thus, the person is told "oh, by the way, these medications will increase your chance of getting cancer or an infection that could kill you."[5,15] Now, if a person knows that the immune system dysregulation has already caused not only an AD but an increased risk of cancer and infections, they may say "this doesn't seem quite right." And our immune system agrees. Our immune system doesn't really want suppression. What it really wants is immune system rebalancing and immune system modulation.

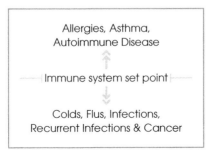

FIGURE 6.2 Immune set point.

Now, there is nothing wrong with using these medications. What is wrong, is thinking that these medications actually fix the problem. What is wrong is thinking that these meds are the only options to treat AD. Only use DMARDs or biologics. Only use NSAIDs. Only use opioids. Only use a combination of all these for ADs. Yes, the DMARDs, biologics, and NSAIDs may protect against tissue damage and changes seen on X-rays. Or, opioids may help patients get out of bed in the morning. But at what cost when they are the only options offered? What is wrong is thinking that the risk/reward profiles of these meds are so much better than other options that even the thought of using other options is nonsensical. (See Case Study 2 for more details.) By the time someone has finally been diagnosed with an AD, their functional abilities and quality of life are oftentimes profoundly compromised. Something has to be done as quickly as possible to help them. These medications can potentially provide this help. But what they really should be doing is buying time to go back and do our due diligence in finding out why this person has developed the AD in the first place. Address the causes identified through testing and allow them to feel even better than they did on the medications alone. Eventually, they could potentially be in a position to not need these medications or use at much lower doses and minimize any side effect potential. Or, given the long history of immune system dysregulation and events that negatively impact the immune system beginning years and decades before the actual diagnosis of an AD, can we not address the problem before these meds are even needed? The Case Studies 1–3 will highlight this.

The unfortunate story of one of rock and roll's greatest icons from the 1970s can illustrate this point. Glenn Frey of the Eagles was diagnosed with rheumatoid arthritis. He used the medications typically used for almost 20 years. When he died in January 2017, did he die from rheumatoid arthritis? No! He died from the "sudden" development of a second AD, ulcerative colitis, and an infection, pneumonia, that no amount of antibiotics could successfully treat.[16] By having a dysregulated immune system and then only using the typical medications that simply suppress the immune system, he was always more likely to get an infection, including an infection that no amount of antibiotics could treat. By not actually rebalancing the immune system, he was more likely to get a second AD on top of his first one. There are also thousands of documented occurrences of these type of medications actually causing a new AD to develop as a side effect.[13,17]

The immune system dysregulation can start very early in life and then only show up decades later as pain and AD. Or it can be so severe that a person develops pain and AD even as a young child. The classic scenario might go as follows. Eczema present since birth. An infection with first antibiotic use at less than one year of age. Recurrent ear infections, sinus infections, or strep throats as a child. Development of allergies or asthma as a child or teenager. Mononucleosis, an Epstein–Barr virus infection, in high school. Or any number of other infections that a young person can get. Already this person's immune system is showing the loss of the set point early in life. Then this disruption just keeps rolling along as the years go by, eventually causing pain and AD.

So, what causes the immune system to lose its set point and move away, both up and down, at the same time? Vitamin deficiencies, hormone deficiencies or imbalances, toxicity, toxic stress, chronic infections, and the gut (Figure 6.3).[18–23] The gut is possibly the central mechanism. When the gut is not functioning

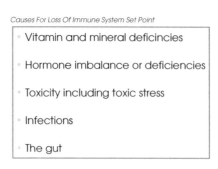

FIGURE 6.3   Causes for loss of immune system set point.

properly, we cannot digest and absorb nutrients from the food we eat, so we develop vitamin and mineral deficiencies. Furthermore, hormone balance can be altered as many hormones undergo enterohepatic circulation.[22] The gut produces important hormones that can impact pain such as melatonin.[24] Low levels of melatonin have been linked to many pain conditions including FM, and endometriosis-related chronic pelvic pain as well as tension, cluster, and migraine headaches.[25] Furthermore, toxic burden can increase when gut function is altered, and there is a major detoxifying pathway in the liver also.[26] This includes environmental toxins as well as toxins produced every day by our own cells as toxic byproducts of metabolism. And when the gut gets thrown off, this will directly affect the immune system because 80% of our immune system actually surrounds the gut.[27] A dysfunctional immune system cannot keep problematic microorganisms out of our bodies, and we develop chronic infections.

Knowing what causes the immune system dysregulation makes it easy then to know what tests to run in order to get the information we need to optimally treat the person with pain and AD. This is because much, if not all, of the pain is being driven by the same exact processes which caused the AD (Figure 6.4).

DIAGNOSTIC TESTING

BLOODWORK

In an effort to delineate the root cause of AD, these initial serology assessments are recommended as outlined in Tables 6.1–6.4.

Nutrients: We want to look very closely at some vitamin and mineral levels. There are tests out there that can look at levels of 80 to 100 different important nutrients. It is quite reasonable though, to test for a few that can typically be done in any hospital or traditional lab. What I tell patients is, "as your gut

```
Tests To Be Run

Always:
    Blood work
    Saliva cortisol
    Digestive stool analysis
    Provocative heavy metal
Usually:
    Food sensitivity test
```

FIGURE 6.4 Diagnostic testing.

TABLE 6.1
Initial Blood Work: Men and Women (Fasting)

General Serology	
CBC	TSH
Chem package	Free T4
Insulin	Free T3
Ferritin	Reverse T3
RBC magnesium	TPO antibodies
RBC zinc	COQ10
Vitamin D (25-OH)	Thyroglobulin antibodies
Homocysteine	DHEA-S
B12	IGF-1
TTG abs	Gliadin abs
Sex hormone binding globulin (SHBG)	

TABLE 6.2

Testing for Systemic Infections

Initial Blood Work: Men and Women (Fasting)

EBV (Epstein–Barr virus)

Lyme antibodies IgG, IgM

Chlamydia (serum) IgG, IgM

Mycoplasma IgG, IgM

Babesia microti antibodies IgG, IgM

Bartonella IgG, IgM

Ehrlichia IgG, IgM

Herpes virus 6 IgG, IgM

Strep pneumonia 23 IgG

Coxsackic virus IgG, IgM

TABLE 6.3

Women Only

Initial Blood Work Women Only: In Addition to Blood Work for Both Sexes

Note: these always need to be run on day 19–21 of the menstrual cycle.

Day 1: first day of menstrual flow

These may be run with initial blood work if convenient or at a later date if menstrual-related issues/sex hormone issues don't clear spontaneously with your interventions.

Estradiol (E2)	TT (total testosterone)
Estrone (E1)	Free T (free testosterone)
Progesterone	DHT (dihydrotestosterone)

TABLE 6.4

Men Only

Initial Blood Work Men Only: In Addition to Blood Work for Both Sexes

TT (total testosterone)

Free T (free testosterone)

DHT (dihydrotestosterone)

Estradiol

health improves and you get better at digesting and absorbing nutrients from the food you eat, you will fix most of these nutritional deficiencies all by yourself." The body is so smart. We don't have to go chasing everything. We just take care of the "biggest fish to fry." The body will take care of the rest all by itself.

Hormones: It is so important, when it comes to hormones, to look at the big picture. A thorough overview is needed of many hormones, all done at the same time. You can think of the hormones like a big symphony orchestra. In a symphony orchestra, all the players individually are very important. But what might be more important is how they are all working together. All it takes is one player to be off and that throws the whole orchestra off. The same is true with hormones. Each hormone is very important. But what might be more important is how they are all working together. All it takes is for one hormone to be off and it throws off all the other hormones. Thus, whenever you see one hormone off, you should wonder about all the others.

If the symphony is off, it needs to be fixed. But you can't just look at the woodwind section and figure out what is going on. You need to look at the whole orchestra at the same time. Then you can say "oh, now I see who is throwing off everybody else." Within this symphony of hormones is a very tight triad (Figure 6.5): cortisol, thyroid, and insulin/blood sugar. Just like any triangle in space, you change one angle and it will change the other two. This is one reason why finding insulin and blood sugar to be off, at least a little bit if not a lot, is so common in AD patients with chronic pain.[28] Cortisol and thyroid are almost always off and create problems with blood sugar control.[20,21]

Chronic infections: These are very common drivers of AD and the related chronic pain.[13,18] As stated earlier, with a dysfunctional immune system, downregulated immune system issues develop at the same time as the upregulated issues. Downregulated immune system issues include colds, flus, infections, recurrent infections, and cancer. More data are accumulating on the role of chronic infections driving chronic disease. An example is an article that came out in 2015. This discussed a new bad microorganism found in the oropharynx of people with schizophrenia but not in healthy controls. The oropharynx microbiome difference between patients and controls could be used to predict who would have the disease.[29]

Now, this should really not have surprised anyone given that we know "the gut is the second brain." What goes on in our gut has such a profound impact on the brain as well as the body as a whole. Most people don't think about this aspect of the gut in regard to the brain though. The gut is really just one long tube though, from the sinuses and mouth all the way down to our rectum. We already know what happens with chronic infections in the large intestine, and in the small intestine with small intestine bacterial overgrowth (SIBO), as well as infections of the stomach like *H. pylori*, bad bugs in our mouths driving gingivitis and increased risk of cardiovascular disease,[30] chronic fungal infections of the sinuses that drive headache pain,[31] and recurrent supra-infections involving bacteria. These bacterial supra-infections of the sinuses occur over and over, with the antibiotics used that disrupt gut function more and more each time. The underlying fungal infection keeps the environment disrupted, and the chronic sinusitis continues between antibiotic courses. Unfortunately, many people end up getting sinus surgery. But because the fungal infection is still present, the sinus symptoms continue. And perhaps they end up having a second sinus surgery, never being able to clear the pain, fullness, post-nasal drip. It is also amazing how often people will test positive for tick-borne illnesses even though they supposedly don't live in an area where "these things occur." These tick-borne illnesses are classic drivers of chronic pain and multi-organ system symptoms and are becoming more and more common.[32]

Testing for celiac disease (CD) always needs to be done. There is an increased risk of CD when a person already has the ADs type 1 diabetes (T1DM), rheumatoid arthritis, Hashimoto's thyroiditis, autoimmune hepatitis, and Sjogren's. When a person has untreated CD, painful conditions can develop (e.g., headaches, migraine headaches, joint pain/arthritis, peripheral neuropathy, and bone fractures). The untreated CD can also cause painful ADs such as T1DM, multiple sclerosis (MS), and dermatitis herpetiformis.[33,34] Only 20% of all people with CD are ever diagnosed. This

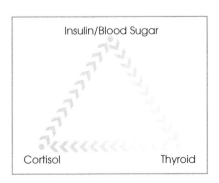

FIGURE 6.5 Insulin-blood sugar cortisol thyroid.

is because only 20% of people have significant GI symptoms, that is, classic CD, while 80% have minimal or no GI symptoms, thus, atypical CD.[33,35]

All the testing done will help us understand why a person has developed their pain and AD, but it will also help show us where the person is going in the future. If they are moving towards something like celiac disease or diabetes, we want to know so we can try and turn them around before they get there. Both TPO and thyroglobulin antibodies need to be checked in all people with an AD to see if they are developing an autoimmune process involving the thyroid (e.g., a true Hashimoto's thyroiditis) or just starting with an early autoimmune thyroiditis.

BLOODWORK: INTERPRETATION

On every blood test report there are three columns. The column on the left-hand side of the page is the name of the test run. The middle column is the specific results for the patient. And on the right side is the reference range. This may also be listed as a "normal range." The reference range is usually treated as the "ideal" range by most practitioners. Patients are often told, "your results are in the reference range. You are good. You are fine. You are healthy. Don't worry." Often times the patient may say "I feel pretty crummy for someone whose labs say they are healthy. What's the deal?" Well, the deal is, the reference range is not where the healthy people are, even though it is usually treated that way. This is why we need to write down for the patient where the healthy people are. If their result is not where the healthy people are, then we will wonder, "if we get them to where the healthy people are, will they feel like a healthy person again?"

So, what makes this so confusing for both patients and doctors? Well, the reference range is not based on where the healthy people are. Instead, it is based on statistics. Testing labs get a lot of different results from all the different people they run any one test on. The distribution of the results looks like a bell-shaped curve (Figure 6.6).

On the left is the lower end of the range and on the right is the higher end. Most results though are in the middle. If we were to test the height of 100 different people, some people would be quite short and some would be quite tall; however most people would be in the middle. Similarly, some people are quite thin while others are quite heavy. But most people are in the middle. The same is true with a grading curve in school. So, the testing labs say "how can we come up with some kind of reference range for reporting lab results? We know! We will use statistics!" And very arbitrarily, the labs say that two standard deviations of the mean will be the reference range we will put on this piece of paper. By definition, 95 out of every 100 results fall within two standard deviations of the mean. That is just the definition of two standard deviations from the mean. It doesn't matter who is being tested. A bunch of sick people. A bunch of healthy people. A bunch of baboons. It is just statistics.

But labs typically tend to test people who aren't feeling so well. So, people tend to get compared to people who don't feel well, when they really want to know "so where am I compared with healthy people? How about those people who climb Mount Everest? Or astronauts? Where are they? I wouldn't mind being where they are." So, if a person ever gets flagged on a specific blood test

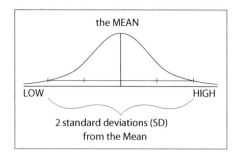

FIGURE 6.6   Standard deviations.

result as being either high or low, they can pretty much say right away that they are one of the 5 worst out of 100. They have gotten a grade of an "F" on this test. If they are not flagged, then they say "oh, I know how this works now. If I am not flagged on this test, it just means that I am not one of the 5 worst out of 100. I am not an 'F'. But what I am left with is that I am somewhere between a D– and an A+." This is a very broad range. A grade of a C or a D is not an F, but it is definitely not an A either. A person wants to be in the A range. This is where human biochemistry and physiology work the best.

So how do we know where the "A" range is for the tests we run? Hundreds if not thousands of studies, some actually done on astronauts and people who have climbed Mount Everest, have told us where the human body needs to be to perform at its highest levels. This is the physiologic range, not the statistical range. As part of this chapter, you will see tables with the ideal ranges for all the tests commonly run (Tables 6.5, 6.6, 6.7). These numbers are always changing as more and more data come out. By the time this book is published, there may need to be some subtle modifications of these ideal numbers. The rule of thumb tends to be, though, that if something is good for us, we want to be in the high end of the range. If it is not good for us, it tends to mean we need to be in the lower end of the range.

This is also why you will see different reference ranges being used by different labs. You can tell a lot about the particular population being tested by a certain lab company by the reference ranges produced. A fasting blood sugar range of 70 to 100 mg/dL is a lot different than one that goes up to 110 mg/dL. The people in the latter community tend to have far higher fasting blood sugar than the

TABLE 6.5
Ideal Physiology Ranges

Ideal Physiological Ranges of Commonly Run Lab Tests (Fasting)

Test	Ideal Range	Usual Reference Range
Blood sugar	Low 70s	70–100 mg/dL
	Always ≤84	
Insulin	4–6	4–10 uU/mL
Ferritin	~100	20–140 ng/mL
RBC mag	6.0–6.4	4.0–6.4 mg/dL
RBC zinc	~1200	900–1500 mg/L
CoQ10	1.6	0.40–1.6 mg/L
Vitamin D	70–80	20–100 ng/mL
Homocysteine	5–7	0.0–15.0 umol/L
B12	≥800–900	200–900 pg/mL
TSH	<2.0	0.4–5.0 uIU/mL
Free T4	>1.0	0.7–1.8 ng/dL
Free T3	≥3.5	2.2–4.2 pg/mL
	≥4.2 very young children	
	≥4.0 young children	
Reverse T3	8–10	8–25 ng/dL
TPO AB	0	0–25 IU/mL
Thyroglobulin AB	0	<1 IU/mL
DHEA-S	>150 women	29.4–220.5 ug/dL
	>350 men	48.9–344.2 ug/dL
IGF-1	>195	68–247 ng/mL
SHBG	~30	10–80 nmol/L
All infections	Negative	Negative

TABLE 6.6
Ideal Physiological Ranges: Women Only

Ideal Physiological Ranges of Commonly Run Lab Tests for Women (Fasting)

Test	Ideal Range	Usual Reference Range
Estradiol (E2)	80–100	12.0–450.0 pg/mL
Estrone (E1)	~30	54–179 pg/mL
Progesterone	≥5–10	0.0–0.73 ng/mL
TT (total testosterone)	40–60	14.0–76.0 ng/dL
Free T (free testosterone)	3–9	0.10–6.40 ng/dL
DHT (dihydrotestosterone)	<5	4–22 ng/dL

TABLE 6.7
Ideal Physiological Ranges: Men Only

Ideal Physiological Ranges of Commonly Run Lab Tests for Men (Fasting)

Test	Ideal Range	Usual Reference Range
TT (total testosterone)	800–1100	200–1100 ng/dL
Free T (free testosterone)	200–300	4.60–22.40 ng/dL
Estradiol	20–40	10.0–40.0 pg/mL
DHT (dihydrotestosterone)	35–85	30.0–85.0 ng/dL

other population. The same is true for a lab with a vitamin D range of 10 to 50 ng/mL compared with a 20 to 80 ng/mL range.

BLOOD WORK: TREATMENT

Red blood cell (RBC) magnesium: Magnesium malate is preferred for muscle-related pain. Magnesium glycinate is preferred if muscle involvement is not a primary component of the patient's symptoms but they have other symptoms of magnesium deficiency such as anxiety, insomnia, constipation, and blood sugar issues.[36] However, proper caution in magnesium use should be taken in patients with cardiac or kidney dysfunction.

RBC zinc: Tissue cannot heal without zinc.[37] RBC zinc levels that are too high without zinc supplementation suggest an inability to clear toxic elements from the body in general.

Ferritin. Ferritin levels being too high without iron supplementation also suggest an inability to clear toxic elements from the body in general. If ferritin levels are low, oxygen cannot be carried to the tissues in our bodies.[38] If the level is actually so low that it is out of the reference range, try and use IV iron once a week for 2 weeks to more quickly fix this deficiency. It can be frustratingly slow to fix low ferritin using oral supplementation. Many insurance plans will cover IV iron infusions when ferritin levels are below the range.

CoQ10: The major source of CoQ10 is biosynthesis.[39] Making CoQ10 is very labor-intensive. So, when a person is not doing well, they tend to not be able to make adequate amounts of CoQ10. CoQ10 is a fuel for the mitochondria, needed to make ATP and power up cells. The muscles, brain, thyroid, heart, and intestines normally contain much of the body's CoQ10 as they require so much ATP to function.[39] Significant issues in these tissues, or overall fatigue in general, may suggest a need to begin supplementing with CoQ10 sooner than later. That being said, many people will start to make more CoQ10 on their own as their bodies heal and may not need supplementation long-term. However it has been said that most people over the age of 40 will have a difficult time making adequate CoQ10 to "power up the body."

Homocysteine: This tends to indicate B vitamin status.[40,41] When homocysteine is high, B vitamin levels are low. Levels can be impacted by other issues as well such as kidney disease. This is a very important test given how important the B vitamins are to our health and well-being. This is made clear when you realize which diseases are more likely to occur when homocysteine levels are higher than ideal: heart attack, stroke, cancer, osteoporosis, mood issues, Alzheimer's, diabetes, gut dysfunction, and ADs to name just a few.[42–52] Of course, B vitamins are extremely important for nerve health. Any neuropathic pain issue needs to have B vitamins to heal.[53–55] A high-quality, fully activated B vitamin complex tablet taken twice daily needs to be used. It is wise to immediately add the amino acid L-glutamine in a powdered form at 3 to 5 grams three times a day if neuropathic pain is the primary complaint or if it is slow to change.[56]

The form of the B vitamins is vitally important. Typically, they must be fully activated, fully methylated B vitamins. MTHFR genetic issues are only one reason, but there are so many more reasons we cannot easily stick a methyl group on the inactive B vitamins we obtain from our foods. The names of the activated B vitamins are for example B12, methylcobalamin not cyanocobalamin; vitamin B2, riboflavin 5'-phosphate; B6, pyridoxal – 5' – phosphate; folate, methyltetrahydrofolic acid. I also particularly like fully activated B complexes that include trimethylglycine, also known as betaine by its common name, as it is a great methyl donor. We need to methylate fat-soluble toxins, turning them into water-soluble toxins, so we can clear them from the body.[57] We need to methylate our DNA to shut down bad genes and turn on good genes if we are to optimize epigenetic influence on health.[58] However, we must monitor methylation status, as over-methylation can increase the risk of cancer.

Vitamin B12: Usually the activated B12 in a high-quality, fully methylated B complex will be adequate. But especially with nerve pain and other chronic nervous system issues, additional B12 may be needed. Even though everyone's B12 levels should be $\geq$800–900, some people need to be a lot higher to achieve optimal benefit.

Vitamin D: Now this is not a true vitamin, as the name implies, but a pro-hormone. The 11,000+ scientific journal articles cited with a simple vitamin D search on PubMed make obvious how much is known about vitamin D's work biochemically and physiologically and its impact on maintaining health and reversing disease. Vitamin D levels should be 50 or greater during pregnancy to decrease the risk of the child ever getting multiple sclerosis by 50%.[59] One study showed dosing 2000 IU of vitamin D per day during an infant's first 12 months of life resulted in a near 90% risk reduction of type 1 diabetes.[60] Women with vitamin D levels greater than or equal to 60 have a breast cancer risk decreased by 82%.[61] Vitamin D deficiency accounts for premature deaths from colon, breast, ovarian, and prostate cancer.[62] And vitamin D and vitamin D receptor activity are important in inflammatory bowel disease and chronic disease in general.[63]

It is so important to optimize vitamin D levels. It is also one of the nutrients that can be optimized relatively quickly compared with others such as oral iron. Most people need between 5000 and 10,000 IU per day of vitamin D to stay in the optimal range, but testing their vitamin D levels is the most important indicator to monitor to achieve an optimal range.

A big mistake you never want to make is thinking that vitamin D only needs to be used temporarily and then the patient can stop. Unfortunately, due to a variety of factors, just about everyone has vitamin D levels that will be much lower than ideal unless they are on vitamin D supplementation long term.[64] Yes, every once in a while, you will see someone who only needs 1000–2000 IU per day to maintain ideal levels. Low vitamin D can also cause low back pain.[65] It is quite an important "vitamin."

Thyroid: Thyroid is called "the great mimicker" as it can present with a variety of symptoms when it is not optimal. Whenever someone has multiple organ system involvement, you need to be very suspicious of thyroid not being optimal.

Often times, a thyroid's contribution to chronic pain and other health issues is missed simply because not enough tests are run, and interpretation is not optimal. TSH is basically based on how a person is doing with T4, but T4 is a relatively inactive hormone. T4 is the primary hormone made by the thyroid gland itself. When TSH levels are high this tends to mean we are low in T4. When T4 levels are low or TSH is high, then T4 medicine might be used to augment what the person's own thyroid can't make on its own. Thus, this person has been identified as a "poor thyroid producer."

In the distant past, T4 dosing was based on symptom resolution. Start low and go up slowly until the person feels their best. Typically, doses needed for optimal symptom resolution were 200–300 micrograms per day. When the TSH test was invented in the late 1970s, dosing of T4 medication began to be based on TSH levels. Doses used dropped almost immediately to 100–150 micrograms. Many people are under-treated when dosing is based on TSH levels alone.[66] But something new has been occurring in the last 20 to 30 years. It is not enough to only look for "poor thyroid producers." Many people are "poor thyroid converters" only or in addition to also being "poor thyroid producers." A person may have optimal T4 and TSH levels on testing while at the same time be finding it very difficult to convert the inactive T4 into the much more active, usable free T3. Instead, they are converting the free T4 excessively to the inactive thyroid hormone called reverse T3 (rT3).[66] Excessive rT3 will block the T3 receptors on every cell of the body so that the available free T3 will not be able to function.

People who have ideal levels of TSH and free T4 while on no thyroid medication may be poor converters and have every single symptom of low thyroid. What causes someone to become a poor thyroid converter? Vitamin and mineral deficiencies, stress, cortisol level dysregulation, environmental toxins, and eating too many carbohydrates and not enough protein just to name a few. This is basically "life in the 21st century." Everyone is vitamin- and mineral-deficient. The nutrient content of our food is depleted.[67] People worldwide spend so much money on products for diarrhea, constipation, reflux, and bloating. Worldwide it is estimated that 10–15% of all people have irritable bowel syndrome.[68] A 2006 study of umbilical cord blood of newborns showed every child is born with mercury, flame retardants, pesticides, and herbicides already in their systems at birth. The reason? They come from the mother through crossing the placenta during gestation.[69] Everyone eats too many carbohydrates and not enough protein. This is the "SAD" diet: the *s*tandard *A*merican *d*iet.

If a person is a poor thyroid converter, it is very hard if not impossible to achieve optimal symptom control when using a T4 medication. They excessively convert the T4 to rT3 rather than converting to free T3. This is when the desiccated thyroid medications come in handy or even using T3 products. Typically, T3 products have a very short half-life of only 4–6 hours, and they are typically dosed two times a day for this reason. But this will leave many hours of the day and night when the active free T3 level is insufficient. Using compounded, sustained-action T3 medications (c-E4M T3) is preferable if at all possible. When poor thyroid conversion is an issue, 100 micrograms of a T4 product could be converted to 60 mg of a desiccated thyroid product for example, or 50 micrograms of a T4 to 30 mg of a desiccated. This would drop the amount of T4, effectively dropping the level of rT3. Because desiccated products actually have T3 in them, this will allow the free T3 levels to stay at or rise to ideal levels.

Some newer information is starting to confirm that people with autoimmune thyroid disease, such as Hashimoto's thyroiditis, may want to avoid the use of porcine-based desiccated thyroid medicines, instead using a compounded non-porcine equivalent to the desiccated products.

Even knowing this information about thyroid restoration, it is necessary to treat cortisol issues for at least a month before anything we do in regard to thyroid will make any difference. That being said, by taking care of the cortisol issues along with treating vitamin and mineral deficiencies, helping the body detoxify better with B vitamins and gut restoration, the person may already be a better thyroid converter and no changes to the T4 medication may need to be made after all.

A handy way to get a sense of how much of an impact thyroid issues may be having on a person's pain and multiple organ system dysfunction is to use something like what I have been using for years, called "The signs and symptoms of low thyroid" (Figure 6.7). This is a list of symptoms that can occur if the thyroid is low. A patient is asked to circle all that applies to them on this list. The more symptoms they circle, the more you can feel comfortable that thyroid is having a great impact on the overall health of the individual, but also, the greater the potential impact that correcting the thyroid issues could have on the patient.

DHEA: This is a hormone made by the adrenal gland. DHEA levels will drop if somebody has been stuck in stress mode for a long time. This causes the chronically elevated cortisol to subsequently drop as well. If you are trying to prevent cortisol from crashing all the way down and starting a "ticking time bomb" for even worse health issues, then DHEA will need to be started immediately. Part of the "ticking time bomb" that occurs when cortisol crashes is actually due to the DHEA crashing. Low DHEA is a major risk factor for heart attack and stroke.[70,71] Also, without DHEA, it is very hard for the body to make anything that is protein-based. This would include

Signs And Symptoms Of Low Thyroid

Depression	Acne	Excess Formation of	Schizoid or Affective
Weight Gain	Swollen Legs, Feet,	Cerumen (Wax) in the	Psychosis
Constipation	Hands and Abdomen	Ear Canal	Congestive Heart
Headaches/Migraine	Low Body Temperature	Dull Facial Expression	Failure
Headaches	Hoarse, Husky Voice	Yellowish Discoloration	Coronary Artery Disease
Brittle, Ridged, Striated,	Low Blood Pressure	of the Skin	or Myocardial
or Thickened Nails	Muscle Weakness	Muscle Cramps	Infarction
Rough, Dry Skin	Agitation/ Irritability	Drooping Eyelids	Coarse or Dry Hair
Menstrual Irregularities	Hypercholesterolemia/	Carpel Tunnel Syndrome	Decreased Cardiac
Fluid Retention	Hyperlipidemia (High	Sleep Apnea	Output
Poor Circulation	Cholesterol)	Endometriosis	Arrhythmias
Elbow Keratosis	Infertility	Down Turned Mouth	Increased Risk of
(Abnormal Skin	PMS	Ear Canal that is Dry,	Developing Asthma
Growth)	Hyperinsulinemia (Insulin	Scaly or Itchy	Hypertension
Slow Speech	Levels >4-6 while	Painful Menstrual Cycles	Mild Elevation of Liver
Nails That are Easily	Fasting)	Tendency to Develop	Enzymes
Broken	Fibrocystic Breast	Allergies	Joint Pain and Stiffness
Anxiety/Panic Attacks	Disease	Loss of the Lateral Third	Low Amplitude Theta
Decreased Memory	Nutritional Imbalances	of Eyebrows, "Queen	and Delta Waves on
Inability to Concentrate	Paresthesia (Pins and	Anne's Sign"	EEG
Muscle and Joint Pain	Needles Sensation)	Fat Pads Above the	Nocturia (Frequent
Reduced Heart Rate	Myxedema (Swelling	Clavicles	Nighttime Urination)
Slow Movements	Due to Increase	Hair Loss in the Front or	Easy Bruising
Morning Stiffness	Connective Tissue)	Back of the Head	Erectile Dysfunction
Puffy Face	Loss of Hair From Legs,	Iron Deficiency Anemia	Hypoglycemia
Swollen Eyelids	Axilla and Arms	B12 Deficiency	Gallstones
Decreased Sexual	Poor Night Vision	Tinnitus (Ringing in the	Bladder and Kidney
Interest	Loss or Decrease of	Ears)	Infections
Cold Intolerances	Eyelashes	Delayed Deep Tendon	Eating Disorders
Cold Hands And Feet	Blepharospasm (Eyelid	Reflexes	Increased Appetite
Insomnia	Twitching)	Recurrent Miscarriages	Muscular Pain
Fatigue	Allergies	Bipolar Disorder	Osteoporosis

FIGURE 6.7 Signs and symptoms of low thyroid.

neurotransmitters, hormones, enzymes, cell walls, etc.[72] So much of our body is protein-based. This includes the DNA being able to make proteins required for proper cell function. Women typically need between 5 and 10 mg of DHEA supplementation daily, and men typically 25 to 50 mg daily. With AD, female doses go up to 25 to 50 mg and men tend to need closer to 50 mg oftentimes. DHEA should be taken on an empty stomach in the morning in order to respect the normal 24-hour cycle of this hormone. If someone is on a thyroid medication before breakfast, then DHEA should be taken 1–2 hours after breakfast.

Sex hormones: As we have noted multiple times already in this chapter, estrogen dominance is a significant issue with women and is a huge driver of AD and disease in general.[73] For men, low testosterone is a huge driver of chronic disease and all by itself can be the cause of back and neck pain.[74,75] Some hormones can be taken orally for hormone restoration therapy. Others only should be used topically. Estrogen is one of those hormones that should never be taken orally. Any oral estrogen, whether bioidentical or non-bioidentical, has a significant negative impact on gut function as well as other side effects which are quite problematic.[76,77] Also, the first-pass metabolism through the liver of estrogen taken orally produces toxic byproducts.[77]

Topical estrogen ideally for women may be BiEst 80/20: 80% estriol and 20% estradiol. When using bioidentical hormone restoration therapy of any kind, the mantra should be "start low and go slow." A reasonable starting dose of BiEst 80/20 could be 0.5 ml of a 1 mg/ml cream daily. Another dose that may be most appropriate could be BiEst 50/50. One of the advantages to compounding is that doses can be personalized to the exact needs of each patient. Typically, with topical use, symptom changes only begin in about 4 to 8 weeks. Dosage can be increased as needed. Ideally, any hormone used topically should be tested for with saliva.[78,79] Thus, when using topical estrogen products, saliva testing should be done. Blood levels will tend to underestimate the levels of hormones truly in the system.[79]

Now why use estriol and not just estradiol alone? Estriol is the weakest of the three estrogens the body produces but has many functions in the body. It is not strong enough to prevent cardiovascular disease and keep the bones strong though, thus the 20% estradiol. Estradiol is powerful enough to produce improvement in cardiovascular risk and bone health but can turn into estrone excessively.[80] Topical estradiol is available in patch form, but great caution needs to be exercised because of its tendency to convert excessively to estrone. Estrogen should never be used without also using progesterone. For one reason, they work together for many processes. Progesterone helps to make good strong bones, and estrogen prevents excessive loss of bone. Also, we do not want excessive estrogen impact on breast tissue without progesterone to protect the breast.[81] The same goes for estrogen dominance and its negative impact on autoimmune disease prevention or reversal.[74]

Progesterone can be taken orally or topically. Both routes of administration work equally well, except oral progesterone tends to be much better at controlling insomnia and anxiety. The full benefit of a particular dose of oral progesterone will be seen much sooner, oftentimes as quick as 2 days or possibly up to 5. Thus, doses can be raised quickly in order to optimize correction of estrogen dominance and other health issues. Topical dosing can be done, but, just as with estrogens, it may take 4 to 8 weeks to see an effect before changing the dose is prudent. Usually starting at 100 mg orally, the lowest dose available through a regular pharmacy, is reasonable. Progesterone is taken near bedtime in order to respect the diurnal rhythm of this hormone. Dosing can be done earlier, 1–2 hours before bedtime if the person feels groggy the next day after initially dosing at bedtime. Dosing of progesterone should be done 1 to 2 hours before bedtime anyway if the person is having a hard time falling asleep. If a person falls asleep OK but can't stay asleep, dosing should be started initially right at bedtime. Sometimes even the 100 mg is more than the person needs. This tends to be relatively infrequent though. Using a compounding pharmacy for a 25 mg capsule going up by 25 mg every 2 to 5 days until optimal symptom control is achieved is a good option for these people.

Pulsing of hormone restoration is important. The body likes to see different amounts of sex hormones on different days. In premenopausal women, topical/oral progesterone use will be cycled. It is extremely rare to ever need to give estrogen to a premenopausal woman. Progesterone is used on days 14–25 of the cycle, and not on days 26–30. If symptoms return to an extent that is unacceptable on the off days, progesterone can be used but at perhaps half the usual dose.

In perimenopausal and post-menopausal women, a pulsing schedule of the BiEst and progesterone can be on Monday through Saturday and off Sunday.

Testosterone: This is another hormone that should never be taken orally. Bioidentical testosterone is an option for both men and women, and injections are a great option for men. The only commercially available testosterone for women, methyl testosterone, should be avoided due to its side effect of increasing liver cancer risk.[82] In women, testosterone should never be taken without also using estrogen at the same time, just like estrogen should never be used without progesterone. Testosterone without estrogen in women will have a negative impact on cardiovascular health.

Dosing of topical testosterone for women might need to start at 0.5 mg and go up slowly. Dosing for men topically can start at 10–20 mg. Topical testosterone has to be done daily and on areas that are relatively hairless. Within the hair follicle, testosterone will be converted into dihydrotestosterone excessively. IM testosterone in the lateral quadriceps muscle for men is ideally done one to two times a week. The advantages of IM dosing include once-a-week dosing and no concerns regarding insufficient absorption though the skin, as well as no tendency to transfer testosterone to others though contact as can be seen with topical use. Nowadays, injectables are typically covered by most insurance companies. When using topicals, cream is far superior to patches as far as absorption.

Celiac testing: Part of the difficulty with completely eliminating gluten is that much of it is in places most people will never know. "Hidden gluten" is found in modified food starches, preservatives and food stabilizers, prescription and over-the-counter medications, vitamin and mineral supplements, herbal and nutritional supplements, lipstick, toothpaste and mouthwash, envelope and stamp glue, and even in the childhood toy Play-Doh.[83]

Infections: Infections are huge drivers of AD and chronic pain. Some infections come into our bodies and we know it right away, such as a cold or pneumonia. We hope the symptoms only last in the short term. Sometimes they create immediate reactions such as the Epstein–Barr virus and mononucleosis, but they remain dormant in the body, creating new problems years or decades later, thus, the more than doubling of the risk of multiple sclerosis when somebody has had mononucleosis.[84,85]

Typically, there will be a combination of viruses, bacteria, funguses, mycoplasma, and possibly even parasites. Thus, a broad antimicrobial agent typically needs to be used in order to get rid of all the bugs, no matter what kind and no matter where they are. Plus, these bugs tend to be very stubborn. Mycoplasma tends to be the most stubborn of all. By the time mycoplasma is cleared, the rest of the bugs will be gone as well. Typically at least 6, 9, or 12 months or even longer on an antimicrobial is required to clear mycoplasma totally. It can be very difficult to clear mycoplasma with traditional antibiotics even if you use them for months or even years at times. But antibiotics will not clear viruses or funguses, and antibiotics will simply disrupt the gut further, creating even more problems. Antimicrobials that can be extremely effective and used for a long duration are available.[86–88] One product is pH structured silver solution. This is a silver formulation that is quite powerful at low doses.[88]

For a very long time, people have used colloidal silver to treat infections. Silver is a great antimicrobial. Colloidal silver, however, is not very powerful and has to be used in high doses. It can never be used for long durations as it can produce toxic levels that can actually turn people blue. This is not good. Silver preparations formulated like the pH structured silver solution, a nanosilver, are able to work well at low doses. Thus, people could use much more every day then we would ever need to use and use it for many decades and never come close to a toxic level. Typically, because mycoplasma likes to create pain issues and brain problems, the recommendation is to continue the nanosilver until the pain and brain issues are gone. If, after stopping the silver solution, the person starts to backslide, including feeling the pain returning, then restart the silver solution immediately. Use it for 2 more months and then try to come off it again. This can be repeated as often as necessary until the person feels fine without it. Then we know all the chronic infections are gone.

Typically, any other infection will be gone by the time the mycoplasma has been cleared. Dosing often times starts at 4 ounces once a day (done as a swish and swallow for 1–2 minutes) for 4 days, then 2 ounces a day.

Another option for long-term antimicrobial therapy is to use the plant-based product Biocidin. Advanced liquid Biocidin is used for GI infections. Liposomal Biocidin is used for systemic infections. Biocidin is so effective at killing microorganisms, a person needs to start at very low doses and titrate up slowly as tolerated. Die-off reactions, or Herxheimer's reactions, as the dose increases, require dropping back down to the previously tolerated doses. Wait 3 to 5 days, and then try to increase the dose again. Because of the profound die-off from the use of Biocidin, typically a second product has to be used in order to bind up the toxins as they are being released and hold onto them until they leave the body, for example, a product such as "G.I. Detox" which is a combination of charcoal and clay. The Biocidin needs to be dosed three times a day on an empty stomach while the G.I. Detox is dosed twice a day, also on an empty stomach. Probiotics need to be taken at bedtime while on this regimen. This is one reason why the pH structured silver solution is an easier regimen as it only needs to be dosed once a day typically.

SALIVARY CORTISOL

SALIVARY CORTISOL: TESTING

One hormone that is not optimally tested in the blood is cortisol. For many reasons, saliva is better than blood. For one, saliva testing was the first way ever developed to test for cortisol.[89] Saliva is a better indicator of intra-cellular levels.[90] What goes on inside the cells tends to be more important than what goes on in the serum, or liquid, part of our blood. Finally, the very worst time to check the level of the "stress hormone" cortisol is right after stabbing the person with a sharp object. And a blood draw is stabbing a person with a sharp object. Immediately, this alters cortisol levels.

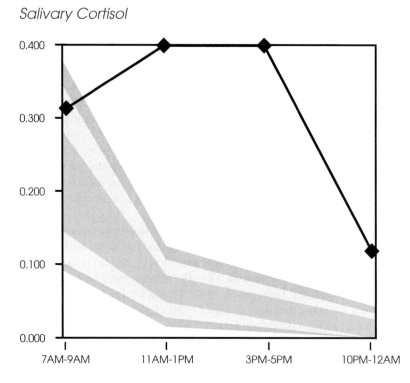

FIGURE 6.8   Salivary control.

Spitting tends to be a lot less stressful for most people. Plus, cortisol levels need to be checked at 8 AM, noon, 5 PM, and 10 PM.[91] Saliva cortisol testing kits are available from several companies (Figure 6.8).

SALIVARY CORTISOL: INTERPRETATION

Cortisol, the "stress hormone," should be highest in the morning and go down as the day progresses, hitting its low point at bedtime.[91] We fall fast asleep easily. Nothing keeps us awake. We get wonderful restorative sleep. Nothing wakes us up. No pain, no bladder, no noise. Nothing. The "sleep of the dead." We then wake up feeling great. Totally energized and refreshed. We then jump out of bed and do it all over again. As you might imagine from this description, many of the chronic pain patients seen will have cortisol issues and may even have the completely opposite rhythm: low all day long and then cannot shut down at night. "Tired and wired" is one way this may present.

Cortisol is designed to go up and down many times a day with any kind of stress. To the body, stress is stress. It doesn't matter if it is emotional, physical, spiritual, or biochemical stress. It is all the same stress to the body. If you stub your toe and hop around in pain, this is physical stress. Driving in a bad snowstorm is emotional stress. But if a person experiences too much or too great a stress or for too long, cortisol can go all the way up and stay in the "on position." They are stuck in the "fight or flight" mode. The "life or death" mode. The "there is a bear chasing me trying to kill me" mode.

Now when the body is stuck with cortisol running high at all times tested, this is called stage 1 adrenal fatigue.[92] (I believe it is important for every physician to know that these terms and concepts have been described in the scientific literature for many decades. This reference here, in the *British Medical Journal*, is from 1950.) The hormone DHEA, like cortisol, will need to stay in an ideal level, or even increase temporarily, in order to allow the person to continue "running from the bear" even though they do not feel very well. If a bear is chasing you, you want to be able to keep running even if you don't feel so well. Stop running and you are dead, or so your body thinks. But because the person is running 24 hours a day, 7 days a week, day after day, month after month, they are feeling worse and worse over time.

This cortisol crash also seems to be a last-ditch effort by the body to protect itself and mainly the brain which is "on fire" and deteriorating rapidly. The most problematic area is the hippocampus, but also, the hypothalamus, prefrontal cortex, and amygdala.[93] The long-term high cortisol levels downregulate the immune system, creating an immunosuppressed state thus allowing the infections to get into the body and establish themselves.

When one out of the four cortisol test results is lower than the ideal and the others are still high, this is called stage 2 adrenal fatigue.[92] When two or more are low, this is stage 3.[92] When a person has crashed all four times in the day this is the worst. This is when a "time bomb" starts ticking for things like a heart attack, stroke, cancer, and diabetes.[91,94]

Some newer terms that may more accurately reflect what is truly occurring are starting to take the place of the older, more traditional terminology: hypercortisolism when levels are high, hypocortisolism when low, and mixed cortisolism when some levels are low and some high.

SALIVARY CORTISOL: TREATMENT

No matter what stage of adrenal dysfunction a person is in, they need calm. The free apps "Insight Timer" and "Calm" may be good options for many patients. The biochemical stressors that we have been discussing in this chapter must also be addressed.

But the most important item to use is a supplement product called an "adrenal adaptogen."[95] This is a combination of several different herbs and some vitamins that create calm in the adrenal gland.

As an "adaptogen," it is not directional. It is balancing. If a person has a cortisol level that is high, it will help to bring it down. If a level is too low, it will come up. If a person has a combination of high and low, all cortisol levels will tend to move towards the ideal.

Eventually, when cortisol curves have normalized, the adrenal adaptogens can be stopped as well.

DIAGNOSTIC STOOL ANALYSIS

DIGESTIVE STOOL ANALYSIS: TESTING

As discussed previously, the gut is a very important mechanism in the maintenance of immune system health. Given that 80% of the immune system surrounds the gut, dysfunction in this organ can directly affect the immune system. The gut dysfunction can then lead to the development of the other drivers of AD.[18–23] As we are seeing more every day, it is a central mechanism for much of chronic disease. When someone has diarrhea, constipation, gastroesophageal reflux disease (GERD), bloating, flatulence, foul-smelling stools, nausea, abdominal pain, undigested food in their stool, and bloody stools it is easy to see the functional issues with the gut. But a person may have none or minimal gut symptoms and still have a very dysfunctional gut. This is why eight out of ten people with celiac disease never get diagnosed. Despite having an AD attacking the small intestine, 80% of celiac patients have minimal or no gut systems.[33]

When the gut is disrupted, food is not digested well, and the nutrients absorbed into the body are compromised. These nutrients are the basic building blocks the body uses for essential daily function. The gut is called the "second brain." The way research is going, the gut may turn out to actually be the "first brain." But let's stick with the gut as the second brain for now. The gut makes items the brain needs to function such as the neurotransmitters serotonin and GABA.[96] Ninety percent of serotonin for example is made in the gut.[96] Now this is not made completely altruistically by the gut for his good friend the brain. The gut uses serotonin itself for purposes such as the regulation of gut motility. Serotonin is known for its effect on mood, but it also has a significant impact on the immune system, sleep, diabetes mellitus, autism spectrum disorder, Parkinson's, and Alzheimer's disease.[96] Thus, disrupted production of serotonin by the gut would affect gut motility, mood, sleep, and the immune system all at once.[96]

The gut is a vital organ for detoxification.[26] Most toxins have to leave the body through defecation. This includes not only the environmental toxins such as lead and mercury but also internally generated toxins such as old, toxic estrogen metabolites.[26] Every cell in our body makes toxic byproducts of metabolism that must be cleared from the body. It is vitally important to be able to clear toxins from the body efficiently and the gut is the primary organ of detoxification. An inability to clear old, toxic estrogens from the body can be one of the causes of estrogen dominance (i.e., too much estrogen compared with progesterone). Estrogen dominance is a big driver of menstrual pain, heavy flows, premenstrual syndrome, PMDD, fibroids, endometriosis, ovarian cysts, and fibrocystic breast disease.[97] Insomnia and anxiety may be impacted by estrogen dominance as well. Many of these can create debilitating pain, and estrogen dominance is such a big driver of AD.[18,20,22,98–101] This is one reason why more women acquire ADs than men.[97]

DIGESTIVE STOOL ANALYSIS: INTERPRETATION

The gut is a huge central mechanism in immune system dysregulation and the associated pain. Information received by the use of a digestive stool analysis is so helpful, and most of it is typically unavailable through hospital or local lab testing (Figure 6.9). Pancreatic elastase levels inform us if the pancreas is still able to produce this important enzyme. It can drop for a variety of reasons including if the pancreas is having to work hard to make higher than ideal levels of insulin due to insulin resistance.[102] Or perhaps even fasting insulin levels have dropped below ideal on their way

Digestive Stool Analysis

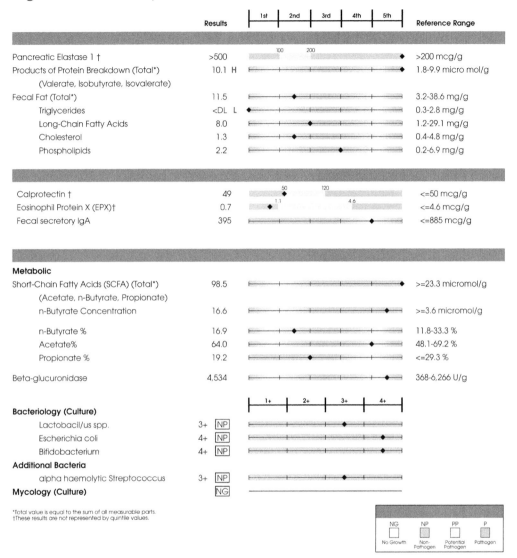

FIGURE 6.9 Digestive stool analysis.

from pre-diabetes to full-blown diabetes. As we discussed earlier, when the important hormone triad of cortisol, thyroid, and insulin/blood sugar is disrupted, insulin resistance will be the result. As cortisol and thyroid are correcting, the insulin resistance and pancreatic elastase production can self-correct.

Fecal fats and fecal protein products are reported. If too high, our body is not digesting them well in order to obtain the nutrients we need to power up our bodies.

Inflammation markers calprotectin, EPX and Sig A are tested. Elevation of calprotectin indicates inflammation and that the patient is moving towards colon cancer and the ADs, such as ulcerative colitis and Crohn's disease.[103] If this number hasn't normalized by the first recheck, a person needs to be referred for colonoscopy. An elevated EPX means some of the foods that are being consumed by the person are having a negative impact on the gut.[104,105] High Sig A means intestinal permeability issues. A low Sig A means that the person has lost the protective mucosal membrane separating the intestinal wall from the contents of the gut.[104,105]

Short-chain fatty acids (SCFAs), including n-butyrate. When n-butyrate is low, so much inflammation is produced that a person has an increased risk of colon cancer.[104,105] The good bacteria in the gut should make these important SCFAs.[104,105]

When beta glucuronidase levels are higher than ideal, this means toxicity.[104,105] When elevated, this also raises the risk of colon cancer.[104,105] Also, when this marker is high, estrogens that need to leave the body are reactivated and reabsorbed into the body, contributing to the estrogen dominance issue.[104,105] The good bacteria should make an enzyme to break beta glucuronidase down and keep levels optimal.[104,105] When the beta glucuronidase level is low, this tends to indicate tolerance issues with carbohydrates, including blood sugar issues.[104,105]

Along with a look at overall intestinal microbiome diversity, the population abundance of at least three very important good bacterial numbers are tested specifically. Levels go from no growth (NG) to 4+; 4+ for each is ideal. Bad bacterial numbers are given as well. Certain bad bacteria are only problematic when they reach levels of 4+. Some are quite problematic even at low numbers and need to be totally removed from the gut if it is ever going to heal. Mold is very similar to the bad bacteria but tends to be very hard to find and diagnose. One of the popular digestive stool analysis companies looks for microscopic mold spores, and this tends to help greatly with identifying the presence of problematic amounts of mold.

DIGESTIVE STOOL ANALYSIS: TREATMENT

There are a couple of different testing companies to use for digestive stool analysis. Some people like one, other people like the other. Several issues noted on testing tend to be the most important to treat and then the body will often take care of all the other areas itself.

Pancreatic elastase (enzymes): This should be >500. If lower, start digestive enzymes 1–2 capsules before each meal, or apple cider vinegar, 2 teaspoons before meals. If high protein products or fecal fats are found in the stool analysis, the patient is not digesting these nutrients well and the treatment suggestions above may be helpful.

Three different inflammation markers are tested.

If calprotectin is high, this is quite concerning. As mentioned before, a person is moving towards diseases such as ulcerative colitis, Crohn's disease, and colon cancer.[103] Simply treating what is found in the rest of our overall testing will work to eliminate this high number. If, upon retesting 3 months after treatment initiation, calprotectin is not yet in the ideal range, then the person will need to have a colonoscopy.[106,107]

EPX: When this is high, it suggests food is bothering the gut. Avoiding the offending foods should drop this number by the next retest. If it is still high, the patient either needs to do better with avoiding offending foods already identified or some additional foods may be problematic and need to be removed from the diet as well. Sometimes, empirically, some foods may need to be removed for a while. An example could be lectin-containing foods or the nightshade family of foods.

Sig A: If high, it suggests intestinal permeability disorder. If low, it suggests the patient has lost the protective membrane that separates the gut wall from the gut contents. If at the time of the retest, perhaps 3 months later, a very low result has now changed to a high result, this is good. The protective membrane has been reestablished, but the intestinal permeability disorder still needs to be corrected. For all these issues, L-glutamine powder needs to be used, on an empty stomach, at 3 to 5 grams TID. This is the best primary agent to use in this situation.

Short-chain fatty acids (SCFAs) and n-butyrate: They should be produced by the good bacteria in the gut. If low, the good bacteria are not doing their job. If n-butyrate is very low, you may want to wait and see if the intestinal microbiome improves enough to self-correct this by the next retest. Or use a butyric acid supplement to start correcting immediately. This important nutrient and its role in the health of the whole body will be discussed further in a minute.

Beta glucuronidase: This tends to self-correct as the good bacteria should make an enzyme to break it down. If they don't start doing this work by the first retest, consider calcium D-glucarate supplementation. Or possibly add a combination insoluble/soluble fiber supplement to bind up the toxins until they can be cleared from the gut and help to feed the good bacteria as a "prebiotic," food for the good bacteria.

Good bacteria: The ideal is 4+ of each and 4+ of all as a good balance, which is so important. High-quality probiotics will always be needed just as vitamin D will always be needed. Which probiotic to use will vary.

Using antibiotics can be quite problematic due to the negative impact on the intestinal microbiome, particularly as they will need to be used for an entire month if the offending bacteria is to be cleared completely. Potentially using probiotics 2 hours after each dose of an antibiotic and continuing the probiotic for at least 2 weeks after antibiotic treatment can minimize the negative impact no matter when we use these medicines.

A quick review is needed of two very important components required for optimal gut health and the body as a whole: vitamin D and vitamin D receptors (VDRs),[63] more specifically, their impact on the intestinal microbiome and overall body inflammation and health. The intestinal mucosa has so many vitamin D receptors. This tells us how important vitamin D is for the gut.[63] VDRs need vitamin D available in the gut in order to function properly. But VDRs need probiotics and n-butyrate for upregulation of the vitamin D receptor sensitivity. All the vitamin D in the gut may not help the situation if the VDRs are downregulated. This is why oral vitamin D optimization, probiotics, and n-butyrate supplementation will be an excellent way to decrease inflammation in the gut, reestablish the intestinal microbiome, and clear even inflammatory bowel disease as well as flares of celiac disease.[63] It will also decrease inflammation in the body as a whole, thus addressing chronic pain problems and chronic disease in general.[63]

PROVOCATIVE HEAVY METAL TEST

PROVOCATIVE HEAVY METAL: TESTING

The increase in environmental toxins in our world seems to be a big driver of the rise in ADs.[108] In 1997, it was estimated that 9 million people in the U.S. had an AD. Now, it is estimated that 50 million people have an AD.[1,109] Nearly 80% are women.[110] Rates are rising in Europe, Scandinavia, and elsewhere just as fast.[111] Rheumatoid arthritis was almost totally unheard of in Japan until only a few years ago and now it is becoming common.[112,113]

Water-soluble toxins are not as big a problem as fat-soluble toxins in general. Water-soluble toxins are relatively easily cleared from the body. Fat-soluble toxins are stored in fat and are leached out slowly into our system, driving chronic disease including pain and the disruption of the immune system. Our brains are 60% fat.[114] Our brains tend to accumulate these fat-soluble toxins. So, often, people with any AD also have memory and concentration issues and co-morbid depression, anxiety, irritability, and many others. Lead is a huge problem when it comes to chronic disease. Recently, a review article suggested that a large percentage of all heart attacks in the U.S. were due to lead toxicity.[115] Lead is so toxic to the cardiovascular system and the body as a whole, that even amounts we typically would not think were significant will have a profoundly negative impact.[116]

Approximately 94% of lead is sequestered in our bones and teeth.[117] So, when menopause or andropause start to cause loss of bone density, the sequestered lead starts to flood into our system, disrupting many organ systems including negatively impacting the immune system and nervous system. Blood testing tends to greatly underestimate the toxic load someone is carrying.[118] If lead can be found in significant levels in serum, you know someone is carrying a very high lead load. Thus, we can test negative for lead or other toxins in the blood and still have a big toxic load in fat and bone stores throughout the body.

Provocative heavy metal tests use a chelating agent to pull these toxins from the fat stores and get them into the urine to be tested. A common chelating agent is DMSA at a dose of 1000 mg 1 hour after the first morning urine. After taking the chelating agent, urine collection is started for a set number of hours and can be done up to 24 hours, but I usually find 6 hours is sufficient to find what you are looking for.[118–121]

Typically, provocative heavy metal testing isn't done right away as part of the initial set of labs. Usually, it is run a few months after blood, saliva, and stool. The reason? The levels of "good" metals in the initial blood work need to be reviewed prior to running the heavy metal test. As we mobilize large amounts of "bad" metals and get them into the urine to be tested, we are doing the same with "good" metals. If someone is low in RBC magnesium, for example, and the provocative heavy metal test is done, they could conceivably get so magnesium-depleted that they could experience heart palpitations and arrhythmias.[122] RBC magnesium is one of the initial blood tests run for a variety of reasons, one being this issue. If RBC magnesium is below the range or at the very low end of the reference range, we should supplement with magnesium for 2 months and then retest levels to see if they are more mid-range.

HEAVY METAL: ASSESSMENT

Some people advocate doing a non-provocative heavy metal test first. A provocative heavy metal test is one that uses an oral chelating agent to mobilize toxins from fat stores into urine for testing. A non-provocative test is one that looks at levels in the urine without having used a chelating agent first. Typically, lead and mercury are not excreted through the kidneys, and they need to be bound by the chelating agent and "dragged" out of the body through the kidneys (Figure 6.10).[123]

Toxic Metals; Urine

TOXIC METALS		RESULTS µg/g creat	REFERENCE INTERVAL	
Aluminum	(Al)	1.9	< 35	
Antimony	(Sb)	0.7	< 0.2	
Arsenic	(As)	11	< 80	
Barium	(Ba)	2	< 7	
Beryllium	(Be)	< dl	< 1	
Bismuth	(Bi)	< dl	< 4	
Cadmium	(Cd)	0.7	< 1	
Cesium	(Cs)	11	< 10	
Gadolinium	(Gd)	0.1	< 0.8	
Lead	(Pb)	13	< 2	
Mercury	(Hg)	1.7	< 4	
Nickel	(Ni)	2	< 10	
Palladium	(Pd)	< dl	< 0.15	
Platinum	(Pt)	< dl	< 0.1	
Tellurium	(Te)	< dl	< 0.5	
Thallium	(Tl)	0.5	< 0.5	
Thorium	(Th)	< dl	< 0.03	
Tin	(Sn)	0.8	< 5	
Tungsten	(W)	0.04	< 0.4	
Uranium	(U)	< dl	< 0.04	

URINE CREATININE		RESULTS mg/dL	REFERENCE INTERVAL	-2SD	-1SD	MEAN	+1SD	+2SD
Creatinine		68.3	30 - 225			•		

FIGURE 6.10 Heavy metal urine.

Heavy Metal: Treatment

Some environmental toxins are so toxic to human beings that even small amounts are problematic.[115,116] Lead is one of them. But there is also mercury, cadmium, nickel, arsenic, and cesium to name a few. The ability to detoxify suffers right along with all of the other important bodily processes when the central mechanisms are off: not enough B vitamins to run detoxification pathways, the inability to activate/methylate the B vitamins, a lack of optimal liver function, a lack of glutathione to keep mitochondria clear of toxins and making ATP, and a lack of gut function as well.

In one respect, it is not so much whether someone avoid environmental toxins as much as whether they get rid of them faster than they are coming in. Our world is so full of environmental toxins, starting in the womb during gestation.[69] When it comes to pain and toxicity, I am usually thinking of neurogenic pain and pain related to mitochondrial dysfunction. But toxicity can really impact any pain process, and formal detoxification needs to occur.

Some people are so full of toxins and so sensitive to their effects, they could feel quite poorly during the days of detoxification. In this case, consider decreasing the daily dose for the same number of days, or maybe only doing 1 or 2 days of detoxification and increasing the dose and number of days as time goes on, with the goal of 3 days on and 4–11 days off; using a multimineral supplement on the "off" days. Maybe consider adding a high-quality fiber supplement to bind up the toxins after they are dumped into the gut, protecting the body until they can be cleared. Retesting can be done after 4–6 months.

It is very important that a person has bowel movements at least daily before starting the formal detoxification. If bowel movements are occurring less often, the mobilized toxins will be dumped into the gut but then reabsorbed back into the system.

FOOD SENSITIVITY TEST

Food Sensitivity Test: Testing

Foods can illicit immediate and delayed hypersensitivity reactions. Immediate hypersensitivity reactions involve IgA and IgE. Delayed reactions involve IgG. Now, if someone wants to start a heated conversation with a more traditional Western allopathic doctor, just mention IgG food testing. This is despite much experience in actual clinical practice that this is of value, as well as studies backing up this form of testing and the profound impact on the gut when these foods are eliminated. One such study was published in the British Medical Journal Open Gastroenterology in 2017.[124] This looked at IgG testing and irritable bowel syndrome (IBS) patients. By eliminating foods identified on IgG testing as being problematic, this notoriously hard-to-treat group of patients was substantially better after only 4 weeks and profoundly better at 8 weeks. No other changes were made other than just to stop eating a few foods which tested positive on a simple IgG test.[124] Immediate hypersensitivity reactions tend to happen fast and dramatically enough that people can figure out the food they are sensitive to. If a child eats a peanut and they have to go to the emergency room due to throat tightness, they should not eat peanuts. This is an IgE immediate hypersensitivity reaction.[125] If someone drinks milk or eats ice cream and within 10 minutes, they are bloated and gassy and have diarrhea, it is obvious that this person has a cow's milk dairy immediate hypersensitivity reaction. This is an IgA reaction.[126] These are the only type of food reactions that are usually tested for and include skin prick testing or blood testing. IgE and IgA testing can be relatively inaccurate at times.[127,128] The tests may say a specific food result is negative, but the person has a bad reaction every time they eat it. Or the test is positive, but the food doesn't cause any immediate reactions after the person eats it. Typically, the patient can do a good job at determining what foods bother them immediately and which ones do not, compared with this type of traditional testing.

Now, foods can also bother us several days or even 3 to 4 weeks after we consume them. These are known as delayed hypersensitivity reactions or IgG reactions.[129,130] These IgG reactions do not cause the dramatic "hit" that the immediate hypersensitivity reactions do. They are not going to send someone to the hospital like an immediate hypersensitivity reaction to peanuts for example. Instead, they tend to create a scenario where the person says "I have all this chronic, smoldering inflammation, crud, just driving my body crazy in so many ways. I do not know what is causing this, but I don't think it is what I am eating. I can actually go a couple weeks without eating a certain food and I don't feel any better. I then eat this food and it doesn't make me feel sick right away. So, I don't think that this food is bothering me." The problem is, by the time they say this, they still haven't gotten "hit" from the last time they ate this food, let alone cleaned up all that chronic, smoldering inflammation, crud that has been going on for years if not decades by now. This is why testing can be so important.

Perhaps the debate on this one will go the way of the "no way an infection can cause stomach ulcers" debate. We now don't think twice about the concept and test for and treat an *H. pylori* bacterial infection of the stomach that causes stomach ulcers all the time. Or the "leaky gut" debate that has morphed into "intestinal permeability disorder," despite all the data on disruption of the intestinal tight junctions and its negative impact not only on gut function but chronic disease in general. There are different companies that provide IgG testing kits. Some kits test for more foods than others. Some testing companies can test up to 500 different foods. In our office, we most often use ones that will test for 96 different foods, grading each food 0–4. These tests provide qualitative measurements of allergenic foods and their degree of severity.

Now with AD, everyone with any autoimmune process for sure will have a delayed hypersensitivity reaction to wheat/gluten proteins and cow's milk dairy proteins.[131] Everyone. No exceptions. These two always need to be eliminated from the diet even if they do not show up as positive on testing.

FOOD SENSITIVITY TEST: ASSESSMENT

The food sensitivity test that I tend to run is one that assesses 96 different foods for an IgG reaction that the foods produce which is the delayed hypersensitivity reaction (Figure 6.11). Each food is graded from 0 to VI. The foods of concern, which need to be eliminated, are the ones graded I to VI. Zeros are zeros. Typically, the problematic foods need to be eliminated for at least 4 to 6 weeks since the half-life of IgG is 21 days.

So much needs to happen to heal the gut once it has been so disrupted that it now sees certain foods as its "enemy," and just eliminating the food for a while is not enough. Celiac is an AD that attacks the small intestine and tends to not only produce abdominal pain and other gut symptoms but also diffuse systemic dysfunction including pain in general.[33] As mentioned previously, having all sorts of systemic symptoms, including pain with minimal or no gut symptoms, occurs in eight out of ten celiac patients.[33] This is one reason four out of five celiac people are never diagnosed but also a great example of what a central mechanism the gut is.[33] Simply eliminating gluten from oral consumption does not allow the gut and immune system to reset, and these patients at times continue to develop new ADs and chronic diseases in general. These include type 1 diabetes, multiple sclerosis, anemia, osteoporosis, infertility, miscarriage, seizures, migraines, intestinal cancers, and dermatitis herpetiformis.[33]

There are also tests that can look at up to 500 different foods. The detail achieved with these tests is amazing. Testing will include things like white pepper, black pepper, sage, oregano, and MSG. When someone sees this kind of detail they may ask "the body really can tell the difference between white pepper and black pepper?" Yes, the body can tell the difference between the proteins in white pepper and black pepper. White pepper may be totally fine while black pepper creates a response. Many people can have sensitivities to foods not included on the 96-foods test. The thing is, most of the self-correcting when we address central mechanisms is done by the body itself. We just want to put the body in a position to be able to start fixing problems on its own. Most of the time people are going to self-correct and clear food sensitivities even if we do not know exactly all that are involved. People of course need to eliminate any foods that produce an immediate hypersensitivity reaction as well.[132–138]

Food Sensitivity Test

GRAINS/LEGUMES/NUTS

Almond, Amaranth, Barley, Bean, Kidney, Bean, Lima, Bean, Pinto, Bean, Soy, Bean, String, Buckwheat, Coconut, Corn, Gliadin, Wheat, Gluten, Wheat, Hazelnut, Lentil, Oat, Pea, Green, Peanut, Pecan, Rice, White, Rye, Sesame Seed, Spelt, Sunflower Seed, Walnut, English, Wheat, Whole

VEGETABLES

Avocado, Beet, Broccoli, Cabbage, Carrot, Cauliflower, Celery, Cucumber, Garlic, Lettuce, Mushroom, Olive, Onion, Pepper, Green Bell, Potato, Sweet, Potato, White, Pumpkin, Readish, Spinach, Squash, Zucchini, Tomato

FRUITS

Apple, Apricot, Banana, Blueberry, Cranberry, Grape, Grapefruit, Lemon, Orange, Papaya, Peach, Pear, Pineapple, Plum, Raspberry, Strawberry

MEAT/FOWL

Beef, Chicken, Egg White, Chicken, Egg Whole, Duck, Egg Yolk, Chicken, Lamb, Pork, Turkey

DAIRY

Casein, Cheese, Cheddar, Cheese, Cottage, Cheese, Mozzarella, Milk, Milk, Goat, Whey, Yogurt

FISH/CRUSTACEA/MOLLUSK

Clam, Cod, Crab, Halibut, Lobster, Red Snapper, Salmon, Scallop, Shrimp, Sole, Tuna

MISC

Cocoa Bean, Coffee Bean, Honey, Bee, Sugar Cane, Yeast, Baker's, Yeast, Brewer's

0	I	II	III	IV	V	VI
No Reaction	Very Low	Low	Moderate	High	Very High	Extremely High

FIGURE 6.11 Food sensitivity test.

Food Sensitivity Test: Treatment

Every person with an AD has a delayed hypersensitivity food reaction to gluten/wheat and cow's milk dairy proteins.[131]

I will typically ask a person with chronic pain along with AD to avoid wheat/gluten and cow's milk dairy products to start with if they have not tried this for at least 4 weeks already. If these are the only two foods bothering them, by the 8-week follow-up office visit, they should feel much improved. If they do not, then other foods are most likely problematic as well. Food sensitivity testing needs to be done and the identified foods eliminated.

After the person's pain and multi-organ system issues are a lot better, there is a good possibility that they have reset the food sensitivities. Now food challenges can be done. This is done by having the patient eat the food being tested two times a day for 3 days straight and then wait the rest of the week. If everything feels just fine, then they have reset the food and can eat it as much as they want. If they feel poorly in any way, such as increased pain or brain fog, stomach issues, or fatigue, etc., they have not reset the food yet and they need to take it out again. They may repeat the food challenge with this food again in 3 to 6 months to see if it has reset by that time. If they still feel badly with a food challenge, they can re-test every 3 to 6 months as often as they want in the hopes of resetting the food eventually. It may take several challenges before someone resets a food or, potentially, they may never reset certain foods despite their best efforts. The reason only one food is tested per week is that we are testing delayed hypersensitivity reactions. Usually people feel poorly if they have not reset a certain food by day 1, 2, or 3. But at times they may only start to feel poorly on days 4 to 7.

A person should keep a diary of the date and the food being tested as well as any reactions they experience.

With AD patients though, they will never fully reset wheat/gluten proteins. These will always need to be avoided if they are to maintain optimal control over the chronic pain and immune system dysregulation.[131] The body actually attacking itself is like going off a cliff. You'll never fully recover from that. But over time, many people will lose much of their sensitivity and they can "cheat," three to four times a year, and only experience mild symptoms of intolerance, rather than the typically severe reactions to these offending foods they experienced early on.

TREATMENT BASED ON EMPIRICAL KNOWLEDGE RATHER THAN LAB RESULTS

Low-dose naltrexone (LDN): Originally, naltrexone was used at relatively high doses. At these dosages, it acts as an immunosuppressant. But at low doses, it was found to act as an immunomodulator.[139] It rebalances the immune system, bringing it back to the "set point." LDN was originally used primarily in multiple sclerosis patients. More recent studies have shown that LDN is an immune modulator and has been studied in a variety of disorders such as inflammatory bowel disease.[140] In adults, dosing of LDN can start at 1.5 mg at bedtime and increase by 1.5 mg weekly to a maximum dose of 4.5 mg, and this is mainly in opioid-naïve patients.

IV glutathione: Glutathione (GSH) is the most important low molecular weight antioxidant synthesized in cells and the most potent free radical scavenger in the body.[141] The liver is a major producer of glutathione, and medications like acetaminophen tend to deplete GSH greatly,[142] thus, the significant downside of using acetaminophen chronically. To give you an example of how important it is for the liver itself to have GSH, consider the case of somebody trying to commit suicide by taking an overdose of acetaminophen. A high dose of acetaminophen depletes glutathione from the liver so dramatically that the liver will die. In the emergency room, the glutathione precursor n-acetylcysteine (NAC) is given IV in an attempt to save the liver. Glutathione is also depleted dramatically by cigarette smoke as well as smoke from forest and brushfires.[143–145]

GSH cannot be taken orally as the stomach acids will break it down. Liposomal products are available. Ideally, IV glutathione is highly preferable. The positive impact for patients with chronic pain as well as fatigue and/or brain fog can be dramatic. IV GSH is typically administered once a week. The first dose is 1000 mg, usually given over 30–45 minutes. Subsequent treatments may use 2500 mg.

Nature: Nature has a profound positive impact on human health and well-being.[146] There are nearly 100 scientific journal articles about nature and its positive impact on human health. This can mean looking at a green space outside the window following gallbladder surgery decreasing the use of antibiotics and decreasing the length of the hospital stay. It can mean observing "charismatic macro fauna," basically, looking at large animals whose personality traits we find appealing. Much of nature's ability to improve human health and well-being comes from its impact on cortisol,[145] and thus, its impact on pain and the immune system. People who work in high-rise office buildings in large cities but have a window that looks down on a green roof have lower cortisol levels and improved immune system function, for example. No matter where a person lives or works, there is always the ability to interact with nature. This can be as simple as having indoor plants in your home, looking out your window at a green space, or actually sitting under a tree. Nature done this way is typically free but profoundly impactful. I have devised a patient education trifold that can be accessed at http://online.flipbuilder.com/cbgg/tosn/html.http://online.flipbuilder.com/cbgg/nxny /html.[147–148]

CASE STUDIES

CASE STUDY 1. AD IN A TRADITIONAL SETTING.

A 55-year-old woman was diagnosed with Hashimoto's thyroiditis in her 20s, psoriasis in her 30s, and rheumatoid arthritis in her 40s. Pre-diabetes has been diagnosed as well as insomnia, fatigue, urinary stress incontinence at times of large amounts, diarrhea, abdominal bloating and pain after meals, gastroesophageal reflux disease, nausea, memory and concentration issues, low mood, excessive anxiety and worry, dysmenorrhea, menorrhagia, premenstrual syndrome, ovarian cyst, breast cysts, fibroids, two miscarriages, dry skin, easy bruising, brittle nails, chronic sinusitis, recurrent vaginal yeast infections, occasional lightheadedness, palpitations, and allergies, and she has had skin cancer once.

Her main complaint includes diffuse joint pain involving the hands, wrists, elbows, knees, and ankles. The left knee and pain in the small joints of the hands are the worst. She has muscle pain involving the lower back and neck with frequent severe calf cramps at night causing her to jump out of bed when they occur. She also has tension headaches four to five times per week and migraine headaches one to two times per month. These migraine headaches used to occur with her menstrual cycles before she had her hysterectomy due to large fibroids. The hysterectomy occurred 18 months before the joint pain started that was later diagnosed as rheumatoid arthritis. She also has tingling, numbness, and burning pain in her feet that used to come and go but is now constant and getting worse. Also, her "sciatica" can be extremely problematic at times but seems to respond to "a steroid shot in my back and some physical therapy but it seems to always want to come back." She also tells you that the menstrual cramps she had for many years prior to her hysterectomy "were just killer."

So here is a "typical" AD patient when it comes to experiencing multiple types of pain and health issues beginning at a young age, with a gradual addition of new types of pain over the years as her immune system dysregulation got worse over time. Multiple organ systems are involved on top of all the pain. This can look like a very confusing picture to many practitioners. But the only way all these organ systems can be thrown off at the same time is if a really important central mechanism has been thrown off, or there are multiple important central mechanisms that are not doing the work that needs to be done.

Because we know she has an AD, we know exactly where to look to find out why. Then, whatever is causing the immune system dysregulation is also causing much if not all of the pain and other issues. Initial tests are run. Issues found are addressed. Retesting occurs at intervals. Fine-tuning of issues still present are taken care of. After proper assessment and addressing root cause, the patient reported dramatic improvement in symptoms. Now, whatever symptoms are still present enough to negatively impact her quality of life can be given more personal attention and addressed specifically. If the issues that still remain are pain problems, the other chapters in this book will give the vital information required to optimize management no matter what type of pain is involved.

CASE STUDY 2. "BILSTROM'S NUCLEARITIS."

What to do with a person who has many of the symptoms and organ systems involved similar to Case Study 1 but no definitive, named ADs yet diagnosed? Antibodies are negative for rheumatoid arthritis and Hashimoto's thyroiditis as well as other ADs. All the issues make people think that AD is a possibility, but repeated testing over and over again keeps coming back negative except for a positive ANA.

A positive ANA up to this point has not had a proper name. The immune system is attacking our own nuclear material, thus, the name anti-nuclear antibody. It is definitely not a good idea to attack our own DNA.

Thus, "Bilstrom's Nuclearitis." Definition: Bilstrom's Nuclearitis. Noun. A chronic autoimmune disease characterized by the production of antibodies which mistakenly attack proteins in the nucleus of cells within the human body including structures such as DNA. First described by American physiatrist, functional medicine and integrative medicine physician David Bilstrom in 2018.

Now we have a named disease to go with a positive ANA. Now treatment can be initiated potentially years earlier, rather than waiting until additional body parts are attacked (new autoantibodies being produced) and the patient's functional status and quality of life are so compromised that medications like immunosuppressants, NSAIDs, and opioids must be the first line of treatment. Thus, the not unsubstantial potential risks of these medications could be avoided when the AD process has a name and is addressed earlier, such as the potential for the immunosuppressants to cause a user to get a new AD as well.[13,17] These medicines will also increase your risk of getting cancer, such as lymphoma, or a life-threatening infection.[15,16,149]

Having a proper name for the disease, which occurs when the ANA is positive, helps to initiate proper treatment earlier than is usually done. Particularly when it is the first antibody to be produced, the autoimmune process can hopefully be reversed before the immune system starts to attack new body structures. If a person is producing thyroid antibodies along with the positive ANA, the TPO and thyroglobulin antibodies can be a nice way to track how well the immune system dysregulation process is being reversed right along with how the person is feeling; the goal being for thyroid antibody numbers to go down to normal levels and the ANA to turn negative.

CASE STUDY 3. LOSS OF IMMUNE SYSTEM SET POINT WITH NO AUTOIMMUNE DISEASE.

How about a person with many different types of pain but no autoimmune processes initiated yet, not even a positive ANA? They have right knee pain, right shoulder pain, bilateral hand pain, low back pain, neck pain, and headaches. This is where the detailed past medical history that has been taken on all patients with chronic disease can be so helpful. This is often the history of the patient type we discussed in case reports numbers 1 and 2 prior to the start of any autoimmune process. Patient birth history is significant for being born 4 weeks early, delivered by C-section, and not breast-fed. Babies delivered by C-section have their intestinal microbiome made up of a microorganism mixture similar to what is on the lighting fixtures in the delivery room and the skin of the nurses present.[150] This is much different than the intestinal microbiome of children delivered vaginally. The intestinal microbiome will also not be well-established without being adequately breast-fed.[151] Being delivered vaginally and breast-fed are the two most important activities to establish early on for a healthy gut microbiome and a healthy immune system. Remember, 80% of our immune system surrounds the gut.

Childhood history includes colic as a baby with intolerance to formula. This person has already developed a dairy protein or the dairy sugar lactose intolerance, possibly due to the disrupted microbiome and too many not good bacteria. First antibiotic was used at two months of age, as early antibiotic use is much more disruptive to the gut.[152] It doesn't even take a whole course.

The child or teenager has recurrent ear infections, sinus infections, and strep throat. These are downregulated immune system issues. They also have developed some allergies and eczema and maybe even asthma. These are upregulated immune system issues. Already we can see the loss of the immune system set point before the age of 18. You can see that this individual is moving towards a future with not only AD and cancer but chronic diseases in general including pain. These may only show up years or decades later, but the process has already started. Now the person also developed mononucleosis in high school. People who have had "mono" more than double their chance of getting multiple sclerosis.[84,85] If this person is a female, menstrual cycles began at age 13 and right away she developed bad flows, bad cramps, and bad premenstrual syndrome. Estrogen dominance is already established, and this is a big driver of AD. This is one reason why women are much more likely to get AD than men; 80% are women in fact.[1]

In her 20s, she developed mild hypertension, probably due to cortisol being stuck in the "on" position. "Running from a bear" tends to cause blood pressure to go up. Here comes an elevated LDL and total cholesterol. The liver, which makes LDL cholesterol, might be trying to feed the steroidogenic hormone production cascade. The liver is making more LDL cholesterol then would typically seem appropriate. With cortisol production high due to being stuck in the "on" position, progesterone levels start to drop, exacerbating the estrogen dominance. The body, always trying to self-correct, is trying to feed the steroidogenic hormone production cascade in order to make more progesterone or DHEA or testosterone, etc., in order to keep the person healthy and well-balanced, despite the cortisol issue. Unfortunately, in this situation, our response to an elevated LDL and total cholesterol might be to give a statin medication. If this is the reason why lipid numbers are running high, these medications will "cut off at the knees" the body's ability to self-correct and fix the hormone deficiency and imbalance problem. This is one reason why we can see cholesterol numbers rise a couple years after statin medications are initiated. The body has found a way around the blockade and is trying to self-correct the hormone issues again. Our typical response? Increase the dose or change to a different statin medication.

Because the estrogen dominance has caused fibroids to be produced on top of the bad flows, the person has a hysterectomy. Unfortunately, a hysterectomy will tend to make the estrogen dominance worse.[153] The person no longer has bad flows and bad cramps or fibroids. But the estrogen dominance will be even worse. The estrogen dominance has also probably produced, usually by the mid-30s if not earlier, insomnia and anxiety. Estrogen is like the "gas pedal" and progesterone is like the "brake pedal." Too much gas or revving of the engine and not enough breaking or calming will cause anxiety and insomnia. Estrogen dominance is so common.

Because of the gut disruption, gastroesophageal reflux disease and constipation become issues. Acid-blocking medicines are started which guarantee vitamin and mineral deficiencies and the inability to digest food optimally.[154] Constipation is now contributing to the inability to clear toxins from the body, both environmental toxins and internally produced toxic byproducts of metabolism. Old toxic estrogens dumped into the gut for removal from the body are instead reactivated and reabsorbed into the body, making the estrogen dominance worse. The gut and immune system issues have now allowed chronic infections to become established not only in the gut but systemically as well. A very common chronic systemic infection in this population is candida or other mold species. Common symptoms of systemic mold include joint pain, muscle pain, brain fog, fatigue, sinus issues, and weight gain. Systemic mycoplasma may be driving the person towards rheumatoid arthritis and all that joint pain they are developing. That chronic Epstein–Barr virus issue may be trying to drive the person towards multiple sclerosis.

So now we are back to the person with the early disruption of the immune system set point. There is multiple organ system involvement, producing many different symptoms including pain. We need to recognize the loss of the immune system set point, do the proper testing, and address what is found. If any pain remains, we have many wonderful interventions to address the pain, whether it is joint, muscle, nerve, central sensitization, or mitochondrial dysfunction.

POTENTIAL TESTING LIMITATIONS

It should be noted that not all patients will have insurance coverage for saliva cortisol and digestive stool analysis testing, while others will have no co-pay at all. Or, even when insurance will cover these tests, the co-pays may be beyond reach. Testing which is never covered by insurance, such as food sensitivity and provocative heavy metal, will tend to have a more reasonable cost, even though it will need to be paid fully as an out-of-pocket expense. The institution may not be ready to use this type of advanced testing and thus only blood work is available. The patient's history, physical exam, and blood work in addition to more traditional testing when necessary, such as EMG and nerve conduction studies, may be the only data available.

CONCLUSION

Treating pain in patients with immune system dysregulation or frank AD has historically been very challenging. As we see here though, simply by addressing the underlying mechanisms involved in the immune system dysregulation, pain problems of all kinds tend to simply "fade away." It is quite satisfying when a practitioner sees this happen. Also, most of the other symptoms that are problematic for the patient are clearing at the same time.

Fortunately, any pain issues that persist, despite optimal management of the immune system dysregulation, can be addressed using the information found in the rest of this book. The information provided in the other chapters of this book will have a profound impact on any pain that remains.

REFERENCES

1. American Autoimmune Related Diseases Association, Inc. Autoimmune diseases statistics, https://www.aardu.org/news-information/statictics/html.
2. Liang X. et al. Bidirectional interactions between indomethacin and murine intestinal microbiota. *eLife* 2015;4. doi:10.7554/eLife.08973.
3. Van Wijak K. et al. Aggravation of exercise-induced intestinal injury by ibuprofen in athletes. *Med Sci Sports Exerc* 2012;44(12):2257–2262.
4. Zoorob R.J., Cender D. A different look at corticosteroids. *Am Fam Phys* 1998;58(2):443–450.
5. Orlicka K. et al. Prevention of infection caused by immunosuppressive drugs in gastroenterology. *Ther Adv Chronic Dis* 2013;4(4):167–185.
6. Klein C.J. et al. Chronic pain as a manifestation of potassium channel-complex autoimmunity. *Neurology* 2012;79(11):1136–1144.
7. Coury F. et al. Rheumatoid arthritis and fibromyalgia: a frequent unrelated association complicating disease management. *J Rhuematol* 2009;36(1):58–62.

8. National Human Genome Research Institute. The human genome project completion: frequently asked questions. https://genome.gov/11006943/human-genome-project-completion-frequently-asked-que stions/html.

9. Belshaw R. et al. Long-term reinfection of the human genome by endogenous retroviruses. *Proc Natl Acad Sci U S A* 2004;101(14):4894–4899.

10. Nelson P.N. et al. Human endogenous retroviruses: transposable elements with potential? *Clin Exp Immunol* 2004;138(1):1–9.

11. Zimmer K. Can viruses in the genome cause disease? *The Scientist* 2019 January 1. https://www.the-scie ntist.com/features/can-viruses-in-the-genome-cause-disease--65212.

12. Brooks W.H., Renaudineau Y. Epigenetics and autoimmune diseases: the X chromosome-nucleolus nexus. *Front Genet* 2015;6:22.

13. Caspi R. Immunotherapy of autoimmunity and cancer: the penalty for success. *Nat Rev Immunol* 2008;8(12):970–976.

14. Boelaert K. et al. Prevalence and relative risk of other autoimmune diseases in subjects with autoimmune thyroid disease. *Am J Med* 2010;123(2):183.e1–183.e9.

15. Barclay L. et al. Rheumatoid arthritis treatment increases cancer risk. *Arthritis Care Res* 2008;59:794–799.

16. https://rheumatoidarthritis.net/living/weighing-the-risks-glenn-frey-and-drugs/html.

17. Araújo-Fernandez S. et al. Drug-induced lupus: including anti-tumour necrosis factor and interferon induced. *Lupus* 2014;23(6):545–553.

18. Anaya J.-m. et al. The autoimmune ecology. *Front Immunol* 2016;7:139.

19. Kivity S. et al. Vitamin D and autoimmune thyroid diseases. *Cell Mol Immunol* 2011;8(3):243–247.

20. Delitala A.P. et al. Thyroid hormones, metabolic syndrome and its components. *Endocr Metab Immune Disord Drug Targets* 2017;17(1):56–62.

21. Joseph J. et al. Diurnal salivary cortisol, glycemia and insulin resistance: the multi-ethnic study of atherosclerosis. *Psychoneuroendocrinology* 2015;62:327–335.

22. Worthington J. The intestinal immunoendocrine axis: novel cross-talk between enteroendocrine cells and the immune system during infection and inflammatory disease. *Biochem Soc Trans* 2015;43(4):727–733.

23. Kabouridis P.S., Pachnis V. Emerging roles of gut microbiota and the immune system in the development of the enteric nervous system. *J Clin Invest* 2015;125(3):956–964.

24. Chen C.Q. et al. Distribution, function and physiological role of melatonin in the lower gut. *World J Gastroenterol* 2011;17(34):3888–3898.

25. Accurate education-melatonin. https://accurateclinic.com/accurate-education-melatonin/.

26. Kieffer DA. et al. Impact of dietary fibers on nutrient management and detoxification organs: gut, liver and kidneys. *Adv Nutr* 2016;7(6):1111–1121.

27. Furness J.B. et al. Nutrient testing and signaling mechanisms in the gut. The intestine as a sensory organ: neural, endocrine, and immune responses. *Am J Physiol* 1999;277(5):6922–6928.

28. Caraba A. et al. Vitamin D status, disease activity, and endothelial dysfunction in early rheumatoid arthritis patients. *Dis Markers* 2017;Article ID 5241012:7 pages.

29. Castro-Nallar E. et al. Composition, taxonomy and functional diversity of the oropharynx microbiome in individuals with schizophrenia and controls. *PeerJ* 2015;3:e1140.

30. Schenkein H.A., Loos B.G.. Inflammatory mechanisms linking periodontal disease to cardiovascular disease. *J Clin Periodont* 2015;40(Suppl 14):s51–s69.

31. Hoggard M. et al. Chronic rhinosinusitis and the evolving understanding of microbial ecology in chronic inflammatory mucosal disease. *Clin Microbiol Rev* 2017;30(1):321–348.

32. Paules C.I. et al. Tickborne diseases-confronting a growing threat. *N Engl J Med* 2018;379(8):701–703.

33. Celiac Disease Foundation. Symptoms of celiac disease. https://celiac.org/about-celiac-disease/sympt oms-of-celiac-disease/html.

34. Celiac Disease Foundation. What is celiac disease. https://celiac.org/about-celiac-disease/what-is-ce liac-disease/.

35. Coeliac Australia. https://coeliac.org.au/.

36. Magnesium in Diet. MedlinePlus(.gov). https://medlineplus.gov/ency/article/002423.html.

37. Tengrup I. et al. Influence on zinc synthesis and the accumulation of collagen in early granulation tissue. *Surg Gynecol Obstet* 1981;152(3):323–326.

38. Gupta P.G. Role of iron (Fe) in body. *IOSR JAC* 2014;7(11).

39. Ernster L., Dallner G. Biochemical, physiological and medical aspects of ubiquinone function. *Biochim Biophys Acta* 1995;1271(1):195–204.

40. Chen K.J. et al. Association of B vitamins status and homocysteine levels in elderly Taiwanese. *Asia Pac J Clin Nutr* 2005;14(3):250–255.

41. Porter K. et al. Causes, consequences and public health implications of low B-vitamin status in aging. *Nutrients* 2016;8(11): 725.

42. Boldyrev A. et al. Why is homocysteine toxic for the nervous and immune systems? *Curr Aging Sci* 2013;6(1):29–36.

43. Perla-Kajan J. et al. Mechanisms of homocysteine toxicity in humans. *Amino Acids* 2007;32(4):561–572.

44. Egnell M. et al. B-vitamin intake from diet and supplements and breast cancer risk in women: results from the prospective NutriNet-Sante cohort. *Nutrients* 2017;9(5).

45. Dai Z., Koh W.P. B-vitamins and bone health: a review of the current evidence. *Nutrients* 2015; 7(5):3322–3346.

46. Kaluzna-Czaplinska J. A focus on homocysteine in autism. *Acta Biochim Pol* 2013;60(2):137–142.

47. Altun H. et al. The levels of vitamin D, vitamin D receptors, homocysteine and complex B vitamin in children with autism spectrum disorders. *Clin Psychopharmacol Neurosci* 2018;16(4):383–390.

48. Oikonomidi A. et al. Homocysteine metabolism is associated with cerebrospinal fluid levls of soluble amyloid precursor protein and amyloid beta. *J Neurochem* 2016;139(2):324–332.

49. McCully K.S. Hyperhomocysteinemia, suppressed immunity, and altered oxidative metabolism caused by pathologic microbes in atherosclerosis and dementia. *Front Aging Neurosci* 2017;9:324.

50. McCully K.S. Homocysteine, infections, polyamines, oxidative metabolism, and the pathogenesis of dementia and atherosclerosis. *J Alzheimers Dis* 2016;54(4):1283–1290.

51. Patterson S. et al. Major metabolic homocysteine-derivative, homocysteine thiolactone, exerts changes in pancreatic beta-cell glucose sensing, cellular signal transduction and integrity. *Arch Biochem Biophys* 2007;461(2):287–293.

52. Gominak S.C. Vitamin D deficiency changes the intestinal microbiota reducing B vitamin production in the gut. The resulting lack of Pantothenic Acid adversely affects the immune system, producing a 'pro-inflammatory' state associated with atherosclerosis and autoimmunity. *Med Hypotheses* 2016;94:103–107.

53. Shandal V., Luo J.J. Clinical manifestations of isolated elevated homocysteine-induced peripheral neuropathy in adults. *J Clin Neuromuscul Dis* 2016;17(3):106–109.

54. Solomon L.R. Vitamin B-12 responsive neuropathies: a case series. *Nutr Neurosci* 2016;19(4):162–168.

55. Solomon L.R. Functional vitamin B-12 deficiency in advanced malignancy: implications for the management of neuropathy and neuropathic pain. *Support Care Cancer* 2016;24(8):3489–3494.

56. Sands S. et al. Glutamine for the treatment of vincristine-induced neuropathy in children and adolescents with cancer. *Support Care Cancer* 2017;25(3):701–708.

57. Manevski N. et al. Phase II metabolism in human skin: skin explants show full coverage for glucuronidation, sulfation, N-acetylation, catechol methylation, and glutathione conjugation. *Drug Metab Dispos* 2015;43(1):126–139.

58. Santos K.F. et al. The prima donna of epigenetics: the regulation of gene expression by DNA methylation. *Braz J Med Biol Res* 2005;38(10):1531–1541.

59. Munger K. et al. Vitamin D status during pregnancy and risk of multiple sclerosis in offspring of women in the Finnish maternity cohort. *JAMA Neurol* 2016;73(5):515–519.

60. Hypponeu E. et al. Intake of vitamin D and type 1 diabetes: a birth-cohort study. *Lancet* 2001; 358(9292):1500–1503.

61. McDonnell S. et al. Breast cancer-risk markedly lower with serum 25-hydroxy vitamin D concentrations > 60 vs <20 ng/ml (150 vs 50 nmol/L): pooled analysis of two randomized trials and a prospective cohort. *PLOS* 2018 June 15. doi:10.1371/journal.pone.0199265.

62. Garland C. et al. The role of vitamin D in cancer prevention. *Am J Public Health* 2006;96(2):252–261.

63. Bakke D., Sun J. Ancient nuclear receptor VDR with new functions: microbiome and inflammation. *Inflamm Bowel Dis* 2018;24(6):1149–1154.

64. Ginde A. et al. Demographic differences and trends in vitamin D insufficiency in the US population, 1988–2004. *Arch Intern Med* 2009;169(6):626–632.

65. Faraj S., Al Mutairi K. Vitamin D deficiency and chronic low back pain in Saudi Arabia. *Spine (Phila Pa 1976)* 2003;28(2):177–179.

66. Peterson S.J. et al. Is a normal TSH synonymous with 'Euthyroidism' in levothyroxine monotherapy? *J Clin Endocrinol Metab* 2016;101(12):4964–4973.

67. Davis D.R. et al. Changes in USDA food composition data for 43 garden crops, 1950 to 1999. *J Am Coll Nutr* 2004;23(6):669–682.

68. International Foundation for Gastrointestinal Disorders. Statistics facts about IBS. https://www.abo utibs.org/facts-about-ibs/statistics.html.

69. Body Burden: The Pollution in Newborns. *A Benchmark Investigation of Industrial Chemicals, Pollutants and Pesticides in Umbilical Cord Blood.* 2005 July 14. Environmental Working Group.

70. Tivesten Å et al. Dehydroepiandrosterone and its sulfate predict the 5-year risk of coronary heart disease events in elderly men. *J Am Coll Cardiol* 2014;64(17):1801–1810.

71. Jimenez M. et al. Low dehydroepiandrosterone sulphate is associated with increased risk of ischemic stroke among women. *Stroke* 2013;44(7):1784–1789.

72. Pluchino N. et al. Neurobiology of DHEA and effects on sexuality, mood and cognition. *J Steroid Biochem Mol Biol* 2015;145:273–280.

73. Hughes G.C., Choubey D. Modulation of autoimmune rheumatic diseases by oestrogen and progesterone. *Nat Rev Rheumatol* 2014;10(12):740–751.

74. Kelly D.M., Jones T.H. Testosterone: a metabolic hormone in health and disease. *J Endocrinol* 2013;217(3):R25–R45.

75. Kaltenboeck A. et al. The direct and indirect costs among US privately insured employees with hypogonadism. *J Sex Med* 2012;9(9):2438–2447.

76. Murkes D. et al. Percutaneous estradiol/oral micronized progesterone has less adverse effects and different gene regulations than oral conjugated equine estrogens/medroxyprogesterone acetate in the breasts of healthy women in vivo. *Gynecol Endocrinol* 2012;28(Suppl 2):21–25.

77. Goodman M.P. Are all estrogens created equal? A review of oral vs transdermal therapy. *J Womens Health (Larchmt)* 2012;21(2):161–169.

78. Du J.Y. et al. Percutaneous progesterone delivery via cream or gel application in postmenopausal women: a randomized cross-over study of progesterone levels in serum, whole blood, saliva and capillary blood. *Menopause* 2013;20(11):1169–1175.

79. O'Leary P. et al. Salivary, but not serum or urinary levels of progesterone are elevated after topical application of progesterone cream to pre and postmenopausal women. *Clin Endocrinol* 2000;53(5):615–620.

80. Mendelsohn M., Karas R.H. The protective effects of estrogen on the cardiovascular system. *N Engl J Med* 1999;340(23):1801–1811.

81. Lyytinen H. et al. Breast cancer risk in postmenopausal women using estrogen-only therapy. *Obstet Gynecol* 2006;108(6):1354–1360.

82. Westaby D. et al. Liver damage from long-term methyltestosterone. *Lancet* 1977;2(8032):262–263.

83. Celiac Disease-Diagnosis and Treatment-Mayo Clinic. https://www.mayoclinic.org/diseases-conditions/celiac-disease/diagnosis-treatment/drc-20352225.

84. Nielsen T.R. et al. Multiple sclerosis after infectious mononucleosis. *Arch Neurol* 2007;64(1):72–75.

85. Handel A.E. et al. An updated meta-analysis of the risk of multiple sclerosis following infectious mononucleosis. *PLOS ONE* 2010 Sep 1;5(9).

86. Railean-Plugaru V. et al. Antimicrobial properties of biosynthesized silver nanoparticles studied by flow cytometry and related techniques. *Electrophoresis* 2016;37(5–6):752–761.

87. Khan S. et al. Nanosilver: new ageless and versatile biomedical therapeutic scaffold. *Int J Nanomed* 2018;13:733–762.

88. Silver as a drinking-water disinfectant. World Health Organization. 2018. https://creativecommans.org/licences/by-nc-sa/3.0/igo.

89. Johnson J. et al. *The* Medico-Chirurgical Review *and* Journal *of* Practical Medicine, vol. 24. New York: Richard George S Wood;1836.

90. Sakihara S. et al. Evaluation of plasma, salivary, and urinary cortisol levels for diagnosis of Cushing's syndrome. *Endocr J* 2010;57(4):331–337.

91. Tsigos C., Chrousos G.P. Hypothalamic-pituitary-adrenal axis, neuroendocrine factors and stress. *J Psychosom Res* 2002;53(4):865–871.

92. Selye H. Stress and the general adaptation syndrome. *Br Med J* 1950;1(4667):1383–1392.

93. McEwen B. Protecting and damaging effects of stress mediators. *N Engl J Med* 2008;338:171–179.

94. Joseph J., Golden S.H. Cortisol dysregulation: the bidirectional link between stress, depression, and type 2 diabetes mellitus. *Ann N Y Acad Sci* 2017;1391(1):20–34.

95. Chandrasekhar K. et al. A prospective, randomized double-blind, placebo controlled study of safety and efficacy of a high-concentration full-spectrum extract of Ashwagandha root in reducing stress and anxiety in adults. *Indian J Psychol Med* 2012;34(3):255–262.

96. de J R De-Paula V et al. Relevance of gut microbiota in cognition, behavior and Alzheimer's disease. *Pharmacol Res* 2018;136:29–34.

97. Patel S. et al. Estrogen: the necessary evil for human health, and ways to tame it. *Biomed Pharmacother* 2018;102:403–411.

98. Cakir M. et al. Musculoskeletal manifestations in patients with thyroid disease. *Clin Endocrinol (Oxf)*;59(2):162–167.

99. Vincent K., Tracey I. Hormones and their interaction with the pain experience. *Rev Pain* 2008;2(2):20–24.

100. Roman-Blas J.A. et al. Osteoarthritis associated with estrogen deficiency. *Arthritis Res Ther* 2009; 11(5):241.

101. Verdi J. et al. The effect of progesterone on expression and development of neuropathic pain in a rat model of peripheral neuropathy. *Eur J Pharmacol* 2013;699(1–3):207–212.

102. Kumar P. et al. Exocrine dysfunction correlates with endocrinal impairment of pancreas in type 2 diabetes mellitus. *Indian J Endocrinol Metab* 2018;22(1):121–125.

103. Menees S.B. et al. A meta-analysis of the utility of C-reactive protein, erythrocyte sedimentation rate, fecal calprotectin, and fecal lactoferrin to exclude inflammatory bowel disease in adults with IBS. *Am J Gastroenterol* 2015;110(3):444–454.

104. Dabritz J. et al. Diagnostic utility of faecal biomarkers in patients with irritable bowel syndrome. *World J Gastroenterol* 2014;20(2):363–375.

105. Parsons K. et al. Novel testing enhances irritable bowel syndrome medical management: the IMMINENT study. *Glob Acv. Health Med* 2014;3(3):25–32.

106. Waugh GE et al. 2013. *Faecal Calprotectin Testing for Differentiating Amongst Inflammatory and Non-Inflammatory Bowel Diseases: Systematic Review and Economic Evaluation*. Chapter 4 discussion. Queen's Printer and Controller of HMSO;2013:1–37.

107. Bjarnason I. The use of fecal calprotectin in inflammatory bowel disease. *Gastroenterol Hepatol N Y* 2017;13(1):53–56.

108. Vojdani A. et al. Environmental triggers and autoimmunity. *Autoimmune Dis* 2014;2014:798029.

109. Autoimmune Registry. Estimates of prevalence for autoimmune disease. http://www.autoimmuneregistry.org/autoimmune-statistics/html.

110. Fairweather D., Rose N.R. Women and autoimmune diseases. *Emerg Infect Dis* 2004;10(11):2005–2011.

111. Lerner A. et al. The world incidence and prevalence of autoimmune diseases is increasing. *Int J Celiac Dis* 2015;3(4):151–155.

112. Machi S. et al. The national burdens of rheumatoid arthritis and osteoarthritis in Japan: projections to the year 2010, with future changes in severity distribution. *Mod Rheum* 2004;14(4):285–290.

113. Yamanaka H. et al. Estimates of the prevalence of and current treatment practices for rheumatoid arthritis in Japan using reimbursement data from health insurance societies and IORRA cohort. *Mod Rheumatol* 2014;24(1):33–40.

114. Chang C.Y. et al. Essential fatty acids and human brain. *Acta Neurol Taiwan* 2009;18(4):231–241.

115. Lanphear B. et al. Low-level lead exposure and mortality in US adults: a population-based cohort study. *Lancet* 2018;3(4):e177–e184.

116. Nawrot T., Staessen J.A. Low-level environmental exposure to lead unmasked as silent killer. *Circulation* 2006;114(13):1347–1349.

117. Agency for toxic substances and disease activity. Lead toxicity. What is the biologic fate of lead in the body? https://atsdr.cdc.gov/csem/csem.asp?csem=4&po=9.html.

118. Pizzorno J. Is challenge testing valid for assessing body metal burden? *Integ Med* 2015;14(4):8–14.

119. Crinnion W.J. The benefits of pre- and post-challenge urine heavy metal testing: part 1. *Altern Med Rev* 2009;14(1):3–8.

120. Crinnion W.J. The benefit of pre- and post-challenge urine heavy metal testing: part 2. *Altern Med Rev* 2009;14(2):103–108.

121. Kubasik N.P., Volosin M.T. Heavy metal poisoning: clinical aspects and laboratory analysis. *Am J Med Technol* 1973;39(11):443–450.

122. Efstratiadis G. et al. Hypomagnesemia and cardiovascular system. *Hippokratia* 2006;10(4):147–152.

123. Masters S.B. et al. *Katzurg and Trevor's Pharmacology: Examination and Board Review*, 18th ed. McGraw Hill Medical;2019:481–483.

124. Ali A. et al. Efficacy of individualized diets in patients with irritable bowel syndrome: a randomized controlled trial. *BMJ Open Gastroenterol* 2017;4(1):e000164.

125. Lozano-Ojalvo D. et al. Immune basis of food allergic reactions. *J Investig Allergol Clin Immunol* 2019;29(1).

126. Justiz Valliant A.A. et al. Hypersensitivity reactions, immediate. StatPearls. Internet. Treasure Island, FL: StatPearls Publishing;2018.

127. Gupta M. et al. Diagnosis of food allergy. *Immunol Allergy Clin North Am* 2018;38(1):39–52.

128. Gordon B.R. Approaches to testing for food and chemical sensitivities. *Otolaryngol Clin North Am* 2003;36(5):917–940.

129. Fell P. et al. High correlation of the Alcat test results with double blind challenge (DBC) in food sensitivity. In 45th Annual Congress of the American College of Allergy and Immunology. Los Angeles: Annals of Allergy;1988.

130. Solomon B. The ALCAT test- A guide and barometer in the therapy of environmental and food sensitivities. *Environ Med* 1992;9(2).

131. Wahls T. 2014. *The Wahls Protocol.* New York: Penguin Group.

132. Cai C. et al. Serological investigation of food specific immunoglobulin G antibodies in patients with inflammatory bowel diseases. *PLOS ONE* 2014;9(11):e112154. doi:10.1371/journal.pone.0112154.

133. Virdee K. et al. Food-specific IgG antibody-guided elimination diets followed by resolution of asthma symptoms and reduction in pharmacological interventions in two patients: a case report. *Glob Adv Health Med* 2015;4(1):62–66.

134. Alpay K. et al. Diet restriction in migraine, based on IgG against foods: a clinical double-blind, randomized, cross-over trial. *Cephalalgia* 30(7):829–837.

135. Guo H. et al. The value of eliminating foods according to food-specific immunoglobulin G antibodies in irritable bowel syndrome with diarrhea. *J Int Med Res* 2012;40(1):204–210.

136. Neuendorf R. et al. Impact of food immunoglobulin G-based elimination diet on subsequent food immunoglobulin G and quality of life in overweight/obese adults. *J Alt Compl Med* 2019;25(2):241–248.

137. Karakula-Juchnowicz H. et al. The food-specific serum IgG reactivity in major depressive disorder patients, irritable bowel syndrome patients and healthy controls. *Nutrients* 2018;10(5):548. doi:10.3390/nu10050548.

138. Tao R. et al. Chronic food antigen-specific IgG-mediated hypersensitivity reaction as a risk factor for adolescent depressive disorder. *Genomics Proteomics Bioinformatics* 2019;17(2):183–189.

139. Brown N., Panksepp J. Low-dose naltrexone for disease prevention and quality of life. *Med Hypotheses* 2009;72(3):333–337.

140. Smith J. et al. Safety and tolerability of low dose naltrexone therapy in children with moderate to severe Crohn's disease: a pilot study. *J Clin Gastroenterol* 2013;47(4):339–345.

141. Forman H. et al. Glutathione: overview of its protective roles, measurement, and biosynthesis. *Mol Aspects Med* 2009;30(1–2):1–12.

142. Comporti M. Glutathione depleting agents and lipid peroxidation. *Chem Phys Lipids* 1987;45(2):143–169.

143. van der Toorn M. et al. Cigarette smoke irreversibly modifies glutathione in airway epithelial cells. *Am J Physiol Lung Cell Mol Physiol* 2007;293(5):L1156–L1162.

144. Maranzana A., Mehlhorn R.J. Loss of glutathione, ascorbate recycling, and free radical scavenging in human erythrocytes exposed to filtered cigarette smoke. *Arch Biochem Biophys* 1998;350(2):169–182.

145. Reid C. et al. Critical review of health impacts of wildfire smoke exposure. *Environ Health Perspect* 2016;124(9):1334–1343.

146. Sandifer P. et al. Exploring connections among nature, biodiversity, ecosystem services, and human health and well-being. Opportunities to enhance health and biodiversity conservation. *Ecosyst Serv* 2005;12:1–15.

147. Bingham Memorial Hospital. Health and healing through nature. Patient educational information. http://online.flipbuilder.com/cbgg/tosn/html.

148. Bingham Memorial Hospital. Health and healing through nature. Physician educational information. http://online.flipbuilder.com/cbgg/nxny/html.

149. Miyazaki T. et al. Remission of lymphoma after withdrwal of methotrexate in rheumatoid arthritis: relationship with type of latent Epstein-Barr virus infection. *Am J Hematol* 2007;82(12):1106–1109.

150. Dominguez-Bello M.G. et al. Delivery mode shapes the acquisition and structure of the initial microbiota across multiple body habitats in newborns. *Proc Natl Acad Sci USA* 2010;107(26):11971–11975.

151. O'Sullivan A. et al. The influence of early infant-feeding practices on the intestinal microbiome and body composition in infants. *Nutr Metab Insights* 2015;(Suppl 1):1–9.

152. Gasparrini A. et al. Antibiotic pertubation of the preterm infant gut microbiome and resistome. *Gut Microbes* 2016;7(5):443–449.

153. Moorman P. et al. Effect of hysterectomy with ovarian preservation on ovarian failure. *Obstet Gynecol* 2011;118(6):1271–1279.

154. Corsonello A. et al. Adverse events of proton pump inhibitors: potential mechanisms. *Curr Drug Metab* 2018;19(2):142–154.

7 Fibromyalgia
A Comprehensive Perspective

Sahar Swidan and Kai-Uwe Kern

CONTENTS

WHAT IS FIBROMYALGIA?

Fibromyalgia is a complex chronic health condition that causes widespread pain and tenderness and a heightened sensitivity to sounds, light, and touch. The pain varies in intensity, migrates around the body, and has been described as stabbing and shooting, with deep muscular aching, throbbing, and twitching.[1] Patients can also experience neurologic pain symptoms such as numbness and tingling or a burning sensation. Other symptoms often present include severe fatigue, sleep problems (waking up unrefreshed), and problems with memory or thinking clearly.[2] Patients will also often have comorbidities including depression or anxiety, migraine or tension headaches, restless legs, skin sensitivity, impaired coordination, digestive problems including irritable bowel syndrome or gastroesophageal reflux disease (GERD), irritable or overactive bladder, pelvic pain, and temporomandibular disorder (TMJ).[2] Fibromyalgia affects 2–4% of people, women much more often than men.

There is no diagnostic test that leads to an objective diagnosis of fibromyalgia. Diagnosis is based on patient-reported pain and symptoms, patient history, and physical examination. Symptoms of fibromyalgia mimic symptoms of other conditions, and additional testing (e.g., blood tests and imaging studies) is commonly performed to rule out other conditions.

Due to the difficulty of diagnosis, some estimates have determined an average of 5 years from the time a patient first reports symptoms to the time a diagnosis of fibromyalgia is made.[3]

According to the 2010 American College of Rheumatology fibromyalgia diagnostic criteria,[4] patients are asked if they have had chronic widespread pain and tenderness, defined as pain and tenderness on both sides of the body, above and below the waist including the axial spine (usually the paraspinal, scapular, and trapezium muscles), over 19 different regions of their body during the past week using the widespread pain index (WPI). The symptom severity (SS) scale is used to quantify problems with fatigue, unrefreshed sleep, cognitive dysfunction, and a number of somatic symptoms over the previous week. A diagnosis of fibromyalgia is made based on the following criteria:

*   WPI score ≥7 and SS scale score ≥5 or WPI score 3–6 and SS scale score >9
*   Symptoms have been present at a similar level for at least 3 months
*   Patient does not have a disorder that could otherwise explain the pain

The causes of fibromyalgia are not clear and can vary among different people. Fibromyalgia is considered its own entity as it does not fit an autoimmune, inflammation, joint, or muscle disorder in the classic sense. Research suggests that the central nervous system in particular plays an active role in fibromyalgia pain.[1] Fibromyalgia likely has a genetic component, making some people more prone to acquiring the disease and other comorbidities. There are also triggers that can worsen symptoms including diet, hormones, schedule, sleep, weather, and physical and emotional stress.[1,2] Patients often experience a decreased quality of life due to discomfort and pain.

A variety of possible mechanisms have been proposed but, because these mechanistic abnormalities are not found in all patients, finding effective treatments has been difficult (Table 7.1). There is increasing evidence that changes in inflammatory mediators and a disturbed balance of pro- and anti-inflammatory cytokines can occur. Fibromyalgia has also been considered a stress-related disorder with dysfunction of the hypothalamic pituitary adrenocortical (HPA) axis. Some researchers have shown increases in oxidative stress and toxic metabolites of lipid peroxidation, while others have studied the idea that fibromyalgia could be a sympathetically maintained neuropathic pain syndrome. It has also been proposed that dorsal root ganglia and peripheral sensory neuron sodium channels may play a major role in fibromyalgia pain transmission.[5]

MICROBIOME COMPOSITION IN PATIENTS WITH FIBROMYALGIA

Gut bacteria may play an active role in promoting and causing fibromyalgia. As our understanding of the interaction between the human microbiota and the central nervous system develops, it is fair to hypothesize that it may affect pain processing and perception. Animal studies have demonstrated that gut microbiota play an important role in the development of visceral pain, of chemotherapy-induced neuropathic pain, and of opioid tolerance. Additionally, patients with chronic fatigue syndrome, which shares some symptomatic features with fibromyalgia, were shown to have altered gut microbiome and metabolomic profiles. Indirect evidence suggests that the gut microbiome may be altered in fibromyalgia patients.[125] Altered small intestinal permeability was reported in a group of fibromyalgia and complex regional pain syndrome (CRPS) patients.[126] Minerbi et al.[125] looked at the microbiome of 77 women with fibromyalgia and compared it to that of 79 control participants using

TABLE 7.1

Summary of Reported Changes in Fibromyalgia

Inflammation and Oxidative Changes in Fibromyalgia	
Mechanism	**Fibromyalgia**
Cytokines	
	Important in FMS[6–8]
	Influence on HPA axis[9–11]
	Mediator of neuropathic pain[12–14]
Proinflammatory	
IL1β	↑[15,16]
IL2	Decreased by therapeutic cryotherapy[17]
IL6	↑[6,18–22]
IL8	↑[6,20,21,23–25]
IL8 intrathecally	↑ Compared to rheumatoid arthritis[20]
TNFα	↑[15,19,26,27]
Anti-inflammatory	
IL1RA	↑[6,20]
IL4	↓[28,29]
	↑Compared to rheumatoid arthritis[20]
IL10	↑[7,16,30–32]
	Unchanged[6,30]
Others	
IL13	↓[29]
IL5	↓[29]
Cellular immunity	↓[33]
NLRP3 inflammasome	Activated[34,35]
Mast cells	↑[36,37]
MCPI	↑[24,38,39]
	Correlation/pain intensity[38]
	↑ in mutation subpopulation[39]
Oxidative stress	
Oxidative stress	↑[40–42]
Oxidative metabolites	↑ (multiple, see below)
Lipid peroxidation	↑[43,44]
Oxidative parameters	
Superoxide	↑[45]
Malondialdehyde	↑[43–47]
Xanthine oxidase	↑ (and correlation with muscle pain)[48]
Antioxidative parameters	
Catalase	↓[44,49]
Glutathione peroxidase	↓[44,49]
Superoxide dismutase	↓[43,47,49]
Nitrosative stress	
Nitrosative stress	↑[41,42]
Nitric oxide	Correlates with FIQ score[50]
	Involved in pathophysiology?[51,52]
	Responsible for pain sensitivity[53]
	Correlation with pain intensity[54]
	Nitric oxide synthase inhibitors needed for therapy[55]

(Continued)

TABLE 7.1 (CONTINUED)
Summary of Reported Changes in Fibromyalgia

Mechanism	Fibromyalgia
Nociceptive and CNS Changes, Cellular Dysfunction in Fibromyalgia	
Muscle pain (common)	Central sensitization[56–58]and long-lasting TTX-r[59]
	Tissue acidosis crucial[60,61]
	ASIC3 essential[62,63]→Na_v1.8 activity↑
	Induction and sensitization by MCP1[38,64]
	Correlation with xanthine oxidase[48]
	Mitochondrial dysfunction in FMS muscles shown and "explanation"[41]
Central sensitization	Involved in FMS[65–67]and chronic muscle pain[56–59,68]
	Chronic widespread pain in FMS animal model Na_v1.8-associated[69]
NP	Involved[70–73]
	Cytokines as mediators[12–14]
Allodynia/hyperalgesia	Common[73,74–76]
Heat hyperalgesia	Reported[73]
Cold hyperalgesia	Reported[77–79]
Mechanical allodynia	Reported[73]
Neurodegeneration	↑ Peripherally[65,71,80,81]
	↑ Also in CNS (eye)[80,81]
Small-fiber pathology	Reported[80,81,82–85]
SNS	Involved[86–89]
Glia	Activation important[21,90–93]
	Activation increases IL8[94]
	IL8[95] and α-synuclein increase activation[96]
Dopamine	↑[97]
	Dysfunction[97,98]
	Impaired neurotransmission[99]
Dysfunction	
Mitochondrial dysfunction	↑ (Skin,[40,58] blood,[40,41,45,100,101] muscle)[41]
	Improvement is therapeutic option[101]
Lysosomal dysfunction	Whole-body cryotherapy helpful[17,102]
Enzymes	↓[43,44,47,49,103]
	Prolyl endopeptidase reduction predictive[103]
Cellular immunity	↓[33]
IFNγ (immunostimulatory)	↑[104]
Cortisone receptor	↓[105]
Relevance of Sodium Channels in Fibromyalgia	
Sodium channels	Important[89,106,107]
Na_v1.7	Polymorphism found in severe FMS,[106] important in DRGs[89]
Na_v1.8	Expressed in (damaged) small C fibers[108–115]
	Important in sensitization[115–119]
	Important for cold pain[109,120] (as in FMS)[77]
	Gain-of-function mutations: FMS-like symptoms[121,115,122–124]

Abbreviations: FIQ, Fibromyalgia Impact Questionnaire; FMS, fibromyalgia syndrome; HPA, hypothalamic–pituitary–adrenocortical; Na_v, voltage-gated sodium; DRGs, dorsal root ganglia.
Adapted from: Kern et al.[5]

16S rRNA gene amplification and whole genome sequencing. Researchers were able to discover an abundance of different species of bacteria and the correlation of severity in patients with fibromyalgia symptoms. The microbiome is being heavily researched, and this may be another potential contributor to fibromyalgia.

CURRENT TREATMENTS FOR FIBROMYALGIA

MEDICATION THERAPIES

There is no cure for fibromyalgia. Treatment is focused on symptom relief and requires a multidisciplinary approach. Choice of treatment is based on patient-specific symptoms and optimally should include medication used in conjunction with non-pharmacologic interventions, both physical and psychological. Over-the-counter medications such as acetaminophen or NSAIDs are peripherally acting and not effective for the symptom management of fibromyalgia pain, but they can be used to treat the pain triggers involved in fibromyalgia.[2] NSAIDs and acetaminophen are most helpful in people who have comorbidities such as arthritis.

As opioid use has increased dramatically in the treatment of chronic pain in the last 20 years, its use has also dramatically increased in this patient population.[127] All current guidelines discourage opioid use for fibromyalgia. Opioid use in this population can actually cause worsening of fibromyalgia, causing greater pain sensitivity or making pain persist.[2]

There are currently three FDA-approved medications for the treatment of fibromyalgia: duloxetine, milnacipran, and pregabalin (Table 7.2).[128] While not completely understood, the effect of duloxetine and milnacipran on chronic widespread pain is thought to be due to direct alteration of serotonin and norepinephrine reuptake at the level of the dorsal horn in the descending pain pathways.[129] Amitriptyline and cyclobenzaprine also have effects on serotonin and norepinephrine and can be used to treat the symptoms of fibromyalgia, but are not FDA-approved. In addition to

TABLE 7.2
Prescription Medications Commonly Used for Fibromyalgia

Name	Therapeutic Class	Dose for Fibromyalgia	Uses in Fibromyalgia	Common Side Effects
Pregabalin*	Antileptic (GABA agonist)	25-75 mg daily with additional 25–75 mg every 1–2 weeks as tolerated	Pain, sleep, anxiety	Dizziness, somnolence, weight gain
Duloxetine HCL*	Antidepressants (SNRI)	30–120 mg daily. Most patients cannot tolerate doses >60 mg	Pain, fatigue, sleep	Headache, palpitations, nausea, flushing
Milnacipran*	Antidepressants (SNRI)	Initiate dose of 25 mg daily and titrate up by 25 mg daily at a minimum of every few days	Pain, fatigue, sleep	Same as duloxetine, may be more stimulating
Amitriptyline	Antidepressant (tricyclic)	10–25 mg taken in early evening, doses above 50 mg seldom tolerated	Pain, sleep, improved sense of well being	Dry mouth, constipation, daytime drowsiness, mental clouding, weight gain
Cyclobenzaprine	Skeletal muscle relaxant	1–4 mg at night	Pain, sleep	Side effects similar to amitriptyline
Tramadol	Analgesic	Studies have used 37.5 mg four times daily	Pain	Drowsiness, dizziness, nausea

*FDA-approved; GABA, gamma-aminobutyric acid; SNRI, serotonin-norepinephrine reuptake inhibitor.

pregabalin, which is involved in pain transmission by binding to voltage-gated calcium channels in several areas of the central nervous system and spinal cord, gabapentin can also be used.[2] Tramadol is a weak opioid analgesic with mild serotonin-norepinephrine reuptake inhibitor (SNRI) effects. Benefits seen with tramadol for fibromyalgia are likely due to its SNRI effects over opioid effects.

To help manage sleep issues associated with fibromyalgia, many of the medications that are used for the treatment of symptoms of pain also have side effects that can promote sleep.[2]

Because fibromyalgia is a heterogeneous disease, medication therapies offer mixed results in terms of efficacy for individual patients. It has been estimated that approximately half of all treated patients experience a 30% reduction in their symptoms with medication therapy.[130]

Additionally, this patient population is often more sensitive to medications and has a higher incidence of adverse effects. Doses are typically lower when used for fibromyalgia as compared to other disease states (Table 7.2). For this reason, and in the context of the opioid crisis, it is important to continue research on practical pharmacotherapy options for fibromyalgia.

MEDICATIONS AND EXPERIMENTAL AGENTS UNDER STUDY FOR FIBROMYALGIA

LOW-DOSE NALTREXONE

It has been proposed that fibromyalgia may represent a state of hypersensitive microglial activity and increased inflammation in the CNS.[131] Known to suppress microglial activity, naltrexone, at doses approximately one-tenth the typical opioid addiction dose, could be a potential treatment for fibromyalgia.[132] Low-dose naltrexone (LDN) exhibits paradoxical properties of analgesia and anti-inflammatory actions that are not seen with higher doses. By suppressing release of proinflammatory factors and antagonizing microglial activity, LDN may reduce pain and other symptoms of fibromyalgia.

In a single blind, cross-over pilot study of ten women with fibromyalgia, LDN (4.5 mg daily) was found to reduce fibromyalgia symptoms for all study patients with a >30% improvement over placebo as measured by daily reports of symptom severity and tests. Twice-monthly tests of mechanical, heat, and cold pain sensitivity demonstrated that mechanical and heat pain thresholds were improved with the drug. Patients with higher erythrocyte sedimentation rates had the greatest reduction in symptoms with LDN. Side effects were rare (including insomnia and vivid dreams) and short-lived. Although this study had promising results, it is important to note that there were several constraints. This study was single blind, included only a small number of patients, was not counterbalanced, and had a short duration of treatment (LDN was administered for 8 weeks).[133]

In a larger randomized, double-blind, placebo-controlled, crossover study, LDN was administered at a dose of 4.5 mg daily for a period of 12 weeks with 4 weeks of placebo taken either before or after the LDN treatment period depending on study arm assignment. This study also included a 2-week baseline period and a 4-week follow-up period for a total length of 22 weeks. All participants were told that they had the option to reduce their daily dosage to 3.0 mg if they experienced side effects. Each participant was given a handheld computer to record their pain, fatigue, and other symptoms on a daily basis, and they continued to record their symptoms for 4 weeks after study medication was stopped. Thirty-one women were enrolled and 28 women had sufficient data to be included in the analyses. Study patients experienced a significantly greater reduction in their pain scores while they were taking the LDN as compared with placebo (28.8% reduction versus 18.0% reduction; $p=0.016$). More participants met criteria for response (defined as a significant reduction in pain plus a significant reduction in either fatigue or sleep problems) during LDN therapy compared to placebo (32% response during LDN versus 11% response during placebo; $p=0.05$). They also reported improved general satisfaction with life and improved mood while taking LDN. However, there was no improvement in fatigue or sleep. All participants tolerated the LDN, with few side effects. Four individuals (three while taking LDN and one while taking placebo) requested the 3.0-mg dosage due to side effects. Side effects resulting in a dose decrease were headaches, heartburn, and irritability. These side effects were reduced by lowering the dosage to 3 mg/day. Low-dose naltrexone may be a great treatment strategy due to its high bioavailability, long history of safe use, low cost, and accessibility.[134]

DOPAMINE AGONISTS

Dopamine is a neurotransmitter that has been shown to have analgesic effects within the central nervous system. There is increasing evidence to support the theory that fibromyalgia is associated with dysfunctional dopaminergic neurotransmission.[135] Neuroimaging studies have shown that patients with fibromyalgia have both a reduction in dopamine synthesis at baseline and a disruption of dopamine release in response to painful stimuli.[135,136] Clinical trial results with dopamine agonists, however, have been mixed. Studies with dopamine agonists demonstrating the greatest efficacy for fibromyalgia are an open trial with ropinirole, which showed a >50% pain reduction in 74% of fibromyalgia patients, and a double-blind randomized placebo-controlled trial with pramipexole, which reported significantly more patients taking pramipexole as having a ≥50% pain reduction (42%) compared with placebo (15%).[137,138] Another double-blind randomized trial found that pramipexole improved restless leg syndrome, a comorbidity commonly found in fibromyalgia.[139] Additional studies are needed to assess the role of dopamine agonists for the treatment of fibromyalgia symptoms.

AMBROXOL

Ambroxol is a secretolytic agent used in the treatment of diseases associated with viscid or excessive mucus. It has the ability to interfere with several of the pathophysiological mechanisms proposed in fibromyalgia due to its multiple modes of action and is being considered as a potential option for treatment. Ambroxol interferes with oxidative stress and influences cytokines and inflammation. It also blocks tetrodotoxin-resistant (TTX-r) sodium channels that are expressed in spinal ganglion cells and in nociceptive sensory neurons. Studies have shown that fibromyalgia patients have an increased number of mast cells, and ambroxol has been shown to inhibit the secretion of mast cells. In addition, ambroxol improved mitochondrial dysfunction and oxidative stress (Table 7.1). It has also been shown to reduce visceral hypersensitivity, which in fibromyalgia could present as irritable bowel syndrome or chronic bladder pain.[5] In a study by Maihöfner et al.[140] topical ambroxol 20% cream was added to standard treatment in eight patients with complex regional pain syndrome (CRPS). The researchers found that the application of topical ambroxol 20% cream reduced spontaneous pain (six patients) and reduced pain on movement (six patients). Other neuropathy-related conditions were reduced, including edema (seven patients), allodynia (six patients), hyperalgesia (seven patients), skin reddening (four patients), motor dysfunction (six patients), and improvement of skin temperature (four patients). In other clinical observations, an application of 20% ambroxol cream or used orally resulted in pain relief in patients with fibromyalgia as well.[5,141]

At this point, the evidence for the use of ambroxol in the treatment of fibromyalgia is not strong enough for clinical recommendation. Although data on effectiveness in humans are limited, ambroxol has great potential in treating painful conditions, such as fibromyalgia. In addition, it has few side effects, is not addictive, and can even be administered topically.

NMDAR INHIBITORS

Activation of the N-methyl-D-aspartate receptor (NMDAR) via the neurotransmitter glutamate results in increased sensitivity of spinal cord and brain pathways that process sensory information, including pain.[142] Imaging studies have shown elevated glutamate levels in the brains of patients with fibromyalgia.[143] Increased glutamate and glycine levels have also been shown in the cerebrospinal fluid of fibromyalgia patients, making the NMDAR receptor a potential target.[144]

Ketamine, a non-competitive NMDAR antagonist, has been evaluated in a limited number of clinical studies with small sample sizes and has demonstrated some efficacy. Three studies were conducted with low-dose ketamine (0.3 mg/kg) infusion in a total of 58 patients with fibromyalgia. Thirty-three (57%) of these patients responded to low-dose ketamine with a reduction in pain of 50% or more.[142,145–147]

Memantine, a NMDAR antagonist typically used to treat dementia in Alzheimer's disease, was studied in 63 patients with fibromyalgia in a double-blind, parallel randomized placebo controlled trial.[148] Memantine was dosed at 20 mg/day after a 1-month titration period, and assessments of pain, global function, clinical impression, depression, anxiety, and quality of life were completed at baseline, post-treatment, and at 3- and 6-month follow-up. Memantine significantly reduced pain and increased pain threshold, and improved all other secondary outcomes with the exception of anxiety at 6 months. Compared with placebo, the absolute risk reduction obtained with memantine was 16.13% (95% confidence interval = 2.0% to 32.6%), and the number needed to treat was 6.2 (95% confidence interval = 3 to 47). Memantine was well-tolerated, with dizziness (eight patients) and headache (four patients) the most common side effects.

A novel oral NMDAR modulator (NYX-2925) currently under development has been shown to activate an NMDA receptor-mediated synaptic plasticity process, which could result in therapeutic potential for a variety of NMDA receptor-mediated central nervous system disorders.[149] Results from a phase II study in patients with fibromyalgia with this compound demonstrated statistically significant changes in neural markers of centralized pain processing via neuroimaging and statistically significant and clinically meaningful improvements on pain, fatigue, and other fibromyalgia symptoms. Across all patients in the study, NYX-2925 was safe and well-tolerated with no serious adverse events.[150]

Larger studies of longer duration are required before recommendations can be made for NMDAR inhibitors in fibromyalgia.

ANTIVIRAL/CYCLOOXYGENASE INHIBITOR COMBINATION (IMC-1)

A novel combination of famciclovir and celecoxib (IMC-1) is currently under development for fibromyalgia under the hypothesis that recurrent reactivation of a tissue-resident herpes virus in genetically susceptible individuals could contribute to the symptoms of fibromyalgia.[151] Both famciclovir and celecoxib have antiviral properties known to suppress herpes simplex virus (HSV).

The first clinical proof-of-concept trial was a 16-week, double-blind, placebo-controlled trial in 143 fibromyalgia patients. At the end of 16 weeks, a significant decrease in fibromyalgia-related pain was observed in the IMC-1-treated group compared to placebo. Response rates on the Patient's Global Impression of Change (PGIC) questionnaire significantly improved in the IMC-1 treatment group. Overall, patient self-reported functioning, as measured by the Revised Fibromyalgia Impact Questionnaire (FIQ-R), was significantly improved, and fatigue, measured by the NIH Patient-Reported Outcomes Measurement Information System (PROMIS), was also significantly improved. There was a lower frequency of AEs and a higher completion rate in the IMC-1 group compared to placebo. If successful, this drug combination could provide a new mechanism for the treatment of fibromyalgia.

CANNABINOIDS

Research on the role of medical cannabis in treating fibromyalgia symptoms is limited, but evidence has suggested that an endocannabinoid deficiency could contribute to the underlying pathophysiology of fibromyalgia.[152] Medical cannabis may be a reasonable therapeutic alternative, especially for those who failed on standard pharmacological therapies.

A randomized, double-blind, placebo-controlled trial was conducted in 40 patients with fibromyalgia to determine the benefit of nabilone, a synthetic form of cannabis, in pain management and quality of life improvement. This study showed significant decreases in VAS (–2.04, p < 0.02), FIQ (–12.07, p < 0.02), and anxiety (–1.67, p < 0.02) in the nabilone group at 4 weeks of treatment compared to no significant differences in the placebo group. There were more side effects in the treatment group per person compared to placebo, but overall the treatment was well-tolerated.[153]

A randomized, double-blind, active-control, equivalency crossover trial in 31 fibromyalgia patients with chronic insomnia compared nabilone (0.5–1.0 mg before bedtime) to amitriptyline (10–20 mg before bedtime). Twenty-nine subjects completed the trial. Nabilone was shown to be superior to amitriptyline for sleep quality (Insomnia Severity Index difference = 3.2; 95% confidence interval = 1.2–5.3) and was marginally better on the restfulness (Leeds Sleep Evaluation Questionnaire difference = 0.5 [0.0–1.0]) but not on wakefulness (difference = 0.3 [–0.2 to 0.8]). No effects on pain, mood, or quality of life were observed. AEs were mostly mild to moderate and were more frequent with nabilone and included dizziness, nausea, and dry mouth. This study concluded that low-dose nabilone given once daily at bedtime may be considered as an alternative to amitriptyline to improve sleep in fibromyalgia patients.[154]

An observational study compared 28 cannabis users with fibromyalgia (smoking, oral, or combined) to 28 non-users. The Fibromyalgia Impact Questionnaire (FIQ), the Pittsburgh Sleep Quality Index (PSQI), and the Short Form 36 Health Survey (SF-36) were used in this study to measure any associated benefits with cannabis. This study showed that, after 2 hours of use, VAS scores showed a significant (p < 0.001) reduction of pain and stiffness (mean reduction of 37.1 mm and 40.7 mm), enhancement of relaxation (change from baseline of 27.6 mm), and an increase in somnolence (change from baseline of 20.0 mm) and feeling of well-being (change from baseline of 40.0 mm). The mental health component summary score of the SF-36 was significantly higher (p < 0.05) in cannabis users than in non-users (mean = 29.6 ± 8.2 in users vs. 24.9 ± 8.9 in non-users). No significant differences were found in the other SF-36 domains, in the FIQ, or the PSQI. This study showed that cannabis did improve some symptoms of fibromyalgia. There were no serious adverse events. The most common side effects were somnolence, dry mouth, sedation, dizziness, tachycardia, conjunctival irritation, and hypotension.[155]

The largest study conducted to date looked at the efficacy of cannabis in fibromyalgia in a prospective, observational study with a 6-month follow-up period that included 367 fibromyalgia patients. Patients completed a variety of intake questionnaires to establish a study baseline and then initially received a low dose of cannabis (below therapeutic effect). The dose was increased gradually in small intervals until therapeutic effect was reached. At 6 months, 81.1% of patients achieved treatment response without experiencing serious adverse events. Of the 193 patients who reported high levels of pain prior to treatment, only 19 reported high pain levels at the end of the study. Overall median pain intensity was significantly reduced from baseline (p < 0.001). Sleep problems improved in 73.4% of patients who reported sleep problems at the beginning of the study and disappeared in 13.2% (p < 0.001). Depression-related symptoms were improved in 80.8% (p < 0.001) of patients who reported these symptoms at baseline. After 6 months of treatment, 148 patients reported their quality of life (five-point Likert Scale) as good or very good (p < 0.001). Additional quality of life factors that improved significantly after 6 months of treatment were sleep quality, appetite, and sexual activity. Mobility, dressing, and concentration did not improve, and quality of daily activities deteriorated at 6 months (p < 0.001). Overall, medical cannabis was well-tolerated. The most comment side effects were dizziness, dry mouth, and nausea/vomiting. Study authors proposed that good tolerability overall might to due to the gradual titration process of cannabis used in this study instead of a fixed dose. Of note, after six months of medical cannabis therapy, a substantial fraction of patients stopped or decreased the dosage of other medical therapies, and 22.2% of opioids users had reduced or ceased the use of opioids.

Overall this study demonstrated a significant improvement in pain intensity and overall quality of life in fibromyalgia patients after 6 months of treatment with cannabis. More studies are needed to establish the role of medical cannabis for fibromyalgia.[156]

HERBALS AND SUPPLEMENTS

5-Hydroxytryptophan (5-HTP)

5-HTP is produced in the body from the essential amino acid L-tryptophan. It is converted to the neurotransmitter serotonin. 5-HTP increases the production of serotonin by the central nervous system. In fibromyalgia, clinical evidence has suggested that taking 100 mg of 5-HTP orally three times daily for 30 to 90 days can help to improve pain, tenderness, sleep, anxiety, fatigue, and morning stiffness.[157,158]

S-Adenosyl-l-Methionine (SAMe)

SAMe is a molecule that is naturally formed in the body from homocysteine and 5-methylene tetrahydrofolate. It is important in the synthesis, activation, and metabolism of many different reactions throughout the body. Research suggests that SAMe used orally helps to improve the symptoms of fibromyalgia. Clinical trials have shown a modest improvement as compared to placebo or compared to transcutaneous electrical nerve stimulation (TENS) therapy.[159] An oral dose of SAMe, 800 mg daily in two divided doses for 6 weeks, has been used.[160] In terms of intravenous use, there is conflicting evidence. Some clinical research shows that 600-mg IV SAMe once daily for 10 days does not appear to help improve symptoms, while other research suggests that 400-mg IV once daily for 15 days significantly reduces pain, the number of tender points, and depression compared to baseline.[161,162]

St. John's Wort

St. John's Wort is a flowering plant that is native to Europe. It primarily grows in sunny, well-drained locations. St. John's Wort does have interactions with many drugs, so this herbal supplement must be used with caution. France has banned the use of St. John's Wort products due to safety concerns. Several other countries including Japan, the United Kingdom, and Canada are in the process of including drug–herb interaction cautionary language on St. John's Wort products.[163]

There is no specific evidence that St. John's Wort is helpful in treating fibromyalgia. Its role in promoting restful sleep and relieving depression is thought to be useful in treating some of the comorbidities that are associated with fibromyalgia.

Magnesium

Magnesium is a chemical element that is important to normal bone structure. It also plays a role in more than 300 cellular reactions.[164] Magnesium hydroxide plus malic acid orally has been found to decrease fibromyalgia-related pain and tenderness among patients.[165] Magnesium citrate 300 mg daily for 8 weeks improved symptoms of fibromyalgia, including number of tender points and comorbidities such as depression as compared to baseline.[166]

Coenzyme Q10

Coenzyme Q10 is a fat-soluble compound with a chemical structure that is similar to vitamin K. Coenzyme Q10 is involved in many biochemical processes throughout the human body. It is found endogenously mostly in the heart, liver, kidney, and pancreas.[167] Clinical research shows that coenzyme Q10 taken orally 300 mg daily for 40 days reduced fibromyalgia pain by 52% to 56%. Fatigue was also reduced by 47%, morning tiredness by 56%, and tender points 44% compared to baseline.[168] It has also been shown that coenzyme Q10 200 mg in combination with ginkgo biloba 200 mg daily by mouth for 12 weeks improves quality of life measures including physical fitness, emotional feelings, social activities, overall health, and pain.[169]

Melatonin

Melatonin is an indole neurohormone compound that is produced in the brain by the pineal gland.[170] The synthesis and release of melatonin in the body are stimulated by darkness and suppressed by light, suggesting that melatonin is involved in circadian rhythm. Melatonin is thought to decrease the severity of pain, as well as the number of painful joints in people with fibromyalgia.[171] Fibromyalgia patients have been shown to have altered levels of melatonin and its precursors, serotonin and tryptophan. Additionally, lower nighttime and higher daytime melatonin levels have been measured in this population. These factors may play a role in the sleep disturbances at night and pain and fatigue during the day that are commonly seen in this population, making melatonin an interesting compound to study for fibromyalgia.[172] The suggested dose of melatonin is 3 mg to 5 mg daily for up to 60 days.[171] Studies exploring the use of melatonin for fibromyalgia have used doses from 3 mg to 15 mg daily for a period of 10 days to 60 weeks.[172]

Panax Ginseng

Panax ginseng is an adaptogen that is native to Asia. The main active components are ginsenosides, which have been shown to have a variety of beneficial effects, including anti-inflammatory, antioxidant, and anticancer effects.[173] For fibromyalgia, clinical research has shown that *Panax ginseng* root extract at 100 mg/day for 12 weeks did not improve pain, fatigue, sleep quality, anxiety, tender point count, or quality of life compared with the placebo.[174] Therefore, it is not recommended as an adjunctive therapy for symptom management with fibromyalgia.

Ribose

Ribose is a building block of RNA, which is one of the two backbone chains in nucleic acids. Ribose is an aldopentose monosaccharide that contains five carbon atoms. In terms of managing fibromyalgia symptoms, clinical research has suggested that taking a ribose supplement, at a dose of 5 grams three times daily, can improve energy and sense of well-being, and decrease pain in patients with fibromyalgia.[175] A duration of therapy has not been specified in preliminary clinical trials for the indication of fibromyalgia.

Vitamin D

Vitamin D is a fat-soluble vitamin. There are several forms of vitamin D. This vitamin is found in dietary sources such as fish, eggs, and fortified milk products and can also be made in the skin during brief exposure to sun light. Preliminary clinical research suggests that taking cholecalciferol reduces pain that fibromyalgia patients experience.[176] The dose is dependent on plasma vitamin D status, with patients taking 2400 IU daily if calcifediol levels were <24 ng/mL or 1200 IU daily if calcifediol levels were 24–32 ng/mL. Supplementation was administered to achieve and maintain blood levels between 32 and 48 ng/mL for 5 weeks. A greater benefit was seen in patients who had low serum levels of vitamin D at baseline compared with placebo. Quality of life was not affected.[176]

Acetyl L-Carnitine

Acetyl L-carnitine is the derivative of the amino acid L-carnitine. L-carnitine is a non-protein amino acid naturally found in the body.[177] The body converts L-carnitine into acetyl-L-carnitine. The main function of L-carnitine is to transfer long-chain fatty acids in the form of their acyl-carnitine esters across the inner mitochondrial membrane before beta-oxidation.[177] One clinical study suggests that taking acetyl L-carnitine 1000 mg per day plus acetyl-L-carnitine 500 mg/day IM for 2 weeks, followed by acetyl-L-carnitine 1500 mg/day orally for 8 weeks can reduce muscle pain and improve mood, general health, and quality of life compared to placebo in patients with fibromyalgia.[178] Another study showed that 1500 mg/day of acetyl-L-carnitine orally in three divided doses for 12 weeks improved depression symptoms, but not pain, quality of life, or anxiety, compared to baseline in patients with fibromyalgia.[179]

CAPSAICIN

Capsaicin is an over-the-counter medication derived from chili peppers and is used topically for a variety of pain syndromes, including fibromyalgia. Repeated use of capsaicin depletes substance P, a neurotransmitter released when axons are stimulated, and can lead to exaggerated nociception to normal stimuli.

Previous research has demonstrated a three-fold elevation in substance P in the cerebrospinal fluid of fibromyalgia patients.[180] There have been a few studies that have assessed capsaicin in fibromyalgia. It is recommended to modestly apply 0.025% or 0.075% capsaicin cream three or four times daily for 4–6 weeks to reduce pain at tender points.[181] Capsaicin must be used consistently in order to decrease the neuronal transmission of pain. Long-term benefits are not known, and more studies needed to further assess capsaicin as a long-term therapy in the symptom management of fibromyalgia.[182]

TURMERIC

Turmeric root is a cooking spice that is traditionally used in curry, mustards, and other foods. Turmeric has anti-inflammatory properties that affect the production of cyclooxygenase-2, prostaglandins, and leukotrienes.[183] There is no reliable clinical evidence that has evaluated turmeric in the treatment of fibromyalgia. Additionally, since fibromyalgia is not considered an inflammatory condition specifically, turmeric is not expected to be of much benefit.[182]

VALERIAN, CHAMOMILE, AND PASSION FLOWER

Valerian, chamomile, and passion flower may help to regulate sleep patterns, as well as ease insomnia and anxiety, all common symptoms associated with fibromyalgia.[182] These herbal supplements have sleep-promoting effects but have not specifically been tested in fibromyalgia patients. They are not recommended at this time for fibromyalgia unless sleep issues are a comorbidity.[182]

ADAPTOGENS

Adaptogens are known for fighting fatigue and stress, which are common symptoms of fibromyalgia. This term "adaptogen" refers to products that help fight environmental stress by helping organisms "adapt" to severe conditions. Many of these herbals are used in traditional Chinese medicine to aid in fighting daily stress, fatigue, colds, infections, and, in general, to improve vitality.[182] *Panax ginseng*, American ginseng, astragalus, and ashwagandha are included among the adaptogens. These agents are commonly used, but there is currently no reliable evidence that they work for the use of symptom management in fibromyalgia patients.[182]

NON-DRUG THERAPIES

Managing fibromyalgia symptoms with medications is only a part of the multidisciplinary approach that is needed to address this disease. Non-drug therapies also play an important role in the overall treatment plan for fibromyalgia. Physical exercise and cognitive behavioral therapy (CBT) are the two most studied non-pharmacologic interventions for fibromyalgia.

Additional interventions that are used include yoga, tai chi, qi gong, mindfulness, acupuncture, and biofeedback.

Physical exercise has been shown to be beneficial for pain control, sleep, mood, and stress and should be used in addition to any drug treatment. Low-impact physical exercises are typically started slowly and increased gradually based on the individual. A meta-analysis of randomized clinical trials looking at the effectiveness of therapeutic exercise in fibromyalgia found evidence to suggest that muscle strengthening and aerobic exercise are most effective in reducing the pain and severity of the disease. Stretching and aerobic exercise produce the largest improvements in health-related quality of life, and combined exercise was the most effective way of reducing symptoms of depression.[184]

Water-based exercises are also beneficial and can decrease pain and improve strength and stamina. A 16-week randomized controlled study assessing the effects of aquatic therapy in patients with heightened fibromyalgia symptoms showed that exercise therapy three times a week in a warm pool improved most symptoms.[185]

Cognitive behavioral therapy focuses on understanding how thoughts and behaviors can affect pain and other symptoms.[2] Cognitive behavioral therapy and related treatment, such as mindfulness, can be helpful for patients for symptom control and to lessen the pain that they experience. A Cochrane review of CBTs for fibromyalgia found that CBTs provided some benefit in reducing pain, negative mood, and disability.[186] Cognitive behavior therapy has also been found to be beneficial in reducing pain catastrophizing in patients with fibromyalgia.[187]

Mind–Body Practices

Yoga is a mind body technique that uses physical postures in combination with breathing techniques and meditation. A meta-analysis of 3 yoga trials in 86 fibromyalgia patients showed positive effects on reducing sleep disturbances, fatigue, depression, improving quality of life, and providing pain relief.[188]

Tai chi is a traditional Chinese practice that combines meditation with deep breathing, relaxation, and gentle movements. A meta-analysis of 6 randomized trials in 657 patients with fibromyalgia demonstrated that tai chi had significant positive benefits for pain, sleep quality index, fatigue, depression, and quality of life as assessed by the Fibromyalgia Impact (FIQ) score.[189] Tai chi could provide an alternative for the management of fibromyalgia symptoms, especially for patients who are unable to tolerate aerobic exercise.

Qi gong is a holistic type of coordinated body posture and movement, breathing, and meditation used for health in Chinese medicine. Preliminary clinical research shows that external qi gong therapy performed by a trained qi gong practitioner might decrease pain and improve functioning in women with fibromyalgia.[190] Other evidence suggests that qi gong sessions three times weekly may improve pain, tender points, and symptom severity in patients with fibromyalgia.[191] Since exercise is the best way to manage fibromyalgia, qi gong is a good complementary option for the management of symptoms in fibromyalgia.

Acupuncture is an ancient Chinese practice that uses needles to stimulate specific points throughout the body in an effort to improve overall function. Studies have shown inconsistent results on the effectiveness of this technique for fibromyalgia symptoms. Kim J et al.[192] conducted a systematic review and meta-analysis of 8 studies comparing verum and sham acupuncture in 579 patients with fibromyalgia and found that verum acupuncture is more effective than sham acupuncture for pain relief, improving sleep quality, and general status posttreatment. A reduction in fatigue was not found.

Biofeedback is a mind body technique that gives a patient visual or auditory feedback on processes such as heart rate, pain perception, muscle tension, and blood flow. This information is then used by the patient to learn to control stress. While biofeedback has been helpful for some people with fibromyalgia, more studies are needed to confirm its effectiveness.

CONCLUSION

Fibromyalgia is a challenging disease with a complex etiology yet to be determined. While advancements are being made to understand the pathophysiology, current treatment is focused on symptom management. A multi-modal, patient-specific approach inclusive of medication, in combination with non-pharmacologic therapies, is a necessary part of the treatment plan. Opioids have proven unhelpful in this patient population and should be avoided as they can cause worsening of pain.

REFERENCES

1. National Fibromyalgia and Chronic Pain Association. Symptoms of fibromyalgia. https://fibroandpain. org/symptoms-2. Accessed 02 December 2019.
2. American College of Rheumatology. Fibromyalgia. https://www.rheumatology.org/I-Am-A/Patient-C aregiver/Diseases-Conditions/Fibromyalgia. Accessed 23 December 2019.
3. National Fibromyalgia and Chronic Pain Association. Diagnosis of fibromyalgia. https://fibroandpain. org/diagnosis-2. Accessed 02 December 2019.
4. Wolfe F., Clauw D.J., Fitzcharles M.A., et al. The American college of rheumatology preliminary diagnostic criteria for fibromyalgia and measurement of symptom severity. *Arthritis Care Res* 2010;62(5):600–610.
5. Kern K.-U., Schwickert M. Ambroxol for the treatment of fibromyalgia: fact or fiction? *J Pain Res* 2017;10:1905–1929.
6. Uçeyler N., Häuser W., Sommer C. Systematic review with meta-analysis: cytokines in fibromyalgia syndrome. *BMC Musculoskelet Disord* 2011;12:245.
7. Rodriguez-Pinto I., Agmon-Levin N., Howard A., Shoenfeld Y. Fibromyalgia and cytokines. *Immunol Lett* 2014;161(2):200–203.
8. Staud R. Cytokine and immune system abnormalities in fibromyalgia and other central sensitivity syndromes. *Curr Rheumatol Rev* 2015;11(2):109–115.
9. Savino W., Mendes-da-Cruz D.A., Lepletier A., Dardenne M. Hormonal control of T-cell development in health and disease. *Nat Rev Endocrinol* 2016;12(2):77–89.
10. Malek H., Ebadzadeh M.M., Safabakhsh R., Razavi A., Zaringhalam J. Dynamics of the HPA axis and inflammatory cytokines: insights from mathematical modeling. *Comput Biol Med* 2015;67:1–12.
11. Gupta D., Morley J.E. Hypothalamic-pituitary-adrenal (HPA) axis and aging. *Compr Physiol* 2014;4(4):1495–1510.
12. DeLeo J.A., Colburn R.W., Nichols M., Malhotra A. Interleukin-6-mediated hyperalgesia/allodynia and increased spinal IL-6 expression in a rat mononeuropathy model. *J Interferon Cytokine Res* 1996;16(9):695–700.
13. Xu X.J., Hao J.X., Andell-Jonsson S., Poli V., Bartfai T., Wiesenfeld-Hallin Z. Nociceptive responses in interleukin-6-deficient mice to peripheral inflammation and peripheral nerve section. *Cytokine* 1997;9(12):1028–1033.
14. Sommer C., Schmidt C., George A. Hyperalgesia in experimental neuropathy is dependent on the TNF receptor 1. *Exp Neurol* 1998;151(1):138–142.
15. Salemi S., Rethage J., Wollina U., et al. Detection of interleukin 1β (IL-1β), IL-6, and tumor necrosis factor-α in skin of patients with fibromyalgia. *J Rheumatol* 2003;30(1):146–150.
16. Imamura M., Targino R.A., Hsing W.T., et al. Concentration of cytokines in patients with osteoarthritis of the knee and fibromyalgia. *Clin Interv Aging* 2014;9:939–944.
17. Banfi G., Lombardi G., Colombini A., Melegati G. Whole-body cryotherapy in athletes. *Sports Med* 2010;40(6):509–517.
18. Hernandez M.E., Becerril E., Perez M., et al. Proinflammatory cytokine levels in fibromyalgia patients are independent of body mass index. *BMC Res Notes* 2010;3(1):156.
19. Tsilioni I., Russell I.J., Stewart J.M., Gleason R.M., Theoharides T.C. Neuropeptides CRH, SP, HK-1, and inflammatory cytokines IL-6 and TNF are increased in serum of patients with fibromyalgia syndrome, implicating mast cells. *J Pharmacol Exp Ther* 2016;356(3):664–672.
20. Kosek E., Altawil R., Kadetoff D., et al. Evidence of different mediators of central inflammation in dysfunctional and inflammatory pain: interleukin-8 in fibromyalgia and interleukin-1 β in rheumatoid arthritis. *J Neuroimmunol* 2015;280:49–55.
21. Kadetoff D., Lampa J., Westman M., Andersson M., Kosek E. Evidence of central inflammation in fibromyalgia-increased cerebrospinal fluid interleukin-8 levels. *J Neuroimmunol* 2012;242(1–2):33–38.

22. Ortega E., Bote M.E., Giraldo E., Garcia J.J. Aquatic exercise improves the monocyte pro- and anti-inflammatory cytokine production balance in fibromyalgia patients. *Scand J Med Sci Sports* 2012;22(1):104–112.

23. Bote M.E., Garcia J.J., Hinchado M.D., Ortega E. Fibromyalgia: anti-inflammatory and stress responses after acute moderate exercise. *PLoS ONE* 2013;8(9):e74524.

24. Bote M.E., Garcia J.J., Hinchado M.D., Ortega E. Inflammatory/stress feedback dysregulation in women with fibromyalgia. *Neuroimmunomodulation* 2012;19(6):343–351.

25. Xiao Y., Haynes W.L., Michalek J.E., Russell I.J. Elevated serum high-sensitivity C-reactive protein levels in fibromyalgia syndrome patients correlate with body mass index, interleukin-6, interleukin-8, erythrocyte sedimentation rate. *Rheumatol Int* 2013;33(5):1259–1264.

26. Iannuccelli C., Di Franco M., Alessandri C., et al. Pathophysiology of fibromyalgia: a comparison with the tension-type headache, a localized pain syndrome. *Ann N Y Acad Sci* 2010;1193:78–83.

27. Bazzichi L., Rossi A., Massimetti G., et al. Cytokine patterns in fibromyalgia and their correlation with clinical manifestations. *Clin Exp Rheumatol* 2007;25(2):225–230.

28. Uceyler N., Valenza R., Stock M., Schedel R., Sprotte G., Sommer C. Reduced levels of anti inflammatory cytokines in patients with chronic widespread pain. *Arthritis Rheum* 2006;54(8):2656–2664.

29. Sturgill J., McGee E., Menzies V. Unique cytokine signature in the plasma of patients with fibromyalgia. *J Immunol Res* 2014;2014:938576.

30. Mendieta D., de la Cruz-Aguilera D.L., Barrera-Villalpando M.I., et al. IL-8 and IL-6 primarily mediate the inflammatory response in fibromyalgia patients. *J Neuroimmunol* 2016;290:22–25.

31. Ranzolin A., Duarte A.L., Bredemeier M., et al. Evaluation of cytokines, oxidative stress markers and brain-derived neurotrophic factor in patients with fibromyalgia: a controlled cross-sectional study. *Cytokine* 2016;84:25–28.

32. Nakamura T., Schwander S.K., Donnelly R., et al. Cytokines across the night in chronic fatigue syndrome with and without fibromyalgia. *Clin Vaccin Immunol* 2010;17(4):582–587.

33. Behm F.G., Gavin I.M., Karpenko O., et al. Unique immunologic patterns in fibromyalgia. *BMC Clin Pathol* 2012;12:25.

34. Cordero M.D., Alcocer-Gómez E., Culic O., et al. NLRP3 inflammasome is activated in fibromyalgia: the effect of coenzyme Q10. *Antioxid Redox Signal* 2014;20(8):1169–1180.

35. Cordero M.D., Alcocer-Gómez E., Marín-Aguilar F., et al. Mutation in cytochrome B gene of mitochondrial DNA in a family with fibromyalgia is associated with NLRP3-inflammasome activation. *J Med Genet* 2016;53(2):113–122.

36. Blanco I., Béritze N., Argüelles M., et al. Abnormal overexpression of mastocytes in skin biopsies of fibromyalgia patients. *Clin Rheumatol* 2010;29(12):1403–1412.

37. Ang D.C., Hilligoss J., Stump T. Mast cell stabilizer (ketotifen) in fibromyalgia: phase 1 randomized controlled clinical trial. *Clin J Pain*. Epub 3 November 2014.

38. Ang D.C., Moore M.N., Hilligoss J., Tabbey R. MCP-1 and IL-8 as pain biomarkers in fibromyalgia: a pilot study. *Pain Med* 2011;12(8):1154–1161.

39. Feng J., Zhang Z., Wu X., et al. Discovery of potential new gene variants and inflammatory cytokine associations with fibromyalgia syndrome by whole exome sequencing. *PLoS ONE* 2013;8(6):e65033.

40. Sánchez-Domínguez B., Bullón P., Román-Malo L., et al. Oxidative stress, mitochondrial dysfunction and, inflammation common events in skin of patients with fibromyalgia. *Mitochondrion* 2015;21:69–75.

41. Meeus M., Nijs J., Hermans L., Goubert D., Calders P. The role of mitochondrial dysfunctions due to oxidative and nitrosative stress in the chronic pain or chronic fatigue syndromes and fibromyalgia patients: peripheral and central mechanisms as therapeutic targets? *Expert Opin Ther Targets* 2013;17(9):1081–1089.

42. Bortolato B., Berk M., Maes M., McIntyre R.S., Carvalho A.F. Fibromyalgia and bipolar disorder: emerging epidemiological associations and shared pathophysiology. *Curr Mol Med* 2016;16(2):119–136.

43. Akbas A., Inanir A., Benli I., Onder Y., Aydogan L. Evaluation of some antioxidant enzyme activities (SOD and GPX) and their polymorphisms (MnSOD2 Ala9Val, GPX1 Pro198Leu) in fibromyalgia. *Eur Rev Med Pharmacol Sci* 2014;18(8):1199–1203.

44. Fatima G., Das S.K., Mahdi A.A. Some oxidative and antioxidative parameters and their relationship with clinical symptoms in women with fibromyalgia syndrome. *Int J Rheum Dis* 2015;20(1):39–45.

45. Cordero M.D., De Miguel M., Fernández A.M., et al. Mitochondrial dysfunction and mitophagy activation in blood mononuclear cells of fibromyalgia patients: implications in the pathogenesis of the disease. *Arthritis Res Ther* 2010;12(1):R17.

46. Toker A., Kucuksen S., Kucuk A., Cicekler H. Serum ischemia-modified albumin and malondialdehyde levels and superoxide dismutase activity in patients with fibromyalgia. *Clin Lab* 2014;60(10):1609–1615.

47. Bagis S., Tamer L., Sahin G., et al. Free radicals and antioxidants in primary fibromyalgia: an oxidative stress disorder? *Rheumatol Int* 2005;25(3):188–190.

48. Ozgocmen S., Ozyurt H., Sogut S., Akyol O., Ardicoglu O., Yildizhan H. Antioxidant status, lipid peroxidation and nitric oxide in fibromyalgia: etiologic and therapeutic concerns. *Rheumatol Int* 2006;26(7):598–603.

49. La Rubia M., Rus A., Molina F., Del Moral M.L. Is fibromyalgia-related oxidative stress implicated in the decline of physical and mental health status? *Clin Exp Rheumatol* 2013;31 (6 Suppl 79):S121–S127.

50. Rus A., Molina F., Gassó M., Camacho M.V., Peinado M.Á., del Moral M.L. Nitric oxide, inflammation, lipid profile, and cortisol in normal- and overweight women with fibromyalgia. *Biol Res Nurs* 2016;18(2):138–146.

51. Fatima G., Das S.K., Mahdi A.A. Oxidative stress and antioxidative parameters and metal ion content in patients with fibromyalgia syndrome: implications in the pathogenesis of the disease. *Clin Exp Rheumatol* 2013;31 (6 Suppl 79):S128–S133.

52. Ozgocmen S., Ozyurt H., Sogut S., Akyol O. Current concepts in the pathophysiology of fibromyalgia: the potential role of oxidative stress and nitric oxide. *Rheumatol Int* 2006;26(7):585–597.

53. Kim S.K., Kim S.H., Nah S.S., et al. Association of guanosine triphosphate cyclohydrolase 1 gene polymorphisms with fibromyalgia syndrome in a Korean population. *J Rheumatol* 2013;40(3):316–322.

54. Sendur O.F., Turan Y., Tastaban E., Yenisey C., Serter M. Serum antioxidants and nitric oxide levels in fibromyalgia: a controlled study. *Rheumatol Int* 2009;29(6):629–633.

55. Cimen O.B., Cimen M.Y., Yapici Y., Camdeviren H. Arginase, NOS activities, and clinical features in fibromyalgia patients. *Pain Med* 2009;10(5):813–818.

56. Arendt-Nielsen L., Fernández-de-Las-Peñas C., Graven-Nielsen T. Basic aspects of musculoskeletal pain: from acute to chronic pain. *J Man Manip Ther* 2011;19(4):186–193.

57. DeSantana J.M., Sluka K.A. Central mechanisms in the maintenance of chronic widespread noninflammatory muscle pain. *Curr Pain Headache Rep* 2008;12(5):338–343.

58. Staud R. Peripheral pain mechanisms in chronic widespread pain. *Best Pract Res Clin Rheumatol* 2011;25(2):155–164.

59. Joseph E.K., Levine J.D. Hyperalgesic priming is restricted to isolectin B4-positive nociceptors. *Neuroscience* 2010;169(1):431–435.

60. Law L.A., Sluka K.A., McMullen T., Lee J., Arendt-Nielsen L., Graven-Nielsen T. Acidic buffer induced muscle pain evokes referred pain and mechanical hyperalgesia in humans. *Pain* 2008;140(2):254–264.

61. Issberner U., Reeh P.W., Steen K.H. Pain due to tissue acidosis: a mechanism for inflammatory and ischemic myalgia? *Neurosci Lett* 1996;208(3):191–194.

62. Sluka K.A., Price M.P., Breese N.M., Stucky C.L., Wemmie J.A., Welsh M.J. Chronic hyperalgesia induced by repeated acid injections in muscle is abolished by the loss of ASIC3, but not ASIC1. *Pain* 2003;106(3):229–239.

63. Yen Y.T., Tu P.H., Chen C.J., Lin Y.W., Hsieh S.T., Chen C.C. Role of acid-sensing ion channel 3 in subacute-phase inflammation. *Mol Pain* 2009;5:1.

64. Alvarez P., Green P.G., Levine J.D. Role for monocyte chemoattractant protein-1 in the induction of chronic muscle pain in the rat. *Pain* 2014;155(6):1161–1167.

65. Cagnie B., Coppieters I., Denecker S., Six J., Danneels L., Meeus M. Central sensitization in fibromyalgia? A systematic review on structural and functional brain MRI. *Semin Arthritis Rheum* 2014;44(1):68–75.

66. Nielsen L.A., Henriksson K.G. Pathophysiological mechanisms in chronic musculoskeletal pain (fibromyalgia): the role of central and peripheral sensitization and pain disinhibition. *Best Pract Res Clin Rheumatol* 2007;21(3):465–480.

67. Desmeules J.A., Cedraschi C., Rapiti E., et al. Neurophysiologic evidence for a central sensitization in patients with fibromyalgia. *Arthritis Rheum* 2003;48(5):1420–1429.

68. Vierck C.J., Wong F., King C.D., Mauderli A.P., Schmidt S., Riley J.L., III. Characteristics of sensitization associated with chronic pain conditions. *Clin J Pain* 2014;30(2):119–128.

69. Chen W.N., Lee C.H., Lin S.H., et al. Roles of ASIC3, TRPV1, and NaV1.8 in the transition from acute to chronic pain in a mouse model of fibromyalgia. *Mol Pain* 2014;10:40.

70. Bazzichi L., Giacomelli C., Consensi A., et al. One year in review 2016: fibromyalgia. *Clin Exp Rheumatol* 2016;34(2 Suppl 96):S145–S149.

71. Lefaucheur J.P. The 'paradox' of neuropathic pain associated with small-fiber lesions in the context of fibromyalgia. *Pain* 2016;157(6):1364–1365.

72. Gauffin J., Hankama T., Kautiainen H., Hannonen P., Haanpää M. Neuropathic pain and use of pain detect in patients with fibromyalgia: a cohort study. *BMC Neurol* 2013;13:21.

73. Koroschetz J., Rehm S.E., Gockel U., et al. Fibromyalgia and neuropathic pain – Differences and similarities: a comparison of 3057 patients with diabetic painful neuropathy and fibromyalgia. *BMC Neurol* 2011;11:55.

74. Littlejohn G. Neuroinflammation in fibromyalgia and CRPS: top-down or bottom-up? *Nat Rev Rheumatol* 2016;12(4):242.

75. Cassisi G., Sarzi-Puttini P., Casale R., et al. Pain in fibromyalgia and related conditions. *Reumatismo* 2014;66(1):72–86.

76. Sumpton J.E., Moulin D.E. Fibromyalgia. *Handb Clin Neurol* 2014;119:513–527.

77. Brusselmans G., Nogueira H., De Schamphelaere E., Devulder J., Crombez G. Skin temperature during cold pressor test in fibromyalgia: an evaluation of the autonomic nervous system? *Acta Anaesthesiol Belg* 2015;66(1):19–27.

78. Gerhardt A., Eich W., Janke S., Leisner S., Treede R.D., Tesarz J. Chronic widespread back pain is distinct from chronic local back pain: evidence from quantitative sensory testing, pain drawings, and psychometrics. *Clin J Pain* 2016;32(7):568–579.

79. Blumenstiel K., Gerhardt A., Rolke R., et al. Quantitative sensory testing profiles in chronic back pain are distinct from those in fibromyalgia. *Clin J Pain* 2011;27(8):682–690.

80. Ramírez M., Martínez-Martínez L.A., Hernández-Quintela E., Velazco-Casapía J., Vargas A., Martínez-Lavín M. Small fiber neuropathy in women with fibromyalgia: an in vivo assessment using corneal confocal bio-microscopy. *Semin Arthritis Rheum* 2015;45(2):214–219.

81. Garcia-Martin E., Garcia-Campayo J., Puebla-Guedea M., et al. Fibromyalgia is correlated with retinal nerve fiber layer thinning. *PLoS ONE* 2016;11(9):e0161574.

82. Kosmidis M.L., Koutsogeorgopoulou L., Alexopoulos H., et al. Reduction of intraepidermal nerve fiber density (IENFD) in the skin biopsies of patients with fibromyalgia: a controlled study. *J Neurol Sci* 2014;347(1–2):143–147.

83. Uçeyler N., Sommer C. Reply: small fibre neuropathy, fibromyalgia and dorsal root ganglia sodium channels. *Brain* 2013;136(9):e247.

84. Doppler K., Rittner H.L., Deckart M., Sommer C. Reduced dermal nerve fiber diameter in skin biopsies of patients with fibromyalgia. *Pain* 2015;156(11):2319–2325.

85. de Tommaso M., Nolano M., Iannone F., et al. Update on laser-evoked potential findings in fibromyalgia patients in light of clinical and skin biopsy features. *J Neurol* 2014;261(3):461–472.

86. Okifuji A., Bradshaw D.H., Olson C. Evaluating obesity in fibromyalgia: neuroendocrine biomarkers, symptoms, and functions. *Clin Rheumatol* 2009;28(4):475–478.

87. Lerma C., Martinez A., Ruiz N., Vargas A., Infante O., Martinez-Lavin M. Nocturnal heart rate variability parameters as potential fibromyalgia biomarker: correlation with symptoms severity. *Arthritis Res Ther* 2011;13(6):R185.

88. Martinez-Lavin M., Vidal M., Barbosa R.E., Pineda C., Casanova J.M., Nava A. Norepinephrine-evoked pain in fibromyalgia: randomized pilot study. *BMC Musculoskelet Disord* 2002;3:2.

89. Martinez-Lavin M., Solano C. Dorsal root ganglia, sodium channels, and fibromyalgia sympathetic pain. *Med Hypotheses* 2009;72(1):64–66.

90. Gür A., Oktayoglu P. Status of immune mediators in fibromyalgia. *Curr Pain Headache Rep* 2008;12(3):175–181.

91. Staud R. Fibromyalgia pain: do we know the source? *Curr Opin Rheumatol* 2004;16(2):157–163.

92. Albrecht D., Protsenko E., Mawla I., et al. Does brain glial activation have a role in fibromyalgia? A PBR28 PET study. Poster presented at 16th World Congress on Pain, 26–30 September 2016; Yokohama, Japan.

93. Kosek E., Martinsen S., Gerdle B., et al. The translocator protein gene is associated with symptom severity and cerebral pain processing in fibromyalgia. *Brain Behav Immun* 2016;58:218–227.

94. Milligan E.D., Watkins L.R. Pathological and protective roles of glia in chronic pain. *Nat Rev Neurosci* 2009;10(1):23–36.

95. Watkins L.R., Maier S.F. Immune regulation of central nervous system functions: from sickness responses to pathological pain. *J Intern Med* 2005;257(2):139–155.

96. Qiao H., Zhang Q., Yuan H., et al. Elevated neuronal α-synuclein promotes microglia activation after spinal cord ischemic/reperfused injury. *NeuroReport* 2015;26(11):656–661.

97. Klein C.P., Sperotto N.D., Maciel I.S., Leite C.E., Souza A.H., Campos M.M. Effects of D-series resolvins on behavioral and neurochemical changes in a fibromyalgia-like model in mice. *Neuropharmacology* 2014;86:57–66.

98. Albrecht D.S., MacKie P.J., Kareken D.A., et al. Differential dopamine function in fibromyalgia. *Brain Imaging Behav* 2016;10(3):829–839.

99. Ledermann K., Jenewein J., Sprott H., et al. Relation of dopamine receptor 2 binding to pain perception in female fibromyalgia patients with and without depression: a [11C] raclopride PET-study. *Eur Neuropsychopharmacol* 2016;26(2):320–330.

100. Cordero M.D., Moreno-Fernández A.M., Carmona-López M.I., et al. Mitochondrial dysfunction in skin biopsies and blood mononuclear cells from two cases of fibromyalgia patients. *Clin Biochem* 2010;43(13–14):1174–1176.

101. Cordero M.D., Díaz-Parrado E., Carrión A.M., et al. Is inflammation a mitochondrial dysfunction-dependent event in fibromyalgia? *Antioxid Redox Signal* 2013;18(7):800–807.

102. Bettoni L., Bonomi F.G., Zani V., et al. Effects of 15 consecutive cryotherapy sessions on the clinical output of fibromyalgic patients. *Clin Rheumatol* 2013;32(9):1337–1345.

103. Culić O., Cordero M.D., Zanić-Grubišić T., et al. Serum activities of adenosine deaminase, dipeptidyl peptidase IV and prolyl endopeptidase in patients with fibromyalgia: diagnostic implications. *Clin Rheumatol* 2016;35(10):2565–2571.

104. Ortega E., García J.J., Bote M.E., et al. Exercise in fibromyalgia and related inflammatory disorders: known effects and unknown chances. *Exerc Immunol Rev* 2009;15:42–65.

105. Geiss A., Rohleder N., Anton F. Evidence for an association between an enhanced reactivity of interleukin-6 levels and reduced glucocorticoid sensitivity in patients with fibromyalgia. *Psychoneuroendocrinology* 2012;37(5):671–684.

106. Vargas-Alarcon G., Alvarez-Leon E., Fragoso J.M., et al.. A SCN9A gene-encoded dorsal root ganglia sodium channel polymorphism associated with severe fibromyalgia. *BMC Musculoskelet Disord* 2012;13:23.

107. Martinez-Lavin M. Small fibre neuropathy, fibromyalgia and dorsal root ganglia sodium channels. *Brain* 2013;136(9):e246.

108. Akopian A.N., Sivilotti L., Wood J.N. A tetrodotoxin-resistant voltage-gated sodium channel expressed by sensory neurons. *Nature* 1996;379(6562):257–262.

109. Zimmermann K., Leffler A., Babes A., et al. Sensory neuron sodium channel Nav1.8 is essential for pain at low temperatures. *Nature* 2007;447(7146):855–858.

110. Blair N.T., Bean B.P. Roles of tetrodotoxin (TTX)-sensitive Na+ current, TTX-resistant Na+ current, and Ca2+ current in the action potentials of nociceptive sensory neurons. *J Neurosci* 2002;22(23):10277–10290.

111. Renganathan M., Cummins T.R., Waxman S.G. Contribution of Na(v)1.8 sodium channels to action potential electrogenesis in DRG neurons. *J Neurophysiol* 2001;86(2):629–640.

112. Kinloch R.A., Cox P.J. New targets for neuropathic pain therapeutics. *Expert Opin Ther Targets* 2005;9(4):685–698.

113. Coggeshall R.E., Tate S., Carlton S.M. Differential expression of tetrodotoxin-resistant sodium channels Nav1.8 and Nav1.9 in normal and inflamed rats. *Neurosci Lett* 2004;355(1–2):45–48.

114. Strickland I.T., Martindale J.C., Woodhams P.L., Reeve A.J., Chessell I.P., McQueen D.S. Changes in the expression of NaV1.7, NaV1.8 and NaV1.9 in a distinct population of dorsal root ganglia innervating the rat knee joint in a model of chronic inflammatory joint pain. *Eur J Pain* 2008;12(5):564–572.

115. Huang J., Yang Y., Zhao P., et al. Small-fiber neuropathy Nav1.8 mutation shifts activation to hyperpolarized potentials and increases excitability of dorsal root ganglion neurons. *J Neurosci* 2013;33(35):14087–14097.

116. Lai J., Gold M.S., Kim C.S., et al. Inhibition of neuropathic pain by decreased expression of the tetrodotoxin-resistant sodium channel, NaV1.8. *Pain* 2002;95(1–2):143–152.

117. Joshi S.K., Mikusa J.P., Hernandez G., et al. Involvement of the TTX-resistant sodium channel Nav 1.8 in inflammatory and neuropathic, but not post-operative, pain states. *Pain* 2006;123(1–2):75–82.

118. Akopian A.N., Souslova V., England S., et al. The tetrodotoxin-resistant sodium channel SNS has a specialized function in pain pathways. *Nat Neurosci* 1999;2(6):541–548.

119. Roza C., Laird J.M., Souslova V., Wood J.N., Cervero F. The tetrodotoxin-resistant Na+ channel Nav1.8 is essential for the expression of spontaneous activity in damaged sensory axons of mice. *J Physiol* 2003;550(3):921–926.

120. Abrahamsen B., Zhao J., Asante C.O., et al. The cell and molecular basis of mechanical, cold, and inflammatory pain. *Science* 2008;321(5889):702–705.

121. Han C., Vasylyev D., Macala L.J., et al. The G1662S NaV1.8 mutation in small fibre neuropathy: impaired inactivation underlying DRG neuron hyperexcitability. *J Neurol Neurosurg Psychiatry* 2014;85(5):499–505.

122. Bagal S.K., Chapman M.L., Marron B.E., Prime R., Storer R.I., Swain N.A. Recent progress in sodium channel modulators for pain. *Bioorg Med Chem Lett* 2014;24(16):3690–3699.

123. Dabby R., Sadeh M., Broitman Y., Yosovich K., Dickman R., Leshinsky-Silver E. Painful small fiber neuropathy with gastroparesis: a new phenotype with a novel mutation in the SCN10A gene. *J Clin Neurosci* 2016;26:84–88.

124. Brouwer B.A., Merkies I.S., Gerrits M.M., Waxman S.G., Hoeijmakers J.G., Faber C.G. Painful neuropathies: the emerging role of sodium channelopathies. *J Peripher Nerv Syst* 2014;19(2):53–65.

125. Minerbi A., Gonzalez E., Brereton N., et al. Altered microbiome composition in individuals with fibromyalgia. *Pain* 2019;160(11):2589–2602.

126. Goebel A., Buhner S., Schedel R., Lochs H., Sprotte G. Altered intestinal permeability in patients with primary fibromyalgia and in patients with complex regional pain syndrome. *Rheumatol Oxf Engl* 2008;47(8):1223–1227.

127. Fitzcharles M.A., Ste-Marie P.A., Gamsa A., Ware M.A., Shir Y. Opioid use, misuse, and abuse in patients labeled as fibromyalgia. *Am J Med* 2011;124(10):955–960.

128. Wright C.L., Mist S.D., Ross R.L., Jones K.D. Duloxetine for the treatment of fibromyalgia. *Expert Rev Clin Immunol* 2010;6(5):745–756.

129. Northcott M.J., Guymer E.K., Littlejohn G.O. Pharmacological treatment options for fibromyalgia. *Clin Pharm* 2017;9(11). doi:10.1211/CP.2017.20203533.

130. Staud R. Pharmacological treatment of fibromyalgia syndrome: new developments. *Drugs* 2010;70(1):1–14.

131. Albrecht D.S., Forsberg A., Sandström A., et al. Brain glial activation in fibromyalgia-a multi-site positron emission tomography investigation. *Brain Behav Immun* 2019;75:72–83.

132. Younger J., Parkitny L., McLain D. The use of low-dose naltrexone (LDN) as a novel anti-inflammatory treatment for chronic pain. *Clin Rheumatol* 2014;33(4):451–459.

133. Younger J., Mackey S. Fibromyalgia symptoms are reduced by low-dose naltrexone: a pilot study. *Pain Med* 2009;10(4):663–672.

134. Younger J., Noor N., McCue R., Mackey S. Low-dose naltrexone for the treatment of fibromyalgia: findings of a small, randomized, double-blind, placebo-controlled, counterbalanced, crossover trial assessing daily pain levels. *Arthiritis Rheum* 2013;65(2):529–538.

135. Wood P.B., Patterson J.C., 2nd, Sunderland J.J., et al. Reduced presynaptic dopamine activity in fibromyalgia syndrome demonstrated with positron emission tomography: a pilot study. *J Pain* 2007;8(1):51–58.

136. Wood P.B., Schweinhardt P., Jaeger E., et al. Fibromyalgia patients show an abnormal dopamine response to pain. *Eur J Neurosci* 2007;25(12):3576–3582.

137. Holman A.J. Ropinirole, open preliminary observations of a dopamine agonist for refractory fibromyalgia. *J Clin Rheumatol* 2003;9(4):277–279.

138. Holman A.J., Myers R.R. A randomized, double-blind, placebo-controlled trial of pramipexole, a dopamine agonist, in patients with fibromyalgia receiving concomitant medications. *Arthritis Rheum* 2005;52(8):2495–2505.

139. Montplaisir J., Nicolas A., Denesle R., Gomez-Mancilla B. Restless legs syndrome improved by pramipexole: a double-blind randomized trial. *Neurology* 1999;52(5):938–943.

140. Maihöfner C., Schneider S., Bialas P., Gockel H., Beer K.G., Bartels M., Kern K.U. Successful treatment of complex regional pain syndrome with topical ambroxol: a case series. *Pain Manag* 2018;8(6):427–436.

141. Martínez-Martínez L.A., Pérez L.F., Becerril-Mendoza L.T., et al. *Clin Rheumatol* 2017;36(8):1879–1884. doi:10.1007/s10067-017-3664-z.

142. Littlejohn G., Guymer E. Modulation of the NMDA receptor activity in fibromyalgia. *Biomedicines* 2017;5(2):15.

143. Harris R.E. Elevated excitatory neurotransmitter levels in the fibromyalgia brain. *Arthritis Res Ther* 2010;12(5):141.

144. Larson A.A., Giovengo S.L., Russell I.J., Michalek J.E. Changes in the concentrations of amino acids in the cerebrospinal fluid that correlate with pain in patients with fibromyalgia: implications for nitric oxide pathways. *Pain* 2000;87(2):201–211.

145. Sörensen J., Bengtsson A., Bäckman E., Henriksson K.G., Bengtsson M. Pain analysis in patients with fibromyalgia: effects of intravenous morphine, lidocaine, and ketamine. *Scand J Rheumatol* 1995;24(6):360–365.

146. Sörensen J., Bengtsson A., Ahlner J., Henriksson K.G., Ekselius L., Bengtsson M. Fibromyalgia—Are there different mechanisms in the processing of pain? A double blind crossover comparison of analgesic drugs. *J Rheumatol* 1997;24(8):1615–1621.

147. Graven-Nielsen T., Aspregen Kendall S., Henriksson K.G., et al. Ketamine reduces muscle pain, temporal summation, and referred pain in fibromyalgia patients. *Pain* 2000;85(3):483–491.

148. Olivan-Blázquez B.B., Herrera-Mercadal P., Puebla-Guedea M., et al. Efficacy of memantine in the treatment of fibromyalgia: a double-blind, randomised, controlled trial with 6-month follow-up. *Pain* 2014;155(12):2517–2525.

149. Khan M.A., Houck D.R., Gross A.L., et al. NYX-2925 is a novel NMDA receptor-specific spirocyclic-β-lactam that modulates synaptic plasticity processes associated with learning and memory. *Int J Neuropsychopharmacol* 2018;21(3):242–254.

150. Biospace. Aptinyx announces results of phase 2 fibromyalgia study of NYX-2925 have been selected for late-breaking presentation at the American college of rheumatology annual meeting. 2019. https://www.biospace.com/article/releases/aptinyx-announces-results-of-phase-2-fibromyalgia-study-of-nyx-2925-have-been-selected-for-late-breaking-presentation-at-the-american-college-of-rheumatology-annual-meeting. Accessed 02 December 2019.

151. Pridgen W.L., Duffy C., Gendreau J.F., Gendreau R.M. A famciclovir + celecoxib combination treatment is safe and efficacious in the treatment of fibromyalgia. *J Pain Res* 2017;10:451–460.

152. Russo E.B. Clinical endocannabinoid deficiency (CECD): can this concept explain therapeutic benefits of cannabis in migraine, fibromyalgia, irritable bowel syndrome and other treatment-resistant conditions? *Neuro Endocrinol Lett* 2008;29(2):192–200.

153. Skrabek R.Q., Galimova L., Ethans K., Perry D. Nabilone for the treatment of pain in fibromyalgia. *J Pain* 2008;9(2):164–173.

154. Ware M.A., Fitzcharles M.A., Joseph L., Shir Y. The effects of nabilone on sleep in fibromyalgia: results of a randomized controlled trial. *Anesth Analg* 2010;110(2):604–610.

155. Fiz J., Durán M., Capellà D., Carbonell J., Farré M. Cannabis use in patients with fibromyalgia: effect on symptoms relief and health-related quality of life. *PLoS ONE* 2011;6(4):e18440.

156. Sagy I., Bar-Lev Schleider L., Abu-Shakra M., Novack V. Safety and efficacy of medical cannabis in fibromyalgia. *J Clin Med* 2019;8(6):807.

157. Sarzi Puttini P., Caruso I. Primary fibromyalgia syndrome and 5-hydroxy-l-tryptophan: a 90-day open study. *J Int Med Res* 1992;20(2):182–189.

158. Caruso I., Sarzi Puttini P., Cazzola M., Azzolini V. Double-blind study of 5-hydroxytryptophan versus placebo in the treatment of primary fibromyalgia syndrome. *J Int Med Res* 1990;18(3):201–209.

159. Tavoni A., Vitali C., Bombardieri S., Pasero G. Evaluation of S-adenosylmethionine in primary fibromyalgia. A double-blind crossover study. *Am J Med* 1987;83(5A):107–110.

160. Jacobsen S., Danneskiold-Samsøe B., Andersen R.B. Oral S-adenosylmethionine in primary fibromyalgia. Double-blind clinical evaluation. *Scand J Rheumatol* 1991;20(4):294–302.

161. Volkmann H., Nørregaard J., Jacobsen S., et al. Double-blind, placebo-controlled cross-over study of intravenous S-adenosyl-L-methionine in patients with fibromyalgia. *Scand J Rheumatol* 1997;26(3):206–211.

162. Tavoni A., Jeracitano G., Cirigliano G. Evaluation of S-adenosylmethionine in secondary fibromyalgia: a double-blind study. *Clin Exp Rheumatol* 1998;16(1):106–107.

163. Rx.list. St. John's Wort. https://www.rxlist.com/st_johns_wort/supplements.htm. Accessed 17 August 2020.

164. Shils M., Olson A., Shike M. *Modern Nutrition in Health and Disease*, 8th ed. Philadelphia, PA: Lea and Febiger, 1994.

165. Russell I.J., Michalek J.E., Flechas J.D., Abraham G.E. Treatment of fibromyalgia syndrome with super malic: a randomized, double blind, placebo controlled, crossover pilot study. *J Rheumatol* 1995;22(5):953–958.

166. Bagis S., Karabiber M., As I., et al. Is magnesium citrate treatment effective on pain, clinical parameters and functional status in patients with fibromyalgia? Rheumatol Int 2013;33(1):167–172.

167. Greenberg S., Frishman W.H. Co-enzyme Q10: a new drug for cardiovascular disease. *J Clin Pharmacol* 1990;30(7):596–608.

168. Cordero M.D., Alcocer-Gómez E., de Miguel M., et al. Can coenzyme Q10 improve clinical and molecular parameters in fibromyalgia? *Antioxid Redox Signal* 2013;19(12):1356–1361.

169. Lister R.E. An open, pilot study to evaluate the potential benefits of coenzyme Q10 combined with Ginkgo biloba extract in fibromyalgia syndrome. *J Int Med Res* 2002;30(2):195–199.

170. Brzezinski A. Melatonin in humans. *N Engl J Med* 1997;336(3):186–195.

171. Citera G., Arias M.A., Maldonado-Cocco J.A., et al. The effect of melatonin in patients with fibromyalgia: a pilot study. *Clin Rheumatol* 2000;19(1):9–13.

172. Lawson K. Is there a role for melatonin in fibromyalgia. *J Clin Med* 2019;8:807.

173. American Family Physician. Panax ginseng. *Am Fam Physician* 2003; 68(8):1539–1542.

174. Braz A.S., Morais L.C., Paula A.P., Diniz M.F., Almeida R.N. Effects of panax ginseng extract in patients with fibromyalgia: a 12-week, randomized, double-blind, placebo-controlled trial. *Rev Bras Psiquiatr* 2013;35(1):21–28.

175. Teitelbaum J.E., Johnson C., St Cyr J. The use of D-ribose in chronic fatigue syndrome and fibromyalgia: a pilot study. *J Altern Complement Med* 2006;12(9):857–862.

176. Wepner F., Scheuer R., Schuetz-Wieser B., et al. Effects of vitamin D on patients with fibromyalgia syndrome: a randomized placebo-controlled trial. *Pain* 2014;155(2):261–268.

177. Vidal-Casariego A., Burgos-Peláez R., Martínez-Faedo C., Calvo-Gracia F., Valero-Zanuy M.Á., Luengo-Pérez L.M., Cuerda-Compés C. Metabolic effects of L-carnitine on type 2 diabetes mellitus: systematic review and meta-analysis. *Exp Clin Endocrinol Diabetes* 2013;121(4):234–238.

178. Rossini M., Di Munno O., Valentini G., et al. Double-blind, multicenter trial comparing acetyl l-carnitine with placebo in the treatment of fibromyalgia patients. *Clin Exp Rheumatol* 2007;25(2):182–188.

179. Leombruni P., Miniotti M., Colonna F., et al. A randomised controlled trial comparing duloxetine and acetyl L-carnitine in fibromyalgic patients: preliminary data. *Clin Exp Rheumatol* 2015;33(1 Suppl 88):S82–S85.

180. Russell I.J., Orr M.D., Littman B., et al. Elevated cerebrospinal fluid levels of substance P in patients with the fibromyalgia syndrome. *Arthritis Rheum* 1994;37(11):1593–1601.

181. McCarty D.J., Csuka M., McCarthy G., et al. Treatment of pain due to fibromyalgia with topical capsaicin: a pilot study. *Semin Arthritis Rheum* 1994;23(6):41–47.

182. Natural Medicines. Natural medicines in the clinical management of fibromyalgia. http://naturaldataba se.therapeuticresearch.com.pitt.idm.oclc.org/ce/CECourse.aspx?cs=naturalstandard&s=ND&pm=5 &pc=17-108. Accessed 27 December 2017.

183. Zhang F., Altorki N.K., Mestre J.R., Subbaramaiah K., Dannenberg A.J. Curcumin inhibits cyclooxygenase-2 transcription in bile acid- and phorbol ester-treated human gastrointestinal epithelial cells. *Carcinogenesis* 1999;20(3):445–451.

184. Sosa-Reina M.D., Nunez-Nagy S., Gallego-Izquierdo T., Pecos-Martín D., Monserrat J., Álvarez-Mon M. Effectiveness of therapeutic exercise in fibromyalgia syndrome: a systematic review and meta-analysis of randomized clinical trials. *BioMed Res Int* 2017;2017:2356346.

185. Munguía-Izquierdo D., Legaz-Arrese A. Assessment of the effects of aquatic therapy on global symptomatology in patients with fibromyalgia syndrome: a randomized controlled trial. *Arch Phys Med Rehabil* 2008;89(12):2250–2257.

186. Bernardy K., Klose P., Busch A.J., Choy E.H., Häuser W. Cognitive behavioural therapies for fibromyalgia. *Cochrane Database Syst Rev* 2013;10(9):CD009796.

187. Alda M., Luciano J.V., Andrés E., et al. Effectiveness of cognitive behaviour therapy for the treatment of catastrophisation in patients with fibromyalgia: a randomised controlled trial. *Arthritis Res Ther* 2011;13(5):R173.

188. Mist S.D., Firestone K.A., Dupree-Jones K. Complementary and alternative exercise for fibromyalgia: a meta-analysis. *J Pain Res* 2013;6:247–260.

189. Cheng C.A., Chiu Y.W., Wu D., Kuan Y.C., Chen S.N., Tam K.W. Effectiveness of Tai Chi on fibromyalgia patients: a meta-analysis of randomized controlled trials. *Complement Ther Med* 2019;46:1–8.

190. Chen K.W., Hassett A.L., Hou F., Staller J., Lichtbroun A.S. A pilot study of external qigong therapy for patients with fibromyalgia. *J Altern Complement Med* 2006;12(9):851–856.

191. Stephens S., Feldman B.M., Bradley N., et al. Feasibility and effectiveness of an aerobic exercise program in children with fibromyalgia: results of a randomized controlled pilot trial. *Arthritis Rheum* 2008;59(10):1399–1406.

192. Kim J., Kim S.-R., Hyangsook L., Dong-Hyun N. Comparing verum and sham acupuncture in fibromyalgia syndrome: a systemic review and meta-analysis. *Evid Based Complement Alternat Med* 2019:8757685. doi:10.1155/2019/8757685.

8 A Functional Approach to Gynecologic Pain

Integrative Gynecology for the Non-Gynecologist

Randy A. Fink

CONTENTS

INTRODUCTION

Gynecologic pain is a frustrating area of practice for many clinicians. The lack of clear understanding of anatomic considerations, inexperience with thorough and meaningful physical examination of the female reproductive system, and a natural discomfort with the intimacy associated with these syndromes lead many non-specialist clinicians to shy away from accurate diagnosis and treatment of gynecologic pain. Additionally, gynecologic pain is often multi-factorial, and a single, well-defined diagnosis may be elusive.

This chapter will seek to provide a basic template for the non-gynecologist to evaluate and treat gynecologic pain, encompassing common treatment options of both mainstream and functional medicine. It should be emphasized that a systematic approach to the accurate diagnosis of pain is critical; generalizing about sources of pain leads to incorrect diagnosis. Incorrect diagnosis both fails to treat the actual source of pain, and also leads to secondary issues. It is in our nature as clinicians to provide answers, but we must avoid the pitfalls of making uncertain diagnoses, especially in gynecologic conditions.

For example, pelvic inflammatory disease (PID) is a frequent diagnosis in emergency departments, but the diagnosis does not necessarily correlate with the actual presence of disease.[1] A reproductive-age woman with pain and vaginal discharge may be diagnosed and treated for PID as a diagnosis of exclusion, for fear that the *missed* diagnosis would be more harmful than the *wrong* diagnosis. But perhaps that patient is in a mutually monogamous married relationship, and is delivered the news that she has an upper genital tract infection due to presumed sexually transmitted disease. The interpersonal outcome from the *incorrect* diagnosis may be just as dire as the sequalae of untreated PID.

A similarly common diagnosis in emergency departments is the "ovarian cyst" as a source of pain. The woman presents with pain, has a CT scan showing a physiologic follicle in the ovary, and perhaps without even a pelvic examination is given the diagnosis of "ovarian cyst." In addition to "ovarian cyst" becoming a part of this patient's medical history forevermore, her actual diagnosis might be missed entirely. Both of these examples are discussed in more detail later.

It should be stressed that this work addresses sources of *non-obstetric* female reproductive pain. The analysis of pregnancy-related pain exceeds the scope of this chapter, so the simple performance of a pregnancy test is a meaningful first step in the evaluation of pain in most reproductive-age women.

EXAMINATION AND IMAGING

The importance of the pelvic examination cannot be understated. There are certainly instances when a pelvic examination is not necessary, but visualization of the reproductive organs by imaging and palpation of the internal pelvis can provide a wealth of information in localizing and defining pain. If the discomfort is of sufficient character to warrant her bringing it to a clinician's attention, then it is deserving of evaluation. Many times, the actual diagnosis may be nebulous or difficult to ascertain. Saying "I don't know" seems inexcusable, but in some cases, the patient only wants the relief of knowing that she does not have a terrible diagnosis, such as cancer. Pelvic pain can be so multifactorial that sometimes "I cannot be sure" is the correct answer.

The proper way of performing a pelvic examination has been covered by other authors *ad nauseum* and is beyond the scope of this text. However, this author wishes to share the following pearls on performing a meaningful exam:

- Be gentle, but do not be afraid. A gruff or inconsiderate examination of the internal or external genitalia must be avoided. The clinician may perform these exams with frequency, and invade the privacy of others as a matter of professional routine. Most patients will only rarely have to expose themselves to a clinician and will probably remember nearly every occasion of doing so for the rest of their lives. Meticulous attention to the patient's comfort, dignity, and humility must be foremost in every circumstance. Gentle means more than avoiding rough handling; it is an overall approach to the patient, acknowledging the emotional and physical discomfort that may result from a pelvic examination and actively taking steps to assure that the experience for the patient is the least negative possible. Obviously, gentle and precise movements can limit the physical discomfort. At the same time, however, excessive timidity in conducting the exam results in a negative experience as well. For example, using a speculum that is too small for the vagina in an effort to avoid discomfort from a larger instrument results in a great deal more manipulation in order to ultimately visualize the cervix. Visualization may still be compromised, and the level of discomfort from moving the small speculum around is increased beyond what would have occurred had a properly sized speculum been used initially. The exam is designed to yield information. The skillful clinician strikes the proper balance between procuring this information and keeping the experience neutral for the patient.
- When possible, conduct the examination on the appropriate furniture. Circumstances arise when a pelvic exam must be performed with the patient's bottom elevated on a bedpan, or the patient in a frog-legged position. This is suboptimal for many reasons. Seek an examination table with stirrups, even if this requires moving the patient to another room.
- During a bimanual examination, the majority of the information is gained from the vaginal hand. The abdominal hand is designed to move the pelvic structures into the vaginal hand, and uterine assessment is often easier than palpation of the adnexa.[2] Nevertheless, careful

- palpation of the adnexa can demonstrate or exclude the ovary as a source of pain, as well as point toward other etiologies of pain, such as the bowel.
- Cervical motion tenderness is usually not a mystery. Everyone is taught that cervical motion tenderness is pathognomonic of pelvic inflammatory disease. Colloquially, this is known as the *chandelier sign*, where the exam evokes such pain that the patient reaches up toward the ceiling for relief.[3] However, remember that the exam itself is uncomfortable. A natural response to painful stimuli is avoidance, so judge any response to pain as relative. In the best of circumstances and without pathology, aggressive motion of the uterus by manipulating the cervix can cause pain. True cervical motion tenderness is usually unmistakable.
- Do not fear the rectum. By the same token, ignore it if you can. Many are taught that the rectovaginal examination is a necessary part of any pelvic examination, however in most cases it does not yield additional information. In general, patients do not like it. However, it is indeed useful to evaluate the posterior pelvis when needed, as well as to rule out certain types of bowel pathology that can masquerade as gynecologic. Do the exam if you need to. But if you do not need to, leave it alone.

The sensitivity of the bimanual examination to diagnose ovarian cancer and to distinguish between benign and malignant lesions is notoriously poor.[4] However, in a non-screening clinical setting it may be useful to localize pain. Both the sensitivity and specificity of ultrasound is much higher than that of physical examination,[5] so the combination of physical examination and imaging should be considered the most reliable.

Pelvic transvaginal ultrasound is the most effective means of evaluating the female reproductive tract, and with no risk of exposure to ionizing radiation, it should be seen as the initial test of choice.[6] Computed tomography (CT scan) is deemed as a secondary modality if sonography is non-diagnostic, however it exposes the patient to an equivalent radiation dose of 200 radiographs.[7] The ready availability of cost-effective ultrasound in the primary care setting also makes sonography a useful diagnostic adjunct. It is able to view the pelvic structures with real-time patient feedback on discomfort, in addition to doppler interrogation of blood flow. Transabdominal ultrasound alone of the pelvic structures is of limited utility and should be avoided unless transvaginal ultrasound is not advisable.

In some acute care settings, sonography is bypassed for CT scan, as the clinician is able to search for pathology in the entire abdomen and pelvis. Ultrasound is deemed an appropriate initial test for appendicitis, for example, but a normal ultrasound does not rule it out. CT scanning has a slightly higher sensitivity for appendicitis,[8] but its diagnostic efficacy is similar to ultrasound in emergency department diagnosis of nephrolithiasis.[9] Many emergency clinicians turn to CT as first line, but for purposes of gynecologic pain, pelvic ultrasound should be the first, and usually the only, imaging modality required.

TYPES OF PAIN

MENSTRUAL

A brief and simplistic understanding of the menstrual cycle is necessary to understand the nature of gynecologic pain that is functional, or cycle-related. The language used here can be used as a template to explain to patients in non-medical terminology.

In reproductive-age women, under normal circumstances, the ovary releases an egg (ovulation), which is taken up by one of the fallopian tubes. Sperm enters the uterus, swims into the fallopian tubes, and can fertilize this egg. If the egg is fertilized, pregnancy has occurred and the fertilized egg (embryo) transits down the tube and implants in the lining of the uterus (endometrium). If the egg is not fertilized, a series of hormone changes signals the brain to instruct the body to slough off the endometrium so that the body can try again for pregnancy next cycle. This is the signal for a normal menstrual period. The uterus is an organ made of muscle. The job of the muscle (myometrium) is to squeeze the baby out when that time comes. As the menstrual bleed ends, the hormones again come on-line, and the glandular endometrium begins to thicken in an effort to provide a hospitable environment for a pregnancy to implant. This thickened endometrium is approximately 10 mm at mid-cycle ovulation.

Application of this template shows where in the menstrual cycle functional pain can arise.

Pain during the Period: Dysmenorrhea

Dysmenorrhea can be of primary or secondary origin. When severe, in addition to impairing quality of life, it interferes with the performance of daily activities, often leading to absenteeism or decreased productivity at school, work, and other responsibilities.[10] The prevalence of primary dysmenorrhea decreases with advancing age while secondary dysmenorrhea tends to develop later in life.[11] A variety of studies demonstrate that the worldwide prevalence of painful menstrual periods is 50–90%.[12]

The anatomic role of the uterus is to provide a hospitable environment for implantation, growth, and ultimately delivery of the pregnancy. At the onset of menses, sloughing of the endometrium causes a release of prostaglandins that induce uterine contractions. Unlike the contractions associated with childbirth, the uterine contractions of menses have dysfunctional and uncoordinated rhythms, and result in high intrauterine pressures. These pressures may be greater than 150–180 mmHg, and sometimes exceed 400 mmHg; they often begin from an elevated basal tone (>10 mmHg), and occur at a high frequency of more than 4–5 per 10 minutes.[13] By comparison, labor contractions are associated with pain when the amplitude is >10 mmHg over baseline, and such contractions are deemed sufficient to cause cervical effacement. Dysmenorrhea can therefore be seen as "mini-labor."

Ischemia results when these uterine pressures exceed that of arterial pressure in the menstruating uterus. Anerobic metabolites accumulate, and these stimulate type C pain fibers. Along with the prostaglandin cascade, the activation of stretch receptors from the contractions themselves results in the clinical syndrome known as dysmenorrhea.

This pain can made worse by secondary conditions.

Adenomyosis occurs when the endometrial glands and stroma grow into the uterine musculature. This growth induces hypertrophy and hyperplasia of the surrounding myometrium, and results in an enlarged, globular presentation of the uterus. The clinical result in addition to uterine enlargement is abnormal bleeding and painful menses. Its origin is unknown, but the two major theories are that it either develops de novo from Müllerian rests, or from endomyometrial invagination of the endometrium.[14] The uterus with adenomyosis takes a characteristic heterogeneous appearance when imaged by ultrasound.

Treatment of dysmenorrhea due to adenomyosis is similar to that of primary dysmenorrhea, though it may be more recalcitrant to standard treatment. Hysterectomy offers the only truly definitive treatment for adenomyosis in women who have completed childbearing, though uterine artery embolization may be a less invasive option. Hormonal options often provide symptomatic relief, but no well-defined herbal treatment has been shown to reverse changes associated with adenomyosis. Keishi-bukuryo-gan (KBG), a traditional Chinese herbal remedy, has been used empirically, and has been shown effective in animal models.[15]

Uterine fibroids may also contribute to dysmenorrhea. Fibroids are the most common pelvic tumor in women and are estimated to occur in up to 80% of females.[16] Fibroids are discussed in more depth later, but often contribute to painful menses as a correlate to heavy menstrual flow and passage of clots. These bleeding irregularities are thought to arise from molecular dysregulation of angiogenic factors leading to abnormalities of the uterine vasculature and impaired endometrial hemostasis.[17]

Endometriosis is defined as endometrial glands and stroma that occur outside the uterine cavity. These lesions are usually within the pelvis, but can occur on the bladder, bowel, abdominal peritoneum, diaphragm, and even in the pleural space. Endometriosis is a common cause of dysmenorrhea, and chronic pelvic pain.

Treatment of Dysmenorrhea

The mainstay of therapy in treating painful menses is to disrupt the prostaglandin cascade. It is the prostaglandins initiated by the sloughing of endometrium that start the process of dysmenorrhea. Non-steroidal anti-inflammatory drugs (NSAIDs) form the basis of this treatment. A meta-analysis including 80 trials reported that NSAIDs were more effective than placebo for patients with primary dysmenorrhea (odds ratio [OR] 4.37, 95% CI 3.76–5.09, 35 trials for comparison).[18] They are inexpensive, are available without a prescription, and are easy to dose. Acetaminophen is an option for those who are unable to take NSAIDs, though the above meta-analysis found NSAIDs to be more effective in reducing pain. Acetaminophen has the significant risk of hepatotoxicity and has been regarded by some to be one of the most dangerous drugs on the market, given its prevalence in the home.

NSAIDs are significantly more effective for pain when used at the onset of menses. It is not uncommon in clinical practice for a patient to state that this class of drug "does not work" for her pain. The use of narcotics for cyclic menstrual pain should generally be avoided, so one must first assess if such a statement is related to drug-seeking behavior. In most cases, however, the patient's poor experience with the NSAID was because it was initiated too late. The most commonly used drugs are phenylpropionic acid derivatives (e.g., ibuprofen, naproxen), which work at the level of inhibiting prostaglandin synthesis. If a high prostaglandin level exists, such as days into the menstrual cycle, inhibition of further synthesis can only modestly bring down pain. If treatment is started at the *onset* of menses, the overall synthesis and exposure to prostaglandin will be lower, and pain symptoms improved. The secondary medications are the fenamates (e.g., mefenamic acid) which, while blocking prostaglandin synthesis, also block prostaglandin action. This may account for their increased efficacy in some studies.[19] While most adverse effects are mild, NSAIDs are notable in having gastrointestinal side effects, concern over bleeding diatheses, and renal metabolic effects.

A reasonable approach to NSAIDs for dysmenorrhea is self-treatment with the phenylpropionic acid derivatives at the higher end of the dosing range starting at the onset of menses. After 2–3 months of ineffective treatment, a trial of the fenamates is indicated.

The other mainstay of traditional medicine treatment is hormonal, specifically the use of hormonal contraceptives. This is especially true for women who require contraception. Estrogen-progesterone-containing contraceptives, such as in a pill or vaginal ring, cause an atrophy of the endometrium over time. The thinned endometrium contains decreased amounts of arachidonic acid, which is the substrate for prostaglandin synthesis. As a result of these changes in the endometrium, estrogen-progestin contraceptives reduce both uterine bleeding flow and uterine contractions occurring during flow, thereby decreasing dysmenorrhea.[20] In general, newer formulations of oral contraceptives with shortened hormone-free intervals result in decreased bleeding, compared to standard 21/7 regimens.

An additional approach is the use of oral tranexamic acid, especially in women with dysmenorrhea who also complain of heavy bleeding. While it requires a prescription in the United States, it is available over the counter in many countries as a self-treatment for heavy menstrual bleeding. By competitively inhibiting multiple plasminogen binding sites, it decreases plasmin formation and fibrinolysis, thus decreasing menstrual bleeding. Less bleeding results in less prostaglandin, thus less pain. The combination of both NSAID and tranexamic acid is an excellent use of pharmacology to address multiple sites of action.

Complementary Approach to Dysmenorrhea

It should be emphasized that the above treatments have been shown to be highly effective in treating menstrual pain. One intervention on the part of the functional medicine clinician is to assure that the NSAID drug is being taken as much as possible *prior to* the onset of acute pain. This simple intervention may make the difference between effective treatment and treatment failure.

The following interventions in complementary and alternative medicine have shown promise.

Both a low-fat, vegetarian diet[21] and an increased dietary intake of dairy[22] have shown meaningful decreases in dysmenorrhea, especially in younger women. This may be due to dietary influences on estrogenic activity. Similarly, exclusion of gluten from the diet results in decreased inflammation overall and a reduction in reported pain from all sources, though the choice to become gluten-free is not one easily made.

Vitamin E (always in non-synthetic form) inhibits the release of arachidonic acid, the substrate in prostaglandin synthesis. It has long been used as an adjunct in the treatment of dysmenorrhea. It is most commonly used at 500 units once daily, or 200 units twice daily beginning 2 days before the expected start of menstruation and continuing for the first 3 days of bleeding.[23] Vitamin B1 (100 mg daily), vitamin B6 (200 mg daily), and fish oil supplement (1080 mg eicosapentaenoic acid, 720 mg docosahexaenoic acid, and 1.5 mg vitamin E) have each been shown to be more effective for reducing pain than placebo.[24]

Ginger powder is also relatively well-studied in treating dysmenorrhea; it has been shown to be as effective as mefenamic acid and ibuprofen in doses ranging from 750 mg to 2 g on days 1 through 3 of the menstrual cycle.[25–26]

Use of *Vitex agnus-castus*, or chasteberry, has been empirically well-established in various gynecologic disorders. Its primary indication is customarily considered to be mood disorders associated with the cycle, such as PMS-related symptoms. When studied for severe primary dysmenorrhea,[27] it was found to be equally efficacious as an ethinyl estradiol/drospirenone oral contractive in managing these symptoms and can be considered a meaningful adjunct to treatment. This is further discussed below.

The Ovarian Cyst

Few diagnoses are more misunderstood by the public than the ovarian cyst. Referring back to the template of the normal menstrual cycle, each month in a reproductive-age woman, the ovary produces an egg, or follicle. More specifically, several follicles emerge in the early cycle, but one continues as the dominant follicle. It is this dominant follicle that is released at ovulation. As the egg prepares for release, it is surrounded by progressively more fluid until such a time that it is ejected from the ovary in search of its fertilization destiny. By sonographic characteristics, the follicle is deemed to be mature when it measures 18 mm. It may commonly be 25 mm before release.

When imaged, this "follicular cyst" may be described to the patient as though it is an abnormal growth on the ovary, rather than a normal, functional part of the menstrual cycle. Indeed, every woman who ovulates will have a "cyst" in the ovary every month. It is rare that a follicular cyst will cause pain, and its presence on imaging should not be construed as pathology. Other sources of pain should be investigated.

Most of the time, routine ovulation of this follicle will be of no clinical significance. Some women have pain with ovulation, and this is known as mittelschmerz. It is usually sharp, one-sided, and self-limited. Once the egg is released, the space left behind becomes the corpus luteum. The cells within the corpus luteum secrete hormone designed to maintain the pregnancy should the egg be fertilized. The corpus luteum can stretch the capsule of the ovary and cause discomfort. Similarly, the space left behind from the ovulation can fill with blood. This is known as a hemorrhagic cyst. The hemorrhagic cyst can quite literally function as a bruise on the ovary and can grow quite large and symptomatic.

In premenopausal women, these physiologic cysts occur monthly. Newly developing simple, physiologic ovarian cysts are also routinely found in post-menopausal women,[28] though it was previously believed that physiologic cysts were exclusive to women of reproductive age. In older women, these are believed to be arrested physiologic follicles from anovulatory cycles. They are usually smaller and encountered with decreasing frequency as the time interval increases from the final menstrual period. They are often found incidentally on ultrasound examination performed for other reasons. If followed by serial ultrasounds, they will be observed to resolve spontaneously like those in the premenopausal ovary.

Polycystic ovarian syndrome (PCOS) is an endocrinopathy characterized by chronic anovulation, hyperandrogenism, and a polycystic morphology of the ovaries on transvaginal ultrasound. These findings are often accompanied by obesity and insulin resistance. The 2003 Rotterdam criteria for ultrasound appearance of polycystic ovaries is that of 12 or more small follicles in an ovary, measuring 2–9 mm. They typically have a "chain of pearls" appearance around the periphery of the ovary, and an increased ovarian volume of >10 mL. Ultrasound diagnosis is not required for PCOS. In fact, more than 50% of normally cycling women may have this sonographic appearance of one or both ovaries.[29] Despite the increase in ovarian volume, PCOS should be considered an endocrine abnormality and not a source of pain.

Aside from these physiologic cysts, cystic structures in the ovary can also be neoplastic. The most common non-physiologic cyst in women of the second and third decades is the mature cystic teratoma, or dermoid. These are nearly always benign,[30] but can become quite symptomatic. The dermoid is considered a developmental cyst, and arises from all three cell lines: endoderm, mesoderm, and ectoderm. As such, it has components of each. Endodermal cells include skin, hair, and sebaceous material. Mesodermal tissue may include muscle and genitourinary cells. And ectodermal contains gastrointestinal and lung. These cysts are bilateral in 10–17% of cases,[31] and morphologically most commonly present as a multi-cystic mass containing hair, teeth, and/or skin that is mixed into sebaceous, thick, sticky, and often foul-smelling material.[32] They are often discovered as incidental findings on pelvic ultrasound, and small dermoids may be followed expectantly and require no intervention. Treatment is exclusively surgical, when indicated. A rapidly growing or changing mass requires exploration to rule out malignancy, and an ovary >5 cm in size must be considered at risk for torsion.

Epithelial ovarian cysts arise from the surface epithelium of the ovary and are known as cystadenomas. They can be serous or mucinous. Serous cystadenomas occur more commonly, while mucinous cystadenomas tend to be larger and are often multiloculated. Cystadenomas are frequently incidental findings on ultrasound, and can be symptomatic by causing pain, bloating, and urinary symptoms. Epithelial ovarian cysts require histologic diagnosis for their subtype, but may be followed expectantly when they are small and asymptomatic. It is generally accepted that a persistently symptomatic cyst or one >5 cm should be removed surgically.

An endometrioma is a collection of ectopic endometrial tissue within the ovary. It contains a thick brown material made of old blood and is also known as a "chocolate cyst." Endometriomas can also grow quite large and may be adherent to other pelvic structures. The endometrioma itself may be painful due to changes within the ovarian cortex or inflammation in surrounding structures, but its mere presence in the ovary suggests endometriosis elsewhere in the pelvis.

It is interesting to note that the expression of endometriosis and the sensation of pain are multifactorial and quite variable from individual to individual. For example, a woman with chronic, debilitating pelvic pain may undergo laparoscopy for diagnostic purposes and show only one or two small endometriosis implants. Conversely, an otherwise asymptomatic woman may undergo a laparoscopy for tubal sterilization and be found incidentally to have severe endometriosis. This suggests a pathological variation in some expression of the disease. Some with endometriosis have chronic pelvic pain and some do not.

Inflammation seems to be the basis of endometriosis pain. The increased inflammatory and pain mediators stimulate peripheral nerve sensitization, acting as a cyclic or even chronic source of nociceptive input through tumor necrosis factor alpha (TNF-α) and related receptors.[33] An imbalance of sensory and sympathetic nerve fibers and dysfunction of these nerves contribute to endometriosis pain.[34–39] Ultimately, this feeds back centrally; the chronic input can lead to changes in regional gray matter volume in areas of the central pain system.[40] These nerve mechanisms are important to acknowledge in endometriosis-related pain, and in fact as a model for other chronic pain syndromes, as well. For example, each level of pathophysiology described practically defines endocannabinoid dysfunction, and opens the door to exciting alternatives in the use of cannabinoids to treat chronic pain. This is especially true in light of data showing the effect of cannabidiol on TNF-α.[41] Use of medical marijuana is not uncommon amongst women with endometriosis, and both marijuana and CBD are reported as moderately to very effective for pelvic pain due to endometriosis in women who have tried them.[42]

Rupture of an ovarian cyst is common in women of reproductive age.[43] Both physiologic cysts and pathologic cysts can rupture, spilling their contents intraperitoneally. Mittelschmerz is likely over-diagnosed as a ruptured ovarian cyst, but the difference may only be semantic. A reproductive-age woman presenting with pelvic pain and a sonogram showing a collapsing cyst and small amount of free fluid in the pelvis shows the signs of a cyst rupture whatever the origin. It is unclear whether the source of pain from the rupture of a simple cyst is due to pain fibers in the ovary itself, or secondary to peritoneal irritation from the fluid. The visceral peritoneum in some women is more sensitive than in others.[44] Physiologic fluid from a ruptured follicle, or fluid from a serous or mucinous cystadenoma is typically non-irritating, and the patient may be asymptomatic despite a large volume of fluid being present in the pelvis. Other women may be wracked with pain due to a small amount of fluid from a ruptured physiologic follicle.

Blood can be very irritating to the peritoneal lining. A ruptured hemorrhagic cyst or a bleeding corpus luteum can even cause hemodynamic instability. A ruptured dermoid cyst is uncommon, but spills sebaceous and other material, potentially including hair, cartilage, and teeth, and can cause an intense, granulomatous chemical peritonitis, resulting in dense adhesions and chronic pain.[45] Rupture of an endometrioma is also associated with bleeding, as well as direct and indirect inflammation in the peritoneum.

The most common presentation of rupture of a physiologic cyst is acute onset of focal lower quadrant pain, often after physical activity such as exercise or sexual intercourse.[46] The pain may be unilateral or referred across and involving the entire pelvis. Cyst rupture occurs more commonly on the right side, as the left is more insulated from trauma by the sigmoid colon.

Ovarian malignancy may also be symptomatic, though the symptoms can be non-specific. The following symptoms are much more likely to occur in women with ovarian cancer than in women in the general population. They include:[47–48] bloating, urinary urgency or frequency, difficulty eating or early satiety, and pelvic or abdominal pain. These symptoms can be associated with gastrointestinal, urologic, or other gynecologic conditions, but are of concern if they are new in onset, occur almost daily, and coexist with other symptoms. Even very early ovarian cancer can present with these symptoms,[49] though the mechanisms are not well understood.

Sonographic characteristics that have been typically associated with an ovarian or fallopian tube malignancy are:[50]

- A solid component that is not hyperechoic and is often nodular or papillary. A solid component is the most significant sonographic gray-scale feature of malignancy.[51]
- Septations that are irregularly thick (>2 to 3 mm). A thick wall can be seen with malignancy, but many benign masses, such as hemorrhagic cysts or endometriomas, can also have a thick wall. Wall thickness alone does not seem to be a reliable feature for distinguishing benign from malignant ovarian masses.
- Color doppler demonstration of flow in the solid component.
- Presence of ascites. Any intraperitoneal fluid in post-menopausal women and more than a small amount of intraperitoneal fluid in premenopausal women is considered abnormal.
- Peritoneal masses, enlarged nodes, or matted bowel.

It is important to note that size of an ovarian cyst has not been shown to necessarily correlate with likelihood of malignancy.

Cysts may also form outside of the ovary, such as paratubal (also known as paraovarian) cysts that develop in the broad ligament. These paratubal cysts are remnants of the Mullerian or Wolffian ducts of embryologic development, and are usually asymptomatic, incidental findings. Occasionally, they can grow large and cause pain, and are subject to torsion similar to an enlarged ovarian cyst. In general, they are managed expectantly and can be considered a normal anatomic feature.

A final consideration of acute ovarian cyst pain is the possibility of torsion. Torsion is a surgical emergency that occurs when the ovary and/or fallopian tube, enlarged due to fluid accumulation such as in the form of a cyst, twists on its ligamentous supports such that its blood supply is compromised. Torsion can occur in women of any age, and even in premenarchal girls with normal-sized ovaries.[52] However, size of the ovary is considered the primary risk factor, and even asymptomatic masses above 5 cm will garner the gynecologic surgeon's attention for intervention to prevent torsion. Torsion typically presents with the patient complaining of the worst pain of her life, often with nausea and vomiting, and findings of an acute abdomen. Ultrasound may demonstrate a mass with absence of blood flow by doppler interrogation. Torsion more often occurs on the right side, due to a longer utero-ovarian ligament on the right and the cushioning presence of the sigmoid colon on the left. Treatment for torsion is surgical.

The Functional Approach to Ovarian Cysts

As most painful ovarian cysts are physiologic, short-term watchful waiting is often the best option. The integrative clinician can play an important role in destigmatizing the ovarian cyst and explaining the normal physiology and helping the patient with short-term pain relief. The standard medical approach to recurrent physiologic cyst formation, and indeed most conditions associated with gynecologic pelvic pain, is in the form of hormonal contraception. Controlling the hypothalamic–pituitary axis and inhibiting ovulation will prevent the formation of most physiologic cysts. However, many integrative clinicians object to the use of the synthetic hormones in birth control.

The use of detailed hormonal testing may play a role in understanding the relationship of the reproductive hormones as they pertain to the cycle and its dysfunction. Bioidentical estrogen and progesterone combinations can be compounded for individual patients to accomplish the same end, though safety and contraceptive efficacy must be weighed carefully.

As previously mentioned, the fruit of the *Vitex agnus-castus* tree, or chasteberry, is used as an effective adjunct for many gynecologic conditions in which hormone dysregulation plays a role. *Vitex agnus-castus* (VAC) is a small deciduous shrub commonly known as monk pepper or chaste tree belonging to the Lamiaceae family of plants that is widely distributed in the Middle East and Mediterranean regions.[53] In additional to the hormonal regulatory function, analysis of the essential oil of the VAC shows that it contains some important monoterpenes and sesquiterpenes such as α-pinene, α-bisabolol, 1,8-cineol, β-caryophyllene, and limonene; these have antinociceptive effects in different models of pain and inflammation.[54] Terpenes are a large class of organic hydrocarbons interactive in the endocannabinoid system, giving further testament to the use of cannabinoids as well in the treatment of gynecologic pain syndromes.

Non-Menstrual Pain

Understanding pelvic pain as it relates to the temporal relation of the menstrual cycle is important in reaching a diagnosis. Pain occurring unrelated to the cycle is often more perplexing, as the differential diagnosis widens outside the reproductive organs. As previously discussed, common GYN sources of non-menstrual pelvic pain are epithelial ovarian cysts, and the sequalae of endometriosis.

Though, as discussed, physiologic ovarian cysts are present in all women of reproductive age, uterine fibroids, or leiomyomas, are a common finding as well. They are a benign, monoclonal growth of cells from the fibroblasts and smooth muscle of the myometrium. They are classified as submucosal (within the uterine cavity), intramural (within the wall), or subserosal (arising at the serosal surface). They are most commonly asymptomatic[55] and in most women should be seen as normal anatomic variants. The prevalence and likelihood of being symptomatic are highly associated with African-American race.[56] When symptomatic, they are associated with abnormal uterine bleeding, and for bulk-related symptoms or discomfort. Bulk-related symptoms arise from an enlarged and irregularly shaped uterus, and may put pressure on the bladder, bowel, or vasculature. Though they may increase dysmenorrhea and dyspareunia, acute pain from fibroids is unlikely outside the scenario of torsion of a pedunculated fibroid, or degeneration of a large fibroid that has outgrown its blood supply. Myomas are frequently visualized on imaging and can be assumed to be benign; the incidence of leiomyosarcoma is fortunately low, and such malignancies are not believed to arise out of benign fibroids.[57]

A variety of complementary and alternative medicine approaches have been proposed for treating uterine fibroids, however there have not been well-constructed trials evaluating these. Traditional Chinese medicine has been modestly successful with certain herbal and acupuncture interventions but these are beyond the reach of most integrative clinicians. Chasteberry, as previously discussed, can decrease symptomatology associated with fibroids, and oral iodine therapy may decrease bulk symptoms due to its anti-estrogenic activity. Indeed, these are reasonable basic interventions, and are commonly offered within our practice. Nutritional intervention toward decreasing inflammatory markers, insulin resistance, and peripheral estrogen conversion, along with micronutrient support are also reasonable long-term interventions, though they may have a nominal effect on acute presentations.

Non-gynecologic pain commonly does present as gynecologic pain. Much as a patient may describe abdominal pain as "my stomach hurts," pain that is localized to the pelvis is commonly presumed to be ovary or uterine pain. In fact, it may be difficult to convince a patient that their pain is non-gynecologic once they have concluded themselves that their pain is reproductive. The two most common types of pain that can masquerade as gynecologic are those of bowel and bladder.

Left-sided pelvic pain may be just as likely bowel as ovarian. While uterine pain is typically crampy in nature, so too might be the contractile forces of bowel that fills the pelvis. Sharp pain may bely the functional nature of the ovary, such as ovulation or a hemorrhagic corpus luteum, but so too might distension of the bowel be perceived as intermittently sharp. With the sigmoid colon present in the left lower quadrant and bowel occupying more space than the reproductive organs, peristaltic activity and distension are a common source of stimulation to the afferent nerves. This might be easily recognizable if history suggests relief of pain with the passage of flatus, or symptoms associated with constipation or diarrhea. A history of irritable bowel syndrome should raise clinical suspicion, as these patients often have underlying bowel motility dysfunction, and visceral hypersensitivity. Nevertheless, even without this history, sometimes the gut just causes pain. Sometimes biologically active systems cause pain without good reason.

More often than not, it is a high index of suspicion, negative imaging, and a physical examination negative for reproductive focus that leads to a diagnosis of gastrointestinal pain in the pelvis. Pelvic examination might reveal generalized discomfort in the adnexa but no focal pain when palpating the ovary, presence of hard stool in the rectum distending the vagina, palpable stool deep in the adnexa from the sigmoid, or copious spongy bowel palpable in either adnexa. Ultrasound often demonstrates distended bowel that may even obscure imaging of the ovaries.

In this author's experience, patients are more apt to conclude their pain is gynecologic than GI, as it is more acceptable to ascribe one's pain to the ovary than it is to flatulence.

Abdominal bloating and distension are commonly believed to be gynecologic. Patients may believe their bloating and distension are actually caused by tremendous swelling of their internal reproductive organs and are sometimes surprised to learn that their organs are of normal size. There is clearly an influence of hormones on gut distension in premenopausal women. Bloating is often cyclic, occurring in the luteal phase and associated with fluid retention. The integrative clinician can address these hormones and their dysregulation with testing. In middle-aged women, it is reasonable to image the pelvis with ultrasound to rule out pathological features associated with ovarian cancer, and sometimes CT scanning of the abdomen is needed to evaluate for partial obstruction or carcinomatosis.

Bloating and distension may be due to conditions causing excessive gas, heightened sensitivity to gaseous distension, or an exaggerated motor response to normal amounts of gas.[58] Mechanisms of gut dysfunction may involve dysbiosis of the gut microbiota and interactions with mucosal surfaces, the immune system, enteric nervous system, and central nervous system.[59] The integrative clinician may be uniquely qualified to evaluate and treat from this perspective. Differing types of probiotic and nutritional interventions may be of relief to the patient and are well in the purview of the integrative clinician. In fact, the functional medicine approach to nutrition, absorption, and the relative health of the microbiome brings the integrative clinician to the forefront in addressing these issues.

Bladder dysfunction can present more obviously with irritative voiding symptoms, but interstitial cystitis/bladder pain syndrome (IC/BPS) is more common in women than men and can be a source of debilitating pain with a significant impact on quality of life.[60] IC/BPS is a frequent comorbidity of endometriosis in women with chronic pelvic pain,[61] as well as other chronic pain syndromes such as irritable bowel syndrome, vulvodynia, and fibromyalgia.[62] There are usually varying degrees of pain or discomfort with filling of the bladder, relieved by voiding. The symptoms are often gradual in onset and may have begun after a triggering event, such as a urinary tract infection, bladder catheterization, or a fall. The pathogenesis is not well-understood, but, similar to endometriosis, there is a neurologic upregulation of pain sensation. Central sensitization and increased activation of bladder sensory neurons during normal bladder filling may result in bladder pain; the increased sensitivity is present both in the bladder itself, and in increased activity and new pathways within the central nervous system.[63] Again, the endocannabinoid system is emerging as integral to the processing and regulation of these pathways, and may hold a key in the management of these chronic pain syndromes.

By understanding IC/BPS as both a local and central response to afferent input, treatment by the integrative clinician can be targeted to both. However, in the absence of specialist training, the initial definitive diagnosis and treatment plan should be made in consultation with a urologist.

INFECTIOUS CAUSES

Pelvic pain presenting with a fever suggests an infectious etiology. This is as important in what it excludes as what it includes. Simple cystitis does not include febrile morbidity, so UTI symptoms with fever suggest a complicated UTI, or one in which infection has extended beyond the bladder. Similarly, simple cervicitis, such as infection with *N. gonorrhea* or *C. trachomatis*, may cause local symptoms but not a fever. The rupture of a common ovarian cyst or cyclic dysmenorrhea should not include fever.

Febrile presentations with pelvic pain suggest upper genital tract or upper urinary tract infections. Upper genital tract infections occur when the normally sterile environment of the uterus becomes infected with cervical pathogens, and this is known as pelvic inflammatory disease (PID). Infection can then spread to the fallopian tubes, the ovary, the peritoneum, the capsule of the liver, and can cause tubo-ovarian abscesses (TOA). Eighty-five percent of cases of PID are caused by sexually transmitted pathogens: *Neisseria gonorrhoeae*, *Chlamydia trachomatis*, and *Mycoplasma genitalium*. Actinomycosis is sometimes implicated, especially in the presence of a foreign body, such as an intrauterine device. Fewer than 15% of acute PID cases are not sexually transmitted and instead are associated with enteric (e.g., *Escherichia coli*, *Bacteroides fragilis*, Group B streptococci, and *Campylobacter* spp.) or respiratory pathogens (e.g., *Haemophilus influenzae*, *Streptococcus pneumoniae*, Group A streptococci, and *Staphylococcus aureus*) that have colonized the lower genital tract.[64] The precise initiating organism may remain elusive, but, regardless, PID is considered to be a mixed polymicrobial event.

PID represents a spectrum of disease. It often can be subacute in onset, with increasing pain over the course of 2 weeks. It is associated with signs of pelvic organ inflammation and may only be noticeable as pain after intercourse or exercise. Most women with PID will have mild to moderate disease, as opposed to those relative few with TOA or intra-abdominal sepsis. Presentation with fever is typically a sign of more severe infection. The pain is rarely localized to one side, as infection typically spreads through both fallopian tubes. Mucopurulent cervicitis is often present, but acute cervical motion, uterine, and adnexal tenderness on bimanual pelvic examination are the defining characteristics of acute symptomatic PID.[65]

The greatest risk factor for a woman is having multiple sexual partners. Younger age (15–25 years being most prevalent)[66], past infection with chlamydia, and previous PID are other risk factors. In fact, one in four women with PID will suffer from recurrence.[67] Barrier contraception is protective against sexually transmitted PID, because the infection is considered to be a liquid-based pathogen that is contained by condom use.

Salpingitis, or infection within the tubes, which has spread to the pelvis can cause perihepatitis (Fitz-Hugh–Curtis syndrome). This is inflammation on the liver capsule and the peritoneal surface anterior to the liver. It is said to occur in 10% of women with acute PID, and causes right upper quadrant pain and tenderness, and no or only mild elevation of liver enzymes.[68] The pain often has a pleuritic component, and can be severe enough that, especially with an acute presentation, it becomes necessary to rule out cholecystitis.

Presentation with acute PID can also mimic other intra-abdominal pathology, particularly appendicitis. Appendicitis often has a different onset in the localization of pain, but in fulminant appendicitis, there may be sufficient inflammation of the visceral peritoneum to cause cervical motion tenderness and significant pelvic pain on bimanual exam. Combined with symptoms of fever, nausea, vomiting, and leukocytosis, imaging takes on an important role. Diverticulitis can also cause acute abdominal signs and symptoms similar to PID, but is typically not in a young woman. PID can still strike women for whom diverticulitis is epidemiologically more common, but imaging typically provides a straightforward diagnosis to diverticular disease.

It is important to note that PID can also affect the pelvis in a sub-acute fashion, and indeed this may be a more common clinical presentation. It is not unusual for a woman to have symptoms so subtle or minimal that they do not require medical care, yet they can have significant sequalae.[69] Every gynecologist has performed laparoscopy and seen adhesions, tubal disease, and even the characteristic Fitz-Hugh–Curtis "violin string" adhesions of the liver to the anterior abdominal wall in a woman who reports no history of PID. Tubal factor is a major cause of infertility in women, and it most often occurs in those with no known history of upper genital tract infection.[70]

PID can lead to scarring and adhesions in the pelvis and is associated with chronic pelvic pain. Adhesions occur after 90% of all abdominal surgeries,[71] but most are clinically silent. Some dense adhesions can limit organ mobility and cause visceral pain. Adhesive disease can be notable to cause partial or even complete bowel obstruction, but laparoscopic adhesiolysis has not been found to cause long-term pain relief in patients with chronic pelvic pain.[72] Scarring in the fallopian tube after the resolution of PID can cause it to become blocked. It can then fill with a sterile physiologic fluid and become enlarged. This is known as a hydrosalpinx. The hydrosalpinx can also occur as a result of prior surgery or adhesions.

The hydrosalpinx is often asymptomatic, and only diagnosed on imaging or as a result of tubal factor infertility. Sometimes it can put a stretch on the tube and lead to visceral pain. Treatment of a persistent hydrosalpinx is usually surgical, though treatment for chronic salpingitis with a prolonged course of doxycycline may cause a resolution of the fluid. This does not repair the damage to the tubal lumen itself, however, and presence of a hydrosalpinx has a negative effect on pregnancy rates and live birth in patients undergoing in vitro fertilization.[73] In such cases, removal of the tube or proximal ligation results in improved outcomes.

VULVAR PAIN SYNDROME

Localized vulvar pain syndrome has previously been referred to by a number of different names, including vulvodynia, vestibulodynia, and vulvar vestibulitis. Consensus panels have recommended a functional approach to this nomenclature: (a) vulvar pain caused by a specific disorder; and (b) vulvodynia (persistent vulvar pain without an identifiable etiology).[74]

The most common sources of vulvar pain due to a specific disorder are infectious or inflammatory causes. Frustratingly, one of the more common presentations in clinical practice of vulvodynia, as defined, is a woman who believes she has persistent symptomatology from an identifiable source. For example, a woman may bring a notebook documenting countless "ineffective" treatments for what she believes was a yeast infection. She has ongoing burning or itch, yet has no evidence of infectious etiology. And she may find it difficult to accept that she does not have a yeast infection. The astute clinician will wonder if there is an inflammatory cause that does not meet the eye, because indeed irritants that cause chronic inflammation may be hard to identify in the history, and may incite their response below the superficial epidermis.

It is important to rule out vulvar dermatoses in these patients, but our discussion here will be limited to those patients without identifiable causes of pain. Vulvodynia can be localized to the vulvar vestibule or may include the clitoris. By definition, it has been present for at least 3 months,[75] and can be elicited by pressure point testing. It may present as persistent itching or burning, or as pain with intercourse, tampon insertion, tight clothes, and prolonged sitting.

The etiology of vulvodynia is likely multifactorial, involving inflammatory and allergic mediators, and can involve hormonal, psychosocial, and personality factors, as well as pelvic floor muscle dysfunction. A leading theory is that an inciting event, such as infection or trauma, leads to a local inflammatory response.[76] In a susceptible woman, this response evokes a proliferation of nerve fibers and a central sensitization to pain.[77] The symptoms can typically wax and wane, but fortunately are amenable to many interventions that are well-understood by the functional clinician.

Behavioral modification is a reasonable initial intervention. The American College of Obstetricians and Gynecologists recommends specific strategies including the wearing of non-constrictive cotton underwear during the day and none during hours of sleep; avoiding pantyhose, tights, and tight pants; using mild soap for bathing and water only for cleansing the vulva; avoiding douches, commercial vaginal wipes, deodorants, bubble bath, deodorants, tampons, or pads; using water-based unscented, non-warming, non-allergic lubricants for intercourse; applying cool gel packs to the vulva before and/or after sex to reduce pain and swelling; and avoiding activities that place pressure directly on the vulva such as bicycling.[78]

Pelvic floor physical therapy is a useful adjunct to all gynecologic pain syndromes. With specific regard to vulvodynia, several factors contribute to muscle restriction and hypertonicity in the pelvic musculature. Many women exhibit myofascial trigger points and increased muscle tension in the pelvis,[79] and numerous studies have demonstrated efficacy in treatment.[80] Pelvic floor physical therapy involves a variety of modalities, including pelvic and core mobilization and stabilization; connective tissue, visceral, and neural mobilization; and internal and external myofascial trigger point release, biofeedback, and electrical stimulation.[81] Given its noninvasive nature, it is also a reasonable first-line therapy. Its cons are the amount of time that must be devoted to treatment, the potential expense of treatment and limitations of visits by managed care, and outcomes tied to the experience of the specialized therapist. A generalist physical therapy practice, such as one used for orthopedic indications, is not well-equipped to deal with pelvic floor issues. Pelvic floor physical therapy should be considered a specialty.

Topical estrogen therapy is indicated for women with genitourinary syndrome of menopause, though some studies also show efficacy in using topical estradiol 0.01% cream or compounded estradiol 0.01% plus testosterone 0.05% or just testosterone cream for vulvodynia in those who are not estrogen-deficient. The use of topical vaginal estrogen is an obvious choice in those with pain secondary to atrophic changes. However, some women will still have pain even after the atrophic changes have been reversed, and there are likely better topical options for those without atrophy.

Topical lidocaine is also widely used for short-term symptom control.[82] Commonly used in a 5% ointment, lidocaine is readily available, generally safe, and low-cost. It can be applied either before or after sexual stimulation and may result in the relief of symptoms. In an office setting, it can be applied for immediate relief and sometimes can be the sole agent allowing an examination to be completed. Its downside is the relatively short duration of action, and the fact that it only blocks pain rather than potentially altering the sensory afferents. Additionally, the removal of most sensation may be an unacceptable choice for some women with sexual pain, and when transferred to the genitalia of a male partner, can delay ejaculation to the point where prolonged intercourse results and becomes even more painful to the woman.

Much like the treatment of other chronic pain syndromes, the mainstay of treatment in Western medicine has been systemic neuromodulators, such as tricyclic antidepressants (TCAs), like amitriptyline, and the newer selective norepinephrine reuptake inhibitors (SNRIs), like duloxetine. These medications should still be considered part of the arsenal of treatments, but their use may be limited by systemic side effects or the patient's desire to avoid systemic medication.

For years, amitriptyline and nortriptyline were considered first-line therapy. They are not approved for the treatment of pain but have been widely used in a variety of pain syndromes to alter neurotransmission, even independent of a diagnosis of a depression. In fact, the TCAs can be used to treat pain at a dose much lower than that required for depression.[83] Amitriptyline can be started at 10 mg at bedtime and increased by 10 mg weekly until either satisfactory effect or dissatisfaction with its anticholinergic side effects. Doses higher than 100 mg have been associated with sudden cardiac death, though it is rare that such a high dose is required with the availability of topical options discussed below. More recently, the SNRIs have taken on a prominent role in the treatment of pain syndromes. Duloxetine is typically started at 20 mg and can be increased as needed to 60 mg, which is the typical treatment dose for depression. Side effects include nausea, headache, and dizziness, as well as the potential for a withdrawal syndrome on stopping the medicine.

There are three anti-epileptic drugs approved for the treatment of neuropathic pain:[84] gabapentin, pregabalin, and carbamazepine. Of these, gabapentin is the best studied, but in our practice, we have never needed to use it orally for vulvodynia.

Our first-line therapy is topical, which is prepared by a compounding pharmacy. Indeed, functional medicine clinicians may be more comfortable with this approach than other clinicians, as the "one-size-fits-all approach" for which allopathic clinicians are trained leads many to a lack of understanding of the availability, usage, and dosing of compounded medications. Both amitriptyline and gabapentin used topically have shown to have high efficacy in treating generalized burning vulvodynia. In our practice, we typically start with 6% gabapentin cream in a transdermal base. It can be applied up to three times daily. Alternatively, topical amitriptyline 2%, or topical amitriptyline compounded with 2% baclofen or 0.5% ketamine have also been shown to have efficacy for the patient with burning pain. Using this topical approach, it is not an unrealistic expectation to have nearly a complete resolution of symptoms with practically no systemic side effects; intercourse can become pain-free.[85–86] Some have proposed using all modalities in a single topical cream, and indeed, with compounding, this is possible. However, most experienced compounding clinicians will report that starting therapy with the most simple, straightforward cream is often the best approach. Additional medications can be added as needed without significantly increasing cost, but using a stepwise approach is sensible to avoid the potential for sensitivity to one of multiple meds in a complex cream. Once the patient has demonstrated a lack of tolerance for a topical, it is more challenging to keep them as a collaborator in their care; it is far easier to add components to their treatment than it is to convince them to continue their treatment on a more limited basis once components are taken away.

Though these topicals are discussed for generalized burning vulvodynia, gabapentin cream remains our first-line therapy even for those presenting with itching. As a second-line treatment for those with itching vulvodynia, topical cromolyn 7–10% in a petrolatum base can stabilize mast cells and result in relief. This can be used either as a primary (solo) treatment, or in combination with gabapentin or amitriptyline.

The use of cannabinoids in these compounds is an emerging therapy. When compounded and applied topically, CBD is utilized as a single isolate. This is because it is less unwieldy and easier to control in terms of weight and accuracy in dosing compared to a full-spectrum product. While its affinity for the CB_1 and CB_2 receptor is high, a single isolate product lacks the entourage effect of a full-spectrum phytocannabinoid mixture. The long-term significance of this is yet to be determined. Nevertheless, in our experience adding CBD to a topical pain cream for musculoskeletal indications results in a synergy with other medications, such that lower concentrations of those other medications are required. For example, in our clinical experience, topical baclofen 2% seems to be inferior to a 3% CBD cream with 0.5–1% baclofen. We do not have extensive experience with topical CBD on the vulva, so obviously further study is needed. We have found that, though CBD can be used topically for dermatologic indications such as psoriasis, it sometimes incites sensitivity in the vulva, especially when the patient is predisposed.

CONCLUSION

Gynecologic pain syndromes can be managed by the clinician when there is a clear understanding of the etiology of the pain, and the anatomic and psychosocial implications thereof. In many instances, the integrative clinician may be better suited to understanding alternative methods of treatment, given the comfort level of using compounds and considering non-mainstream approaches. It is always advisable to have input from a consulting gynecologist, especially when surgical interventions are included within the differential diagnosis. Nonetheless, a functional approach to gynecologic pain may offer treatment considerations not previously offered to the patient, but with a scientific basis just as strong as a mainstream approach.

REFERENCES

1. Bartlett E.C. Pelvic inflammatory disease. *BMJ* 2013;346:f3189.
2. Padilla L., Radosevich D., Milad M. Limitations of the pelvic examination for evaluation of the female pelvic organs. *Int J Gynecol Obstet* 2005;88:84–88.
3. Gomella L.G., Haist S.A. (2007). Chapter 13. Bedside procedures. *Clinician's Pocket Reference: The Scut Monkey* (11th ed.). McGraw-Hill.
4. Bloomfield H.E., Olson A., Greer N., Cantor A., MacDonald R., Rutks I., Wilt T.J. Screening pelvic examinations in asymptomatic, average-risk adult women: an evidence report for a clinical practice guideline from the American college of physicians. *Am J Prev Med* 2015;48(3):350–356.
5. Brown T., Herbert M.E. Medical myth: bimanual pelvic examination is a reliable decision aid in the investigation of acute abdominal pain or vaginal bleeding. *Can J Emerg Physicians* 2003;5:120–122.
6. Vandermeer F.Q., Wong-You-Cheong J.J. Imaging of acute pelvic pain. *Clin Obstet Gynecol* 2009;52(1):2–20.
7. Laméris W., van Randen A., van Es H.W., et al. OPTIMA study group. Imaging strategies for detection of urgent conditions in patients with acute abdominal pain: diagnostic accuracy study. *BMJ* 2009;338:b2431.
8. Wu, Jing, et al. Diagnostic value of ultrasound and CT in acute appendicitis. *Int J Clin Exp Med* 2017;10(10):14377–14385.
9. Brisbane, W., et al. An overview of kidney stone imaging techniques. *Nat Rev Urol* 2016;13(11):654–662.
10. Schoep M.E., Adang E.M.M., Maas J.W.M., De Bie B., Aarts J.W.M., Nieboer T.E. Productivity loss due to menstruation-related symptoms: a nationwide cross-sectional survey among 32,748 women. *BMJ Open* 2019;9(6):e026186. Epub June 27, 2019.
11. Sundell G., Milsom I., Andersch B. Factors influencing the prevalence and severity of dysmenorrhoea in young women. *Br J Obstet Gynaecol* 1990;97(7):588.
12. Ju H., Jones M., Mishra G. The prevalence and risk factors of dysmenorrhea. *Epidemiol Rev* 2014;36:104. Epub November 26, 2013.
13. Dawood M.Y. Primary dysmenorrhea: advances in pathogenesis and management. *Obstet Gynecol* 2006;108(2):428.
14. Ferenczy A. Pathophysiology of adenomyosis. *Hum Reprod Update* 1998;4(4):312.
15. Mori, Takao, et al. Suppression of spontaneous development of uterine adenomyosis by a chinese herbal medicine, Keishi-Bukuryo-Gan, in mice. *Planta Med* 1993;59(4):308–311.

16. Baird D.D., Dunson D.B., Hill M.C., Cousins D., Schectman J.M. High cumulative incidence of uterine leiomyoma in black and white women: ultrasound evidence. *Am J Obstet Gynecol* 2003;188(1):100.

17. Stewart E.A., Nowak R.A. Leiomyoma-related bleeding: a classic hypothesis updated for the molecular era. *Hum Reprod Update* 1996;2(4):295.

18. Marjoribanks J., Ayeleke R.O., Farquhar C., Proctor M. Nonsteroidal anti-inflammatory drugs for dysmenorrhoea. *Cochrane Database Syst Rev* 2015;2015(7):CD001751. doi: 10.1002/14651858.CD001751. pub3.

19. Budoff P.W. Use of mefenamic acid in the treatment of primary dysmenorrhea. *JAMA* 1979;241(25): 2713.

20. Smith R.P., Kaunitz A.M. *Dysmenorrhea in Adult Women: Treatment*. Edited by Barbieri R.L. Waltham, MA: UpToDate Inc. https://www.uptodate.com (Accessed May 3, 2019).

21. Barnard N.D., Scialli A.R., Hurlock D., Bertron P. Diet and sex-hormone binding globulin, dysmenorrhea, and premenstrual symptoms. *Obstet Gynecol* 2000;95(2):245.

22. Abdul-Razzak K.K., Ayoub N.M., Abu-Taleb A.A., Obeidat B.A. Influence of dietary intake of dairy products on dysmenorrhea. *J Obstet Gynaecol Res* 2010;36(2):377.

23. Ziaei S., Zakeri M., Kazemnejad A. A randomised controlled trial of vitamin E in the treatment of primary dysmenorrhoea. *BJOG* 2005;112(4):466.

24. Proctor M.L., Murphy P.A. Herbal and dietary therapies for primary and secondary dysmenorrhoea. *Cochrane Database Syst Rev* 2001;(3):CD002124. doi: 10.1002/14651858.CD002124.

25. Daily J.W., Zhang X., Kim D.S., Park S. Efficacy of ginger for alleviating the symptoms of primary dysmenorrhea: a systematic review and meta-analysis of randomized clinical trials. *Pain Med* 2015;16(12):2243. Epub July 14, 2015.

26. Ozgoli G., Goli M., Moattar F. Comparison of effects of ginger, mefenamic acid, and ibuprofen on pain in women with primary dysmenorrhea. *J Altern Complement Med* 2009;15(2):129.

27. Ayse, Nur Aksoy, et al. Evaluation of the efficacy of fructus agni casti in women with severe primary dysmenorrhea: a prospective comparative doppler study. *J Obstet Gynaecol Res* 2014;40(3): 779–784.

28. Healy D.L., Bell R., Robertson D.M., Jobling T., Oehler M.K., Edwards A., Shekleton P., Oldham J., Piessens S., Teoh M., Mamers P., Taylor N., Walker F. Ovarian status in healthy postmenopausal women. *Menopause* 2008;15(6):1109–1114.

29. Johnstone E.B., Rosen M.P., Neril R., Trevithick D., Sternfeld B., Murphy R., Addauan-Andersen C., McConnell D., Pera R.R., Cedars M.I. The polycystic ovary post-rotterdam: a common, age-dependent finding in ovulatory women without metabolic significance. *J Clin Endocrinol Metab* 2010;95(11):4965–4672. Epub August 18, 2010.

30. Ayhan A., Bukulmez O., Genc C., Karamursel B.S., Ayhan A. Mature cystic teratomas of the ovary: case series from one institution over 34 years. *Eur J Obstet Gynecol Reprod Biol* 2000;88(2):153.

31. Hackethal A., Brueggmann D., Bohlmann M.K., Franke F.E., Tinneberg H.R., Münstedt K. Squamous-cell carcinoma in mature cystic teratoma of the ovary: systematic review and analysis of published data. *Lancet Oncol* 2008;9(12):1173.

32. Talerman A. Germ cell tumours of the ovary. In: *Blaustein's Pathology of the Female Genital Tract*, Kurman R.J. (ed.). New York: Springer Verlag;1994:849.

33. Wheeler M.A., Heffner D.L., Kim S., Espy S.M., Spano A.J., Cleland C.L., Deppmann C.D. TNF-α/TNFR1 signaling is required for the development and function of primary nociceptors. *Neuron* 2014;82(3):587–602.

34. Anaf V., Simon P., El Nakadi I., Fayt I., Buxant F., Simonart T., Peny M.O., Noel J.C. Relationship between endometriotic foci and nerves in rectovaginal endometriotic nodules. *Hum Reprod* 2000;15(8):1744.

35. Wang G., Tokushige N., Markham R., Fraser I.S. Rich innervation of deep infiltrating endometriosis. *Hum Reprod* 2009;24(4):827. Epub January 16, 2009.

36. Tran L.V., Tokushige N., Berbic M., Markham R., Fraser I.S. Macrophages and nerve fibres in peritoneal endometriosis. *Hum Reprod* 2009;24(4):835. Epub January 9, 2009.

37. Matsuzaki S., Darcha C. Involvement of the Wnt/β-catenin signaling pathway in the cellular and molecular mechanisms of fibrosis in endometriosis. *PLoS One* 2013;8(10):e76808. Epub October 4, 2013.

38. McKinnon B.D., Bertschi D., Bersinger N.A., Mueller M.D. Inflammation and nerve fiber interaction in endometriotic pain. *Trends Endocrinol Metab* 2015;26(1):1–10. Epub November 19, 2014.

39. Arnold J., Barcena de Arellano M.L., Rüster C., Vercellino G.F., Chiantera V., Schneider A., Mechsner S. Imbalance between sympathetic and sensory innervation in peritoneal endometriosis. *Brain Behav Immun* 2012;26(1):132–141. Epub August 25, 2011.

40. As-Sanie S., Harris R.E., Napadow V., Kim J., Neshewat G., Kairys A., Williams D., Clauw D.J., Schmidt-Wilcke T. Changes in regional gray matter volume in women with chronic pelvic pain: a voxel-based morphometry study. *Pain* 2012;153(5):1006–1014.

41. Petrosino S., Verde R., Vaia R., Allara M., Iuvone T., DiMarzo V. Anti-inflammatory properties of cannabidiol, a nonpsychotropic cannabinoid, in experimental allergic contact dermatitis. *J Pharmacol Exp Ther* 2018;365(3):652–663.

42. Reinert A.E., Hibner M. Self-reported efficacy of cannabis for endmetriosis pain. *J Min Inv Gynaecol* 2019;26(7):S72.

43. Bottomley C., Bourne T. Diagnosis and management of ovarian cyst accidents. *Best Pract Res Clin Obstet Gynaecol* 2009;23(5):711–724. Epub March 18, 2009.

44. Sharp, H.T. *Evaluation and Management of Ruptured Ovarian Cyst.* Edited by Levine D. Waltham, MA: UpToDate Inc. https://www.uptodate.com (Accessed September 03, 2019).

45. Koshiba H. Severe chemical peritonitis caused by spontaneous rupture of an ovarian mature cystic teratoma: a case report. *J Reprod Med* 2007;52(10):965.

46. Kim J.H., Lee S.M., Lee J.H., Jo Y.R., Moon M.H., Shin J., Kim B.J., Hwang K.R., Lee T.S., Bai K.B., Jeon H.W. Successful conservative management of ruptured ovarian cysts with hemoperitoneum in healthy women. *PLoS One* 2014;9(3):e91171.

47. Goff B.A., Mandel L.S., Melancon C.H., Muntz H.G. Frequency of symptoms of ovarian cancer in women presenting to primary care. *JAMA* 2004;291:2705.

48. Olson S.H., Mignone L., Nakaraseive C., et al. Symptoms of ovarian cancer. *Obstet Gynecol* 2001;98:212.

49. Vine M.F., Ness R.B., Calingaert B., et al. Types and duration of symptoms prior to diagnosis of invasive or borderline ovarian tumor. *Gynecol Oncol* 2001;83:466.

50. International Ovarian Tumour Analysis. IOTA Simple Rules and SRrisk calculator to diagnose ovarian cancer. https://www.iotagroup.org/iota-models-software/iota-simple-rules-and-srrisk-calculator-diagnose-ovarian-cancer (Accessed March 20, 2019).

51. Brown D.L., Doubilet P.M., Miller F.H., Frates M.C., Laing F.C., DiSalvo D.N., Benson C.B., Lerner M.H. Benign and malignant ovarian masses: selection of the most discriminating gray-scale and doppler sonographic features. *Radiology* 1998;208(1):103.

52. Tsafrir Z., Azem F., Hasson J., Solomon E., Almog B., Nagar H., Lessing J.B., Levin I. Risk factors, symptoms, and treatment of ovarian torsion in children: the twelve-year experience of one center. *J Minim Invasive Gynecol* 2012;19(1):29–33. Epub October 20, 2011.

53. Stojkovic D., Sokovic M., Glamoclija J., Dzamic A., Ciric A., Ristic M., Grubišic D. Chemical composition and antimicrobial activity of vitex agnus-castus L. fruits and leaves essential oils. *Food Chem* 2011;128:1017–1022.

54. Guimarães A.G., Quintans J.S., Quintans L.J. Monoterpenes with analgesic activity–a systematic review. *Phytother Res* 2013;27(1):1–15.

55. Lee D.W., Gibson T.B., Carls G.S., Ozminkowski R.J., Wang S., Stewart E.A. Uterine fibroid treatment patterns in a population of insured women. *Fertil Steril* 2009;91(2):566–574.

56. Marshall L.M., Spiegelman D., Barbieri R.L., Goldman M.B., Manson J.E., Colditz G.A., Willett W.C., Hunter D.J. Variation in the incidence of uterine leiomyoma among premenopausal women by age and race. *Obstet Gynecol* 1997;90(6):967.

57. Hodge J.C., Morton C.C. Genetic heterogeneity among uterine leiomyomata: insights into malignant progression. *Hum Mol Genet* 2007;16 Spec No 1:R7.

58. Tomlin J., Lowis C., Read N.W. Investigation of normal flatus production in healthy volunteers. *Gut* 1991;32(6):665.

59. Lin H.C. Small intestinal bacterial overgrowth: a framework for understanding irritable bowel syndrome. *JAMA* 2004;292(7):852.

60. Konkle K.S., Berry S.H., Elliott M.N., Hilton L., Suttorp M.J., Clauw D.J., Clemens J.Q. Comparison of an interstitial cystitis/bladder pain syndrome clinical cohort with symptomatic community women from the RAND interstitial cystitis epidemiology study. *J Urol* 2012;187(2):508.

61. Chung M.K., Chung R.R., Gordon D., Jennings C. The evil twins of chronic pelvic pain syndrome: endometriosis and interstitial cystitis. *JSLS* 2002;6(4):311–314.

62. Clemens J.Q., Meenan R.T., O'Keeffe Rosetti M.C., Kimes T.A., Calhoun E.A. Case-control study of medical comorbidities in women with interstitial cystitis. *J Urol* 2008;179(6):2222.

63. Nazif O., Teichman J.M., Gebhart G.F. Neural upregulation in interstitial cystitis. *Urology* 2007;69 (4 Suppl) Suppl:24.

64. Brunham R.C., Gottlieb S.L., Paavonen J. Pelvic inflammatory disease. *N Engl J Med* 2015;372(21): 2039–2048.
65. Peipert J.F., Ness R.B., Blume J., Soper D.E., Holley R., Randall H., Sweet R.L., Sondheimer S.J., Hendrix S.L., Amortegui A., Trucco G., Bass D.C. Pelvic inflammatory disease evaluation and clinical health study investigators. clinical predictors of endometritis in women with symptoms and signs of pelvic inflammatory disease. *Am J Obstet Gynecol* 2001;184(5):856.
66. Forslin L., Falk V., Danielsson D. Changes in the incidence of acute gonococcal and nongonococcal salpingitis. A five-year study from an urban area of central Sweden. *Br J Vener Dis* 1978;54(4):247.
67. Weström L. Effect of acute pelvic inflammatory disease on fertility. *Am J Obstet Gynecol* 1975;121(5):707.
68. Bolton J.P., Darougar S. Perihepatitis. *Br Med Bull* 1983;39(2):159–162.
69. Wiesenfeld H.C., Sweet R.L., Ness R.B., Krohn M.A., Amortegui A.J., Hillier S.L. Comparison of acute and subclinical pelvic inflammatory disease. *Sex Transm Dis* 2005;32(7):400.
70. Wølner-Hanssen P. Silent pelvic inflammatory disease: is it overstated? *Obstet Gynecol* 1995;86(3):321.
71. ten Broek R.P., Strik C., Issa Y., Bleichrodt R.P., van Goor H. Adhesiolysis-related morbidity in abdominal surgery. *Ann Surg* 2013;258(1):98–106.
72. van den Beukel B.A., de Ree R., van Leuven S., Bakkum E.A., Strik C., van Goor H., ten Broek R.P.G. Surgical treatment of adhesion-related chronic abdominal and pelvic pain after gynaecological and general surgery: a systematic review and meta-analysis. *Hum Reprod Update* 2017;23(3):276.
73. Camus E., Poncelet C., Goffinet F., Wainer B., Merlet F., Nisand I., Philippe H.J. Pregnancy rates after in-vitro fertilization in cases of tubal infertility with and without hydrosalpinx: a meta-analysis of published comparative studies. *Hum Reprod* 1999;14(5):1243–1249.
74. Bornstein J., Goldstein A.T., Stockdale C.K., Bergeron S., Pukall C., Zolnoun D., Coady D. Consensus vulvar pain terminology committee of the International Society for the Study of Vulvovaginal Disease (ISSVD), the International Society for the Study of Women's Sexual Health (ISSWSH), and the International Pelvic Pain Society (IPPS). 2015 ISSVD, ISSWSH and IPPS consensus terminology and classification of persistent vulvar pain and vulvodynia. *Obstet Gynecol* 2016;127(4):745–751.
75. Akopians A.L., Rapkin A.J. Vulvodynia: the role of inflammation in the etiology of localized provoked pain of the vulvar vestibule (Vestibulodynia). *Semin Reprod Med* 2015;33(4):239–245.
76. Bonham A. Vulvar vestibulodynia: strategies to meet the challenge. *Obstet Gynecol Surv* 2015;70(4): 274–278.
77. Wesselmann U., Bonham A., Foster D. Vulvodynia: current state of the biological science. *Pain* 2014; 155(9):1696–1701.
78. http://www.acog.org/Patients/FAQs/Vulvodynia (Accessed September 15, 2019).
79. American College of Obstetricians and Gynecologists'Committee on Gynecologic Practice, American Society for Colposcopy and Cervical Pathology (ASCCP). Committee opinion no 673: persistent vulvar pain. *Obstet Gynecol* 2016;128(3):e78.
80. De Andres J., Sanchis-Lopez N., Asensio-Samper J.M., Fabregat-Cid G., Villanueva-Perez V.L., Monsalve Dolz V., Minguez A. Vulvodynia–an evidence-based literature review and proposed treatment algorithm. *Pain Pract* 2016;16(2):204.
81. Kellogg-Spadt S., Kingsberg S. *Treatment of Vulvodynia (Vulvar Pain of Unknown Cause)*. Edited by Barbieri R.L. Waltham, MA: UpToDate Inc. https://www.uptodate.com. (Accessed October 13, 2019).
82. Goldstein A.T., Pukall C.F., Brown C., Bergeron S., Stein A., Kellogg-Spadt S. Vulvodynia: assessment and treatment. *J Sex Med* 2016;13(4):572–590.
83. Janakiraman R., Hamilton L., Wan A. Unravelling the efficacy of antidepressants as analgesics. *Aust Fam Physician* 2016;45(3):113–117.
84. Dobecki D.A., Schocket S.M., Wallace M.S. Update on pharmacotherapy guidelines for the treatment of neuropathic pain. *Curr Pain Headache Rep* 2006;10(3):185.
85. Pagano R., Wong S. Use of amitriptyline cream in the management of entry dyspareunia due to provoked vestibulodynia. *J Low Genit Tract Dis* 2012;16(4):394–397.
86. Boardman L.A., Cooper A.S., Blais L.R., Raker C.A. Topical gabapentin in the treatment of localized and generalized vulvodynia. *Obstet Gynecol* 2008;112(3):579.

9 Headache Disorders

Todd D. Rozen

CONTENTS

Headache is one of the most common medical complaints. At present there are more than 300 recognized forms of headache in the recent iteration of the International Classification of Headache Disorders (ICHD-3) criteria.[1] It is probably surprising to note that we understand more about the pathogenesis of primary headache disorders than we do about most other neurologic conditions. This knowledge is changing the landscape of headache therapy. The goal of this chapter is to discuss some of the better and lesser known primary headache disorders and their treatment.

MIGRAINE

Migraine is a very common medical disorder, affecting more than 30 million individuals in the United States alone. It is the most typical headache condition that presents to the physician's office. Migraine is considered an episodic disorder, but in reality it is a brain-based chronic disease state that can affect multiple body systems. According to the Global Burden of Disease Study in 2013, migraine is one of only eight chronic medical conditions that affect more than 10% of the population worldwide.[2]

Diagnosis

The International Headache Society has formulated diagnostic criteria (ICHD-3) for most primary and secondary headache disorders. The current ICHD-3 criteria for migraine is as follows:

- At least five attacks fulfilling criteria B–D
- Headache attacks lasting 4–72 h (untreated or unsuccessfully treated)
- Headache has ≥2 of the following characteristics:
  ◦ Unilateral location
  ◦ Pulsating quality
  ◦ Moderate or severe pain intensity
  ◦ Aggravation by or causing avoidance of routine physical activity (e.g., walking, climbing stairs)
- During headache ≥1 of the following:
  ◦ Nausea and/or vomiting
  ◦ Photophobia and phonophobia

In most instances, migraine can be easily diagnosed, but there are some clinical issues that medical personnel should recognize that may help in making a correct diagnosis if "typical symptomatology" is not present.

- Location: we think of migraine as a one-sided headache; the criteria say it is, but many times it is not. Kelman looked at 1283 patients and hemi-cranial location was noted in 66.6% of patients while 23.7% had headache bilaterally.[3] Multiple other cite references state that in about 40% of migraineurs headache is bilateral.[3–5]
- Quality: pulsating pain has been stated to occur in 47–82% of migraineurs.[6–8] However, patients may misunderstand the terms "throbbing" and "pulsating." It has been suggested using the expression "throbbing with your heartbeat" could be a better representation of the pain.
- Intensity: moderate to severe pain is a hallmark of migraine and has been documented in 85–91% of patients in population-based studies.[6] However, we recognize that mild migraine exists.
- Associated symptoms: many patients may deny light or sound sensitivity during a migraine headache when indeed they have photophobia or phonophobia. This may relate to the way the questions about these symptoms are posed to the patient. Evans et al.[9] used a more detailed close-ended question as part of their routine headache history to test this issue. They first would query "Does light bother you during a headache?" If the patient answered "No" then a follow-up question was asked: during a headache would you prefer to be in bright sunlight or in a dark room?" They then asked "Does noise bother you during a headache?" If the patient answered "No" then the follow-up question was: "During a headache would you prefer to be in room with loud music or in a quiet room?" Eighty-five patients were questioned. For light sensitivity, patients (26%) said "No" on initial questioning but on the follow-up question 91% preferred being in a dark room. For sound sensitivity, 22 patients (26%) again said "No" to the initial question, but 95.5% preferred a quiet room after further questioning. The authors stated that there was underreporting of light and sound sensitivity in 24% of patients via routine questioning with 93% having *awareness* on more direct questioning.
- Age of patient: there is also an issue when we ask about quality, sidedness, and associated symptoms in patients of different ages. Bigal et al.[10] looked at a study sample of 145,335

participants. The prevalence of unilateral and throbbing pain peaked at intermediate ages and declined after that. Photophobia and phonophobia declined with age in addition. Kelman studied 1009 patients,[11] and in regard to the associated symptoms of photophobia and phonophobia these decreased with age while nausea, vomiting, and osmophobia showed no significant differences with aging. Headache quality showed decreasing throbbing, pressure, and stabbing with age. The 50+ age group tended to have less dizziness, photophobia, phonophobia, nausea, vomiting, temporal location, throbbing, pressure, stabbing, headache days, moderate days, severe days, aggravation of headache by activity, and recurrence but tended to have more mild days, greater ability to function during headache, and greatest response to acute medication.

So how good are the established migraine criteria for diagnosis? Diagnosis depends on the presence of a specific group of symptoms, but we recognize that the symptoms in the established criteria (unilateral pain, pulsatile quality, moderate to severe pain, and the associated symptoms) either are not present in a number of sufferers or are history-dependent or age-dependent. Field testing has suggested that the presence of associated symptoms provides the greatest discrimination between migraine without aura and other headache subtypes. The criteria are definitely not age-sensitive criteria.

There may be a simpler way to diagnose migraine by just asking about three issues. If the patient presents with nausea, photophobia, and disability (two of three), the sensitivity, specificity, and positive predictive value of making a correct diagnosis of migraine is extremely high.[12] However, what if a patient tells us that they have migraine? Is that good enough? Schürks et al.,[13] utilizing the Women's Health Study in which 1675 of the sample reported migraine, found that over 87% could then be classified as "migraine without aura" or "probable migraine" without aura, applying ICHD criteria. Qiu et al.[14] looked at 500 women and could confirm self-reported migraine in 81.6% when applying ICHD criteria.

PATHOGENESIS

Migraine is actually made up of multiple phases and is not just a head pain condition. Each phase has its own distinct pathogenesis and treatment. Not every migraineur has every phase, but their recognition will allow better treatment options.

- Prodrome: the migraine prodrome, or premonitory phase, can occur several hours to several days prior to a headache. The main symptoms of this phase include excessive yawning which is probably related to a hyperdopaminergic state and food cravings which suggests a hypothalamically modulated stage. Recent functional imaging has actually shown hypothalamic activation during the prodrome as well as activation in the periaqueductal gray and pons.[15] This phase of the migraine attack can actually be treated. Taking a mild dopamine receptor antagonist like metoclopramide (10 mg one dose only) as early into the prodrome as possible can prevent the onset of a migraine attack in a significant number of patients. It is actually one of the better acute treatments for migraine.
- Migraine aura: migraine should not be defined by aura as it occurs in only about 20% of sufferers. However the aura when present should have a distinct clinical presentation based on symptoms and duration. Auras should last between 5 minutes and 60 minutes.[1] If auras are of a shorter duration or more prolonged a secondary issue should be looked for. Auras of prolonged duration are the most concerning as they are a risk factor for migraine-induced stroke and have been linked to coagulopathies, carotid or vertebral dissection, underlying mitochondrial disorders, and from a true stroke. There are various forms of aura with visual (spreading scotoma, fortification spectra) and sensory (spreading paresthesias or numbness typically going from hand to ipsilateral face and half of tongue) being the most common. Other aura types include language (typically aphasia) and brainstem (bilateral

visual disturbances, vertigo, bilateral paresthesias which can involve arms and legs, and sometimes true syncope). Hemiplegic migraine can be diagnosed if a patient has true motor weakness during an aura phase regardless of the duration of the aura. The aura phase is caused by a dynamic brain-based event called cortical spreading depression (CSD) which involves a slow wave of neural depolarization, leading to changes in brain glial activity with alteration of cerebral blood flow. During CSD there is an initial increase in cerebral blood flow along with enhanced cortical activity, and this correlates with the positive aura phenomena (bright scintillations) but is then followed by a reduction in cerebral blood flow with resultant negative phenomena like loss of vison, scotoma, and motor weakness.[16]

Treatment of the aura: although the typical migraine aura is somewhat unpleasant for the patient, it does not require treatment because of its short duration and very small, if any, risk of causing permanent neurologic dysfunction. During an aura, regional cerebral blood flow is reduced by about 30%. A prolonged aura may reflect a continuous state of cortical spreading depression, but along with this, a persistent reduction in cerebral blood flow with a remote risk of migrainous infarction. Patients who present with a prolonged aura should be evaluated for a migrainous infarction, but, if imaging is negative for ischemia, a strong effort should be made to terminate the aura. Various treatments have shown efficacy in alleviating or shortening a prolonged migraine aura, including oral divalproex,[17] oral acetazolamide,[18] and intranasal ketamine;[19] however, several other IV therapies (furosemide,[20] magnesium sulfate combined with a dopamine receptor antagonist[21]) may be more available, especially if patients are presenting to the emergency department (ED). There are also certain oral preventive medications that can work not only on reducing headache frequency but also to reduce aura frequency. These include divalproex sodium, calcium channel antagonists (both verapamil and flunarizine), topiramate (in first multicenter trial for migraine prevention [CAPSS-155] patients who had migraine with aura showed a significant reduction in aura frequency on topiramate versus placebo), lamotrigine (several studies have demonstrated the efficacy of lamotrigine to reduce aura frequency and duration, and this is probably the preventive of choice to reduce aura; sadly it is much less effective as a migraine preventive versus topiramate and valproic acid), and oral magnesium (which in essence is a NMDA receptor antagonist and thus blocks glutamate).[22] In the lab glutamate as well as potassium are the main triggers of CSD.[16]

- Headache phase: the headache itself is a brain-based disorder which involves activation of the trigeminovascular system with the release of various neurotransmitters including CGRP, substance P, and neurokinin A, leading to an inflammatory cascade involving the meninges, meningeal arteries and veins, and cortical substance.[16] In essence migraine is a focal meningitis and focal cerebritis with minimal vascular-based pathology. Thus referring to migraine as a primary vascular headache is truly a misnomer. Activation of the trigeminal system can lead to central sensitization, which produces symptoms of allodynia (painful response to a non-painful stimulus). One of the recent advances in migraine research has been the identification of possible biomarkers in migraineurs. Glutamate, CGRP, β-endorphin, and nerve growth factor (NGF) levels have all been found to be significantly increased or decreased in cerebrospinal fluid (CSF) and blood (with the exception of NGF, which has only been shown to be elevated in CSF).[16] Glutamate has been implicated in the pathogenesis of cortical spreading depression; NGF and β-endorphin are thought to affect analgesia pathways. However, the optimal use of biomarkers for diagnosis, prognosis, and treatment is still to be determined. What is exciting is that our knowledge of migraine headache pathogenesis has led to effective therapies for this disabling condition, first the triptans in the 1990s and now monoclonal antibody therapy introduced in 2018 (see below).
- Postdrome: the least studied of the migraine phases but one that should be looked into further as it is truly part of the migraine disability cascade is the prodrome. This phase typically includes non-headache symptoms such as malaise, fatigue, or gastrointestinal complaints.

Migraine Treatment

Most treatments for migraine (acute and preventive) are well-known to treating physicians. Sadly, these were unchanged for decades until recently.

Acute treatment: the current American Headache Society evidence assessment for acute therapy states that all triptans in all formulations as well as dihydroergotamine (nasal spray) have Level A effectiveness. Level A evidence requires at least two Class I studies.[23] Ergotamine and other forms of dihydroergotamine are probably effective with Level B evidence. Level B evidence requires one Class I or two Class II studies. Nonspecific medications showing Level A evidence include acetaminophen, nonsteroidal anti-inflammatory drugs (aspirin, diclofenac, ibuprofen, and naproxen), opioids (butorphanol nasal spray), sumatriptan/naproxen, and the combination of acetaminophen/aspirin/caffeine. Level B evidence has been noted for ketoprofen, intravenous and intramuscular ketorolac, intravenous magnesium (in migraine with aura), isometheptene compounds, codeine/acetaminophen, and tramadol/acetaminophen. Antiemetics including prochlorperazine, droperidol, chlorpromazine, and metoclopramide are Level B. There is inadequate evidence for butalbital and butalbital combination, butorphanol or meperidine injections, intranasal lidocaine, and corticosteroids.[23]

Preventive treatment: the most recent guidelines for the prevention of episodic migraine by the American Headache Society/American Academy of Neurology, the Canadian Headache Society, and the European Federation of Neurological Societies were published in 2012.[24] The medications with Level A evidence included sodium valproate, topiramate, propranolol, timolol, metoprolol, and frovatriptan (prevention of menstrual migraine). There is Level B evidence for amitriptyline, venlafaxine, atenolol, and nadolol as well as naratriptan and zolmitriptan for short-term menstrual migraine prevention. Level C (possibly effective) evidence was noted for lisinopril, candesartan, clonidine, guanfacine carbamazepine, nebivolol, and pindolol. Finally Level U (conflicting or inadequate evidence) was noted for gabapentin, fluoxetine, fluvoxamine, protriptyline, nicardipine, nifedipine, nimodipine, verapamil, and acetazolamide.

New Thoughts on Treatment

With the rise of complementary and alternative medicine worldwide, an increasing number of supplements and vitamins have been suggested as effective migraine treatments. Many of these treatments have shown benefit, leading to varying degrees of endorsement in migraine guidelines for butterbur, feverfew, coenzyme Q10, and others.[25] Butterbur, however, has since been associated with rare but severe hepatotoxicity, so the headache societies have suggested to avoid its usage.

Botulinum toxin type A is approved by the Food and Drug Administration (FDA) for use in the preventive treatment of chronic migraine. A recent study using insurance claims data demonstrated that botulinum toxin therapy significantly reduced headache-related emergency department visits and hospitalizations when compared to other oral migraine preventative medications.[26] Botulinim toxin is typically reserved for patients who have failed two to three preventative medications and are experiencing chronic migraine per ICHD criteria.[1]

Non-invasive brain stimulation is a broad term that includes transcutaneous magnetic stimulation (TMS) and transcutaneous direct current stimulation (tDCS). These modalities, which have been studied as both preventative and acute treatments, offer the advantage of being non-medicinal, non-invasive, typically painless, and rapidly administered. There are currently two main commercially available tDCS devices that have been studied in migraine: Cefaly (supraorbital/supratrochlear stimulation) and gammaCore (external vagal nerve stimulation). Both devices deliver low-dose electric current and have been approved by the FDA for use in migraine. Few data are available from randomized sham-controlled studies to evaluate the efficacy of tDCS devices; however, subgroup analysis from a recent meta-analysis of non-invasive brain stimulation found moderate quality evidence suggesting that tDCS reduced pain intensity, number of migraines, and acute medication intake.[27] The Cefaly device has been shown in randomized controlled trials (RCTs) to be of benefit for both abortive and preventative therapy and is FDA-approved for the prevention of episodic migraine. The gammaCore device (a peripheral vagal nerve stimulator) has shown efficacy in randomized controlled trials as an acute treatment for episodic and chronic migraine.[28] TMS, which applies magnetic impulse to the cerebral cortex, has shown some benefit for use as an abortive treatment for migraine. The open-label, multicenter ESPOUSE study, published in January 2018, suggested that TMS is safe and effective for the prevention of migraine.[29] The previously mentioned systematic review and meta-analysis revealed that non-invasive brain stimulation, including TMS and tDCS, had a low to very low quality of evidence and no clear benefit over sham treatment in a review of studies up to January 2016; open-label studies since that time have been generally positive, so the true benefit of these therapies remains to be seen in clinical practice.

New Developments in Migraine Treatment

Several touted "migraine-specific" agents have been recently developed, including CGRP receptor antagonists (for abortive use) and monoclonal antibodies targeting CGRP receptors or the protein itself (preventive use). These medications represent a great advancement in current treatment of migraine to a more specific, tailored therapy based on known pathophysiologic mechanisms. Several oral CGRP receptor antagonists in development have shown promising efficacy in treating migraine with superiority to placebo and comparability to triptans, but many of the trials have been discontinued due to concerns of hepatotoxicity after taking the drug for multiple consecutive days. A phase II RCT published in 2016 found that ubrogepant, a CGRP receptor antagonist, yielded modest results as an abortive agent in the indicator single migraine freedom at two hours after medication administration when compared to placebo; there were no signs of hepatotoxicity within 1 week of drug administration.[30] These agents are on track for possible FDA approval.

In recent years, four monoclonal antibodies targeting CGRP or the CGRP receptor have been tested in humans for the prevention of migraine: galcanezumab, eptinezumab, erenumab, and fremanezumab.[31] High-quality RCTs have demonstrated the efficacy of these antibodies in decreasing migraine days in episodic migraine as well as chronic migraine. Fremanezumab showed efficacy in reducing monthly migraines in a phase III trial of 1130 patients with chronic migraine.[32] Erenumab—the only monoclonal antibody that targets the CGRP receptor—demonstrated similar efficacy for episodic migraine in addition to chronic migraine.[33] The reported reduction in monthly migraine has been approximately three to six episodes per month and significantly greater than placebo. Of note, patients with chronic migraine were excluded from the previously cited studies if they had failed preventative treatment with two to three prophylactic medications. Despite the promising results of these positive trials, additional studies are needed to determine the long-term efficacy, safety, and cost-effectiveness of monoclonal antibodies. An analysis of a 5-year study of erenumab revealed sustained treatment effect and safety at week 64, with 25% of patients reporting 100% reduction in monthly migraine days.[34] Erenumab, galcanezumab, and fremanezumab are all currently FDA-approved for migraine prevention. The long-term safety is still questioned, as well as the role of these agents as first-line treatments or only after multiple medications failures. As CGRP is an essential vasodilatory protein for cerebral and coronary arteries, its potential contraindication in patients with coronary artery disease, past stroke, or uncontrolled hypertension for example has not been well-studied but should be taken into consideration when there is a thought of prescribing these agents.

Another breakthrough in the treatment of migraine is the development of 5-HT1F receptor antagonists Particularly, this drug class binds more specifically to the serotonin 1F receptor than triptans which bind to the 5HT1b/d receptors with the potential for vasoconstriction.[35] This new drug class called ditans may be highly valuable for an aging population that is no longer eligible for triptan therapy because of cardiovascular and cerebrovascular risk factors or in those with known coronary artery disease.

Role of Opiates in Migraine Treatment

A crisis exists in the United States and other countries around the world with the inordinate amount of opioids being used for non-cancer-related pain syndromes. One of the largest culprits is the use of opioids for migraine, especially in the ED. Although consensus guidelines have advised against the use of opioids for migraine, a recent publication noted a 70% increase in the use of hydromorphone, morphine, and oxycodone in U.S. emergency departments from 2001 to 2010.[36] Looking at the data, opioids are typically less effective or, at most, equally effective as multiple non-opioid acute migraine treatments, including ketorolac,[37] DHE,[38] corticosteroids,[39] and dopamine receptor antagonists.[40] In addition, opioids have the distinction of being associated with abuse and habituation. Opioids drain medical resources, as they have been shown to lead to an increase in headache relapse and need for a return to the ED for further treatment.[41] A recent study has shown that if patients in the ED are administered opioids, it results in longer ED stays than if non-opioid compounds are utilized.[42] Opioids should only be used on infrequent occasions for migraine therapy, including pregnancy, in patients with multiple risk factors to non-opioid medications, and in the rare patient who presents to the ED with no history of abuse (opioid or other drugs or alcohol) and has multiple documented medical contraindications to almost every other class of acute migraine medication that can be delivered in the ED for status migrainosus; thus on very rare occasions. All opioids for home use as an acute headache treatment should be limited at maximum to 2 days a week and with a limited number of pill amounts being given on the prescription which automatically limits abuse and medication overuse potential.

Migraine and the Emergency Department

The general principles of treating migraine in the ED include: (a) adequately hydrate all patients with IV fluids if no contraindication exists; (b) treat headache with non-opioid medications if options to do so are available; (c) provide rapid relief with IV medications; and (d) establish the correct expectations for the patient. If, for example, a patient with a 10-year history of chronic daily headache presents with an exacerbation of pain, the goal of ED treatment is to provide adequate relief for that single exacerbation, not to try to make someone pain free who has not had a pain-free moment in many years. However, if the patient has only episodic migraine, the goal of ED treatment is sustained pain freedom for that particular headache.

Medication Choices for Acute Treatment of Migraine in the Emergency Department:

- Intravenous fluids. It seems clear that the patient with migraine who has vomited before coming to the ED would need fluid rehydration, but in reality all patients in status migrainosus (persistent migraine) should receive IV hydration. In the author's experience, IV fluids alone can sometimes be as successful in reducing pain intensity as medication. To date, no studies have looked at the efficacy of IV fluids alone for treating acute migraine; however, a study by Harden and colleagues[43] compared the efficacy of ketorolac 60 mg, meperidine 50 mg plus promethazine 25 mg, and normal saline all given by IM injection and noted that all treatments produced a significant reduction in head pain ($p < 0.0001$), but that pain reduction did not differ among the treatments. This could indicate that saline was as effective as ketorolac and meperidine for migraine or that there was an equally robust placebo effect for all.
- Magnesium sulfate. Magnesium sulfate may exert a therapeutic effect on migraine through its antagonism of N-methyl-D-aspartate (NMDA) receptors, its blockade of cortical spreading depression, or both. It can be used for both status migrainosus and for treating prolonged auras. Studies have shown mixed evidence of effectiveness for acute migraine in the ED. Two placebo-controlled trials evaluated the efficacy of IV magnesium sulfate, and while one showed no improvement versus placebo, the other demonstrated a significant difference favoring magnesium sulfate in a migraine with aura subgroup.[44] In the

original open-label trial of IV magnesium sulfate in acute migraine, 35 of 40 patients treated achieved 50% or greater reduction in pain intensity. Low serum ionized magnesium levels appeared to predict sustained treatment response to IV magnesium, as 86% of patients (18 of 21 subjects) with serum ionized magnesium levels below 0.54 mmol/L had pain relief lasting over 24 hours compared with only 16% (3 of 19 subjects) with ionized magnesium levels at or above 0.54 mmol/L (p < 0.001).[45]

- Dopamine receptor modulators. Dopamine receptor antagonists are readily utilized in the ED for status migrainosus. Their antiemetic effects are useful for the nausea and vomiting that accompany a severe migraine headache. Dopamine antagonism may also provide relief of both pain and aura symptoms. Finally, their antihistaminic and anticholinergic properties provide a sedative effect, and for most patients with migraine, sleep has therapeutic value. The three subclasses of dopamine receptor antagonists include metoclopramide, phenothiazines (prochlorperazine, promethazine, and chlorpromazine), and the butyrophenones (droperidol and haloperidol). In the author's opinion, the higher the degree of CNS dopamine receptor blockade, the greater the efficacy in providing migraine relief, but also the higher the potential for adverse side-effects (in descending order of degree of dopamine receptor blockade and efficacy in providing migraine relief: haloperidol, chlorpromazine, droperidol, prochlorperazine, promethazine, metoclopramide). Based on a recent systematic review of the entire literature on the use of drugs for the treatment of migraine in the ED, prochlorperazine and metoclopramide have received a strong recommendation supporting their use based on high and moderate levels of evidence, respectively.[46] Chlorpromazine received a weak recommendation, despite a moderate level of evidence, on the basis of a more significant adverse event profile. Regardless of which dopamine receptor antagonist is chosen, IV fluid boluses should be administered as a pretreatment because of the potential for hypotension. In addition, an ECG with QTc interval measurements should be obtained prior to administering butyrophenones and chlorpromazine, as these agents can prolong QT intervals and are contraindicated if a patient has a baseline prolonged QT interval. Low dosages should be used initially, as superior efficacy for some dopamine receptor antagonists, including metoclopramide, droperidol, and prochlorperazine, has been demonstrated at lower doses compared to higher doses.[47–49] Lower doses of dopamine receptor antagonists also have a better side effect profile. Prior to administering antidopaminergic drugs, patients should be cautioned about their potential side effects. Pretreatment with IV diphenhydramine is recommended to minimize or avoid extrapyramidal side effects, especially with dopamine receptor antagonists that have a high incidence of posttreatment akathisia and dystonia. Akathisia, a common adverse event secondary to dopamine receptor antagonists, can eliminate any positive headache response from these medications, because it can be as disabling to the patient as the pain itself. Akathisia can occur almost immediately after dosing with some antidopaminergic medications but can also be a delayed reaction, especially with droperidol, starting many hours after medication administration and thus after the patient has left the ED. IV diphenhydramine should eliminate this side effect and may itself have migraine-alleviating properties.[50]

- Nonsteroidal anti-inflammatory drugs. A recent systematic review looked at 34 studies, including 8 trials, assessing the efficacy of ketorolac for the acute treatment of migraine.[51] The overall assessment was that this NSAID is effective, with similar pain relief to meperidine (with less addictive potential), and more efficacious than sumatriptan, but not as effective as phenothiazines and metoclopramide. The Canadian Headache Society strongly recommends IM or IV ketorolac for migraine treatment in the ED based on a systematic review of the literature, clinical experience, and a favorable side effect profile.[46] Typical dosing is 30 mg IV, but 60 mg IV can have efficacy rates up to 80%.

- Corticosteroids. It is very common to see the addition of IV corticosteroids to a migraine treatment regimen in the ED. In a recent meta-analysis, 25 studies involving 3989 patients indicated the potential benefit of using IV dexamethasone to prevent headache recurrence up to 72 hours after discharge from the ED.[52] However, evidence suggests that IV dexamethasone is not effective for the acute treatment of migraine in the ED.[46] All patients who receive corticosteroids must recognize the potential risk of avascular necrosis of the hip, which is exceedingly rare with single dosing but has been known to arise with short courses of treatment. In the author's experience, patients may respond to IV methylprednisolone 100 mg to 200 mg or dexamethasone 4 mg to 16 mg in the ED; if no contraindications are present (concomitant infection, diabetes mellitus, history of tuberculosis) and first-line treatments are unsuccessful, the author will prescribe this therapy.
- IV antiepileptic drugs. IV sodium valproate (typical dosing 500 mg to 1000 mg) has some support for its use in open-label studies and some recent support in comparator trials, but no placebo-controlled studies have evaluated its efficacy in patients with status migrainosus or intractable migraine.[53] Based on the author's clinical experience, however, this medication can be helpful for status migrainosus and could be tried if more conventional treatments (e.g., IV NSAIDs, dopamine receptor antagonists) have failed and the patient has no medical contraindications, including liver dysfunction, failure, or transplant, or pregnancy. Surprisingly, the author has seen hyperammonemia with encephalopathy develop acutely after a single dose of IV sodium valproate when given to patients with migraine who are on oral topiramate for migraine prevention. It is known that oral combination therapy with valproic acid and topiramate can cause this metabolic response, but it is somewhat alarming that it can occur after a single IV dose of medication.[54] Intravenous levetiracetam has not been thoroughly studied for the treatment of status migrainosus, although one single case has been reported in the literature stating its efficacy.[55]
- Vasoconstrictors. In the author's opinion, the use of migraine-specific vasoconstrictive compounds (triptans and DHE) in an ED setting can be problematic. This does not relate at all to the effectiveness of these medications. Injectable sumatriptan has shown efficacy rates higher than 70% in an ED setting,[56] while DHE has shown a 60% reduction in head pain at 1 hour with IV administration in the ED.[57] The issue is in giving medications that can constrict cardiac and cerebral arteries to patients whose background cardiovascular and neurovascular history the physician is not fully aware of. As so many non-vasoconstrictive medication choices are available, why even take the chance of administering DHE or sumatriptan in the ED with the risk of causing a myocardial infarction or a stroke, or even exacerbating vasospasm in a missed case of reversible cerebral vasoconstriction syndrome (which is more likely to occur in a patient with a history of migraine), if, by chance, a thunderclap onset of headache was missed in the history? Triptans or DHE should typically only be administered in the ED setting if the treating physician is very familiar with the patient's medical and migraine history or has personally spoken with the patient's treating physician, who requests for these medications to be given. Contraindications to the use of triptans and DHE include uncontrolled hypertension, past stroke or myocardial infarction, peripheral vascular disease, presence of aneurysms, and certain types of aura, including hemiplegic aura and prolonged (more than 1 hour) aura.
- Nerve blockade. If IV therapy in the ED has failed and the patient continues to have unabated head pain, then a greater occipital nerve block can be helpful. Other procedures, including supraorbital, auriculotemporal, and supratrochlear nerve injections, may also be beneficial.[58]

TRIGEMINAL AUTONOMIC CEPHALALGIAS

The trigeminal autonomic cephalalgias (TACs) are a group of headache disorders marked by trigeminal-based head pain and prominent cranial autonomic-associated symptoms of both cranial parasympathetic activation (conjunctival injection, lacrimation, nasal congestion and/or rhinorrhea, eyelid edema) and sympathetic dysfunction (ptosis, miosis—partial or full Horner's syndrome).[1] This subgroup of headache syndromes is also marked by their severity (many times off the pain scale), repetitive attacks per day of typically short duration, and seasonal and diurnal predilection indicating a possible hypothalamic/circadian influence over the syndromes. Currently recognized TACs include cluster headache (CH), paroxysmal hemicrania, SUNCT syndrome, and hemicrania continua.

Diagnosis

To make a proper diagnosis of a TAC the key is to look at the frequency of attacks and headache attack duration (Table 9.1). Many of these syndromes have migrainous-associated symptoms but they would not be migraine based on the duration and frequency of attacks.

Cluster Headache

ICHD-3 diagnostic criteria:

- At least five attacks fulfilling criteria B–D
- Severe or very severe unilateral orbital, supraorbital, and/or temporal pain lasting 15–180 min (when untreated)
- Either or both of the following:
    ○ At least one of the following ipsilateral symptoms or signs:
        – Conjunctival injection and/or lacrimation
        – Nasal congestion and/or rhinorrhea
        – Eyelid edema
        – Forehead and facial sweating
        – Forehead and facial flushing
        – Sensation of fullness in the ear
        – Miosis and/or ptosis
    ○ A sense of restlessness or agitation
- Frequency from 1/2 d to 8/d for > half the time when active

Cluster headache is a stereotypic episodic headache disorder marked by frequent attacks of short-lasting, severe, unilateral head pain with associated cranial autonomic symptoms.[1] A cluster

TABLE 9.1
Clinical Characteristics of the TACs

Characteristics	Cluster	Paroxysmal Hemicrania	SUNCT	Hemicrania Continua
Frequency	1–3 attacks/day	5–24 attacks/day	>25 attacks/day	Daily low-grade pain with severe exacerbations lasting 1–3 days
Duration	15–180 minutes	2–30 minutes	1–600 seconds	Constant
Gender	M > F	F > M	M > F	F > M
Indomethacin-responsive	No	Yes	No	Yes

headache is defined as an individual attack of head pain, while a cluster period or cycle is the time in which a patient is having daily cluster headaches. Most cluster patients have episodic cluster headache, indicating that they will have remission periods in between cluster cycles, while a few unfortunate individuals have chronic cluster headache where cycles occur for more than 1 year without remission or with remission periods lasting <1 month.[1]

The typical cluster headache location is retro-orbital, periorbital, and occipitonuchal. Cluster headache intensity is almost always severe. The one-sided nature of cluster headaches is a trademark. Cluster sufferers will normally experience cluster headaches on the same side of the head their entire life. The duration of individual cluster headaches is between 15 minutes and 180 minutes with more than 75% attacks being shorter than 60 minutes. Attack frequency is between one and three attacks per day with most patients experiencing two or fewer headaches in a day. Cluster period duration normally lasts between 2 and 12 weeks, and patients generally experience one or two cluster periods per year. Remission periods (headache-free time in between cluster cycles) average 6 months to 2 years. Cluster headache is marked by its associated autonomic symptoms that typically occur on the same side as the head pain but can be bilateral. Lacrimation is the most common associated symptom followed by conjunctival injection, nasal congestion, nasal rhinorrhea, and a partial Horner's syndrome in 16–84%. Symptoms generally attributed to migraine can also occur during a cluster headache including nausea, vomiting, photophobia, and phonophobia. This typically occurs more in female cluster headache patients. During an individual cluster headache, patients are unable to sit or stand completely still. Cluster is really a state of agitation, as remaining still appears to make the pain worse. Many patients will develop their own routine during a cluster attack which may include self-injurious behavior including banging their heads against the wall or hitting themselves in the head.

Pathogenesis: the circadian periodicity of CH (attacks occur at the same time every day, cycles begin at the time of the clock change or solstice) suggests that the hypothalamus in some manner is involved in CH pathogenesis but in what capacity is as yet not understood.[59,60] It may act as the primary generator or as an area of susceptibility. What has been documented via functional neuroimaging studies is that the posterior hypothalamus, in the region of the suprachiasmatic nucleus (our circadian clock) ipsilateral to the headache, becomes active during attacks. Again the generator or modulator is unknown at present.

Treatment

All cluster headache patients require treatment. Other primary headache syndromes can sometimes be managed non-medicinally but in regard to cluster headache, medication, sometimes even polypharmacy, is indicated. Cluster headache treatment can be divided into three classes. Acute therapy is treatment given at the time of an attack to treat that individual attack alone. Transitional preventive therapy can be considered an intermittent or short-term preventive treatment. An agent is started at the same time as the patient's true maintenance preventive. The transitional therapy will provide the cluster patient attack relief while the maintenance preventive is being built up to a therapeutic dosage. Maintenance preventive therapy consists of daily medication, which is supposed to reduce the frequency of headache attacks, lower attack intensity, and lessen attack duration. The main goal of cluster headache preventive therapy should be to make a patient cluster-free on preventives even though they are still in a cluster cycle. As most cluster headache patients have episodic cluster headache, medications are only utilized while a patient is in cycle and stopped during remission periods.

- Acute Therapy
  The goal of abortive therapy for cluster headache is fast, effective, and consistent relief. There is no role for over-the-counter agents or butalbital-containing compounds and little if any need for opiates. Abortives need to show effect usually within 20 minutes as the attacks are short in duration.

○ Sumatriptan

Subcutaneous sumatriptan is the most effective medication for the symptomatic relief of cluster headache. In a placebo-controlled study, 6 mg of injectable sumatriptan was significantly more effective than placebo, with 74% of patients having complete relief by 15 minutes compared with 26% of placebo-treated patients.[61] In long-term, open-label studies, sumatriptan is effective in 76% to 100% of all attacks within 15 minutes even after repetitive daily use for several months.[62] Sumatriptan is contraindicated in patients with uncontrolled hypertension, and past history of myocardial infarction or stroke. As almost all cluster patients have a strong history of cigarette smoking, the physician must closely monitor cardiovascular risk factors in these patients.

Sumatriptan nasal spray (20 mg) has been shown to be more effective than placebo in the acute treatment of cluster attacks. In over 80 patients tested, intranasal sumatriptan reduced cluster headache pain from very severe, severe, or moderate to mild or no pain at 30 minutes in 58% of sumatriptan users versus 30% of patients given placebo on the first attack treated, while the rates were 50% (sumatriptan) versus 33% (placebo) after the second treated attack.[63] Sumatriptan nasal spray appears to be efficacious for cluster headache but less effective than subcutaneous injection. Sumatriptan nasal spray should be considered as a cluster headache abortive in patients who cannot tolerate injections or when situationally (e.g., an office setting)injections would be considered socially unacceptable.

In many instances cluster headache patients may need to use sumatriptan more than one time in a day for days to weeks at a time. There is still controversy over whether cluster headache patients can develop medication overuse headache. Even though daily sumatriptan may be benefiting a cluster headache patient the goal should be to have them cluster-free on preventive medication and not using abortives to achieve cluster-free status.

○ Inhaled Oxygen

Oxygen inhalation has been a well-known therapy for cluster headache dating back to the 1950s. What has changed is dosing, where now high-flow oxygen up to 15 liters per minute (LPM) is the norm, whereas for many years the dosing schedule was only 7–10 LPM. Typical dosing is 100% oxygen given via a non-rebreather face-mask at 12–15 liters per minute for 20 minutes.[64,65] In some patients, oxygen is completely effective at aborting an attack if taken when the pain is at maximal intensity, while in others, the attack is only delayed rather than completely alleviated. It is not uncommon for a cluster patient to be headache-free while on oxygen but immediately re-develop headache when the oxygen is removed. Oxygen is overall a very attractive therapy as it is completely safe and can be used multiple times during the day.

See Table 9.2 for acute treatment options. In patients with known coronary artery disease or past stroke or myocardial infarction #s 2, 6–13 can be alternative treatment options.

• Transitional Therapy

Transitional cluster therapy is a short-term preventive treatment that bridges the time between cluster diagnosis and the time when the true traditional maintenance preventive agent becomes efficacious. Transitional preventives are started at the same time the maintenance preventive is begun. The transitional preventive should provide the cluster patient with almost immediate pain relief and allow the patient to be headache-free or near headache-free while the maintenance preventive medication dose is being tapered up to an effective level. When the transitional agent is tapered off the maintenance preventive will have kicked in; thus, the patient will have no gap in headache preventive coverage.

TABLE 9.2

Acute Treatment Options for Cluster Headache

1. Sumatriptan injection or nasal spray
2. 100% oxygen: via non-rebreather face mask at 12–15 LPM
3. Zolmitriptan: 10 mg > 5 mg PO or nasal spray
4. DHE injection
5. Ergotamine: PO, suppository
6. Intranasal lidocaine (4%)
7. Olanzapine: 2.5–10 mg PO
8. GON block: if in office or ED
9. Chlorpromazine supp 25–100 mg
10. Indomethacin supp 50 mg repeat q 30 minutes
11. Rare opiates or butorphanol
12. Subcutaneous octreotide 100 μg
13. External vagal nerve stimulator

○ Corticosteroids

A short course of corticosteroids is the most recognized transitional therapy for cluster headache. Typically within 24 to 48 hours of administration patients become headache-free and by the time the steroid taper has ended the patient's maintenance preventive agent has hopefully started to become effective. Prednisone or dexamethasone are the most typically used corticosteroids in cluster headache. A typical taper would be 80 mg of prednisone for the first 2 days followed by 60 mg for 2 days, 40 mg for 2 days, 20 mg for 2 days, 10 mg for 2 days, then stopping the agent.

○ Dihydroergotamine

Intravenous DHE is an attractive transitional treatment but is more labor-intensive because patients either need to be admitted or brought to an outpatient infusion center for therapy. Typically within 1 or 2 days of repetitive DHE treatment cluster attacks stop and will not return for days to months. This allows time for a maintenance preventive agent to be started, and when the effects of the DHE wear off the true maintenance preventive's effects have already kicked in.

○ Occipital Nerve Blockade

Greater occipital nerve blockade using a combination of an anesthetic (e.g., lidocaine) and steroid (e.g., triamcinolone) can prevent cluster headaches attacks. They may be used to try to abort an episodic cluster headache cycle or be used as a transitional or even maintenance preventive in some. Either typical GON-based or suboccipital-located injections appear helpful.[66–68]

• Preventive Therapy

Preventive agents are absolutely necessary in cluster headache patients unless the cluster periods last for less than 2 weeks. Preventive medications are only used while the patient is in cycle and they are tapered off once a cluster period has ended. If a patient decides to remain on a preventive agent even after they have gone out of cycle this typically does not appear to prevent a subsequent cluster period from starting. The maintenance preventive should be started at the time a transitional agent is given. Most physicians treating cluster headache will increase the dosages of the preventive agents very quickly to get a desired response. Very large dosages, much higher than that suggested in the PDR, are sometimes necessary when treating cluster headache. A well-recognized trait of cluster patients is that they can tolerate medications much better than non-cluster patients. Most of the recognized cluster preventives can be used in both episodic and chronic cluster headache (Table 9.3).

TABLE 9.3

Cluster Headache Preventives "Big 7"

- Verapamil short-acting preferred—may need to push doses to high levels (800 mg plus); EKG with every dose change above 480 mg
- Lithium carbonate (300 mg): 300 mg TID or higher depending on serum levels
- Valproic acid (250 mg): 1000–3000 mg (ER formulation)
- Daily corticosteroids—if short cluster periods (1–3 weeks)
- Topiramate-average dose is 75–100 mg*
- Melatonin—9 mg QHS
- Methylergonovine—must come off every 6 months for testing (0.2–0.4 mg TID)—only have DHE as abortive

*May work better in female cluster.

New Cluster Headache Therapies

Acute

- Demand Valve Oxygen
  A demand valve delivers oxygen to the user as soon as they try to inhale from an attached mask; thus dosage is controlled by respiration rate and tidal volume. If the user inhales more deeply, more oxygen will flow in response to the increased demand, hence the name. Unlike a continuous-flow oxygen regulator (CFO), a demand valve is capable of delivering 100% oxygen from 0 to 160 LPM. One benefit of a demand valve is that it can also support hyperventilation. CFO regulators are typically limited to 15 LPM, thus incapable of supporting hyperventilation. Hyperventilation leads to a state of hyperoxia and hypocapnia. Based on its mechanics, a demand valve assures the delivery of 100% oxygen without dilution by room air, which plagues delivery via nasal cannula and non-rebreather face masks. Two studies have now suggested that demand valve oxygen therapy may be superior to CFO via non-rebreather face mask for time to pain relief, complete pain freedom rates, and a possible preventive effect for cluster headache. The need for hyperventilation with a demand valve versus non-hyperventilatory breathing needs further study.[69,70]
- External vagal nerve stimulator: now FDA-approved for the acute treatment of episodic but not chronic cluster headache. Provides a non-medicinal treatment option.[71]
- Sphenopalatine ganglion stimulation is an implantable wireless stimulator which has shown both a positive effect to acutely abort a cluster headache but also appears to have a maintenance preventive effect when used as a prn abortive. At time of this writing it is not yet FDA-approved.[72]

Preventive

- Clomiphene Citrate
  Small studies have shown that clomiphene citrate, a hypothalamic estrogen modulator, can be a unique CH preventive agent in treatment refractory CH cases.[73–75] Clomiphene citrate appears to act as an estrogen agonist via ER alpha and as an estrogen antagonist via ER beta on human hypothalamic receptors. Clomiphene citrate potentially acts as a CH preventive by modulating orexin, as estrogen and ER alpha receptors co-localize with orexin in the hypothalamus.
  Dosing: 50 mg QD for 2 weeks, then if no improvement 75 mg QD × 2 weeks, then if no improvement 100 mg QD × 2 weeks—do not go higher on dosing if patients fails 100 mg.

Only suggested in males and post-menopausal females.

Risks: potential clotting issues (especially in females) and a heightened risk of testicular cancer and prostate hypertrophy—so if treatment is long term, yearly testicular and prostate/PSA exams will be needed.

- Monoclonal CGRP antibodies: the same agents that are now FDA-approved for migraine prevention may end up showing efficacy in episodic but not chronic cluster headache based on phase 3 trials.

INDOMETHACIN-RESPONSIVE TACS

Chronic paroxysmal hemicrania (CPH) and hemicrania continua (HC) are defined by their response to indomethacin. A short discussion on these two syndromes will be followed by treatment suggestions.

Chronic Paroxysmal Hemicrania

ICHD-3 diagnostic criteria:
- At least 20 attacks fulfilling criteria B–E
- Severe unilateral orbital, supraorbital, and/or temporal pain lasting 2–30 minutes
- Either or both of the following:
  - At least one of the following symptoms or signs, ipsilateral to the headache:
    - Conjunctival injection and/or lacrimation
    - Nasal congestion and/or rhinorrhea
    - Eyelid edema
    - Forehead and facial sweating
    - Miosis and/or ptosis
  - Sense of restlessness or agitation
- Occurring with a frequency of >5 per day
- Prevented absolutely by therapeutic doses of indomethacin

Chronic paroxysmal hemicrania is a rare syndrome marked by headaches of short duration, a high frequency of attacks, and associated autonomic symptoms. CPH pain location is normally orbital, temporal, and above or behind the ear and is one-sided. The pain is severe in intensity. Normal headache duration is between 2 and 30 minutes and frequency is greater than five attacks per day. Unlike cluster headache, there is no predilection for nocturnal attacks, although attacks can certainly awaken a patient from sleep. Associated symptoms are marked by autonomic phenomena. CPH attacks can sometimes be triggered by rotating the neck or flexing the head to the side of the headaches, or by applying external pressure to the transverse processes of C4–C5 or the C2 nerve root on the symptomatic side. This syndrome used to be termed female cluster headache but it is not cluster headache based on the frequency and duration of attacks, and a misdiagnosis can lead to continued disability as indomethacin is not suggested for CH but is for CPH.

Hemicrania Continua

ICHD-3 diagnostic criteria:
- Unilateral headache fulfilling criteria B–D
- Present for >3 months, with exacerbations of moderate or greater intensity
- Either or both of the following:
  - At least one of the following symptoms or signs, ipsilateral to the headache:
    - Conjunctival injection and/or lacrimation
    - Nasal congestion and/or rhinorrhea
    - Eyelid edema

- Forehead and facial sweating
- Miosis and/or ptosis
∘ A sense of restlessness or agitation, or aggravation of the pain by movement
• Responds absolutely to therapeutic doses of indomethacin

Initially hemicrania continua was felt to be a very rare syndrome although it is now felt to be more common and probably routinely misdiagnosed. Hemicrania continua, like CPH, has a female predominance. There are two recognized forms of HC: non-remitting (typically daily from onset), which occurs in about 85% of patients (no remission periods), and the remitting form. The non-remitting form can evolve from the remitting form. In regard to the clinical characteristics of HC there are two patterns of headache. Hemicrania continua patients will experience a continuous daily head pain which is present 24 hours per day, 7 days per week and then pain exacerbation periods which occur with varying frequency from multiple times per week to every third month or less. The daily continuous pain is usually of mild to moderate intensity. It is always present on the same side of the head. There are some reports of the pain of HC switching sides or being bilateral but that would be a rarity. The pain exacerbation periods are marked by moderate to severe pain lasting hours to days in duration with associated symptoms that are seen in migraine and cluster headache. Migrainous symptoms include nausea, vomiting, photophobia, and phonophobia. Cranial autonomic symptoms include unilateral lacrimation, ptosis, nasal congestion and rhinorrhea, and agitation. Other key symptoms that are commonly seen during a pain exacerbation period include eyelid swelling, eyelid twitching, and "stabbing" headaches. Some HC patients will also complain of a foreign body sensation in the eye on the same side as their headaches such as a feeling as if there is a piece of sand in the eye or an eyelash. HC patients can also experience auras typically occurring just prior to a pain exacerbation period.

Pathogenesis: as TAC spectrum disorders, a hypothalamic involvement is suggestive for CPH and HC as is noted for cluster headache even though the indomethacin-responsive TAC syndromes do not have the same circadian rhythmicity as CH. Functional neuroimaging for CPH notes activation of the contralateral posterior hypothalamus and contralateral ventral midbrain, while for HC there is noted contralateral posterior hypothalamus and ipsilateral dorsal rostral pons activation.[76,77]

Indomethacin Treatment

The normal starting dosage of indomethacin for both CPH and HC is one 25 mg tablet three times a day for 3 days; this dose can be increased to two tablets (50 mg) three times a day if there is not total relief of pain. Most individuals will respond by 150 mg a day, and the response can be dramatic, with quick dissipation of headache symptoms regardless of how long the patient had suffered with head pain. A beneficial effect will normally be seen within 48 hours after the correct dosage has been found. Some individuals need a dose as high as 300 mg of indomethacin per day, but there is a true safety issue with this high of a dose, so going above 225 mg per day is not suggested. If there is no response at 150 mg a day, and the physician still suspects CPH or HC, an extra 25 mg dose of indomethacin can be added every 3 days, to a total of 225 mg a day or the onset of side effects. If the patient does not respond at 75 mg three times a day, one should consider an alternative diagnosis. There are both gastrointestinal and renal potential side effects with chronic indomethacin usage. After 3 months of doing well on indomethacin the medication should be tapered to see if still needed. Many patients cannot come off indomethacin without headache recurrence, however.

Other Potential Non-Indomethacin Treatments[78]

• COX-2 inhibitors: both CPH and HC have shown some positive response to celecoxib. The dosing is typically high from 200 mg BID to QID. At these doses the gastrointestinal protection these agents afford may be lost. In addition, the safety of COX-2 inhibitors when used on a continuous basis is in question.

- Melatonin: melatonin has a similar chemical structure to indomethacin and has been shown to have anti-inflammatory and anti-nociceptive properties. The pain-relieving mechanisms of melatonin are not completely understood, but reports have suggested that melatonin can increase the release of endogenous beta-endorphins and its anti-hyperalgesic effect appears to involve both nitric oxide and opiate pathways. Melatonin has now been shown to help alleviate the pain of hemicrania continua and primary stabbing headache, and in some cases patients become pain-free on melatonin. Melatonin should be tried on all patients with indomethacin-sensitive headaches, including those who are doing well on indomethacin, to try and either lower the indomethacin dose or come off indomethacin entirely or in those who have contraindications to indomethacin. Recently the author did a larger study of melatonin in patients with CPH and HC.[78] Less than 20% achieved pain freedom on melatonin alone, but as an add-on therapy about 45% had substantial reduction in pain with the ability to reduce their baseline indomethacin dose. Melatonin dosing: start at 3 mg at bed for 5 nights, then increase every 5 nights by 3 mg up until 5 tabs (15 mg at bed) and re-assess with physician. Can continue dosing up to 30 mg if tolerated.
- The author and colleague have documented the long-term efficacy of radiofrequency lesioning of the C2 dorsal root ganglia, C2 ventral ramus, and/or sphenopalatine ganglia in indomethacin-responsive headaches. Post-procedure most patients can come off indomethacin without pain recurrence.[79]

SUNCT Syndrome

ICHD-3 diagnostic criteria:

- At least 20 attacks fulfilling criteria B–D
- Moderate or severe unilateral head pain, with orbital, supraorbital, temporal, and/or other trigeminal distribution, lasting for 1–600 seconds and occurring as single stabs, series of stabs, or in a saw-tooth pattern
- At least one of the following five cranial autonomic symptoms or signs, ipsilateral to the pain:
  - Conjunctival injection and/or lacrimation
  - Nasal congestion and/or rhinorrhea
  - Eyelid edema
  - Forehead and facial sweating
  - Miosis and/or ptosis
- Occurring with a frequency of at least one a day

The syndrome of short-lasting unilateral neuralgiform headache attacks with conjunctival injection and tearing (SUNCT) is one of the rarest of the primary headache disorders. SUNCT is comprised of brief attacks of moderate to severe head pain with associated autonomic symptoms of conjunctival injection, tearing, rhinorrhea, or nasal obstruction. SUNCT pain is normally localized to an orbital or periorbital distribution, although the forehead and temple can be the main site of pain. Head pain can radiate to the temple, nose, cheek, ear, and palate. The pain is normally side-locked and remains unilateral throughout an entire attack. In rare instances SUNCT pain can be bilateral. Pain duration is extremely short, lasting between 1 and 600 seconds, with an average duration of 10 to 60 seconds. This extremely brief pain duration sets SUNCT apart from other primary headache syndromes (e.g., cluster headache, chronic paroxysmal hemicrania, and migraine). Pain onset is abrupt, with maximum intensity being reached in 2 to 3 seconds. SUNCT pain normally plateaus at a maximum intensity for several seconds and then quickly abates. SUNCT can occur at any time of the day and does not show a tendency toward nocturnal attacks. Attack frequency varies greatly between sufferers and within an individual sufferer. The usual attack frequency ranges anywhere from 1 to more than 80 episodes a day. Individuals can experience from fewer than 1 attack an hour to more than 30 an hour. Most SUNCT patients will be pain-free between attacks, although there are isolated reports of patients experiencing low background pain interictally. SUNCT is an episodic disorder that presents in a relapsing or remitting pattern. Each symptomatic period can last from several days to several months, and a person with SUNCT will typically have one to two symptomatic periods a year. SUNCT can arise spontaneously, but many sufferers have identified triggering maneuvers, including mastication, nose blowing, coughing, forehead touching, eyelid squeezing, neck movements (rotation, extension, and flexion), and ice cream eating. In SUNCT there is no refractory period between pain attacks, so if a trigger zone is stimulated during the ending phase of a previous attack, a new one can begin immediately. This is unlike the refractory period of trigeminal neuralgia. There may indeed be an overlap between trigeminal neuralgia and SUNCT. SUNCT has recently been linked to trigeminal nerve/vessel compression which has been a known etiology for trigeminal neuralgia. All patients with SUNCT should have neuroimaging to look for vessel/nerve contact near the trigeminal root entry zone. In addition, looking for an underlying secretory pituitary tumor (growth hormone, prolactin) is also mandatory by lab work and imaging. Suggested treatments that have shown efficacy in SUNCT include lamotrigine, gabapentin, topiramate, and clomiphene citrate in refractory cases. Decompression of a nerve contact point may also have efficacy.[80,81]

Pathogenesis: data suggest that there is indeed posterior hypothalamic activation in many SUNCT patients on functional neuroimaging and this is bilateral in many even though headaches are one-sided, but it also can be ipsilateral or contralateral to the side of the pain.

OTHER LESS COMMON PRIMARY HEADACHE SYNDROMES

PRIMARY EXERCISE HEADACHE[1,82]

Description: headache precipitated by any form of exercise in the absence of any intracranial disorder.

ICHD-3 diagnostic criteria:

- At least two headache episodes fulfilling criteria B and C
- Brought on by and occurring only during or after strenuous physical exercise
- Lasting <48 hours
- Not better accounted for by another ICHD-3 diagnosis.
  *On first occurrence of this headache type it is mandatory to exclude subarachnoid hemorrhage, arterial dissection, and reversible cerebral vasoconstriction syndrome (RCVS).

Key clinical points: primary exercise headache is more common in females. The location is typically bilateral but can be one-sided. The quality can be throbbing, pulsatile, and should be non-explosive. Duration is normally 5 minutes to 48 hours.

Triggers include prolonged physical exertion, and the pain typically starts at the peak of exertion. Associated symptoms outside of head pain are typically lacking although migrainous symptoms can occur in those with a history of migraine. The key is that the age of onset is normally below age 50 years. It can occur in athletes and non-athletes.

Treatment:
Acute: Abortives are not very useful as the induced pain normally alleviates on its own or becomes low level when exercise is stopped. Additionally, patients normally want to prevent pain rather than treat it when it happens.

Preventive

- Non-Medicinal
  - ◦ Avoiding activity is a preventive maneuver of choice but may not be acceptable for the patient
  - ◦ Improve warm-up routine prior to exertion
- Medicinal

Pretreat Activity

- Indomethacin short-acting formulation: dosing 25 mg to 250 mg has been published—no controlled trials
  Suggested strategy: pretreat event by 30–60 minutes with 25–50 mg
- Tripans: pretreat event by 60 minutes—although has not been studied

PRIMARY COUGH HEADACHE[1,82]

ICHD-3 diagnostic criteria:

- At least two headache episodes fulfilling criteria B–D
- Brought on by and occurring only in association with coughing, straining, and/or other Valsalva maneuver
- Sudden onset
- Lasting between 1 second and 2 hours

Clinical features: the headache arises immediate after cough, reaches peak almost instantaneously, then subsides over several seconds to a few minutes; sometimes peak pain can last several seconds. Most patients are pain-free in between attacks, but some have pain that lingers for hours after triggered attack. Migrainous-associated symptoms are rare. Attacks are typically bilateral but can be one-sided. For age of onset primary cough headache normally starts after age 50 years versus primary exercise headache which normally begins younger than age 50. If a patient presents with these headaches but in the wrong age range then evaluation for secondary causes is mandatory although in reality primary cough headache needs at least a brain MRI to rule out secondary disorders.

Treatment:
- Acute: abortive therapy not utilized secondary to short duration of attacks.
- Preventive
  - ◦ Indomethacin—most frequent choice. Would suggest extended-release formulation 75 mg to 150 mg per day.
  - ◦ Acetazolamide (125–500 mg per day).
  - ◦ Lumbar puncture: typically remove CSF volume until cough headache ceases. This can be a very effective treatment if medicines are not helpful or tolerated.

PRIMARY HEADACHE ASSOCIATED WITH SEXUAL ACTIVITY[1,82]

ICHD-3 diagnostic criteria:

- At least two episodes of pain in the head and/or neck fulfilling criteria B–D
- Brought on by and occurring only during sexual activity
- Either or both of the following:

- ○ Increasing in intensity with increasing sexual excitement
  - ○ Abrupt explosive intensity just before or with orgasm
- Lasting from 1 minute to 24 hours with severe intensity and/or up to 72 hours with mild intensity
  *On the first onset of headache with sexual activity, it is mandatory to exclude subarachnoid hemorrhage, intra- and extracranial arterial dissection, and reversible cerebral vasoconstriction syndrome (RCVS). Multiple explosive headaches during sexual activities should be considered as RCVS until proven otherwise.

Clinical presentation: typical headache duration is minutes to a few hours to a day. The intense pain normally occurs in the first 5–15 minutes, and then subsides, although duration may be longer if pain comes at orgasm versus before orgasm. The headache is bilateral in two-thirds and unilateral in one-third of cases and is diffuse or occipitally located.[15] Associated symptoms are rare. The course of these headaches over time can be unpredictable, and thus can be regular for periods of time occurring with every coital event and then become sporadic or alleviate all together.

Treatment:
Short-term or mini Prevention—thus treating just prior to activity:

- Indomethacin: 25–50 mg dosed 1–2 hours prior to coitus

Acute treatment at time of headache:

- Indomethacin 25–50 mg and or a triptan but only after ruling out secondary vascular issues for triptan use

New Daily Persistent Headache

ICHD-3 diagnostic criteria:

- Persistent headache fulfilling criteria B and C
- Distinct and clearly remembered onset, with pain becoming continuous and unremitting within 24 hours
- Present for >3 months

This is a unique form of chronic daily headache that is hallmarked by a daily headache from onset (typically in individuals who do not have a prior headache history), and most individuals can name the date or at least the month their headache began.[83] There is a remitting form in which the headache can go away up to 2 years after onset and a refractory form in which the headache will continue for years unabated. It is recognized as one of the most treatment-refractory of all headache subtypes. Known triggers include post-infection, post-stressful life event, and post-surgical procedure, although 50% plus cannot recognize a triggering event. Clinical characteristics include female predominance noted in almost all studies with a younger age of onset in women. Typical age of onset is mid- to late teens to early twenties in most, but this also depends on triggering event (for example post-surgical is an older age class, 50–60s). Location is bilateral in most and pain intensity is typically moderate to severe. Pain is constant. Migrainous-associated symptoms are common in NDPH, but this is not migraine. Pathogenesis is unknown, but it appears NDPH is not one entity but multiple disparate conditions that can present as a daily headache from onset.[84] Possible etiologies include changes in CSF pressure high or low, hyperimmune response to infectious agents, typically viruses, and possible cerebral artery vasospasm if the first headache is a thunderclap headache (pain reaches maximum intensity without latency). Finally the majority of these patients have an underlying hypermobility disorder and thus this may play a role in headache pathogenesis; the main theory is that cervical hypermobility leads to upper cervical facet irritation and chronic daily headache. At present there are no known specific treatments for this syndrome. Possibly effective treatments include doxycycline, mexiletine, high-dose IV corticosteroids, gabapentin, and topiramate.[83]

Secondary Disorders Mimicking NDPH

All patients with a daily headache from onset must be ruled out for secondary underlying conditions. The most frequent mimics are cerebral vein thrombosis and a spinal fluid leak. Other possible causes include elevated CSF pressure, nasal contact syndrome, sphenoid sinusitis, and neoplasm. If NDPH is one-sided/side-fixed, the differential diagnosis includes cerebral vein thrombosis or vein occlusive syndrome, sphenoid sinus lesion (sinusitis, fungal, mass), spinal fluid leak, cervicogenic-based headache, nasal contact syndrome, cavernous sinus lesion, aneurysm, carotid dissection, and giant cell arteritis. Primary headache syndromes must be considered including hemicrania continua and trochlear headache.

Key Points in Regard to NDPH

- Always rule out a secondary cause of the daily headache.
- Try to determine a triggering event for NDPH if possible as that may help to establish an underlying pathogenesis theory and treatment (post-infectious, post-surgical, post-stressful life event).
- Always ask about the first ever headache and temporal profile of that headache onset. There is a distinct form of NDPH that starts with a thunderclap headache, and in that setting the evaluation is different (include arterial studies with imaging), and one may consider nimodipine as a preventive choice if no secondary cause is noted.
- Utilize the Trendelenburg test to help with diagnosis. If a patient improves in head down tilt position, consider evaluation for a CSF leak, or if they rapidly worsen then consider utilizing a medication that lowers CSF pressure/volume.
- Evaluate for cervical hypermobility as, if there is no triggering event and significant cervical irritation on exam, the predisposing cause of the headaches is probably related to hypermobility issues.
- Be aggressive with therapy up front, especially if you meet an individual within 1 year of headache onset. Treating with infusion therapy or inpatient therapy with intravenous medications (even with standard migraine protocols) may help break the cycle. This is less effective years into the syndrome.

SUMMARY

In summary, headaches are a fascinating condition. The key is to make a proper diagnosis which will then lead to effective treatment. The pathogenesis of many headache syndromes is now understood, and this has led to new treatments.

REFERENCES

1. Headache classification committee of the International Headache Society (IHS). The international classification of headache disorders, 3rd edition. *Cephalalgia* 2018;38(1):1–211. doi:10.1177/0333102417738202.
2. Global, regional, and national incidence, prevalence, and years lived with disability for 301 acute and chronic diseases and injuries in 188 countries, 1990–2013: a systematic analysis for the global burden of disease study 2013. *Lancet* 2015;386(9995):743–800.
3. Kelman L.. Migraine pain location: a tertiary care study of 1283 migraineurs. *Headache* 2005;45(8): 1038–1047.
4. Campbell J.F., Mitch A., Brisebois Hughes N.M.G.. Spatial distribution of head pain as a factor in migraine experience. *Headache* 1987;27(3):134–137.

5. Lance J.W., Anthony M. Some clinical aspects of migraine. A prospective survey of 500 patients. *Arch Neurol* 1966;15(4):356–361.

6. Rasmussen B.K., Jensen R., Olesen J. A population-based analysis of the diagnostic criteria of the international headache society. *Cephalalgia* 1991;11(3):129–134.

7. Olesen J. Some of the clinical features of the acute migraine attack. An analysis of 750 patients. *Headache* 1978;18(5):268–271.

8. Russell M.B., Rasmussen B.K., Fenger K., Olesen J. Migraine without aura and migraine with aura are distinct clinical entities: a study of four hundred and eighty-four male and female migraineurs from the general population. *Cephalalgia* 1996;16(4):239–245.

9. Evans R.W., Seifert T., Kailasam J., Mathew N.T. The use of questions to determine the presence of photophobia and phonophobia during migraine. *Headache* 2008;48(3):395–397.

10. Bigal M.E., Liberman J.N., Lipton R.B. Age-dependent prevalence and clinical features of migraine. *Neurology* 2006;67(2):246–251.

11. Kelman L. Migraine changes with age: IMPACT on migraine classification. *Headache* 2006;46(7):1161–1171.

12. Lipton R.B., Dodick D., Sadovsky R., et al. A self-administered screener for migraine in primary care: the ID migraine validation study. *Neurology* 2003;61(3):375–382.

13. Schürks M., Buring J.E., Kurth T. Agreement of self-reported migraine with ICHD-II criteria in the women's health study. *Cephalalgia* 2009;29(10):1086–1090.

14. Qiu C., Williams M.A., Aurora S.K., et al. Agreement of self-reported physician diagnosis of migraine with international classification of headache disorders-II migraine diagnostic criteria in a cross-sectional study of pregnant women. *BMC Womens Health* 2013;13:50.

15. Maniyar F.H., Sprenger T., Monteith T., Schankin C., Goadsby P.J. Brain activations in the premonitory phase of nitroglycerin-triggered migraine attacks. *Brain* 2014;137(1):232–241.

16. Dodick D.W. A phase-by-phase review of migraine pathophysiology. *Headache* 2018;58(Suppl 1):4–16.

17. Rothrock J.F. Successful treatment of persistent migraine aura with divalproex sodium. *Neurology* 1997;48(1):261–262.

18. Haan J., Sluis P., Sluis L.H., Ferrari M.D. Acetazolamide treatment for migraine aura status. *Neurology* 2000;55(10):1588–1589.

19. Afridi S.K., Giffin N.J., Kaube H., Goadsby P.J. A randomized controlled trial of intranasal ketamine in migraine with prolonged aura. *Neurology* 2013;80(7):642–647.

20. Rozen T.D. Treatment of a prolonged migrainous aura with intravenous furosemide. *Neurology* 2000;55(5):732–733.

21. Rozen T.D. Intravenous prochlorperazine with magnesium sulfate can abort a prolonged migrainous aura during pregnancy. *Headache* 2003;43(8):901–903.

22. Viana M., Afridi S. Migraine with prolonged aura: phenotype and treatment. *Naunyn Schmiedebergs Arch Pharmacol* 2018;391(1):1–10.

23. Marmura M.J., Silberstein S.D., Schwedt T.J. How to apply the AHS evidence assessment of the acute treatment of migraine in adults to your patient with migraine. *Headache* 2015;55(1):3–20.

24. Loder E., Burch R., Rizzoli P. The 2012 AHS/AAN guidelines for prevention of episodic migraine: a summary and comparison with other recent clinical practice guidelines. *Headache* 2012;52(6):930–945.

25. Rajapakse T., Pringsheim T. Nutraceuticals in migraine: a summary of existing guidelines for use. *Headache* 2016;56(4):808–816.

26. Hepp Z., Rosen N.L., Gillard P.G., et al. Comparative effectiveness of onabotulinumtoxinA versus oral migraine prophylactic medications on headache-related resource utilization in the management of chronic migraine: retrospective analysis of a US-based insurance claims database. *Cephalalgia* 2016;36(9):862–874.

27. Shirahige L., Melo L., Nogueira F., Rocha S., Monte-Silva K. Efficacy of noninvasive brain stimulation on pain control in migraine patients: a systematic review and meta-analysis. *Headache* 2016;56(10):1565–1596.

28. Tassorelli C., Grazzi L., de Tommaso M., et al. Noninvasive vagus nerve stimulation as acute therapy for migraine: the randomized Presto study. *Neurology* 2018;91(4):e364–e373.

29. Starling A.J., Tepper S.J., Marmura M.J., et al. A multicenter, prospective, single arm, open label, observational study of sTMS for migraine prevention (ESPOUSE study). *Cephalalgia* 2018;38(6):1038–1048. doi: 10.1177/333102418762525.

30. Voss T., Lipton R.B., Dodick D.W., et al. A phase IIb randomized, double-blind, placebo-controlled trial of ubrogepant for the acute treatment of migraine. *Cephalalgia Int J Headache* 2016;36(9):887–898.

31. Dodick D.W. Migraine. *Lancet* 2018;391(10127):1315–1330.

32. Silberstein S.D., Dodick D.W., Bigal M.E., et al. Fremanezumab for the preventive treatment of chronic migraine. *N Engl J Med* 2017;377(22):2113–2122.
33. Tepper S., Ashina M., Reuter U., et al. Safety and efficacy of erenumab for preventive treatment of chronic migraine: a randomised, double-blind, placebo-controlled phase 2 trial. *Lancet Neurol* 2017;16(6):425–434.
34. Ashina M., Dodick D., Goadsby P.J., et al. Erenumab (AMG 334) in episodic migraine: interim analysis of an ongoing open-label study. *Neurology* 2017;89(12):1237–1243.
35. Vila-Pueyo M. Targeted 5-HT1F therapies for migraine. *Neurotherapeutics* 2018;15(2):291–303.
36. Mazer-Amirshahi M., Dewey K., Mullins P.M., et al. Trends in opioid analgesic use for headaches in us emergency departments. *Am J Emerg Med* 2014;32(9):1068–1073.
37. Davis C.P., Torre P.R., Williams C., et al. Ketorolac versus meperidine-plus-promethazine treatment of migraine headache: evaluations by patients. *Am J Emerg Med* 1995;13(2):146–150.
38. Carleton S.C., Shesser R.F., Pietrzak M.P., et al. Double-blind, multicenter trial to compare the efficacy of intramuscular dihydroergotamine plus hydroxyzine versus intramuscular meperidine plus hydroxyzine for the emergency department treatment of acute migraine headache. *Ann Emerg Med* 1998;32(2):129–138.
39. Taheraghdam A.A., Amiri H., Shojaan H., et al. Intravenous dexamethasone versus morphine in relieving of acute migraine headache. *Pak J Biol Sci* 2011;14(12):682–687.
40. Friedman B.W., Kapoor A., Friedman M.S., et al. The relative efficacy of meperidine for the treatment of acute migraine: a meta-analysis of randomized controlled trials. *Ann Emerg Med* 2008;52(6):705–713.
41. Colman I., Rothney A., Wright S.C., et al. Use of narcotic analgesics in the emergency department treatment of migraine headache. *Neurology* 2004;62(10):1695–1700.
42. Tornabene S.V., Deutsch R., Davis D.P., et al. Evaluating the use and timing of opioids for the treatment of migraine headaches in the emergency department. *J Emerg Med* 2009;36(4):333–337.
43. Harden R.N., Gracely R.H., Carter T., Warner G. The placebo effect in acute headache management: ketorolac, meperidine, and saline in the emergency department. *Headache* 1996;36(6):352–356.
44. Bigal M.E., Bordini C.A., Tepper S.J., Speciali J.G. Intravenous magnesium sulphate in the acute treatment of migraine without aura and migraine with aura. A randomized, double-blind, placebo-controlled study. *Cephalalgia* 2002;22(5):345–353.
45. Mauskop A., Altura B.T., Cracco R.Q., Altura B.M. Intravenous magnesium sulphate relieves migraine attacks in patients with low serum ionized magnesium levels: a pilot study. *Clin Sci (Lond)* 1995;89(6):633–636.
46. Orr S.L., Aubé M., Becker W.J., et al. Canadian headache society systematic review and recommendations on the treatment of migraine pain in emergency settings. *Cephalalgia* 2015;35(3):271–284.
47. Friedman B.W., Mulvey L., Esses D., et al. Metoclopramide for acute migraine: a dose-finding randomized clinical trial. *Ann Emerg Med* 2011;57(5):475–482.
48. Saadah H.A. Abortive headache therapy in the office with intravenous dihydroergotamine plus prochlorperazine. *Headache* 1992;32(3):143–146.
49. Silberstein S.D., Young W.B., Mendizabal J.E., et al. Acute migraine treatment with droperidol: a randomized, double-blind, placebo-controlled trial. *Neurology* 2003;60(2):315–321.
50. Swidan S.Z., Lake A.E., III, Saper J.R. Efficacy of intravenous diphenhydramine versus intravenous DHE-45 in the treatment of severe migraine headache. *Curr Pain Headache Rep* 2005;9(1):65–70.
51. Taggart E., Doran S., Kokotillo A., et al. Ketorolac in the treatment of acute migraine: a systematic review. *Headache* 2013;53(2):277–287.
52. Colman I., Friedman B.W., Brown M.D., et al. Parenteral dexamethasone for acute severe migraine headache: meta-analysis of randomised controlled trials for preventing recurrence. *BMJ* 2008;336(7657):1359–1361.
53. Shahien R., Saleh S.A., Bowirrat A. Intravenous sodium valproate aborts migraine headaches rapidly. *Acta Neurol Scand* 2011;123(4):257–265.
54. Deutsch S.I., Burket J.A., Rosse R.B. Valproate-induced hyperammonemic encephalopathy and normal liver functions: possible synergism with topiramate. *Clin Neuropharmacol* 2009;32(6):350–352.
55. Farooq M.U., Majid A., Pysh J.J., Kassab M.Y. Role of intravenous levetiracetam in status migrainosus. *J Headache Pain* 2007;8(2):143–144.
56. Akpunonu B.E., Mutgi A.B., Federman D.J., et al. Subcutaneous sumatriptan for treatment of acute migraine in patients admitted to the emergency department: a multicenter study. *Ann Emerg Med* 1995;25(4):464–469.
57. Callaham M., Raskin N. A controlled study of dihydroergotamine in the treatment of acute migraine headache. *Headache* 1986;26(4):168–171.

58. Ashkenazi A., Young W.B. The effects of greater occipital nerve block and trigger point injection on brush allodynia and pain in migraine. *Headache* 2005;45(4):350–354.

59. Hoffmann J., May A. Diagnosis, pathophysiology, and management of cluster headache. *Lancet Neurol* 2018;17(1):75–83.

60. May A., Bahra A., Büchel C., Frackowiak R.S., Goadsby P.J. Hypothalamic activation in cluster headache attacks. *Lancet* 1998;352(9124):275–278.

61. Ekbom K. Treatment of acute cluster headache with sumatriptan. *N Eng J Med* 1991;325(5):322–326.

62. Ekbom K., Krabbe A., Micieli G., et al. Cluster headache attacks treated for up to three months with subcutaneous sumatriptan (6mg) (sumatriptan long-term study group). *Cephalalgia* 1995;15(3):230–236.

63. van Vliet J.A., Bahra A. Martin V. Intranasal sumatriptan is effective in the treatment of acute cluster headache-a double-blind placebo-controlled crossover study. *Cephalagia* 2001;21(4):267–272.

64. Rozen T.D. High oxygen flow rates for cluster headache. *Neurology* 2004;63(3):593.

65. Cohen A.S., Burns B., Goadsby P.J. High-flow oxygen for treatment of cluster headache: a randomized trial. *JAMA* 2009;302(22):2451–2457.

66. Lambru G., Abu Bakar N., Stahlhut L. et al. Greater occipital nerve blocks in chronic cluster headache: a prospective open-label study. *Eur J Neurol* 2014 ;21(2):338–343.

67. Gantenbein A.R., Lutz N.J., Riederer F., Sándor P.S. Efficacy and safety of 121 injections of the greater occipital nerve in episodic and chronic cluster headache. *Cephalalgia* 2012;32(8):630–634.

68. Rozen T.D. High volume anesthetic suboccipital nerve blocks for treatment refractory chronic cluster headache with long term efficacy data: an observational case-series study. *Headache* 2019;59(1):56–62. doi:10.1111/head.13394.

69. Rozen T.D., Fishman R.S. Demand valve oxygen: a promising new oxygen delivery system for the acute treatment of cluster headache. *Pain Med* 2013;14(4):455–459.

70. Petersen A.S., Barloese M.C., Lund N.L., Jensen R.H. Oxygen therapy for cluster headache: a mask comparison trial. A single-blinded, placebo-controlled, crossover study.*Cephalalgia* 2017;37(3):214–224.

71. Holle-Lee D., Gaul C. Noninvasive vagus nerve stimulation in the management of cluster headache: clinical evidence and practical experience. *Ther Adv Neurol Disord* 2016;9(3):230–234.

72. Fontaine D., Santucci S., Lanteri-Minet M.J. Managing cluster headache with sphenopalatine ganglion stimulation: a review. *Pain Res* 2018;11:375–381.

73. Rozen T. Clomiphene citrate for treatment refractory chronic cluster headache. *Headache* 2008;48(2):286–290.

74. Rozen T.D. Clomiphene citrate as a preventive treatment for intractable chronic cluster headache: a second reported case with long-term follow-up. *Headache* 2015;55(4):571–574.

75. Nobre M.E., Peres M.F.P., Filho M.P.F., Leal A.J. Clomiphene treatment may be effective in refractory episodic and chronic cluster headache. *Arq Neuro Psiquiatr* 2017;75(9):620–624.

76. Matharu M.S., Cohen A.S., Frackowiak R.S.J., Goadsby P.J. Posterior hypothalamic activation in paroxysmal hemicrania. *Ann Neurol* 2006;59(3):535–545.

77. Matharu M.S., Cohen A.S., McGonigle D.J., Ward N, Frackowiak RS, Goadsby PJ. Posterior hypothalamic and brainstem activation in hemicrania continua. *Headache* 2004;44(8):747–761.

78. Rozen T.D. How effective is melatonin as a preventive treatment for hemicrania continua? A clinic based study. *Headache* 2015;55(3):430–436.

79. Beams J.L., Kline M.T., Rozen T.D. Treatment of hemicrania continua with radiofrequency ablation and long-term follow-up. *Cephalalgia* 2015;35(13):1208–1213.

80. Rozen T.D. Complete alleviation of treatment refractory primary SUNCT syndrome with clomiphene citrate (A medicinal deep brain hypothalamic modulator). *Cephalalgia* 2014;34(12):1021–1024.

81. Hassan S., Lagrata S., Levy A., Matharu M., Zrinzo L. Microvascular decompression or neuromodulation in patients with SUNCT and trigeminal neurovascular conflict? *Cephalalgia* 2018;38(2):393–398.

82. Bahra A. Other primary headaches. *Ann Indian Acad Neurol* 2012;15(Suppl 1):S66–S71.

83. Rozen T.D. New daily persistent headache: a clinical perspective. *Headache* 2011;51(4):641–649.

84. Rozen T.D. Triggering events and new daily persistent headache: age and gender differences and insights on pathogenesis-a clinic-based study. *Headache* 2016;56(1):164–173.

10 Biotensegrity

Advancing Pain Diagnosis and Treatment by Rethinking Anatomy and Biomechanics

Bradley D. Fullerton

CONTENTS

INTRODUCTION*

Regardless of specialty, clinicians need anatomic models as a context for the diagnosis and treatment of pain complaints. This chapter argues that the fundamental mis-framing of musculoskeletal anatomy has impeded our ability to diagnose and treat myofascial pain and traditional orthopedic pathologies. Biotensegrity theory and recent advances in fascial anatomy provide a context for understanding all other anatomic structures in new ways. This reframing of anatomy helps explain the persistence of myofascial pain and the effectiveness of alternative treatments, such as prolotherapy, manual fascial therapies, and manipulation. A detailed case example illustrates the clinical application of biotensegrity and dynamic ultrasound in the context of orthopedic injury and neuromuscular dysfunction.

> MPS [myofascial pain syndrome] is actually a complex form of neuro- muscular dysfunction associated with functional deficits and broader symptomatology.
>
> **Jay Shah, et al.**[1]

---

* Numbered videos available at https://vimeo.com/showcase/7087178 with password BF57%$81

MYOFASCIAL PAIN AS AN INTRODUCTION TO UNDERSTANDING CHRONIC PAIN AND SPORTS INJURY

The "trigger point" has become common knowledge among pain sufferers and athletes; foam rollers and other devices for the self-treatment of trigger points are now present in most gyms and available at most big box stores. Chiropractors and physical therapists now commonly provide dry needling for symptomatic trigger points. So, what are these trigger points, and why are they so prevalent and persistent? To acknowledge the role of muscle and fascial elements in this pathology, the proper name is myofascial trigger points (MTrP). MTrPs are exquisitely tender nodules within a taut band of muscle which reproduce the patient's symptoms with sustained pressure. They are associated with a twitch response when palpated in a "strumming" fashion, perpendicular to the muscle fibers. Active MTrPs correlate with spontaneously reported symptoms, while latent MTrPs do not produce spontaneous symptoms, though they may affect muscle function. The pain perceived can be local with specific referral patterns as outlined in *The Trigger Point Manual*.[2] The myofascial pain syndrome (MPS) is a local or regional phenomenon of pain and other signs and symptoms, including autonomic symptoms, muscle stiffness, altered muscle control, and referred pain that can imitate radicular patterns. MPS is covered in Chapter 11 of this text, including mechanisms of central and peripheral sensitization. These important concepts help explain how a focal muscle pathology can spread via neurologic and inflammatory mechanisms. In a recent review article, the authors state "the development of successful treatment approaches depends upon identifying and targeting the underlying mechanisms of pain and dysfunction and addressing the perpetuating factors that maintain this common pain syndrome."[1] Yet, the etiology and perpetuating factors are often unclear. Perhaps, an overly mechanistic view of anatomy and biomechanics blurs our vision.

The eye sees only what the mind is prepared to comprehend.

Robertson Davies[3]

NOT ALL FEEDBACK AND CONTROL ARE NEUROLOGIC

In the research model of the decerebrate cat, scientists have explored the neurologic control of locomotion.[4] The focus has been on the neurologic anatomy behind oscillating, controlled movement that is unconscious. With the cerebrum disconnected, a cat can walk, trot, and run if provided with external stimulus from a treadmill. A video of this model is available on YouTube.[5] Whether trained in science or not, we tend to look at videos like this and wonder about the complex neurologic control that makes it possible. We are less likely to wonder about the complex myofascial anatomy that makes it possible.

In many ways, musculoskeletal anatomy is defined by the bones of our ancestors. This is what is left behind after life. Thousands of years of the collective unconscious have witnessed these bones and interpreted our form based on them. As an embryo, however, we have no bones. We are soft-bodied organisms, yet stable and capable of movement as seen in the mobility of both sperm and egg before they meet. Human anatomy began to be understood once dissection became culturally sanctioned. The reductionism of science involved cutting and separating structures so that the internal anatomy could be understood, surgeries developed, and suffering relieved. Our first imaging modality, X-ray, implies the obvious: the skeleton is the frame of our body. Muscles then are defined by where they originate and insert on bone. This allows us to picture shortening of a muscle and what that shortening would do to an adjacent joint. This model then becomes an unconscious visual pattern. The grasping of a weight or the process of locomotion involves the shortening of muscles to allow bending of joints and pulling of bones in a direction we desire. And biomechanics becomes a mapping of levers, joint angles, and force transfer controlled by neurologic signaling. Yet, our patients' stories are always more than the sum of these parts.

THE CASE OF A BODYBUILDER WITH DEGENERATIVE ARTHROSIS

A 41-year-old bodybuilder presents with >6-month history of left upper quadrant/shoulder pain after a weight lifting injury. While performing a 565-pound Hatfield squat, he felt the bar on his shoulders shift to the left and he heard a "very loud pop" in the left shoulder as he was going down and up. Since then, his powerlifting has been limited due to pain and poor active range of motion with abduction/external rotation. He is unable to lift weights and experiences pain "even with lifting a bottle of water." Physical exam is remarkable for pain to palpation at the posterior glenohumeral joint and infraspinatus trigger points, 4/5 strength in the left shoulder extensor and adductor groups, limited AROM in flexion (145 degrees) (Figure 10.1) and abduction (150 degrees). Abnormal orthopedic tests include O'Brien's (weakness and pain felt deep in the joint when testing strength in 90 degree forward flexion, 15 degree adduction, and extremity internal rotation/pronation), apprehension (posterior pain with limited passive abduction/external rotation) (Figure 10.2), modified Hawkins–Kennedy (pain with passive 90 degree abduction/internal rotation), and Speed's test (weakness without pain when testing strength from 90 degree flexion in supination/external rotation and pronation/internal rotation) (Figures 10.3 and 10.4). The patient declined MR arthrogram of the shoulder; MRI of the shoulder (>6 months after injury) revealed focal chondral thinning at superomedial aspect of humeral head (suspicious for previous impaction trauma) (Figure 10.5), degenerative arthrosis of the glenohumeral joint, degenerative changes at the superior labrum near the biceps anchor, and distal supraspinatus tendinopathy.

AN ADVANTAGE OF DYNAMIC ULTRASONOGRAPHY

At follow-up to review the MRI results, the posterior joint was observed with dynamic ultrasonography during passive abduction/external rotation. The humeral head translates and pivots near

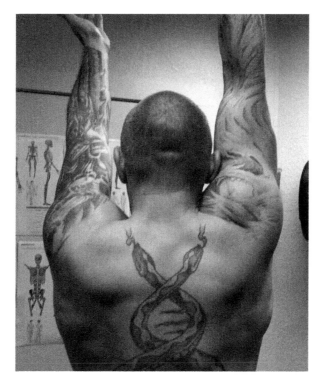

FIGURE 10.1 A weight lifter with glenohumeral arthrosis and limited AROM into flexion at initial exam. Still photograph capture from video 1.

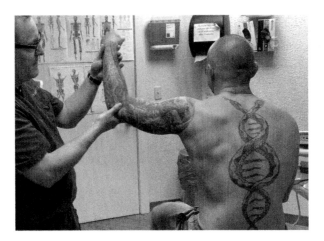

FIGURE 10.2   Apprehension test with posterior pain and limited PROM into external rotation at 90 degrees abduction (see video 2).

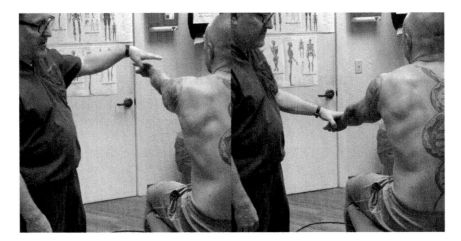

FIGURE 10.3   Speed's test from supinated/externally rotated position reveals weakness without pain (see video 3).

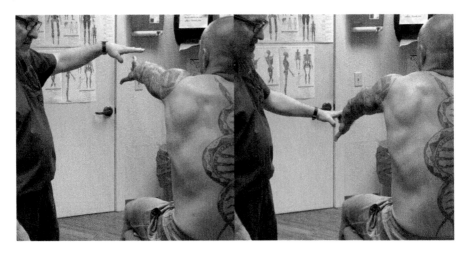

FIGURE 10.4   Speed's test from pronated/internally rotated position reveals weakness without pain (see video 4).

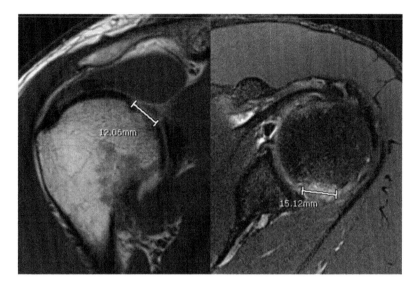

FIGURE 10.5 MRI (proton density, coronal on left; fat saturation axial on right) with evidence of previous impaction injury to posterior, superior humeral head, and cartilage degeneration of the glenoid.

the impact site, resulting in impingement of the posterior joint capsule and the deep surface of the infraspinatus tendon (Figure 10.6); the patient confirms this as the location of his posterior pain.

This posterior joint pain has now been reproduced at two appointments and two imaging studies correlate with his pain. Referral to orthopedic surgery appears to be the next step.

Questions:

1. What is the pain generator? The answer appears clear from the MRI, yet, is this even the right question?
2. The impaction injury likely occurred during the weight lifting injury. Did the arthrosis/chondromalacia pre-date this injury?
3. This patient suffered a unilateral injury while performing a symmetric exercise. Why did this happen?
4. Could biotensegrity theory, fascial anatomy, and the science of myofascial pain lead to new answers to these questions, new diagnoses, and a different treatment approach?

The value of the tensegrity model is that it provides a better means to visualize the mechanics of the body in the light of new understanding's about functional anatomy.

Graham Scarr, DO[4]

TENSEGRITY: THE TENSION IS THE FRAME

Tensegrity theory was developed at the intersection of art and science at Black Mountain College in North Carolina during the 1940s.[6] Inspired by the geometry lectures of futurist and scientist Buckminster Fuller, Kenneth Snelson, an art student and eventually world-famous sculptor, presented a work which he described as floating compression. Professor Fuller observed the sculpture and saw continuous tension. The term tensegrity points to the fact that the integrity of the structure depends on the continuity of tension within the structure, as in this 1968 work by Snelson shown in Figure 10.7. The rods, which resist compression, did not float in stability until the tension in the cables was balanced and continuous. The energy used to tension these cables remains in the structure to this day; thus, Snelson referred to his sculptures as "forces made visible."[7] Tensegrity theory now influences numerous sciences including architecture, cell biology, robotics, and others.[8–10] Some of the characteristics of tensegrity structures were recently summarized in a companion textbook to this volume[11] and are included here.

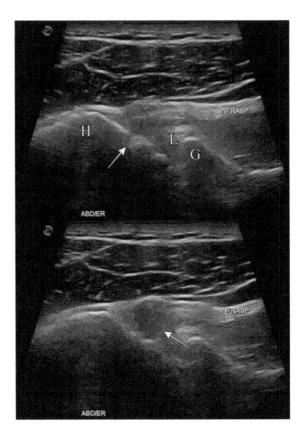

FIGURE 10.6 Posterior/internal impingement at posterior shoulder. Axial images at the posterior glenohumeral joint (still images from dynamic ultrasonography; see video 5) during PROM into external rotation at 90 degrees abduction. Top image: just before impact of the labrum (L) at the deep surface of the infraspinatus tendon and joint capsule. Arrow indicates pitting from chronic impingement. Irregular signal medial and deep to the arrow corresponds to the impaction site seen on the MRI. Bottom image: moment of impact and pain at maximum external rotation with deformation of the infraspinatus tendon indicated by arrow. H—humerus; G—glenoid.

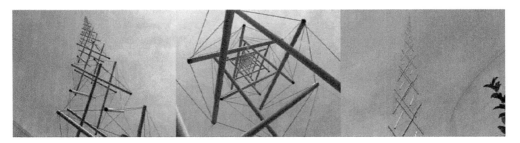

FIGURE 10.7 Tensegrity sculpture: "Needle Tower" 1968 by Kenneth Snelson. Photographs by the author at the Hirshhorn Museum and Sculpture Garden in Washington D.C., United States.

TENSEGRITY structures…:

1. …are a closed, stable system of only two forces: tension and compression.
2. …maintain structural integrity via *continuous* tension and *discontinuous* compression.
3. …store energy as pre-stress in the tension elements.
4. …create maximum stability with minimal mass.

5. …*instantaneously* diffuse outside forces through the *entire* structure.
6. …naturally produce oscillations without dissipating stored energy.

Since the early 1980s, orthopedic surgeon Stephen Levin M.D. has argued that traditional bio-mechanics can never explain biologic motion with stability.[12] Dr. Levin originated the term bio-tensegrity to emphasize the unique qualities of biologic structures which cannot be explained by traditional biomechanics. His concern was that tensegrity applications in human-made materials are fundamentally different than biology. The most highly developed biological application of tensegrity theory was initiated by Donald Ingber to develop the science of mechanotransduction.[13] If cellular mechanics follow tensegrity theory, perhaps biologic structures also follow tensegrity rules at the organism level. In discussing the hierarchical nature of tensegrity application from the cellular to tissue to organism level, Ingber et al. state "the shape stability and immediate mechanical responsiveness of all these structures depends on the pre-stress that is transmitted across their structural elements."[9] If this is true, our understanding of "musculoskeletal anatomy" would conform to the following characteristics amongst others, see below.

BIOTENSEGRITY-BASED ANATOMY AND BIOMECHANICS: A SUMMARY

1. The most rapid communication in the body occurs via the pre-stressed collagen fibers of the myofascial system.
2. Muscles are *not* structures that "pull" on bones to cause movement.
3. Bones float in a *variable tension network* consisting of muscle and fascial elements.
4. Fascial continuity provides *passive* tension and stored energy in the form of pre-stress.
5. Muscle fibers within the fascial continuity provide *dynamic* tension.
6. Thus, bones move (or, in the setting of outside forces, remain stable) when the tension around them changes.

FASCIA AS A BODY-WIDE SIGNALING MECHANISM

The Fascia Research Congress (FRC) brings together manual and movement therapists from varied schools of thought with connective tissue researchers to facilitate creative advances.[14] This collaboration has led to both a narrow and a broad definition of fascia, a kind of "tree and forest" view.[15] The term "A Fascia" is used to describe specific "aggregations of connective tissue that forms beneath the skin to attach, enclose, separate muscles and other internal organs," for example, the individually named parts and layers of the thoracolumbar fascia (TLF).[16] This specific definition facilitates communication between researchers. The term "The Fascial System" refers to "a network of interacting, interrelated, interdependent tissues forming a complex whole, all collaborating to perform a movement." This broad definition facilitates communication of the tactile knowledge of body workers and movement therapists.

Prior to the first FRC in 2008, Langevin proposed that fascia could act as a body-wide signaling mechanism through three possible mechanisms: electrical, cellular, and tissue remodeling.[17] Tensegrity theory would take this signaling function a step further, arguing that the body-wide signaling is inherent to the structure itself. All of the tissues of the musculoskeletal system derive from mesoderm. The embryologic fascia develops before the other tissues and becomes the context for development of muscles, bones, ligaments, and tendons.[18] Thus, all of these "separate tissues" derive from a continuity. If the tension in the mesokinetic system (a term from Levin and Scarr[6]) is continuous, a physical stress to the structure instantly changes the shape of the *entire* structure. Thus, the stress is communicated through the entire structure instantaneously. If there has been injury with loss of pre-stress in the past (i.e., an injury without full repair of the fascial structure), the instantaneous communication would be altered at the area of injury and the body would adjust its shape to reestablish communication. How can this theory be applied clinically?

CLINICAL APPLICATION OF BIOTENSEGRITY PRINCIPLES IN PAIN MEDICINE: A SUMMARY

1. Construct—focus on tensional continuity, which provides instantaneous, body-wide communication.
2. History—past trauma (acute or repetitive) is a loss of pre-stress in the tensegrity system.
3. Signs/Symptoms—a loss of pre-stress results in muscle dysfunction (e.g., spasm, poor control, inability to strengthen, development of trigger point) as the body attempts to compensate.
4. Diagnosis—use dynamics (in physical exam and ultrasonography) to find a loss of tensional continuity in the myofascia.
5. Treatment—stimulate repair at the loss of tensional continuity.

In the biotensegrity construct, the etiology and perpetuating factors of muscle dysfunction can be the same: injury to tensional elements (collagen/fascia) through repetitive stressors or acute trauma. With a loss of tensional continuity, the dynamic tensors (muscle) must "take up the slack," resulting in excessive and prolonged muscle contraction, which sets up the patient for repeat episodes of active trigger point symptoms. Remote injury (i.e., loss of pre-stress) results in recurring latent or active trigger point development, which responds to manual therapies and adjustments. If the repair of tensional fibers after injury is short of full integrity, the trigger point symptoms reoccur. The neuromuscular dysfunction that results from trigger point development predisposes patients to recurring injury under specific stressors based on the specific fascial fibers that did not fully repair.

BIOTENSEGRITY-INFORMED HISTORY

If past injury represents a potential loss of tensional continuity (i.e., an alteration of instantaneous communication in the body), a thorough history of past injury becomes a prime concern. On further questioning, our weight lifter reports that he was involved in a motor-vehicle accident (MVA) 12 years prior. He was a seat-belted driver, when another vehicle accelerated around a turning vehicle, striking his car directly at the driver's door at high speed. Disoriented by the smoke from the airbags, he tried to reach with the left hand to open the driver's door. He realized the door was immovable and his left arm was useless due to pain. Using the right hand, he was able to break through the shattered glass of the driver's door and use the right arm to pull himself through the window and fall to the ground on his left side. He recalls days to weeks of left-sided pain after this; however, no significant lasting deficits. When questioned about more subtle symptoms of latent trigger points, he reports odd sensations on the left side which have persisted since this accident. An intermittent feeling, similar to a vague itching, starts in the left low back and spreads a feeling of tightness to the muscles around the left scapula. This leads to a request to mimic the moment of impact.

> One must be able to imagine a possible world before it can be tested.
>
> **Root-Bernstein**[19]

BIOTENSEGRITY-INFORMED PHYSICAL EXAM

When he demonstrates the moment of impact, the diffusion of forces can be seen as his left brachium is driven into the ribs and the left scapula is driven medially with some glenoid depression and counter-clockwise rotation of the scapula. This leads to more detailed examination of the left flank, which reveals taut bands and latent trigger points in the lower latissimus dorsi (LD), lower serratus anterior, and adjacent external oblique fibers at the low ribs. Focal pressure at the rib entheses results in pain response as well. If his remote injury in this area did not fully repair, the connective tissue here would be lax. The taut muscle fibers in this region could be a response to connective tissue laxity. Could passive tension be returned to the system temporarily through more diffuse palpation? How would this change his examination? When support is applied to this region, with the intent of restoring some of the pre-stress lost in the accident, two remarkable changes occur:

1. The apprehension test now has full, painless PROM into abduction/external rotation (Figure 10.8).
2. Speed's testing in supination and pronation now displays normal strength and stability (Figures 10.9 and 10.10).

Movement is not bending of hinges, but expansion, repositioning and contraction of tensegrities.

Levin and Martin[20]

With pre-stress added back into the system, the quality of active muscle contraction during Speed's testing changes from an attempt at "pulling" the upper extremity into position to "an expansion" of the upper extremity and trunk into the applied downward force. The movement is now a "complex whole" rather than an uncoordinated contraction of parts (videos 7 and 8). To confirm these observations, the tests are repeated without the pre-stress applied to the left flank. They revert back to the uncoordinated contraction of parts and pain with limited PROM. Let's explore these observations in the context of fascial anatomy and trigger point science.

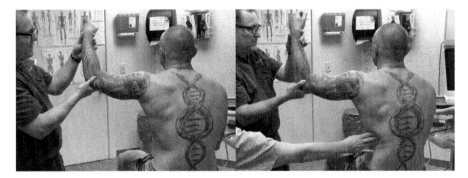

FIGURE 10.8 Biotensegrity-informed physical exam: left image same as Figure 10.3. Right image same test performed; however, prior to beginning the test, tension (pre-stress) is added via palpation pressure at an area of remote trauma. PROM normalizes, and he has no posterior pain (see video 6).

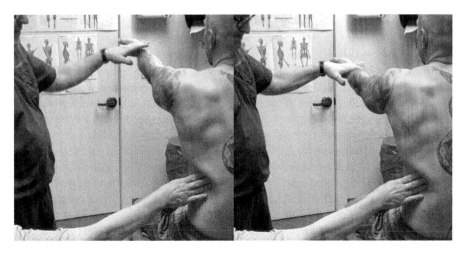

FIGURE 10.9 Biotensegrity-informed Speed's test in supination: with the arm resting on his lap, pressure is applied at left low ribs/LD/SPI; then, test is repeated with full strength (see video 7).

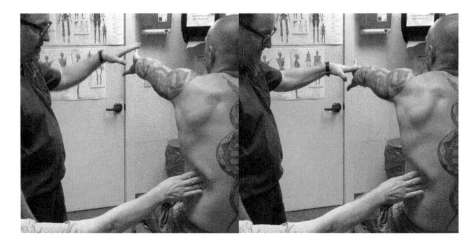

FIGURE 10.10   Biotensegrity-informed Speed's test in pronation: with the arm resting on his lap, pressure is applied at left low ribs/LD/SPI; then, test is repeated with full strength (see video 8).

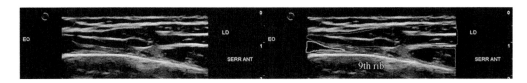

FIGURE 10.11   Ultrasound imaged uncompressed: probe is long axis on the ninth rib with three muscles visualized. Left image is unlabeled; right with muscles outlined LD in red, SA in blue, and EO in green.

THE FALSE CONCEPT OF LIGAMENTS AS THE ONLY CONTROLLERS OF PROM

In musculoskeletal anatomy, ligaments (including joint capsules) are conceived as the passive controllers of joint motion. Tests of ligamentous and capsular integrity focus on forces applied to a joint while the patient is relaxed, such as this apprehension test designed to evaluate joint stability. If there is posterior impingement with this test in an overhead athlete, the conceptual explanation then becomes laxity in the anterior capsule versus tightness in the posterior, inferior joint capsule which pushes the humeral head anterior, creating posterior impingement.[21] Yet, in our patient, adding tension by applying pressure at the flank improves the passive dynamics at the shoulder joint.

Van Der Wal[22] has argued that the radial collateral and annular ligaments of the lateral elbow do not exist as separate structures from the myofascial continuity of the extensor forearm mechanism. He argues that the appearance of a ligament structure in this location is an artifact of the dissection process. Ultimately, Van Der Wal argues that muscle tendon units are more commonly in series with ligamentous tissue rather than in parallel as most anatomic drawings illustrate. Numerous examples of muscle to tendon to joint capsule have been described in the knee,[23] hip,[24] and shoulder.[25]

The muscle–fascial continuity, then, is a pre-stressed controller of PROM, just as the ligaments and joint capsules have been described. In fact, Masi et al. have described the resting tone of muscles as a significant contributor to dynamic control.[26] This broadly extended, impossibly complex continuity of tension has been described by Levin et al. as a multi-bar kinematic mechanism of biologic movement.[27] So, what part of this mechanism was injured in our patient during the MVA? At the ninth rib, three muscles partially blend with each other: serratus anterior (SA), external oblique (EO), and latissimus dorsi (LD). Dynamic ultrasonography with compression at this location reveals the poor definition and instability of this blending (Figures 10.11 and 10.12). Serratus anterior translates toward the inferior angle of the scapula which reveals incompetence of the muscle as it blends with the periosteum of the rib and the adjoining external oblique. LD also compresses easily and

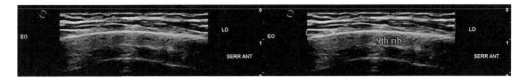

FIGURE 10.12 Ultrasound imaged with compression showing loss of tensional integrity (see video 9): probe is long axis on the ninth rib with three muscles visualized. Left image is unlabeled; right with muscles outlined LD in red, SA in blue, and EO in green.

translates toward the scapula (video 9). Similar weakness is seen at the serratus posterior inferior (SPI) and LD insertions at ribs 10 through 12.

BIOTENSEGRITY-INFORMED TREATMENT

If remote injury without full repair represents a loss of tensional integrity, repair at that location (or locations) would restore tensional continuity in the fascial structures and allow muscles to contract only when needed as a fine-tuning mechanism. Ease of movement would return. These are the clinical observations of prolotherapists through the decades since Hackett defined prolotherapy as an injection technique for strengthening "the weld of disabled ligaments and tendons to bone by stimulating the production of new bone and fibrous tissue cells".[28] For 36 years, the American Association of Orthopedic Medicine has educated physicians in the clinical application of prolotherapy (www.aaomed.org). Since the early 2000s, the University of Wisconsin in Madison with the Hackett Hemwall Patterson Foundation has hosted a comprehensive course on prolotherapy. For years the title of the course was "Prolotherapy in the Treatment of Myofascial Pain." An annual research conference was added in 2005 and a dedicated research collaboration established.[29] Prolotherapy technique involves the injection of various agents (most commonly 15% dextrose) at numerous entheses; often these are locations where there is no pathology recognized by mainstream medicine. To many, the broad pattern of injection has been a sign that the diagnosis is imprecise. Yet, if loss of tension in the myofascial continuity is the diagnosis, only a broad intervention would address the pathology. The technique described below is an attempt to "split the difference" between widespread injection guided by palpation (as in traditional prolotherapy technique) and specific tissue pathology targets guided by ultrasound.

In our patient, the treatment applied will be simultaneously diagnostic as well as therapeutic. Injection of 0.3% lidocaine, 15% dextrose is performed under ultrasound diagnosis at:

1. Blending of EO/LD/SA at the ninth rib.
2. SA attachments at the ninth rib.
3. Ninth to tenth intercostal fascia (overlying the intercostal muscle).
4. SPI and LD attachments at ribs 10–12.

A total of 10–15 ml solution was used at these locations. By spreading the solution through this region of myofascial continuity, there is potential for blocking nociceptive signals which inhibit muscle contraction while also using fluid pressure as a temporary establishment of tensional continuity to enhance the function of this "multibar kinematic mechanism of biologic movement" (Figure 10.13). As in the physical exam above, the injections produce rapid improvement in strength, muscle coordination, and ROM. Within 5 minutes of injection at the ribs, Speed's test is normal (Figure 10.14) and AROM has improved to near normal (Figure 10.15).

Once information is gained from these post-injection tests, autologous leukocyte poor platelet-rich plasma (LP-PRP) is injected at the same locations. The hypothesis for this patient is that the remote injury to the left flank contributed to altered scapulohumeral rhythm during weight lifting

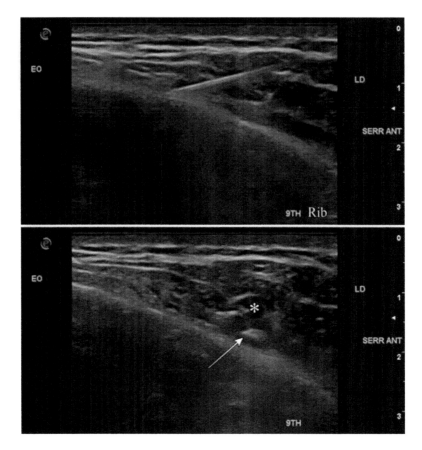

FIGURE 10.13 Ultrasound of injections at ninth rib. Top image: needle tip at periosteum of ninth rib, deep to LD. Bottom image: arrow points to needle tip. The * indicates injected fluid contained within the myofascial continuity; thus, using fluid pressure to produce temporary increase in tension within the continuity (see video 10).

since the accident, leading to abnormal pressure/shear forces at the glenohumeral joint and supraspinatus impingement at the subacromial space. The poor coordination between the abdominal wall and upper extremity under the extreme load of more than 500 pounds allowed the weight to shift left, causing the impaction injury at the humeral head. To address both remote and recent injuries, other locations were treated with the same solutions the same day:

1. Posterior glenohumeral joint capsule and the overlying infraspinatus tendon.
2. Intraarticular glenohumeral joint.
3. Junction of lower and middle trapezius near the medial scapula.
4. Supraspinatus tendon (a small tear was confirmed during injection).
5. Acromioclavicular joint and capsule.

RESTORATION OF TENSIONAL INTEGRITY: CLINICAL AND TISSUE IMPROVEMENTS 3 MONTHS POST-PROCEDURE

To allow normal tissue repair response over the next 2–3 months, anti-inflammatory medications are forbidden.[30] Activity is to tolerance with no attempts at weight lifting until 4 weeks at which a self-guided, gradual introduction of exercise is allowed. No formal therapies were performed. At 3-month follow-up, the patient reports that he has been able to return to weight lifting and can

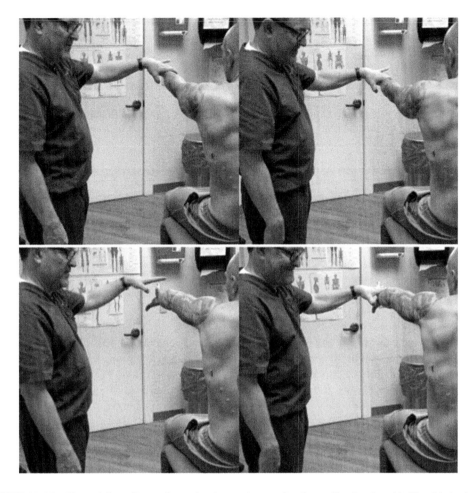

FIGURE 10.14 Normal Speed's test in supination and pronation immediately after 10–15 ml injection of 0.3% lidocaine, 15% dextrose at ribs 9–12. Note injection sites at left flank (see videos 11 and 12).

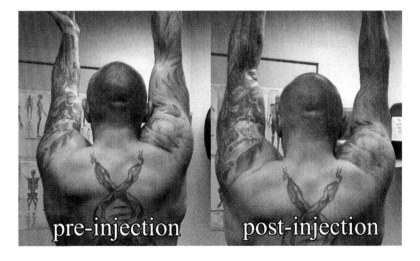

FIGURE 10.15 Pre-injection (left) and post-injection at ribs (right) AROM in flexion. (See video 13.) [FYI: Videos 14, 15 and 16 are described in the text of the article. There are no still images/figures from these videos.]

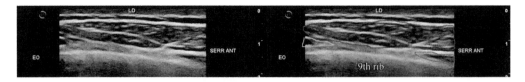

FIGURE 10.16 Ultrasound imaged uncompressed 4 months after treatment with improved myofascial definition: probe is long axis on the ninth rib with three muscles visualized. Left image is unlabeled; right with muscles outlined LD in red, SA in blue, and EO in green.

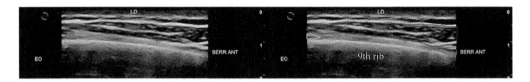

FIGURE 10.17 Ultrasound images with compression 4 months after treatment with improved resistance to compression indicating a return of tensional integrity (see video 17): probe is long axis on the ninth rib with three muscles visualized. Left image is unlabeled; right with muscles outlined LD in red, SA in blue, and EO in green.

deadlift 475 pounds "with ease"; overall he feels "70% improvement." He has full AROM in flexion and abduction, normal strength, normal Speed's test in supination and pronation, and normal apprehension test with full PROM into abduction/external rotation (see videos 14, 15, 16). Tissue definition and dynamic compression at the ninth rib have markedly improved (Figures 10.16 and 10.17).

CONCLUSION

Biotensegrity-informed anatomy, biomechanics, and patient evaluation help us to see the patient as a whole, integrating their life experience of physical trauma/stress and arriving at previously unrecognized diagnoses. Body workers, movement therapists, osteopathic physicians, prolotherapists, and others have recognized these injuries for decades through tactile knowledge without clear diagnosis. Improved knowledge of the fascial system as an integrative tissue, awareness of specific fascial anatomic structures as crucial forms of communication, dynamic ultrasonography for the diagnosis/treatment of these structures, and biotensegrity theory as a guiding principle combine to clarify the importance of "soft tissue" injury in perpetuating chronic pain.

REFERENCES

1. Shah, J.P., Thaker, N., Heimur, J., Aredo, J.V., Sikdar, S., and Gerber, L.H. (2015). Myofascial trigger points then and now: a historical and scientific perspective. *PM R* 7(7), 746–761.
2. Simons, David G., Travell, Janet G., and Simons, Lois S. (1999). *Myofascial Pain and Dysfunction: The Trigger Point Manual, Vol 1, Upper Half of Body*. London: Lippincott Williams and Wilkins.
3. Davies, R. (1951). *Tempest-Tost*. Harmondsworth, Middlesex, England: Penguin Books.
4. Whelan, P.J. (1996). Control of locomotion in the decerebrate cat. *Progress in Neurobiology* 49(5), 481–515.
5. Decerebrate cat walks and exhibits multiple gait patterns. https://www.youtube.com/watch?v=wPiLLplofYw. Accessed February 26, 2019.
6. Scarr, G. (2018). *Biotensegrity: The Structural Basis of Life*, 2nd ed. Pencaitland, Scotland: Handspring.
7. Heartney, E. (2009). *Kenneth Snelson: Forces Made Visible*. Burlington, VT: Hudson Hills.
8. Skelton, R.E., Fraternali, F., Carpentieri, G., and Micheletti, A. (2014). Minimum mass design of tensegrity bridges with parametric architecture and multiscale complexity. *Mechanics Research Communications* 58, 124–132.

9. Ingber, D.E., Wang, N., and Stamenović, D. (2014). Tensegrity, cellular biophysics, and the mechanics of living systems. *Reports on Progress in Physics 77*(4), 046603.

10. Iscen, A., Agogino, A., SunSpiral, V., and Tumer, K. (2013, July). Controlling tensegrity robots through evolution. In: *Proceedings of the 15th Annual Conference on Genetic and Evolutionary Computation* (pp. 1293–1300). ACM.

11. Fullerton, B. (2018). Biotensegrity: how ultrasound diagnostics guide regenerative orthopedic therapies to restore biomechanical function. In: *Metabolic Therapies in Orthopedics*, 2nd ed. (pp. 93–111). Boca Raton, FL: CRC Press.

12. Levin, S.M. (1981). The icosahedron as a biologic support system. In: *34th Annual* Conference *Alliance for* Engineering *in* Medicine *&* Biology. Bethesda, MD: Alliance for Engineering in Medicine & Biology.

13. Ingber, D.E. (2008). Tensegrity and mechanotransduction. *Journal of Bodywork and Movement Therapies 12*(3), 198–200.

14. https://fasciacongress.org/congress/about-the-congress/. Accessed February 26, 2019.

15. Stecco, C., and Schleip, R. (2016). A fascia and the fascial system. *Journal of Bodywork and Movement Therapies 20*(1), 139–140.

16. Willard, F.H., Vleeming, A., Schuenke, M.D., Danneels, L., and Schleip, R. (2012). The thoracolumbar fascia: anatomy, function and clinical considerations. *Journal of Anatomy 221*(6), 507–536.

17. Langevin, H.M. (2006). Connective tissue: a body-wide signaling network? *Medical Hypotheses 66*(6), 1074–1077.

18. Willard, F.H. (2012). Somatic fascia. In: *Fascia: The Tensional Network of the Human Body*, eds Schleip, R., Findley, T.W., Chaitow, L., and Huijing, P.A. (pp. 11–17). New York: Elsevier.

19. Root-Bernstein, R. (1989). *Discovering: Inventing and Solving Problems at the Frontiers of Science and Knowledge*, 1st ed. Cambridge, MA: Harvard University Press.

20. Levin, S., and Martin, D. (2012). Biotensegrity, the mechanics of fascia. In: *Fascia: The Tensional Network of the Human Body*, eds Schleip, R., Findley, T.W., Chaitow, L., and Huijing, P.A. (pp. 137–142). New York: Elsevier.

21. Burkhart, S.S., Morgan, C.D., and Kibler, W.B. (2003). The disabled throwing shoulder: spectrum of pathology part I: pathoanatomy and biomechanics. *Arthroscopy: The Journal of Arthroscopic and Related Surgery 19*(4), 404–420.

22. van der Wal, J. (2009). The architecture of the connective tissue in the musculoskeletal system–an often overlooked functional parameter as to proprioception in the locomotor apparatus. *International Journal of Therapeutic Massage and Bodywork 2*(4), 9–23.

23. Dalmau-Pastor, M., Fargues-Polo, B., Casanova-Martínez, D., Vega, J., and Golanó, P. (2014). Anatomy of the triceps surae: a pictorial essay. *Foot and Ankle Clinics 19*(4), 603–635.

24. Walters, B.L., Cooper, J.H., and Rodriguez, J.A. (2014). New findings in hip capsular anatomy: dimensions of capsular thickness and pericapsular contributions. *Arthroscopy: The Journal of Arthroscopic and Related Surgery 30*(10), 1235–1245.

25. Rahu, M., Kolts, I., Põldoja, E., and Kask, K. (2017). Rotator cuff tendon connections with the rotator cable. *Knee Surgery, Sports Traumatology, Arthroscopy 25*(7), 2047–2050.

26. Masi, A.T., and Hannon, J.C. (2008). Human resting muscle tone (HRMT): narrative introduction and modern concepts. *Journal of Bodywork and Movement Therapies 12*(4), 320–332.

27. Levin, S., de Solórzano, S.L., and Scarr, G. (2017). The significance of closed kinematic chains to biological movement and dynamic stability. *Journal of Bodywork and Movement Therapies 21*(3), 664–672.

28. Hackett, G.S. (1958). *Ligament and Tendon Relaxation Treated by Prolotherapy*, 3rd ed. Springfield, IL: Charles C Thomas.

29. https://www.fammed.wisc.edu/prolotherapy/. Accessed February 26, 2019.

30. Lee, K.S., Wilson, J.J., Rabago, D.P., Baer, G.S., Jacobson, J.A., and Borrero, C.G. (2011). Musculoskeletal applications of platelet-rich plasma: fad or future? *American Journal of Roentgenology 196*(3), 628–636.

11 Myofascial Trigger Points, Sensitization, and Chronic Musculoskeletal Pain

Evaluation and Management

Vy Phan, Jay P. Shah, and Pamela Stratton

CONTENTS

SUMMARY

Chronic musculoskeletal pain is highly prevalent and presents a major burden to individuals and society. Myofascial pain syndrome (MPS) is one of the most common musculoskeletal disorders and encompasses the surrounding fascia and connective tissue. MPS can be either acute or chronic and is highly associated with myofascial trigger points (MTrPs) in the affected muscles. Active (spontaneously painful) MTrPs, which comprise the gold standard for the diagnosis of myofascial pain, are one of the major peripheral pain generators for musculoskeletal pain conditions. The continual nociceptive bombardment from primary afferent activity over time leads to abnormal functional and structural changes in the dorsal root ganglia and dorsal horn, a phenomenon known as central sensitization. Sensitization is consistently associated with musculoskeletal pain states, underscoring its significance. Moreover, the sensitized spinal segments and somatic dysfunction may be explained, in part, by viscerosomatic convergence and viscerosomatic reflex; both highlighting the contributions of visceral pathologies to somatic structure pain. In addition, the limbic forebrain and hypothalamus likely play a role in myofascial pain. For example, the limbic system has a bidirectional relationship with negative affect, which may contribute to the amplification or maintenance of the pain. These central factors illustrate the importance of a systematic evaluation in addition to palpation of the skeletal muscle for the objective physical findings of active MTrPs. Comprehensive management of MPS focuses on deactivating painful MTrPs and addressing sensitization at both the peripheral and central level through the use of manual therapies, dry needling, paraspinous injection blocks, electrical modalities, local botulinum toxin injection, centrally acting pharmacologic agents, and biofeedback, among others.

INTRODUCTION

Myofascial pain is the most common component of musculoskeletal pain conditions. As a form of muscle pain, myofascial pain can often be described as aching, cramping, deep, and difficult to localize. Several biological processes differ between muscle and cutaneous pain. For example, muscle pain involves nociceptive-specific neurons in the brainstem and spinal cord to a greater extent than observed in cutaneous pain.[1,2] In addition, muscle pain activates midbrain areas that are associated with affective or emotional components of pain.[3] Although muscle nociception is inhibited more intensely by descending pain-modulating pathways,[4,5] persistent muscle nociception is more effective than cutaneous nociception at inducing maladaptive neuroplastic changes within the dorsal horn.[6] Such neuroplastic changes underlie the clinical observation that chronic muscle pain is often persistent and difficult to resolve.

Myofascial pain syndrome (MPS) is a term used to describe a pain condition which can be acute (less than 3 months in duration) or, more commonly, chronic, and stems from the muscle and its surrounding connective tissue and fascia. For many clinicians and investigators, a necessary component to the diagnosis of MPS is the finding of one or more MTrPs. An MTrP is palpable on physical examination as a discrete hyperirritable nodule in a taut band of skeletal muscle (Figure 11.1). The pain experienced with MPS is associated with but not necessarily caused by an active MTrP. An active MTrP is associated with spontaneous pain in the surrounding tissue and with referred pain. Strong digital pressure on the active MTrP intensifies the patient's pain and mimics the patient's typical pain experience. MTrPs can also be latent, such that the MTrP is present but not associated with spontaneous pain. However, pressure on a latent MTrP often elicits pain at the nodule even in individuals who are not experiencing pain in that region. Both latent and active MTrPs can be associated with muscle dysfunction, muscle weakness, and limited range of motion.

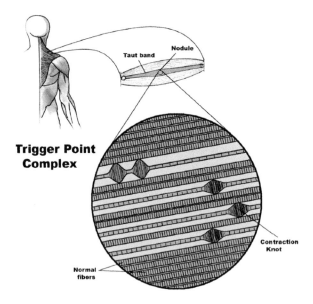

FIGURE 11.1   Schematic of a trigger point complex. A trigger point complex in a taut band of muscle is composed of multiple contraction knots. (Adapted from Simons, D.G., Travell, J.G. *Myofascial Pain and Dysfunction: The Trigger Point Manual*, vol. 1; second ed., and Användare: Chrizz.)

ORIGIN AND HISTORY OF MPS

The clinical study of MPS and its associated MTrPs has spanned the past two centuries in which scientists and physicians have striven to characterize MPS, proposing distinguishing characteristics and associations for the disorder. However, the scientific literature appears disjointed and confusing, as the terminology, theories, concepts, and diagnostic criteria are inconsistent, incomplete, and, at times, controversial. As a result, MPS and its relationship to MTrPs are not fully understood.

The term "myofascial" conveys that both muscle and fascia likely contribute to the symptoms. In the past, "chronic muscle pain" and nomenclature such as "fibrositis" reflected inflammation of connective tissue lining muscle. These terms have been replaced by the term "myofascial pain."

The study of myofascial pain and dysfunction was pioneered by the U.S. physician Janet Travell, whose work is arguably the most comprehensive to date. Travell and Rinzler coined the term "myofascial trigger point" in the 1950s, reflecting their finding that the nodules can be present and refer pain to both muscle and overlying fascia.[7] The two-volume book, *Myofascial Pain and Dysfunction: The Trigger Point Manual*, which she co-authored with her colleague, David Simons, represents decades of keen observations and study of myofascial pain and MTrPs.[8]

This manual, along with over 40 papers Travell published, remains crucial in defining and popularizing the diagnosis and treatment of MPS and MTrPs within the healthcare community, which includes physical therapists, allopathic and osteopathic physicians, chiropractors, dentists, pain specialists, massage therapists, and myofascial trigger point therapists. Among the various allopathic medical specialties, physiatrists currently have the most comprehensive understanding of MTrPs, in part because physiatrists see MPS and the MTrP as related to muscle and musculoskeletal dysfunction. Physiatrists are perhaps unique among the medical specialties as they do not regard muscle as an "orphan organ." Simons used this term to describe the medical community's lack of understanding and consideration of muscle as a contributor to non-articular musculoskeletal pain syndromes. Now, Simons' comments along with Travell's myofascial pain concepts are gaining ground in mainstream medicine.

The contemporary use of the term "MPS" implies a specific condition which is distinguished from other soft tissue pain disorders such as fibromyalgia, tendonitis, or bursitis.[9] For instance, unlike fibromyalgia, which is widespread, symmetrically distributed, and frequently affects sleep and mood, MPS presents as local or regional pain, sometimes with referred pain, and is often accompanied by increased tension and decreased flexibility. The pain of MPS may present independently of mood or sleep abnormalities and has been reported with other diseases and syndromes associated with pain, such as rheumatologic diseases and fibromyalgia.[10] Other pain conditions associated with MPS include radiculopathies, joint dysfunction, disk pathology, tendonitis, craniomandibular dysfunction, migraines, tension type headaches, carpal tunnel syndrome, computer-related disorders, whiplash-associated disorders, spinal dysfunction, pelvic pain and other urologic syndromes, post-herpetic neuralgia, and complex regional pain syndrome.[10] In addition, MTrPs have been associated clinically with a variety of medical conditions including those of metabolic, visceral, endocrine, infectious, and psychological origin.[11]

MPS has generally been characterized by a physical finding and symptom cluster that lacked demonstrable pathology and attracted little research attention until recently. Additionally, characteristics such as pain quality, distribution, and whether the pain radiates have never been required for the diagnosis of MPS. The inter-subject variability and subjective nature of each individual's symptoms present a challenge for standardization and validation if these are to be used as diagnostic criteria, outcome measures of improvement, or in clinical trials. However, the nature of the symptoms of muscle pain in general is highly dependent upon the individual's perception of its intensity, distribution, and duration. Centralized mechanisms have been suggested to be involved in MPS, potentially altering the pain threshold, pain intensity, and emotional affect.[12] Thus, it is recommended that examiners take a systematic approach to evaluating the individual's pain perception along with related central factors when diagnosing and treating MPS.

CHRONIC MUSCULOSKELETAL PAIN AND SENSITIZATION: IMPLICATIONS FOR EVALUATION AND TREATMENTS

AIMS AND OBJECTIVES

- To gain a deeper understanding of the mechanisms of central and peripheral sensitization, and to investigate the critical role of these neuroplastic changes in perpetuating chronic musculoskeletal pain.
- To recognize the associated affective manifestations and limbic system dysfunction, and the relevance of factors influencing quality of life in the evaluation of chronic musculo-skeletal pain.
- To summarize the reproducible physical manifestations of spinal segmental sensitization (SSS) associated with chronic musculoskeletal pain.
- To review how improved quantitative and objective diagnostic techniques are used to determine the spinal segments involved in SSS (including dermatomes, myotomes, and sclerotomes), and how such investigations are applicable in the palpatory diagnosis and management treatment of chronic musculoskeletal pain.
- To discuss and demonstrate modalities and needling techniques used to desensitize the involved segments, eliminate chronic myofascial trigger points, and alleviate chronic *neuro*-musculoskeletal pain.

MPS, SENSITIZATION, AND VISCEROSOMATIC INTERACTIONS

Sensitization is the lowering of the activation threshold for nociceptors, which then increases neuronal activity in the central nervous system. Through sensitization, chronic pain syndromes, such as MPS, exhibit profound neuroplastic changes, altering neuronal excitability in the pain pathways including the spinal cord, thalamic nuclei, cortical areas, amygdala, and periaqueductal gray area. This dynamic process can fundamentally alter the pain threshold, pain intensity, and emotional affect.[12] Common manifestations of sensitization are hyperalgesia (increased pain to a normally painful stimulus), and allodynia (pain to a normally non-painful stimulus).

Signaling in the pain matrix may begin with activation of polymodal nociceptors by a noxious stimulus. These peripheral structures can be sensitized by substances released from damaged tissue and the nociceptor terminals themselves. Peripheral tissue damage arising from muscle trauma and tissue inflammation triggers the release of numerous substances from damaged muscle, such as adenosine triphosphate (ATP), bradykinin (BK), serotonin (5-HT), prostaglandins, protons, and potassium. This inflammatory pool of biochemicals sensitizes and/or activates local nociceptors, an event known as peripheral sensitization.

Under normal circumstances, activation of primary afferent nociceptors in the dorsal horn is modulated by inhibitory mechanisms either locally or via descending pathways from the cerebral cortex or brainstem. However, persistent nociceptive afferent input may result in inhibitory neuronal cell death, wind-up, and sensitization of second-order neurons in the dorsal horn. This continual bombardment over time leads to abnormal functional and structural changes in the dorsal root ganglia and dorsal horn, a process known as central sensitization, and results in the co-release of L-glutamate and substance P (SP). Released together, these two substances can lower thresholds for synaptic activation and open previously ineffective synaptic connections in wide dynamic range (WDR) neurons.[13,14] In turn, the bombardment of nociceptive stimuli will lead to spinal facilitation, an increase in spinal cord neuronal activity.[15] Circuits in the spinal cord (including the dorsal horn, ventral horn, and lateral horn) may develop lowered thresholds of activation, causing them to be more easily activated by minimal or no input at all.

The ensuing spinal facilitation is characterized by:

1) Increased ventral horn outflow that stimulates anterior motor horn cells, resulting in increased muscle tone in the myotome corresponding to its segmental level of afferent barrage.

2) Increased lateral horn outflow which results in autonomic reflexes that enhance nociceptive activity.

3) Increased dorsal horn outflow that causes antidromic (retrograde) electrical activity along a sensory nerve.

Dorsal root reflexes activate dorsal root ganglion cell bodies to increase the production and release of vasoactive neuropeptides (e.g., SP, calcitonin gene-related peptide, and somatostatin) both centrally and peripherally. These neuropeptides cause leaky blood vessels and trigger the release of inflammatory mediators into the tissue, causing inflammation *de novo*, a condition known as neurogenic inflammation.[13] However, when inflammation is already present, the release of these vasoactive neuropeptides further exacerbates it. The resultant local tissue tenderness and mechanical hyperalgesia either begin or worsen, and may underlie the clinical findings of active MTrPs.

An understanding of segmental distribution of sensory nerve fibers is a vital component in proper pain management.[16] Innervation patterns of the skin, muscles, and deep structures occur at an early stage of human fetal development, and little variability exists among individuals.[14] As each spinal cord segment has a consistent segmental relationship to its spinal nerves, clinicians can attribute the pattern of dermatomal, myotomal, and sclerotomal hyperalgesia to dysfunction in the corresponding spinal segment.[16,17]

Spinal segmental sensitization (SSS) is a hyperactive state of the dorsal horn caused by bombardment of nociceptive impulses from sensitized or damaged tissue including somatic structures (such as active MTrPs) or visceral structures (such as the gall bladder or pelvic organs). Afferent nociception from viscera to spinal segments leads to two features related to central sensitization: viscerosomatic convergence and the viscerosomatic reflex. As less than 10% of all afferent fibers synapsing onto the spinal cord are visceral afferents, spinal neurons predominately receive input from somatic structures like muscle and skin. Viscerosomatic convergence is the process in which the spinal neurons receive both visceral and somatosensory input, and contributes to pain referred from visceral pathologies to somatic structures since both are innervated by the same spinal segments. Moreover, visceral afferent fibers extend over adjacent spinal segments and can sensitize multiple areas of the spinal cord. This "viscerosomatic reflex" may result in "referred" pain, which is pain experienced in areas remote from the affected visceral organ. At times, this convergence of inputs leads to broad areas of allodynia and hyperalgesia, making it challenging to distinguish and localize the sensory information. The viscerosomatic reflex may increase muscle tone and spasm in somatic structures that, in turn, may result in the development or activation of MTrPs.[16,18] Active MTrPs may then refer pain from the somatic structures back to the visceral organ or become a self-sustaining source of pain after the visceral pathology has resolved.[18] Ultimately, myofascial pain and manifestations related to sensitization may become widespread.

Manifestations from the sensitized spinal segment include dermatomal allodynia, sclerotomal tenderness, and myotomal MTrPs,[16,19] and often hyperalgesia. For example, in one study, hyperalgesia was present in 61% of patients suffering from arthrosis-related pain. This observation suggests that both central and peripheral mechanisms contribute to maintaining a chronic pain state in these individuals. Initially, hypersensitivity occurs at an affected site, but central sensitization can begin and persist independent of the peripheral process.[20] Further, segmental sensitization occurs through the upregulation of excitatory neurons, prohyperalgesic peptides, and neurotransmitters at the dorsal horn. Pain and inflammation are independent events and are not indicative of each other.

The sensitization of primary afferents is responsible for the transition from normal to aberrant pain perception in the central nervous system that outlasts the noxious peripheral stimulus. A possible explanation for expanded referral pain patterns is increased synaptic efficacy through the activation of previously silent synapses at the dorsal horn. This concept was demonstrated in a rat myositis model in which experimentally induced inflammation unmasked receptive fields remote from the original field, indicating that dorsal horn connectivity expanded beyond the original neurons involved in nociceptive transmission.[21] Ultimately, nociceptive input resulted in central hyperexcitability, suggesting that referred pain patterns are common to myofascial pain syndrome.

Central sensitization may facilitate additional responses from other receptive fields because of convergent somatic and visceral input at the dorsal horn[22] via WDR neurons. Furthermore, afferent fibers can sprout new spinal terminals that broaden synaptic contacts at the dorsal horn and may also contribute to expanded pain receptive fields.[23] This change in functional connectivity may occur within a few hours, even before metabolic and genetic alterations occur in dorsal horn neurons.[24]

THE ROLE OF THE LIMBIC SYSTEM

After stimulating WDR neurons, afferent input from active MTrPs then ascends the spinothalamic tract to reach higher brain centers, activating the limbic system. The limbic system plays a critical role in modulating muscle pain and the emotional or affective component of persistent pain.[3] Increased activity in the limbic system leads to greater fear, anxiety, and stress. For example, Niddam et al. demonstrated increased anterior insula activity in patients with upper trapezius myofascial pain syndrome.[13] Insular activity is associated with fear, anxiety, and depression along with fibromyalgia, somatization, and subjective feelings of pain (Figure 11.2).[25]

The limbic system is part of the brainstem's descending pain modulatory network leading to myofascial pain. Recent neuroimaging studies have suggested the brain regions associated with several cognitive factors altering pain perception. For example, attention appears to modulate the pain experience through the activity of the amygdala[26] and may explain the prevalence of hypervigilance in many chronic pain patients. The anticipation of pain worsens the pain experience and may become maladaptive in chronic pain patients, contributing to avoidance behavior and anxiety.[25] In fact, anticipatory anxiety appears to influence pain perception through increased activity in the entorhinal cortex, which subsequently increases activity in other affective pain-processing regions in the brain.[26] Even in healthy individuals, anticipation of pain is positively correlated with pain intensity.[25] Catastrophizing can intensify pain through rumination, helplessness, and magnification.[25]

The interrelationship between depression and pain is observed. Experimentally induced pain studies have shown a correlation between the negative mood and an increase in pain perception.

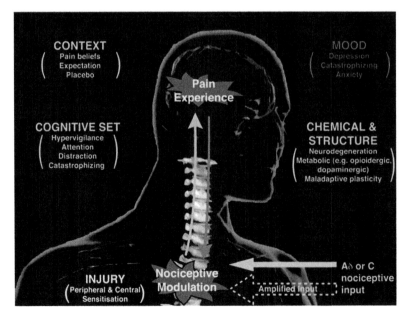

FIGURE 11.2 Centralized factors that influence the pain experience. (Adapted from Tracey I., and Mantyh P.W. The cerebral signature for pain perception and its modulation. *Neuron.* 2007; 55: 377–391.)

Individuals with chronic musculoskeletal pain conditions and concomitant depression have activation of brain regions related to emotions including the amygdala, anterior insula, and medial prefrontal cortex upon painful stimulation. Behavioral and animal studies suggest that heightened hyperalgesia in those with chronic pain and comorbid depression may be influenced by a lack of descending pain inhibition.[25]

In addition to influencing the limbic system, negative affect and hormonal fluctuations may then modulate the periaqueductal gray (PAG) in the midbrain and influence the rostral ventral medulla (RVM), contributing to maladaptive neuroplastic changes and neurogenic inflammation (Figure 11.3). The RVM, a relay area between the PAG and the spinal dorsal horn, contains a population of ON cells, which can increase pain perception, and OFF cells, which can decrease pain perception. These ON/OFF cells are part of the descending inhibitory pain system. Following initial tissue injury, the ON cells serve a useful and protective purpose to prevent further damage. Under ordinary circumstances, tissue healing would lead to a decrease in ON cell activity and an increase in OFF cell activity.[13] However, in chronic musculoskeletal pain conditions, there appears to be a shift to a decrease in inhibition, presumably due to an imbalance of ON cell and OFF cell activity.[27] Thus, over time, maladaptive neuroplastic changes may result in disinhibition in the spinal dorsal horn. As a result, dorsal root reflexes can create a neurogenic inflammation, which then leads to local tissue tenderness, even in the absence of ongoing tissue injury or nociception.

Given the interrelationship among sensitization, the limbic system, and chronic pain in conditions like MPS, clinicians are broadening their focus from not only obtaining pain relief and increasing function, but also to improving the patient's quality of life. For example, in a study of adults with MPS and active MTrPs compared to those without pain, Gerber et al. assessed quality of life and function, disability, sleep, mood, and range of motion in addition to pain.[28] Those with MPS significantly differed from those without MPS not only in their physical findings and self-reported pain levels but also quality of life factors like sleep disturbance, disability, health status, and mood.[28] Specifically, significant disability using the Oswestry Disability Scale was associated with

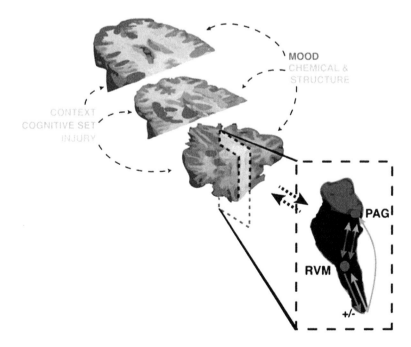

FIGURE 11.3 Role of periaqueductal gray (PAG) and rostral ventromedial medulla (RVM) in the descending modulatory system in response to noxious stimulus. (Adapted from: Tracey I., and Mantyh P.W. The cerebral signature for pain perception and its modulation. *Neuron*. 2007; 55: 377–391.)

active MTrPs, supporting a relationship between MPS and global activity.[28] Similarly, Kaergaard and Andersen's research on female sewing machine operators suggested an increased likelihood of shoulder/neck pain with increased length of employment and decreased social support.[29] Such studies emphasize the importance and relevance of assessing daily routines, mood, and health status in addition to physical symptoms to improve pain management.

POSSIBLE PHYSIOLOGICAL MECHANISMS

Simons' Integrated Trigger Point Hypothesis, introduced in 1999, may explain the role of peripheral and central sensitization. Due to abnormal endplate activity, high levels of acetylcholine (ACh) are released, which bind to receptors on the muscle membrane and initiate excessive release of calcium from the sarcoplasmic reticulum. When excessive calcium binds to troponin on the muscle fibers, the fibers enter a state of persistent contracture, leading to MTrP development. In order to release the contraction, ATP is needed to cause the conformational change of the muscle fibers and actively pump calcium back into the sarcoplasmic reticulum. Thus, the sustained contracture near an abnormal endplate leads to compressed capillary circulation which reduces blood flow, forming local hypoxic conditions, and a polarized membrane potential. Consequently, this results in a lack of ATP, perpetuating an increased metabolic demand and reduced supply. The increased demand for and reduced supply of ATP form an energy crisis, which may provoke the release of neuroactive substances and metabolic byproducts like BK, SP, and 5-HT that could sensitize peripheral nociceptors.[30] Simons' hypothesis explains how sensitizing neuroactive substances may be responsible for the pain associated with active MTrPs. This hypothesis is supported by Shah et al., who demonstrated that active MTrPs have elevated levels of inflammatory mediators, neuropeptides, catecholamines, and cytokines—biochemicals associated with inflammation, pain, sensitization, and intercellular signaling.[14,20,31]

Remarkably, key tenets of Simons' Integrated Trigger Point Hypothesis overlap with the role of muscle in MTrP development suggested by the Cinderella Hypothesis.[32] Musculoskeletal disorder symptoms may arise from muscle recruitment patterns during sub-maximal level exertions with moderate or low physical load among office workers, musicians, and dentists, in which myalgia and MTrPs have been commonly reported.[29] According to Henneman's size principle, smaller type I muscle fibers are recruited first and de-recruited last during static muscle exertions. As a result, these "Cinderella" fibers are continuously activated and metabolically overloaded, in contrast to larger motor muscle fibers that spend less time being activated and do not work as hard. This property makes these fibers more susceptible to muscle damage and calcium dysregulation, key factors in the formation of MTrPs.[33] Treaster et al. demonstrated that low-level static continuous muscle contractions during 30 minutes of typing induced the formation of MTrPs, supporting the Cinderella Hypothesis.[34]

MTrPs can also develop with muscle overuse in cervical and postural muscles during the low-intensity activities.[29,34] A possible mechanism occurs during sustained low-level muscle contractions in tasks requiring precision and postural stability which may then result in a decrease in intramuscular perfusion. Thus, a vicious cycle of ischemia, hypoxia, and insufficient ATP synthesis may occur in type I motor unit fibers and result in increasing acidity, Ca^{2+} accumulation, and subsequent sarcomere contracture. As a result, several sensitizing substances may be released, leading to local and referred pain and muscle tenderness, the clinical hallmarks of MPS.

Sikdar et al. used ultrasound imaging techniques to distinguish MTrPs from the surrounding tissue. Thirty-three sites in the upper trapezius of nine subjects were assessed and classified as active MTrP, latent MTrP, or normal by using gray-scale and color variance ultrasound imaging to distinguish palpable nodules and normal myofascial tissue based on relative stiffness and echogenicity (Figure 11.4). These findings not only confirmed the underlying morphological changes associated with MTrPs, but also suggested that the structure and characteristics of normal muscle fibers are disrupted, possibly by increased muscle contraction, injury, or ischemia. Additionally, blood flow waveform patterns differed between active and latent MTrPs, with active MTrPs associated with retrograde flow in diastole, suggesting that pain at these active sites may result indirectly from decreased blood flow to the region.[35]

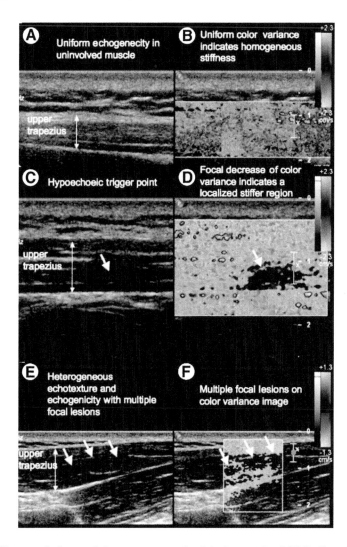

FIGURE 11.4 Ultrasound of normal tissue versus myofascial trigger point (MTrP). (A and B) Normal upper trapezius muscle. (C and D) Muscle with a palpable MTrP in a single hypoechoic region. (E and F) Muscle with a palpable MTrP in multiple hypoechoic regions. (Sikdar S., Shah J.P., Gebreab T., et al. 2009. Novel applications of ultrasound technology to visualize and characterize myofascial trigger points and surrounding soft tissue. *Arch Phys Med Rehabil*, 90(11):1829–1838.)

Other researchers have studied the "neighborhood" of the MTrP to explain the symptom complex and physical findings. Specifically, Stecco focused on three anatomical layers: the deep fascia, the layer of loose connective tissue housing the highest concentration of hyaluronic acid, and the epimysium layer below it. Hyaluronic acid (HA), an anionic, non-sulfated glycosaminoglycan, is distributed widely throughout various tissues, and is a chief component of the extracellular matrix. Normally, HA functions as a lubricant that helps muscle fibers glide against each other without friction. However, Stecco theorized that because of muscle overuse or traumatic injury, the sliding layers start to produce immense amounts of HA, which then aggregate into supramolecular structures, changing HA's configuration, viscoelasticity, and viscosity. Due to its increased viscosity, HA can no longer function as an effective lubricant, which increases resistance in the sliding layers and leads to densification of fascia, or abnormal sliding in muscle fibers. Interference with sliding can impact range of motion and movement including quality of movement and stiffness. In addition, the friction results in increased neural hyperstimulation (irritation), which then hypersensitizes mechanoreceptors and nociceptors embedded within this densified fascia. This hypersensitization correlates with a patient's experience of pain, allodynia, paresthesia, abnormal proprioception, and altered movement. Very few objective studies have been conducted to validate or elucidate these concepts. Given the current limited knowledge regarding the pathophysiology of MPS, research is needed to determine not only the role of the MTrP, but also its surrounding environment.[36]

CLINICAL EVALUATION OF THE MTrP AND SENSITIZED SEGMENTS

A comprehensive evaluation of MPS assesses the patient not only for MTrPs, but also for sensitized spinal segments. The requisite examination skills are easy to learn and fundamentally important to the evaluation and management of the chronic pain patient. Furthermore, examination before and after treatment that is aimed at desensitizing the involved spinal segment provides the clinician and patient with meaningful, objective, and reproducible physical findings to guide future treatment.

Palpation of the skeletal muscle for the objective physical findings of active and latent MTrPs is the gold standard for the diagnosis of myofascial pain. Identifying and adequately treating active and, at times, latent MTrPs may have very important implications for the resolution of a patient's pain. Active MTrPs can be a common source of peripheral nociceptive bombardment, which, in turn, may lead to central sensitization and perpetuation of pain. If left untreated, active MTrPs or other peripheral pain generators can re-sensitize the dorsal horn, resulting in the re-emergence of segmental findings of allodynia and hyperalgesia, and the same pain pattern even after treatment. Latent MTrPs, under certain conditions, can become active MTrPs and merit identification. To review, light-touch palpation of a latent MTrP induces pain locally and in remote areas.[37] Latent MTrPs send excitatory, sub-threshold potentials to the dorsal horn. Excitatory sub-threshold potentials from latent MTrPs can summate with sub-threshold potentials from active MTrPs to surpass the threshold necessary for SSS to occur. Once the myotome is sensitized, all MTrPs in that myotome may become active.

The related spinal segments may be severely sensitized, and, should be assessed at the dermatomal, myotomal, and sclerotomal levels for MPS. Adjacent dermatomal levels are examined paraspinally by checking for allodynia and hyperalgesia. Allodynia is assessed by picking up the skin between the thumb and forefinger and rolling the tissue underneath, also known as a pinch and roll test (Figure 11.5). The patient is instructed to simultaneously report any sensation of pain, which is indicative of allodynia, a finding that is the most sensitive indicator for the diagnosis of sensitization. Hyperalgesia is assessed by scratching the skin with the sharp edge of a paper clip or Wartenberg pinwheel. The patient is instructed to simultaneously report any sharpening or dulling in the sensation of pain during the procedure. An increased painful response is indicative of hyperalgesia.

Myotomal levels are examined by palpating segmentally related musculatures for tender spots, taut bands, and MTrPs and measuring the pressure pain threshold (PPT) using a pressure algometer along the myotome. The PPT is the minimum pressure that elicits pain and is considered abnormal if it is at least 2 kg/cm² lower than the value expected for a healthy subject.

Sclerotomal levels are examined by palpating segmentally related tendons, entheses, bursae, and ligaments, and measuring the PPT along these structures with an algometer.

These objective and quantitative findings help the clinician to identify the tissues and likely pain mechanisms involved in their patients' chronic pain. The segmental findings are not only reproducible but are often indicative of the severity of the sensitized state and may provide important information about the underlying pain syndrome.

PRINCIPLES AND METHODS OF TREATMENT

TREATING THE MTrP

Muscle, fascia, and their cellular components are important contributors to both MPS and the formation of the MTrP. Clinician-investigators recommend that treatments focus not only on the

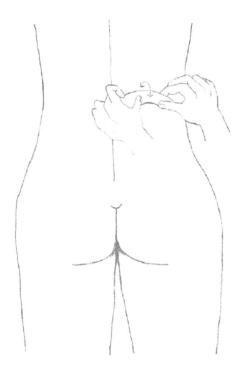

FIGURE 11.5 Pinch and roll test for allodynia. The skin and subcutaneous tissue are gently pinched between the thumb and forefinger and rolled vertically across dermatomal borders. Elicitation of a painful response is indicative of allodynia. (Original art work.)

MTrP, but also on the surrounding environment, with the goals to reduce the size of the MTrP, correct underlying contributors to the pain, and restore the normal working relationship between the muscles of the affected functional units. According to Dommerholt, all treatments fall into one or both of two categories: a pain-control phase and a deep conditioning phase. During the pain-control phase, trigger points are deactivated, improving circulation, decreasing pathological nociceptive activity, and eliminating the abnormal biomechanical force patterns. During the conditioning phase, the intra- and inter-tissue mobility of the functional unit is improved, which may include specific muscle stretches, neurodynamic mobilizations, joint mobilizations, orthotics, and muscle strengthening.[38]

Current approaches for the management of MPS include pharmacological and non-pharmacological interventions. Among the pharmacological approaches are anti-inflammatory, analgesic, topical creams, and trigger point injections, which are now safer and more effective. Non-pharmacological interventions include manual therapies, such as post-isometric relaxation, counterstrain method,[39] trigger point compression, muscle energy techniques, and myotherapy,[40] along with other treatments like laser therapy,[41] dry needling, and massage.[42,43]

Among the invasive therapies, dry needling, and injection of anesthetic, steroids, or botulinum toxin-A (BTA) into the MTrP have all been shown to provide pain relief in peer-reviewed clinical studies. Regardless of the method used, elicitation of a local twitch response (LTR), an involuntary spinal cord reflex that may be visually observable within a taut band, produces more immediate and longer-lasting pain relief than no elicitation of an LTR.[44–49] Within minutes of a single induced LTR, Shah et al. found that the initially elevated levels of SP and calcitonin gene-related peptide within the active MTrP in the upper trapezius muscle decreased to levels approaching that of normal, uninvolved muscle tissue. The reduction of these biochemicals in the local muscle area may be due to a small, localized increase in blood flow or nociceptor and mechanistic changes associated with an augmented inflammatory response.[13,31]

Beyond the MTrP: Spinal Segmental Sensitization

Sometimes treating active MTrPs is insufficient. In these situations, segmental sensitization may be present and is determined by findings of allodynia, hyperalgesia, and measurable pressure pain sensitivity over the sensory, motor, and skeletal areas supplied by a particular spinal segment.

All forms of manual therapy include some form of mechanical pressure and are commonly employed as a first line of treatment before attempting more invasive therapies.[50] While recent reviews and meta-analyses have focused on dry needling, manual therapy may be just as effective.[50] For example, osteopathic manipulative medicine, and "spray and stretch" with pentafluoropropane or tetrafluoroethane are commonly used to treat myofascial pain and SSS.

Additionally, various forms of electrical stimulation including microcurrent, transcutaneous electrical nerve stimulation (TENS), and percutaneous electrical nerve stimulation (PENS) may alleviate SSS. Laser and ultrasound are also effective for pain management, but the effectiveness of these technologies for the deactivation of MTrPs is uncertain. Biofeedback and other relaxation techniques, like hypnotherapy, help patients with pain management. Other effective (but more invasive) treatments for SSS include paraspinous injection block techniques and paraspinous needling, as discussed below.

The paraspinous injection block technique and paraspinous needling are used particularly in chronic cases in which the physical examination reveals severe and persistent allodynia and hyperalgesia, suggesting multi-segmental dermatomal, myotomal, and sclerotomal manifestations of SSS (Figure 11.6). Often, these findings coincide segmentally, making diagnosis of the sensitized level relatively straightforward. However, when they do not, or if pain relief is only partial/persists after treatment, the affected segmental levels most closely aligned with the principal pain can be treated

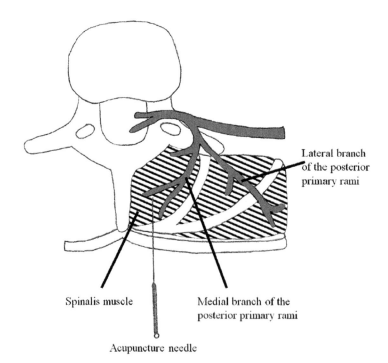

Lateral branch of the posterior primary rami

Spinalis muscle

Medial branch of the posterior primary rami

Acupuncture needle

FIGURE 11.6 Paraspinal needling. An acupuncture needle is inserted sagittally into the spinalis muscle and then manipulated as described. Multiple acupuncture needles may be inserted to create a paraspinous block at each affected segmental level. (Original art, but has been published in the textbook *Fisioterapia Invasiva del Síndrome de Dolor Miofascial: Manual de punción seca de puntos gatillo (Spanish Edition)* by Orlando Mayoral del Moral [ISBN-13: 978-8498351033].)

first with a technique such as paraspinous needling, which addresses the centrally sensitized component of pain. If the patient experiences little or no pain relief, adjacent segmental levels may be treated until the patient reports a decrease in pain. This subjective decrease in pain is typically accompanied by an objective improvement in segmental findings.

Effective management involves the identification and treatment of both the peripheral and central components of sensitization which includes any foci responsible for initiating or perpetuating the centrally sensitized segmental findings.

Paraspinal muscles can be facilitated by active MTrPs elsewhere in the body. However, MTrPs within paraspinal muscles can act as a source of peripheral nociceptive input, further sensitizing the paraspinal muscles. To desensitize the muscles along a specific segment, Fischer et al.'s (2002) paraspinous injection block technique utilizes a 1% lidocaine injection and a 25-gauge needle, of sufficient length to reach the deep layers up to the vertebral lamina.[51] Once the affected levels are identified by physical examination, injection is performed between the spinous process levels. The needle is inserted in the sagittal plane through the paraspinal muscle to a maximal depth but before contacting the vertebral lamina. After aspiration confirms blood vessels were avoided, approximately 0.1 mL of anesthetic is injected. Next, the needle is withdrawn to a subcutaneous level and redirected in the caudal direction, about 5 mm from the initial anesthetic solution. One continues this procedure, going as far as the needle reaches. The same procedures are repeated going in the cephalad direction. The result of this technique is multi-segmental desensitization, by effectively blocking the medial branch of the posterior primary rami at the affected segmental levels.[51]

Many practitioners have observed improvement in pain levels after paraspinous block and paraspinous dry needling. However, randomized, double-blinded, placebo-controlled clinical trials examining the effects of paraspinous block and paraspinous dry needling are needed to assess its efficacy.

PERPETUATING FACTORS OF MPS

Many conditions may act as perpetuating factors of chronic MPS including nutritional deficiency states, such as iron insufficiency and vitamin B12 deficiency, hormonal disorders such as hypothyroidism, and trauma such as cervical strain injury. For example, vitamin D deficiency is associated with musculoskeletal pain, loss of type 2 muscle fibers, and proximal muscle atrophy.[52,53] One study found that 89% of subjects with chronic musculoskeletal pain were deficient in vitamin D. The deficient state can be treated, but up to 6 months may be required for vitamin D levels to return to normal levels. Iron deficiency in the muscle may also play a role in the development or maintenance of MTrPs. Hypothyroidism also produces a hypometabolic state, which may augment MTrP formation.[52]

Perpetuating factors may be structural, postural, or ergonomic if co-morbid conditions such as scoliosis, leg length discrepancy, pelvic torsion, or hypomobility or hypermobility of joints, among others, are present. Co-morbid conditions, whether of a medical or mechanical nature, may initiate or interfere with the treatment or recovery process. Thus, in cases of chronic MPS, a thorough history and physical examination as well as a targeted laboratory exam can be beneficial.[52]

CONCLUSION

Chronic musculoskeletal pain, specifically MPS, is associated with MTrPs and sensitization. Therefore, it is essential that pain management practitioners perform a comprehensive evaluation to assess these factors and incorporate them into the management of MPS. While the etiology of MPS is uncertain, advances in the characterization of the MTrP and the surrounding environment have increased the knowledge regarding the mechanism and provided some translational insights into the potential role of MTrP in MPS. There remains a lack of consensus on the definition and diagnostic criteria for MPS, hindering a standardized approach to the clinical examination of this common disorder. Additionally, while a variety of pharmacological and non-pharmacological treatments have shown efficacy and improvement in pain associated with MPS, these findings are typically limited to self-reported pain levels pre- and post-treatment. Although such measures are valid, the outcomes are subjective and thus difficult to quantify in the context of the variable presentations of MPS. Moreover, to date, few randomized, placebo-controlled trials have been undertaken, and most have limited sample size. Thus, in addition to the development of standardized diagnostic criteria, studies of sufficient size and power with quantitative outcome measures are sorely needed in order to improve the treatment of chronic musculoskeletal pain and MTrPs.

A CASE SCENARIO

Bethany is a 30-year-old woman who has been living for 15 years with chronic pelvic pain that is primarily focused in her left lower quadrant. She is frustrated and discouraged because her pelvic pain is still present, despite having undergone four laparoscopic procedures for endometriosis over the last few years. She is puzzled by having been told that the endometriosis lesions were in locations different from her most intense areas of pain. This observation along with her continued exhaustion from pain even during recovery after each surgery and the lack of long-lasting pain relief prompted Bethany to seek other medical specialists' opinions, including that of a physiatrist. To develop an effective approach to treatment for Bethany, the physiatrist reviews her medical and pain history, including eliciting any emotional aspects, and performs a pain-focused physical examination. This strategy enables Bethany's physiatrist to organize and synthesize her complex 15-year pain history into a pattern of interconnected pain conditions.

During her first visit, the physiatrist focuses on the history and pattern of her painful symptoms. She reports having severe, doubling over midline pelvic cramping during her menstrual cycles that is often accompanied by low back pain. Initially she thought that these symptoms were normal with menstruation and endometriosis as her mother and sisters each had similar pain symptoms. A few years ago, she was diagnosed with irritable bowel syndrome and experiences both constipation and bloating.

For many years before she was diagnosed with endometriosis and irritable bowel syndrome, Bethany had gone from doctor to doctor looking for a diagnosis and a strategy to manage her symptoms. Some clinicians did not acknowledge the severity of her chronic pelvic pain and did not consider the diagnosis of endometriosis, especially since her symptoms occurred primarily during menses. They conveyed a belief that these painful symptoms were normal with menstruation. In fact, Bethany was told by at least four doctors that her symptoms were "in her head" and imaginary. This minimizing of the severity of her symptoms delayed referral to a gynecologist specializing in chronic pelvic pain. Because of this lack of understanding, Bethany alternated between believing her physicians and feeling frustrated and depressed. Over time, her chronic pain worsened and occurred at other times of the menstrual cycle. She found she frequently had negative thoughts and reported a sense of diminished self-worth. She was unable to function well at work and found her feeling began to impact her family and intimate relationships.

After almost ten years of pain, Bethany was first surgically diagnosed with endometriosis at age 25. After her first laparoscopy, the gynecologist told her that he had burned off some endometriosis lesions in her region of pain but left some others that he did not think were related to her pain. Within a year, she switched gynecologists and underwent another laparoscopy, this time with an endometriosis specialist surgeon who resected all the endometriosis lesions she could find. Just before the second surgery, the gynecologist surgeon placed Bethany on 6 months of hormonal therapy with GnRH agonists to suppress endometriosis growth. While Bethany got relief for about 6 months, the pain returned when the hormonal therapy was stopped. The combination of surgery with hormonal management only provided temporary relief of her chronic pain. She tried other hormones including cyclic birth control pills and now uses a progestin-releasing IUD that suppresses her menstrual flow. Over time, she underwent two more similar surgical procedures. Now, at age 35 she still feels the same pain even after a recent endometriosis surgery 6 weeks ago at which all endometriosis lesions were resected. *Could Bethany's continued pain be explained and/or maintained by other factors beyond the pelvic floor? Could potential stressors in her life exacerbate her pain symptoms?*

After listening to Bethany's medical history, the physiatrist explains that active MTrPs in the pelvic floor and abdomen may refer pain to other pelvic regions as well as her lower back and abdomen. Widespread pain might be generated from the active MTrPs and could be a result of central sensitization. This sort of pain would not be addressed by surgical or hormonal therapies that only target the ectopic endometrial lesions.

To determine the additional factors that could maintain Bethany's pain, the physiatrist conducts a thorough *neuro*-musculoskeletal pain examination to assess for signs of widespread pain, central sensitization, and myofascial dysfunction. He begins by assessing the dermatomes for allodynia and hyperalgesia bilaterally. He brushes the skin with a thin microfilament, approximately 2.5 cm lateral to each spinal process, in order to assess for allodynia. He then uses a Wartenberg pinwheel to scratch the skin and assess for hyperalgesia. As suspected, Bethany exhibits allodynia and hyperalgesia in more than half of the spinal segments, suggesting widespread sensitization.

Next, the physiatrist assesses the myotome for the presence of MTrPs, measuring the PPT over each MTrP. Digital pressure on the active MTrP reproduces her pain. Bethany has active MTrPs in over half of the assessed regions, and a low PPT (<4 kg/cm^2) suggests a lowered pressure-pain threshold. This neuro-musculoskeletal exam allows the physiatrist to evaluate the distribution of Bethany's myofascial dysfunction and the extent of her sensitization. At times, active MTrPs might be a somatic manifestation of an underlying visceral problem like endometriosis. To assess whether Bethany also has MTrPs throughout her pelvic floor muscles, the physiatrist refers her to a gynecologist who understands the complex interaction between myofascial dysfunction, sensitization, and chronic pelvic pain.

The physiatrist conveys the findings of Bethany's neuro-musculoskeletal exam and her medical and pain history to the gynecologist who then also performs a history and evoked-pain gynecologic examination. The gynecologist examines the abdominopelvic region for allodynia, tenderness, number of MTrPs, and severity of pain elicited upon palpation of the active abdominal wall MTrPs. Bethany did not have abdominal wall allodynia but did experience tenderness in her lower left quadrant and suprapubic region.

Next, the superficial perineal muscles are palpated externally for muscle spasm and tenderness using a single digit. The gynecologist then performed an intravaginal assessment of the pelvic floor muscles to identify the presence of active MTrPs, taut bands, or tenderness. Bethany was found to have active MTrPs in the pubococcygeus, iliococcygeus, and obturator internus on the left side that reproduced her pain, and an active MTrPs in the right iliococcygeus. Bethany also had bladder, urethral, and uterosacral tenderness on gentle single-digit palpation but no forniceal tenderness or uterosacral nodularity. On bimanual exam, she has central uterine tenderness. Bethany reported her pattern of pelvic tenderness to be diffuse with the worst pain in the pelvic floor.

The gynecologist and Bethany also discussed potential topics of emotional and physical stress. Bethany indicated that she had recently been involved in a car accident and now had panic attacks when she had to drive on the highway. She explained that she always strives to do her best and has recently transitioned to a fast-paced, high-stress job.

The gynecologist agrees with the physiatrist that Bethany's continuing pain after complete surgical resection of ectopic endometrial lesion may be maintained by the presence of MTrPs. This thorough assessment for tenderness throughout the pelvis provides insight on the pattern of the pain as well as potential triggers.

Considering all of Bethany's symptoms and dysfunction, what is the best course of treatment? The comprehensive neuro-musculoskeletal exam and the gynecological evoked pain assessment together provide a thorough assessment of the patient with chronic pelvic pain. After obtaining the gynecologist's clinical assessment and impression of Bethany's condition and results of her pelvic exam, the physiatrist offers Bethany a dry needling treatment in order to deactivate active and latent

MTrPs in the periphery and paraspinous dry needling to desensitize the spinal segments along her areas of pain as a potentially beneficial form of treatment. In addition, the physiatrist recommends trigger point injections with lidocaine on the active MTrPs in Bethany's abdominal wall.

He also recommends that Bethany supplement the dry needling treatments with myofascial release techniques, biofeedback therapy, cognitive behavioral therapy, or mindfulness-based stress reduction techniques to address both the physiological and psychological components of chronic myofascial pain. This combined approach may also alleviate the pain associated with active MTrPs, improve her strength and flexibility, and provide Bethany with useful coping strategies during a painful episode.

After the paraspinous dry needling sessions in the L3-L4 and T6 segments, Bethany's low back pain decreased, and her clinical findings of allodynia and hyperalgesia also decreased. Moreover, the lidocaine injections in her abdominal wall provided pelvic pain relief. When an algometer is once again used to measure tenderness along the affected myotomes, there is an increase in PPT, suggesting that the area is no longer sensitized.

In the months following her treatment, Bethany reports that her mood and quality of life have improved significantly. For the first time in years, she is achieving a full night's rest without waking up in the middle of the night in pain. Even years after her treatment, Bethany's improvements are sustained, reinforcing the importance of identifying and treating symptoms and signs of peripheral and central sensitization commonly found in chronic pain syndromes such as chronic pelvic pain.

REFERENCES

1. Sessle B.J., Acute and chronic craniofacial pain: brainstem mechanisms of nociceptive transmission and neuroplasticity, and their clinical correlates. *Critical Reviews in Oral Biology & Medicine*, 2000;11(1): 57–91.
2. Arendt-Nielsen L., Graven-Nielsen T., Deep tissue hyperalgesia. *Journal of Musculoskeletal Pain*, 2002;10(1–2): 97–119.
3. Svensson P., Minoshima S., Beydoun A., Morrow T.J., Casey K.L., Cerebral processing of acute skin and muscle pain in humans. *Journal of Neurophysiology*, 1997;78(1): 450–460.
4. Yu X.M., Mense S., Response properties and descending control of rat dorsal horn neurons with deep receptive fields. *Neuroscience*, 1990;39(3): 823–831.
5. Fields H.L., Basbaum A.I., Central nervous system mechanisms of pain modulation. In: *Textbook of Pain*, R.Melzack, P.D. Wall, eds. Edinburgh: Churchill Livingstone; 1999: 309–329.
6. Wall P.D., Woolf C.J., Muscle but not cutaneous *c*-afferent input produces prolonged increases in the excitability of the flexion reflex in the rat. *Journal of Physiology*, 1984;356: 443–458.
7. Travell J.G., Rinzler S.H., The myofascial genesis of pain. *Postgraduate Medicine*, 1952;11(5): 425–434.
8. Travell J.G., Simons D.G., *Myofascial Pain and Dysfunction: The Trigger Point Manual*. Baltimore, MD: Williams & Wilkins; 1983.
9. Bennett R., Myofascial pain syndromes and their evaluation. *Best Practice & Research. Clinical Rheumatology*, 2007;21(3): 427–445.
10. Borg-Stein J., Simons D.G., Focused review: myofascial pain. *Archives of Physical Medicine & Rehabilitation*, 2002;83(3 Suppl 1): S40–7, S48–9.
11. Hong C., Pathophysiology of myofascial trigger point. *Journal of the Formosan Medical Association = Taiwan Yi Zhi*, 1996;95(2): 93–104.
12. Zieglgänsberger W., Berthele A., Tölle T.R., Understanding neuropathic pain. *CNS Spectrums*, 2005;10(4): 298–308.
13. Willard F., 'Basic Mechanisms of Pain.' Future trends in CAM research. In: *Integrative Pain Medicine: The Science and Practice of Complementary and Alternative Medicine in Pain Management*, J.F.Audette, A. Bailey, eds. Totowa, NJ: Humana Press Inc.; 2008.
14. Shah J.P., Gilliams E.A., Uncovering the biochemical *milieu* of myofascial trigger points using *in vivo* microdialysis: an application of muscle pain concepts to myofascial pain syndrome. *Journal of Bodywork & Movement Therapies*, 2008;12(4): 371–384.
15. Romero Ventosilla P., *Consecuencias clínicas de la Estimulación Sensorial persistente: Sensibilización Espinal Segmentaria*. 2010.

16. Waldman S.D., *Physical Diagnosis of Pain: An Atlas of Signs and Symptoms*, 1st ed., S.D.Waldman, ed. Philadelphia, PA: Saunders & Elsevier; 2006.
17. Fischer A.A., Imamura M., New concepts in the diagnosis and management of musculoskeletal pain. In: *Pain Procedures in Clinical Practice*, T.A.Lennard, ed. Philadelphia, PA: Henley & Belfus; 2000: 213–229.
18. Aredo J.V., Heyrana K.J., Karp B.I., Shah J.P., Stratton P., Relating chronic pelvic pain and endometriosis to signs of sensitization and myofascial pain and dysfunction. *Seminars in Reproductive Medicine*, 2017;35(1): 88–97.
19. Imamura M., Imamura S.T., Kaziyama H.H.S., et al., Impact of nervous system hyperalgesia on pain, disability, and quality of life in patients with knee osteoarthritis: a controlled analysis. *Arthritis Care & Rheumatology*, 2008;59(10): 1424–1431.
20. Shah J.P., Phillips T.M., Danoff J.V., Gerber L., An *in vivo* microanalytical technique for measuring the local biochemical *milieu* of human skeletal muscle. *Journal of Applied Physiology*, 2005;99(5): 1977–1984.
21. Hoheisel U., Koch K., Mense S., Functional reorganization in the rat dorsal horn during an experimental myositis. *Pain*, 1994;59(1): 111–118.
22. Sato A., Somatovisceral reflexes. *Journal of Manipulative & Physiological Therapeutics*, 1995;18(9): 597–602.
23. Sperry M.A., Goshgarian H.G., Ultrastructural changes in the rat phrenic nucleus developing within 2 h after cervical spinal cord hemisection. *Experimental Neurology*, 1993;120(2): 233–244.
24. Mense S., Hoheisel U., Central nervous sequelae of local muscle pain. *Journal of Musculoskeletal Pain*, 2004;12(3–4): 101–109.
25. Tracey I., Mantyh P.W., The cerebral signature for pain perception and its modulation. *Neuron*, 2007;55(3): 377–391.
26. Wiech K., Tracey I., The influence of negative emotions on pain: behavioral effects and neural mechanisms. *NeuroImage*, 2009;47(3): 987–994.
27. Niddam D.M., Chan R.C., Lee S.H., Yeh T.C., Hsieh J.C., Central modulation of pain evoked from myofascial trigger point. *Clinical Journal of Pain*, 2007;23(5): 440–448.
28. Gerber L.H., Sikdar S., Armstrong K., et al., A systematic comparison between subjects with no pain and pain associated with active myofascial trigger points. *PM R*, 2013;5(11): 931–938.
29. Kaergaard A., Andersen J.H., Musculoskeletal disorders of the neck and shoulders in female sewing machine operators: prevalence, incidence, and prognosis. *Occupational & Environmental Medicine*, 2000;57(8): 528–534.
30. Gerwin R.D., Dommerholt J., Shah J.P., An expansion of Simons' integrated hypothesis of trigger point formation. *Current Pain & Headache Reports*, 2004;8(6): 468–475.
31. Shah J.P., Danoff J.V., Desai M.J., et al., Biochemicals associated with pain and inflammation are elevated in sites near to and remote from active myofascial trigger points. *Archives of Physical Medicine & Rehabilitation*, 2008;89(1): 16–23.
32. Hägg G., ed., Static work load and occupational myalgia: a new explanation model. In: *Electromyographical Kinesiology*, P.Anderson, Hobart D., Danoff J., eds. Amsterdam: Elsevier; 1991: 141–144.
33. Henneman E., Somjen G., Carpenter D.O., Excitability and inhibitability of motoneurons of different sizes. *Journal of Neurophysiology*, 1965;28(3): 599–620.
34. Treaster D., Marras W.S., Burr D., Sheedy J.E., Hart D., Myofascial trigger point development from visual and postural stressors during computer work. *Journal of Electromyography & Kinesiology*, 2006;16(2): 115–124.
35. Sikdar S., Shah J.P., Gebreab T., et al., Novel applications of ultrasound technology to visualize and characterize myofascial trigger points and surrounding soft tissue. *Archives of Physical Medicine & Rehabilitation*, 2009;90(11): 1829–1838.
36. Stecco C., Stern R., Porzionato A., et al., Hyaluronan within fascia in the etiology of myofascial pain. *Surgical & Radiologic Anatomy*, 2011;33(10): 891–896.
37. Mense S., How do muscle lesions such as latent and active trigger points influence central nociceptive neurons? *Journal of Musculoskeletal Pain*, 2010;18(4): 348–353.
38. Saal J. *Rehabilitation of the Patient. Conservative Care of Low Back Pain. A. White and R. Anderson.* Baltimore, MD: Williams and Wilkins; 1991: 21–34.
39. Myers H.L. *Clinical Application of Counterstrain.* Tucson, AZ: Osteopathic Press; 2006.
40. Cantu R.I., Grodin A.J., *Myofascial Manipulation: Theory and Clinical Application*, 2nd ed. Gaithersburg, MD: Aspen Publishers; 2001.

41. Uemoto L., Nascimento de Azevedo R., Almeida Alfaya T., Nunes Jardim Reis R., Depes de Gouvêa C.V., Cavalcanti Garcia M.A., Myofascial trigger point therapy: laser therapy and dry needling. *Current Pain & Headache Reports*, 2013;17(9): 357.

42. Simons D., Understanding effective treatments of myofascial trigger points. *Journal of Bodywork & Movement Therapies*, 2002;6(2): 81–88.

43. Dommerholt J., Huijbregts P., *Myofascial Trigger Points: Pathophysiology and Evidence-Informed Diagnosis and Management*. Sudbury, MA: Jones and Bartlett Publishers; 2011.

44. Majlesi J., Unalan H., Effect of treatment on trigger points. *Current Pain & Headache Reports*, 2010;14(5): 353–360.

45. Peloso P., Gross A., Haines T., et al., Medicinal and injection therapies for mechanical neck disorders. *Cochrane Database of Systematic Reviews*, 2007;3(3): CD000319.

46. Ho K.Y., Tan K.H., Botulinum toxin a for myofascial trigger point injection: a qualitative systematic review. *European Journal of Pain*, 2007;11(5): 519–527.

47. Lang A.M., Botulinum toxin therapy for myofascial pain disorders. *Current Pain & Headache Reports*, 2002;6(5): 355–360.

48. Birch S., Jamison R.N., Controlled trial of Japanese acupuncture for chronic myofascial neck pain: assessment of specific and nonspecific effects of treatment. *Clinical Journal of Pain*, 1998;14(3): 248–255.

49. Chu J., Dry needling (intramuscular stimulation) in myofascial pain related to lumbar radiculopathy. *European Journal of Physical Medicine & Rehabilitation*, 1995;5: 106–121.

50. Rayegani S.M., Bayat M., Bahrami M.H., Raeissadat S.A., Kargozar E., Comparison of dry needling and physiotherapy in treatment of myofascial pain syndrome. *Clinical Rheumatology*, 2014;33(6): 859–864.

51. Fischer A.A., New injection techniques for treatment of musculoskeletal pain. In: *Myofascial PAIN & Fibromyalgia: Trigger Point Management*, E.S.Rachlin, I.S. Rachlin, eds. Mosby; 2002: 403–419.

52. Gerwin R.D., A review of myofascial pain and fibromyalgia--Factors that promote their persistence. *Acupuncture in Medicine*, 2005;23(3): 121–134.

53. Tague S.E., Clarke G.L., Winter M.K., McCarson K.E., Wright D.E., Smith P.G., Vitamin D deficiency promotes skeletal muscle hypersensitivity and sensory hyperinnervation. *Journal of Neuroscience*, 2011;31(39): 13728–13738.

12 Mycotoxins and Tick-Borne Disease
Increasingly Common Causes of Unexplained Chronic Pain

Ellen Antoine and Scott Antoine

CONTENTS

In the modern medical system, the search for the cause and cure for chronic pain often begins and ends with the consideration of a structural lesion as the sole etiology. Although these structural causes may be identifiable targets for intervention in many cases, there is a growing number of patients with chronic pain syndromes caused by *environmentally acquired illnesses*. Exposure to some infections and environmental toxins cause pain through unique biochemical pathways. Two of the most common (and increasingly seen) causes of chronic pain among the environmentally acquired illnesses are Lyme disease and mycotoxin exposure from contact with toxic mold species.

LYME DISEASE

HISTORY

"Lyme arthritis" was first identified in Lyme, Connecticut, in 1975 after a cluster of cases of what was thought to be juvenile rheumatoid arthritis was reported.[1,2] It was subsequently noted that additional symptoms were often present in patients with this disorder including a characteristic rash, neurologic signs and symptoms, and other constitutional symptoms such as fever, headache, fatigue, and myalgias. For this reason, the disorder eventually became known as "Lyme disease." A few years later, investigators discovered[3] that the cause of Lyme disease was infection with the spirochete, *Borrelia burgdorferi*, and improvement was seen in some patients with antibiotic treatment.[4]

Lyme disease ("Borreliosis") was not a new phenomenon, however. Tick-borne disease has been well-described in the world medical literature since the early part of the 1900s. In 2011, National Geographic published[5] an article detailing findings of the autopsy the 5300-year-old mummy, Ötzi. The article notes that *Borrelia burgdorferi* DNA was found in his tissue.

EPIDEMIOLOGY

Currently, the Centers for Disease Control (CDC) note that there are about 30,000 cases of Lyme disease reported yearly, although conservative estimates[6] indicate that this might reflect under-reporting with the true number of cases being about 10-fold higher. Once thought to be a disease entity confined only to the Northeastern United States, current reports from the CDC indicate that Lyme disease has been reported in every state except Hawaii.[7] Lyme disease has also been reported in over 50 countries.[8] Recently, researchers have compiled borrelial DNA data[9] from over 11 million tick samples from the 48 contiguous United States and have used these data along with information on forestation and topography to compose a map (called a Bayesian model), to help provide a *risk forecast* for pet owners which would predict the risk of Lyme disease transmission to pets based upon current location. As expected, the risk is greatest in the northeastern United States and in Michigan, but the maps show some southern and western spread in contiguous areas with some isolated high-prevalence areas noted in the western United States. As with human testing, it is difficult to tell with tick testing whether current numbers reflect true epidemiological differences in prevalence versus biases due to under-reporting or under-testing.

PAIN AS A CLINICAL PRESENTATION

Lyme disease is traditionally described as having three forms: early localized Lyme disease (3–30 days from the bite), early disseminated Lyme disease (3–5 weeks from the bite), and late Lyme disease.[8] In early localized Lyme disease, patients may present with (or without) a known tick bite and a characteristic rash (erythema migrans). They may also have some constitutional symptoms such as a headache, myalgias, neck stiffness, and a fever. In the early disseminated form, patients may have multiple erythema migrans rashes, cranial nerve palsies (like bell's palsy), carditis with cardiac arrhythmia, or meningitis. Conjunctivitis is seen as well. In late Lyme disease, patients often develop monoarticular arthritis of a large joint. Even after treatment with antibiotics, some patients with Lyme arthritis continue to have pain. It has been proposed that an autoimmune mechanism is responsible.[10] Encephalitis, encephalopathy, and polyneuropathy may be seen as well. The original paper[11] describing these entities notes the fact that patients may improve with antibiotics and that later the symptoms may reoccur. It is the pattern of persistent, multi-system, and recurring symptoms in some patients which has resulted in Lyme disease being called "the great imitator."

Longitudinal studies of patients with confirmed Lyme disease indicate that these patients are 35% more likely to have complaints of chronic joint and muscle pain as well as other constitutional symptoms.[12] Because Lyme disease has such a varied clinical presentation and diagnosis is challenging (see below), patients may be diagnosed with a plethora of other conditions including depression, cognitive impairment, chronic fatigue syndrome, and fibromyalgia.

MOLECULAR MECHANISMS OF PAIN IN LYME DISEASE

Molecular mechanisms for pain as a result of infection with *Borrelia* have been studied previously in patients with Lyme neuroborreliosis.[13] Pain is due to chemokines from *Borrelia* which stimulate an inflammatory response. Elevated levels of IL-6, IL-8, chemokine ligand 2, and CXCL13 and white blood cell pleocytosis have been noted in this same group of patients.[14] Lymphokines from liberated T-cells may also contribute to inflammation and pain.[15]

DIAGNOSIS OF LYME DISEASE

The definitive diagnosis of Lyme disease can be daunting for several reasons. As mentioned previously, the clinical manifestations can be varied in timing and may involve multiple bodily systems. The presence of a classical erythema migrans rash following a tick bite is considered pathognomonic, but the rash may vary in appearance. About 70–80% of patients develop this rash, but the appearance may vary, and it is recognized that only about 10% of patients with erythema migrans get a classic "target lesion."[16] The incubation between tick bite and the lesion may be as long as 30 days. It is also well known that only 50–70% of patients recall being bitten by a tick prior to diagnosis.[17]

Laboratory diagnosis of Lyme disease is also challenging. The *Borrelia* spirochete is notoriously hard to culture, may take 6 weeks to recover, and results of the culture process are fair at best.[8] There are several reasons for this. First, the Lyme spirochete is only present in the bloodstream transiently.[18] Skin biopsy of the periphery of the erythema migrans lesion recovers spirochetes in 80% of cases with 100% specificity but is rarely used since special culture media (Barbour–Stoenner–Kelly medium) and prolonged culture observation are required.[18]

The most common method currently used to support the diagnosis of Lyme disease involves measuring antibodies to *Borrelia* using some combination of ELISA or IFA testing and Western Blot testing (IgM and IgG).[18] The current testing sequence recommended by the Centers for Disease Control (CDC) in the United States starts with an ELISA test or IFA test. These tests are reportedly very sensitive but not specific. In addition, the timing of testing may alter the sensitivity of the testing. The CDC recommends no further testing if the IFA or ELISA are negative. If positive, the CDC recommends Western Blot IgG and IgM testing for confirmation. Like IFA and ELISA testing, the sensitivity of the Western Blot tests can be affected by the timing of the test and other factors. A large meta-analysis on the subject of Lyme testing accuracy[19] found that the current "two-tier" testing approach demonstrated a sensitivity of 57% across all stages of Lyme disease. This number increased to a sensitivity of about 99% for stage 3 Lyme disease detection. Specificity for the detection of *Borellia burgdorferi* was close to 99% for the commercially available IgG and IgM Western Blot. Other tests are available from various specialty laboratories which have higher sensitivities (from 70 to 90%) including immunoblot testing, PCR, and C6 peptide testing. Often, if patients have a positive IgM for Lyme and the exposure to the tick bite has been more than 30 days prior, the test is labeled a "false positive" and the patient is told they do not have Lyme disease. However, the peer-reviewed infectious disease literature confirms persistent positivity of the IgM antibody test for as long as 10–20 years in at least 10% of patients with proven Lyme disease.[20] Further complicating testing is the fact that the two-tiered test was originally designed for population surveillance of the disease and was not intended to be used as the sole criteria to make a diagnosis.[21] The ability of current two-tier testing to detect newer species of *Borrelia* is unknown.[22] The most current *Testing and Diagnostics Subcommittee's Report to the Tick-Borne Disease Working Group*[23] from the U.S. Department of Health and Human Services reiterated the fact that some patients fail to make antibodies in high enough titers to be measured by current testing.

ANTIBIOTIC TREATMENT OF LYME DISEASE

As difficult as testing for Lyme disease is, treatment may be even more challenging. As previously mentioned, patients with Lyme disease have varied clinical presentations as well as varied periods from initial infection to discovery of the disease. Oral antibiotic therapy is used for most Lyme patients. Initial recommendations from the Infectious Disease Society of America (IDSA)[24] include doxycycline or a penicillin such as amoxicillin or cefuroxime. The recommended duration of treatment is 14–21 days. Intravenous antibiotics are recommended in cases of neuroborreliosis and for cardiac manifestations of the disease. There have been concerns, however, about the IDSA process for professional guideline development for Lyme disease diagnosis and treatment.[25] Among the concerns is the fact that persistence of symptoms is often seen after discontinuation of antibiotic treatment.[26] The conventional viewpoint is that these symptoms either do not occur or are immunologic phenomena unrelated to the persistence of infection. Researchers at Johns Hopkins have recently published an article[27] affirming the occurrence of "post-treatment Lyme disease syndrome" (PTLDS). In addition, studies have found that this persistence of infection can occur.[28,29] It has also been shown that Lyme spirochetes have various mechanisms of immune evasion including the production of cystic forms and microcolonies.[30] For this reason, Lyme patients may require treatment with several antibiotics concomitantly or for prolonged periods of time.[31] In this way, *Borrelia* is very similar to tuberculosis, for which multi-drug therapy is now routine.

The International Lyme and Associated Disease Society (ILADS) is a literature-based organization composed of physicians, researchers, and other clinicians who study and treat Lyme disease. ILADS has been at the forefront of advances in the diagnosis and treatment of Lyme disease and tick-borne co-infections. ILADS favors diagnosis and treatment based upon clinical responses and advocates individualizing treatment. The organization has published evidence-based diagnostic and treatment guidelines.[32]

HERBAL TREATMENT OF LYME DISEASE

Various products are commercially available for herbal treatment of Lyme disease. There is growing evidence for the efficacy of herbal preparations for treatment.[33–35] Efficacy for these compounds has been demonstrated through in vitro studies. These products are still not considered first-line therapies by most physicians, as efficacy in patient populations (in vivo) has not been formally studied.

A NOTE ON CO-INFECTIONS

It is well-known that co-infections of ticks with various pathogens including *Babesia*, *Bartonella*, and ehrlichiosis occur.[36] The CDC has listed several other co-infections and *Borrelia* variants on their website.[37] It is interesting to note that the CDC acknowledges that variant strains of *Borrelia*, such as *Borrelia miyamotoi*, *Borrelia hermsii*, *B. parkerii*, and *B. turicatae*, are not identified by current two-tier testing. The presence of co-infections often causes differences in clinical presentation and laboratory testing and may make treatment of the patient more challenging. Additional antimicrobials or a longer period of treatment is often required.

MYCOTOXIN ILLNESS

Mold exposure (in genetically susceptible patients) is one of the most misunderstood causes of chronic disease. It is known by various names such as mycotoxin illness, biotoxin illness, chronic inflammatory response syndrome (CIRS), and, simply, mold illness. None of these titles, however, takes into account that there are multiple "antigens" (molecules which cause our immune system to react) well beyond the mold itself.[38,39] Mold illness itself can be an elusive and persistent cause of chronic pain.

It is estimated that one in two homes in the United States has evidence of water intrusion.[40] This intrusion often goes unnoticed unless telltale signs are present such as stains on ceilings or around windows or the presence of visible mold. Although the length of exposure and amount of mold present are generally directly proportional to the severity of patient illness, in our practice patients who have been cleared of mycotoxins and subsequently re-exposed can develop symptoms (often a headache, brain fog, or nausea) within minutes of re-exposure. Our food supply can also contain harmful mycotoxins,[41] especially in grains which often mold while being stored after harvest.

Pain is only one symptom of mycotoxin illness. Patients also present with confusion, headaches, seasonal allergies, recurrent respiratory infections, mood disorders, insomnia, and digestive issues. Most often, patients experience multiple symptoms concurrently. It is important to note that the symptom overlap for mycotoxin illness and tick-borne disease is nearly 100%.

MOLECULAR MECHANISMS OF PAIN IN MYCOTOXIN ILLNESS

Mycotoxin exposure activates the innate immune system and elicits an inflammatory response.[42] This inflammatory response may impair the body's immune system which leaves the patient with a depressed immune function. This immune system depression can lead to various infections.[43] Pain due to mycotoxin exposure is often a result of direct neurotoxicity.[44]

ENVIRONMENTAL DIAGNOSIS

The diagnosis of mycotoxin illness begins with a careful inventory of possible exposures. Exposure to organic environmental pathogens and antigens can occur in the home, school, the workplace, or even in automobiles.[45] Water leaks in homes can often be identified when damp areas are noted or when water stains from past exposure appear on walls and baseboards. Visible mold can vary from white residue to black patches of mold on walls, ceilings, and belongings. It is important to note that significant microbial growth may be present without any visible evidence as it may be behind walls, inside cabinets, in ventilation ducts or furnaces, or under horizontal surfaces of furniture. In addition, although a "musty" smell (due to volatile organic compounds produced by molds) often indicates microbial growth, many mycotoxins are odorless. There are known to be over 200 different types of mycotoxins.

Currently there are several commercial assays available to detect mycotoxins in the environment. These range from swab sampling methods to the analysis of air handler filters. Polymerase chain reaction (PCR) testing of fabric samples for mold DNA is sometimes used, but this testing is controversial as the literature supporting its use is not very strong and many environmental engineers do not feel the limited initial sample of homes used to establish the test can be generalized across the United States to other homes. Tape samples are also helpful to speciate molds.

PATIENT DIAGNOSIS

Although the detection of actual molds in patients is not possible (except in the case of fungemia noted in blood cultures in immunosuppressed patients), several commercial tests exist to document mycotoxins in patients. These tests are commonly run on urine and test for various mycotoxins.[46]

There are additional labs which are commonly run to test for alterations in hormonal health, inflammation, and activation of the innate immune system. These include MSH, complement C4a, complement C3a, and human TGFβ-1. Additional markers such as tests for ADH, osmolarity, HLA haplotypes, leptin, and PAI-1 are sometimes used. However, in our clinical experience they may remain elevated after patients recover and are sometimes normal in sick patients with confirmed mycotoxin exposures, which greatly limits their diagnostic utility and their use to track therapeutic progress.

Visual contrast sensitivity testing may be used to help track recovery from mycotoxin illness; however normalization of this test may lag behind clinical improvement.

TREATMENT OF MYCOTOXIN ILLNESS

The first and most important step in treating a patient with mycotoxins is to remove the patient from the exposure. If the exposure is occurring at the patient's home or work, complete avoidance of the location may be necessary until proper remediation is performed. The next step involves stopping water intrusion events, sealing leaks, and properly managing crawl space and basement utility. The removal of visible microbial growth and water damage is next. Finally, the removal of mold and mycotoxins from surfaces, air, and belongings is undertaken. This may be accomplished with enzyme sets, cleaning by hand, and ultra-fine particulate vacuuming. Small-particle air filtration is also required on an ongoing basis. The specifics of remediation of water-damaged buildings and belongings is beyond the scope of this book. One fundamental point which must be emphasized, however, is that it is never appropriate to have a sick patient remediate their own space, as the particulate matter inevitably stirred up during this process may exacerbate current symptoms. Avoidance of some dried fruits, grains, and coffees not specifically noted to be "mold-free" may also be helpful.

Once a safe space is assured, the patient may begin treatment for mycotoxin illness. The removal of mycotoxins is accomplished with binders. Several binders have been studied for their ability to remove mycotoxins. Cholestyramine was shown in rats and mice to lower levels of mycotoxins obtained from a dietary source.[47,48] Alfalfa has also been shown to increase mycotoxin excretion in rats and swine.[49] Zeolite,[50] activated charcoal, and several other binders[51] including bentonite clay and beta-glucans have also shown efficacy in vitro and in animals. No good human studies have specifically looked at mycotoxin removal. In clinical practice, cholestyramine has begun to fall out of favor as it appears most active against a single mycotoxin (aflatoxin). In our current practice, we use activated charcoal in combination with zeolite and aloe vera with success. Glutathione (the body's master detoxifier) is also used to enhance the removal of mycotoxins. Oral glutathione is not well absorbed, so IV glutathione or liposomal forms of glutathione should be used.[52] A deficiency in glutathione production has also been identified[53] in patients with mycotoxin illness. N-acetyl cysteine is a precursor to glutathione and may be used as well.

PAIN MANAGEMENT IN ENVIRONMENTALLY ACQUIRED ILLNESS

As the primary inciting event (tick-borne infection or mycotoxin exposure) is being managed, the treatment of the patient's chronic pain may begin. The pain associated with environmentally acquired illness is usually caused by inflammation, oxidative stress, direct neurotoxicity, and immune dysregulation as noted above. Good strategies for pain management often require the physician to address all of these areas concomitantly.

Common natural herbal anti-inflammatories providing excellent pain relief include *Boswellia* and curcumin. *Boswellia* (also called Indian frankincense) comes from the plant *Boswellia serrata*. It has been used for thousands of years in Africa and Asia by indigenous people for religious and medicinal purposes. It contains four main boswellic acids. One of the four, acetyl-11-keto-β-boswellic acid, is a potent inhibitor of the 5-lipoxygenase inflammatory pathway.[54] Rat studies have shown inhibition of glioma (brain tumor growth) when extracts of gum resin from *Boswellia* are used.[55] *Boswellia* has also been shown to preserve the intestinal epithelial barrier and prevent oxidative stress.[56] This is notable since most patients with environmentally acquired illness have some degree of increased intestinal permeability. Animal studies have demonstrated that boswellic acids may protect the liver from chemotherapy-induced damage.[57] Dosage is typically 350 mg twice daily. Curcumin is a phenol and comes from the turmeric plant (*Curcuma longa*). It is also a powerful anti-inflammatory compound. The molecular mechanism of action involves the ability of curcumin to inhibit multiple inflammatory compounds including TNF-α, IL-1β, NF-κB, and IL-8.[58,59] In addition to its benefits in inflammatory conditions such as arthritis,[60] curcumin has anti-neoplastic[61,62] effects including induction of apoptosis, regulation of expression of micro-RNA, and inhibition of metastasis and tumor invasion. Typical dosing is 350–700 mg twice daily. Bioavailability can be an issue with curcumin so it is typically administered with black pepper extract (piperine) or administered in a phospholipid to enhance bioavailability. Note that black pepper extract will enhance the absorption of other items such as medications so monitoring is important for drug interactions.

Alpha-lipoic acid, the only fat- and water-soluble antioxidant in the body, is very helpful for neuropathic pain. In a meta-analysis of current studies, alpha lipoic acid was shown to significantly improve neuropathic pain.[63–65] It also helps with insulin resistance.[67] Typical dosing is 600–1200 mg twice daily.

Naloxone is an injectable or inhaled rescue medication for cases of narcotic overdose in the out-of-hospital or emergency setting or in cases iatrogenic respiratory depression during medical procedures where narcotics are administered. It binds to narcotic receptors and nearly instantaneously reverses the effects of opiates. Naloxone is not absorbed well orally. Subsequently, naltrexone was developed for oral use and is most commonly used as a preventative in patients who are undergoing treatment for addiction. At doses of 50–150 mg daily, it prevents euphoric feelings when narcotics are taken. An injectable form of naltrexone is also used to treat alcoholism. The mechanism here is not known, but it is suspected that it helps increase dopamine in the brain which is similar to the effects of consuming alcohol. In very low doses (1.5–4.5 mg) daily, naltrexone ("low-dose naltrexone" [LDN]) increases endogenous endorphin production which helps with chronic pain.[66] Various studies have demonstrated the benefits of LDN in Crohn's disease,[67,68] multiple sclerosis,[69] fibromyalgia,[70,71] and for the normalization of immune system function.[72] It is known to be effective at decreasing microglial activation (a neurologic inflammatory condition)[73] and decreasing neuropathic pain.[74] LDN is also helpful in the treatment of complex regional pain syndrome.[75] In our clinical practice, LDN may help promote sleep as it is mildly sedating. In rare cases, it stimulates patients and causes unusual dreams. In these cases it is moved to daytime dosing. Naltrexone is available commercially in 50 mg tablets. LDN must, therefore, be compounded. Typically, adult patients start at 1.5 mg at bedtime and titrate slowly up to a top dose of 4.5 mg over a month. Sensitive patients may need to start lower and titrate slower. We have used LDN in children as well.

A relatively new addition which is quite useful for chronic pain is palmitoylethanolamide ("PEA"). PEA has been well-studied in Europe[76] for use in relieving pain. First identified in 1957,[77] PEA is a biologically active lipid which is naturally found in egg yolk. In addition to good data for its use to relieve pain,[78,79] PEA has also been found to be helpful in cases of eczema and to prevent neurodegeneration.[80] Other studies show that PEA can downregulate mast cell activation.[81,82] The dental literature also contains studies showing significant pain reduction and improved mouth opening in patients with TMJ syndromes.[83]

In our practice, we also use stress-reduction techniques (breathing, meditation, prayer, and visualization), pulsed electromagnetic therapy (PEMF), massage, and essential oils very successfully in a multi-modal approach to help patients recover and manage pain without the use of narcotics.

SUMMARY

Although environmentally acquired illness can be a challenge to diagnose, once these disorders have been correctly identified, removal of the primary inciting cause and treatment aimed at reducing inflammation and oxidative stress are very helpful to eliminate pain in most cases. A root-cause approach and therapies directed at the interruption of pain at the molecular level are most effective in these patients.

REFERENCES

1. Mast W.E., Burrows W.M. Erythema chronicum migrans and 'Lyme arthritis'. *JAMA* 1976;236(21):2392.
2. Steere A.C., Malawista S.E., Snydman D.R., Shope R.E., Andiman W.A., Ross M.R., Steele F.M. Lyme arthritis: an epidemic of oligoarticular arthritis in children and adults in three Connecticut communities. *Arthritis Rheum* 1977;20(1):7–17.
3. Burgdorfer W. Discovery of the Lyme disease spirochete and its relation to tick vectors. *Yale J Biol Med* 1984;57(4):515–520.

4. Steere A.C., Hutchinson G.J., Rahn D.W., Sigal L.H., Craft J.E., DeSanna E.T., Malawista S.E. Treatment of the early manifestations of Lyme disease. *Ann Intern Med* 1983;99(1):22–26.

5. Hall Stephen S. Iceman autopsy. *National Geographic* 2011. Archived from the original on 19 October 2011.

6. Mead P.S. Epidemiology of Lyme disease. *Infect Dis Clin North Am* 2015;29(2):187–210.

7. https://www.cdc.gov/lyme/stats/tables.html (accessed 15 October 2018).

8. Shapiro Eugene D., Gerber Michael A. Lyme disease. *Clin Infect Dis* 2000;31(2):533–542.

9. Watson S.C., Liu Y., Lund R.B., Gettings J.R., Nordone S.K., McMahan C.S., Yabsley M.J. A Bayesian spatio-temporal model for forecasting the prevalence of antibodies to *Borrelia burgdorferi*, causative agent of Lyme disease, in domestic dogs within the contiguous United States. *PLOS ONE* 2017;12(5).

10. Steere A.C., Dwyer E., Winchester R. Association of chronic Lyme arthritis with HLA-DR4 and HLA-DR2 alleles. *N Engl J Med* 1990;323(4):219–223.

11. Logigian E.L., Kaplan R.F., Steere A.C. Chronic neurologic manifestations of Lyme disease. *N Engl J Med* 1990;323(21):1438–1444.

12. Seltzer E.G., Gerber M.A., Cartter M.L., Freudigman K., Shapiro E.D. Long-term outcomes of persons with Lyme disease. *JAMA* 2000;283(5):609–616.

13. Rupprecht T.A., Koedel U., Fingerle V., Pfister H.W. The pathogenesis of Lyme neuroborreliosis: from infection to inflammation. *Mol Med* 2008;14(3–4):205–212.

14. Ramesh G., Didier P.J., England J.D., et al. Inflammation in the pathogenesis of Lyme neuroborreliosis. *Am J Pathol* 2015;185(5):1344–1360.

15. Singh S.K., Girschick H.J. Lyme borreliosis: from infection to autoimmunity. *Clin Microbiol Infect* 2004;10(7):598–614.

16. Smith R.P., Schoen R.T., Rahn D.W., et al. Clinical characteristics and treatment outcome of early Lyme disease in patients with microbiologically confirmed erythema migrans. *Ann Intern Med* 2002;136(6):421–428.

17. Bratton Robert L., Whiteside J.W., Hovan M.J., Engle R.L., Edwards F.D. Diagnosis and treatment of Lyme disease. *Mayo Clin Proc* 2008;83(5):566–571.

18. Bunikis Jonas, Barbour Alan G. Laboratory testing for suspected Lyme disease *Medical Clinics* 2002;86(2):311–340.

19. Waddell L.A., Greig J., Mascarenhas M., Harding S., Lindsay R., Ogden N. The accuracy of diagnostic tests for Lyme disease in humans, A systematic review and meta-analysis of North American research. *PLOS ONE* 2016;11(12):e0168613. doi:10.1371/journal.pone.0168613

20. Kalish Robert A., McHugh Gail, Granquist John, Shea Barry, Ruthazer Robin, Steere Allen C. Persistence of immunoglobulin M or immunoglobulin G antibody responses to *Borrelia burgdorferi* 10–20 years after active Lyme disease. *Clin Infect Dis* 2001;33(6):780–785.

21. Aucott John, Morrison Candis, Munoz Beatriz, Rowe Peter C, Schwarzwalder Alison, West Sheila K. Diagnostic challenges of early Lyme disease: lessons from a community case series. *BMC Infect Dis* 2009;9(1):1–8.

22. Pritt B.S., Mead P.S., Johnson D.K.H., et al. Identification of a novel pathogenic Borrelia species causing Lyme borreliosis with unusually high spirochaetaemia: a descriptive study. *Lancet Infect Dis* 2016;16(5):556–564.

23. https://www.hhs.gov/ash/advisory-committees/tickbornedisease/reports/testing-and-diagnostics-2018-5-9/index.html (accessed 24 February 2019).

24. Wormser G.P., Dattwyler R.J., Shapiro E.D., et al. The clinical assessment, treatment, and prevention of Lyme disease, human granulocytic anaplasmosis, and babesiosis: clinical practice guidelines by the infectious diseases society of America. *Clin Infect Dis* 2006;43(9):1089–1134.

25. Johnson L., Stricker R.B. The infectious diseases society of America Lyme guidelines: a cautionary tale about the development of clinical practice guidelines. *Philos Eth Humanit Med* 2010:5–9.

26. Melia Michael T., Auwaerter Paul G. Time for a different approach to Lyme disease and long-term symptoms. *N Engl J Med* 2016;374(13):1277–1278.

27. Rebman Alison W., Bechtold Kathleen T., Ting Yang, Mihm Erica A., Soloski Mark J., Novak Cheryl B., Aucott John N. The clinical, symptom, and quality-of-life characterization of a well-defined group of patients with posttreatment Lyme disease syndrome. *Front Med* 2017;4:1–10.

28. Middelveen M.J., Sapi E., Burke J., et al. Persistent Borrelia infection in patients with ongoing symptoms of Lyme disease. *Healthcare (Basel)* 2018;6(2):33. doi:10.3390/healthcare6020033

29. Feng J., Auwaerter P.G., Zhang Y. Drug combinations against *Borrelia burgdorferi* persisters *in vitro*: eradication achieved by using daptomycin, cefoperazone and doxycycline. *PLOS ONE* 2015;10(3):e0117207.

30. Sharma Bijaya, Brown Autumn V., Matluck Nicole E., Hu Linden T., Lewis Kim. *Borrelia burgdorferi*, the causative agent of Lyme disease, forms drug-tolerant persister cells. *Antimicrob Agents Chemother* 2015;59(8):4616–4624.

31. Stricker Raphael B. Counterpoint: long-term antibiotic therapy improves persistent symptoms associated with Lyme disease. *Clin Infect Dis* 2007;45(2):149–157.

32. Cameron Daniel J., Johnson Lorraine B., Maloney Elizabeth L. Evidence assessments and guideline recommendations in Lyme disease: the clinical management of known tick bites, erythema migrans rashes and persistent disease. *Expert Rev Anti-Infect Ther* 2014;12(9):1103–1135.

33. Feng Jie, Shi W., Miklossy J., Tauxe G.M., McMeniman C.J., Zhang Y. Identification of essential oils with strong activity against stationary phase Borrelia burgdorferi. *Antibiotics* 2018;7(4):89.

34. Feng J., Zhang S., Shi W., Zubcevik N., Miklossy J., Zhang Y. Selective essential oils from spice or culinary herbs have high activity against stationary phase and biofilm *Borrelia burgdorferi*. *Front Med* 2017;4:169.

35. Goc A., Rath M. The anti-borreliae efficacy of phytochemicals and micronutrients: an update. *Ther Adv Infect Dis* 2016;3(3–4):75–82.

36. Swanson S.J., Neitzel D., Reed K.D., Belongia E.A. Coinfections acquired from ixodes ticks. *Clin Microbiol Rev* 2006;19(4):708–727.

37. https://www.cdc.gov/ticks/diseases/index.html (accessed 23 February 2019).

38. Douwes J., Thorne P., Pearce N., Heederik D. Bioaerosol effects and exposure assessment: progress and prospects. *Annals Occup Hygeine* 2003;47(3):187–200.

39. Rao C.Y., Riggs M.A., Chew G.L., et al. Characterization of airborne molds, endotoxins, and glucans in homes in New Orleans after hurricanes Katrina and Rita. *Appl Environ Microbiol* 2007;73(5):1630–1634.

40. Wu F., Jacobs D., Mitchell C., Miller D., Karol M.H. Improving indoor environmental quality for public health: impediments and policy recommendations. *Environ Health Perspect* 2007;115(6):953–957.

41. Wayne L. Bryden PhD, mycotoxins in the food chain: human health implications. *Asia Pac J Clin Nutr* 2007;16 (Suppl 1):95–101.

42. Maresca Marc, Yahi N., Younès-Sakr L., Boyron M., Caporiccio B., Fantini J. Both direct and indirect effects account for the pro-inflammatory activity of enteropathogenic mycotoxins on the human intestinal epithelium: stimulation of interleukin-8 secretion, potentiation of interleukin-1beta effect and increase in the transepithelial passage of commensal bacteria. *Toxicol Appl Pharmacol* 2008;228(1):84–92.

43. Oswald I.P., Marin D.E., Bouhet S., Pinton P., Taranu I., Accensi F. Immunotoxicological risk of mycotoxins for domestic animals. *Food Addit Contam* 2005;22(4):354–360.

44. Doi K., Uetsuka K. Mechanisms of mycotoxin-induced neurotoxicity through oxidative stress-associated pathways. *Int J Mol Sci* 2011;12(8):5213–5237.

45. Ahearn Donald, Simmons R.B., Crow S.A., Rose L.J. Volatile organic compounds associated with microbial growth in automobile air conditioning systems. *Curr Microbiol* 2000;41(3):206–209.

46. https://www.greatplainslaboratory.com/gplmycotox (accessed 23 February 2019).

47. Solfrizzo M., Visconti A., Avantaggiato G., Torres A., Chulze S. *In vitro* and *in vivo* studies to assess the effectiveness of cholestyramine as a binding agent for fumonisins. *Mycopathologia* 2001;151(3):147.

48. Underhill K.L., Rotter B.A., Thompson B.K., Prelusky D.B., Trenholm H.L. Effectiveness of cholestyramine in the detoxification of zearalenone as determined in mice. *Bull Environ Contam Toxicol* 1995;54(1):128.

49. James L.J., Smith T.K. Effect of dietary alfalfa on zearalenone toxicity and metabolism in rats and swine. *J Anim Sci* 1982;55(1):110–118.

50. Smith T.K. Effect of dietary protein, alfalfa, and zeolite on excretory patterns of 5',5',7',7'-[3H]zearalenone in rats. *Can J Physiol Pharmacol* 1980; 58(11):1251–1255. doi: 10.1139/y80-191.

51. https://www.biofuelscoproducts.umn.edu/sites/biodieselfeeds.cfans.umn.edu/files/cfans_asset_413777.pdf (accessed 23 February 2019).

52. Schmitt B., Vicenzi M., Garrel C., Denis F.M. Effects of N-acetylcysteine, oral glutathione (GSH) and a novel sublingual form of GSH on oxidative stress markers: a comparative crossover study. *Redox Biol* 2015;6:198–205.

53. Guilford F.T., Hope J. Deficient glutathione in the pathophysiology of mycotoxin-related illness . *Toxins* 2014;6(2):608–623.

54. Siddiqui M.Z. Boswellia serrata, a potential antiinflammatory agent: an overview. *Indian J Pharm Sci* 2011;73(3):255–261.

55. Winking M., Sarikaya S., Rahmanian A., Jödicke A., Böker D.K. Boswellic acids inhibit glioma growth: a new treatment option? *J Neurooncol* 2000;46(2):97.

56. Catanzaro D., Rancan S., Orso G., et al. *Boswellia serrata* preserves intestinal epithelial barrier from oxidative and inflammatory damage. *PLOS ONE* 2015;10(5):e0125375.

57. Barakat Bassant M., Ahmed Hebatalla I., Bahr Hoda I., Elbahaie Alaaeldeen M. Protective effect of boswellic acids against doxorubicin-induced hepatotoxicity: impact on Nrf2/HO-1 defense pathway. *Oxid Med Cell Longev* 2018;Article ID 8296451:10.

58. Abe Y., Hashimoto S., Horie T. Curcumin inhibition of inflammatory cytokine production by human peripheral blood monocytes and alveolar macrophages. *Pharmacol Res* 1999;39(1):41–47.

59. Singh S., Aggarwal B. Activation of transcription factor NF-κB is suppressed by curcumin (diferuloyl-methane). *J Biol Chem* 270(42):24995–25000.

60. Nakagawa Y., Mukai S., Yamada S. et al. Short-term effects of highly-bioavailable curcumin for treating knee osteoarthritis: a randomized, double-blind, placebo-controlled prospective study. *J Orthop Sci* 2014;19(6):933.

61. Zhou S., Zhang S., Shen H., et. al. Curcumin inhibits cancer progression through regulating expression of microRNAs. *Tumour Biol* 2017;39(2).

62. Kunnumakkara A.B., Anand P., Aggarwal B.B. Curcumin inhibits proliferation, invasion, angiogenesis and metastasis of different cancers through interaction with multiple cell signaling proteins. *Cancer Lett* 2008;269(2):199–225.

63. Mijnhout G.S., Alkhalaf A., Kleefstra N., Bilo H.J. Alpha lipoic acid: a new treatment for neuropathic pain in patients with diabetes? *Neth J Med* 2010;68(4):158–162.

64. Agathos E., Tentolouris A., Eleftheriadou I., et al. Effect of α-lipoic acid on symptoms and quality of life in patients with painful diabetic neuropathy. *J Int Med Res* 2018;46(5):1779–1790.

65. Nascimento O.J., Pessoa B.L., Orsini M., et al. Neuropathic pain treatment: still a challenge. *Neurol Int* 2016;8(2):6322.

66. Younger J., Parkitny L., McLain D. The use of low-dose naltrexone (LDN) as a novel anti-inflammatory treatment for chronic pain. *Clin Rheumatol* 2014;33(4):451–459.

67. Smith J.P., Bingaman S.I., Ruggiero F., Mauger D.T., Mukherjee A., McGovern C.O., Zagon I.S. Therapy with the opioid antagonist naltrexone promotes mucosal healing in active Crohn's disease: a randomized placebo-controlled trial. *Dig Dis Sci* 2011;56(7):2088–2097.

68. Smith J.P., Stock H., Bingaman S., Mauger D., Rogosnitzky M., Zagon I.S. Low-dose naltrexone therapy improves active Crohn's disease. *Am J Gastroenterol* 2007;102(4):820–828.

69. Cree B.A., Kornyeyeva E., Goodin D.S. Pilot trial of low-dose naltrexone and quality of life in multiple sclerosis. *Ann Neurol* 2010;68(2):145–150.

70. Younger J., Noor N., McCue R., Mackey S. Low-dose naltrexone for the treatment of fibromyalgia: findings of a small, randomized, double-blind, placebo-controlled, counterbalanced, crossover trial assessing daily pain levels. *Arthritis Rheum* 2013;65(2):529–538.

71. Younger J., Mackey S. Fibromyalgia symptoms are reduced by low-dose naltrexone: a pilot study. *Pain Med* 2009;10(4):663–672.

72. Bihari B. Bernard Bihari, MD: low-dose naltrexone for normalizing immune system function. *Altern Ther Health Med* 2013;19(2):56–65.

73. Hutchinson M.R., Zhang Y., Brown K., et al. Non-stereoselective reversal of neuropathic pain by naloxone and naltrexone: involvement of toll-like receptor 4 (TLR4). *Eur J Neurosci* 2008;28(1):20–29.

74. Lewis S.S., Loram L.C., Hutchinson M.R. *et al.* (+)-Naloxone, an opioid-inactive toll-like receptor 4 signaling inhibitor, reverses multiple models of chronic neuropathic pain in rats. *J Pain* 2012;13(5):498–506.

75. Chopra P., Cooper M.S. Treatment of complex regional pain syndrome (CRPS) using low dose naltrexone (LDN). *J Neuroimmune Pharm* 2013;8(3):470–476.

76. D'Agostino G., La Rana G., Russo R., *et al.* Central administration of palmitoylethanolamide reduces hyperalgesia in mice via inhibition of NF-κB nuclear signalling in dorsal root ganglia. *Eur J Pharmacol* 2009;613(1–3):54–59.

77. Kuehl F., Jacob T., Ganley O., Ormond R., Meisinger M. The identification of *N*-(2-hydroxyethyl)-palmitamide as a naturally occurring anti-inflammatory agent. *J Am Chem Soc* 1957;79 (20):5577–5578.

78. Paladini A., Fusco M., Cenacchi T., Schievano C., Piroli A., Varrassi G. Palmitoylethanolamide, a special food for medical purposes, in the treatment of chronic pain: a pooled data meta-analysis. *Pain Phys* 2016;19(2):11–24.

79. Gatti A., Lazzari M., Gianfelice V., Di Paolo A., Sabato E., Sabato A.F. Palmitoylethanolamide in the treatment of chronic pain caused by different etiopathogenesis. *Pain Med* 2012;13(9):1121–1130.

80. Gabrielsson L., Mattsson S., Fowler C.J. Palmitoylethanolamide for the treatment of pain: pharmacokinetics, safety and efficacy. *Br J Clin Pharmacol* 2016;82(4):932–942.

81. Aloe L., Leon A., Levi-Montalcini R. A proposed autacoid mechanism controlling mastocyte behaviour. *Agents Actions* 1993;39(Spec No):C145–C147.

82. Mazzari S., Canella R., Petrelli L., Marcolongo G., Leon A. *N*-(2-hydroxyethyl) hexadecamide is orally active in reducing edema formation and inflammatory hyperalgesia by down-modulating mast cell activation. *Eur J Pharmacol* 1996;300(3):227–236.

83. Marini I., Bartolucci M.L., Bortolotti F., Gatto M.R., Bonetti G.A. Palmitoylethanolamide versus a nonsteroidal anti-inflammatory drug in the treatment of temporomandibular joint inflammatory pain. *J Orofac Pain* 2012;26(2):99–104.

13 Regenerative Medicine in Pain Management

Sharon McQuillan and Rafael Gonzalez

CONTENTS

INTRODUCTION

Regenerative medicine offers an entirely new approach to repairing, replacing, maintaining, or enhancing organ or tissue function that has been lost due to disease, injury, or aging. By combining biomedical, biochemical, and biomechanical technologies, regenerative medicine strives to improve cellular migration, replication, and remodeling.[1] Treatment approaches include cell therapies, tissue engineering, gene therapy, immunomodulation therapy, and biomedical engineering.

Presently, clinical practice within the United States focuses mainly on approved autologous therapies utilizing platelet-rich plasma (PRP) or bone marrow aspirate (BMAC). Here, we will review various stem cell therapies for pain management based on in vitro and clinical studies.

MESENCHYMAL STEM CELLS

Adult stem cells are found throughout the body. The primary role of these cells is to maintain and repair the tissue in which they are found. Adult stem cells possess two very important properties—self-renewal and differentiation. Adult stem cells are multipotent, meaning they can be differentiated into subsets of cell types. Stem cells have been used for many different disease states as they also have the capacity to change the local environment via their paracrine effect, which may render them capable of disease modification.

Mesenchymal stem cells (MSCs) arise from pericytes released from broken and inflamed blood vessels. Once released, the MSCs exhibit an immunomodulatory as well as a regeneration zone of influence. Additionally, they have an angiogenic and antibiotic effect. Caplan et al. describe the immunomodulatory zone as a curtain of bioactive molecules that prevent the body from mounting a chronic autoimmune reaction.[2,3] MSCs address the regeneration zone, or the damaged tissue, by secreting a different set of bioactive molecules that have trophic functions. This results in four basic actions: apoptosis inhibition, inhibition of scar formation, angiogenesis, and mitogenesis. Lastly MSCs possess antimicrobial properties that can sense and address infection.[4,5]

Sources of MSCs include bone marrow, adipose, peripheral blood, amniotic, umbilical, and placental tissue. Most clinical studies involve the use of autologous sources of MSCs due to their accessibility and low risk of infection. In terms of clinical practice, the most popular types are derived from bone marrow aspirate or lipoaspirate.

The International Society for Cellular Therapy (ISCT) set forth minimum criteria to define human MSCs: (a) plastic adherence in standard culture; (b) positive for endoglin, CD73, and CD90, and negative for CD45, CD34, CD14 or CD11, CD97-alpha or CD19, and HLADR surface markers; (c) in vitro differentiation into osteoblasts, adipocytes, and chondroblasts.[6]

BONE MARROW-DERIVED STEM CELLS

Bone marrow-derived stem cells are the most commonly used source and are permitted by the FDA and other governing bodies. Bone marrow aspirate has been approved and used safely for many years for the treatment of blood cancers and other hematological disorders. Bone marrow is the primary site of new blood cell production. Two main cell types are produced in bone marrow: hematopoietic cells (myelopoietic, erythropoietic, lymphocytes, plasma, reticular, monocytes, magakaryocytes, hematopoietic stem cells) and stromal cells (fibroblasts, macrophages, adipocytes, osteoblasts, osteoclasts, endothelial cells, MSCs). The frequency of stem cell production decreases proportionately with age.

Bone marrow MSCs are obtained via bone marrow aspiration of the iliac crest (most commonly) under sterile conditions. The aspirate is then typically washed and centrifuged to remove the plasma and buffy coat until the final "cell pellet" is obtained; in some instances, a separation medium may be utilized. This pellet is commonly referred to as bone marrow aspirate concentrate (BMAC). A milliliter of bone marrow aspirate yields approximately 6×10^6 nucleated cells; only 0.01% are bone marrow stem cells.[7]

Bone marrow MSCs are a population of cells found in bone marrow that are different from blood cells in a variety of ways. They are multipotent stem cells, giving them the ability to differentiate into bone, cartilage, and fat cells. Additionally, they can support the formation of new blood cells. Two types of stem cells originate in bone marrow—hematopoietic stem cells and MSCs. There are also endothelial progenitor cells that have the capacity to form new vasculature. Hence, they have similar capabilities to stem cells.

Bone marrow-derived MSCs regenerate injured or damaged tissue via the following pathways—fibrinogenesis, osteogenesis, adipogenesis, and chondrogenesis.[4] Bone marrow-derived MSCs home to injury sites via migratory properties in bone marrow, bone, and cartilage.[8] Additionally, BMAC contains the following growth factors—basic fibroblast growth factor (b-FGF), platelet-derived growth factor (PDGF-BB), vascular endothelial growth factor (VEGF), transforming growth factor-beta (TGF-ß), and bone morphogenetic protein-2 (BMP-2), to name a few.[9]

While the number of stem cells found in BMAC is relatively low compared to those found in lipoaspirate, the growth factors and platelets contained in BMAC are believed to enhance their therapeutic ability. A study by Schafer et al. found that BMAC increases the concentration of PDGF-BB and VEGF in mononuclear cells.[10] Both PDGF-BB and VEGF contribute to angiogenesis.[11,12]

ADIPOSE-DERIVED STEM CELLS

Adipose-derived stem cells are a population of cells found in adipose tissue that have adipogenic, myogenic, neurogenic, chondrogenic, and osteogenic differentiation potential. Additionally, they possess angiogenic and vasculogenic tendencies.[8] Human adipose stem cells were first character-ized by Zuk et al., in 2001.[13] In adipose tissue, MSCs originate in perivascular locations and can be found in the stromal vascular fraction (SVF). The regenerative components of SVF include preadi-pocytes, endothelial progenitor cells, macrophages, monocytes, pericytes, and MSCs.[2]

Rodbell and Jones pioneered the initial methods to isolate stem cells from adipose tissue in the 1960s.[14] Current methods of adipose stem cell isolation involve tumescent liposuction which pro-duces the minced adipose tissue fragments, depending on the size of the harvesting cannula used. This is followed by cell washing to remove some red blood cells, enzymatic digestion, centrifuga-tion, and further cell wash steps to isolate the SVF.

The regenerative capacity of the SVF is likely a result of the "sum of its parts." This multi-com-ponent cellular result provides numerous pathways and mechanisms for regeneration to occur.[2] Pre-adipocytes are the most plentiful component of SVF and share many characteristics and markers of MSCs.[15] Endothelial progenitor cells release VEGF and insulin-like growth factor-1 (IGF-1), which activate angiogenesis.[16] Macrophages contained in SVF have demonstrated immunomodulatory properties via cytokine expression, as well as plastic adherence, multilineage differentiation, and immunosuppression via T-cell modulation.[17] Pericytes produce extracellular matrix components capable of improving cellular adhesion, migration, and cell interaction.[18]

Cell surface markers, including clusters of differentiation (CD), are critical for cell–cell and cell–environment interactions and are used to define mixed cell populations. Despite an enor-mous amount of research, there is little consensus with regard to CD characterization of the SVF. Table 13.1 shows a comparison of SVF-defined cell surface markers.[15,19–25] Table 13.2 provides a comparison of cell surface markers between bone marrow and adipose-derived stem cells.[20]

It is important to note that, as of this publication, the FDA currently views the standard method of adipose-derived stem cell isolation as manufacturing a drug; therefore this is not permissible in clinical practice in the United States. Bone marrow aspirate concentration (BMAC) using density centrifugation methods is permissible so long as the procedure is carried out the same day.

MSCs IN PAIN MANAGEMENT

It is well-established that the effectiveness of MSCs is mainly due to their paracrine effects to pro-mote a regenerative localized environment, rather than their direct effect or replacing tissue. For chronic pain and neuroinflammation, data suggest MSCs secrete the following noteworthy factors: transforming growth factor beta, interleukin-10, tumor necrosis factor-stimulated gene-6, hepato-cyte growth factor 1, and matrix metalloproteinases.

Transforming growth factor beta (TGF-β) controls many functions in the cellular environment, including growth, propagation, differentiation, and apoptosis. TGF-β possesses both powerful immunosuppressive and neuromodulatory properties. It is thought that TGF-β may reduce chronic pain by inhibiting the activation and propagation of nerve-injury-induced microglia and astrocytes.[26] TGF-β also decreases the secretion of pro-inflammatory cytokines. However, the mechanisms of TGF-β inhibition of neuropathic as well as chronic pain need further elucidation.[26–28]

Interleukin-10 (IL-10) is known to be a powerful anti-inflammatory cytokine affecting inflam-mation and immunoregulation. The role of IL-10 remains elusive in pain management, with con-flicting study results. A study by Li et al. demonstrated that the effects of MSCs were reversed by TGF-β and IL-10 antibody neutralization.[29] These data suggest that IL-10 plays a critical role in reducing pain and inflammation.

Tumor necrosis factor stimulated gene-6 (TSG-6) is an immunomodulatory protein secreted by MSCs. Animal studies using various disease models suggest that MSCs show dependence on TSG-6 for therapeutic effect. TSG-6 may shift cells such as macrophages from a pro-inflammatory state to an anti-inflammatory state. Injection of TSG-6 in mice with ulcerative colitis reduces the severity of colitis and the number of inflammatory cells.[30]

TABLE 13.1
SVF Cell Surface Markers

	MSCs (ADSCs)	Pericytes	Endothelial Progenitor Cells	Pre-Adipocytes	Transitional Cells	Macrophage/Monocyte
Bourin et al., 2013	CD45− CD31− CD13− CD73− CD90+ CD105+ CD34+ (unstable) CD45+ (<50%) CD31− (<20%)	CD13+ CD29+ CD44+ CD73+ CD90+ (>40%)	CD34+ (<40%)			
Zimmerlin et al., 2013		CD45− CD31− CD146+	CD45− CD31+ CD34+	CD45− CD31− CD146− CD34+	CD146+ CD31− CD34+	
Hager et al., 2013			CD133+ CD146+ CD34+ CD31+			
Bianchi et al., 2013	CD90+ CD29+ CD34−	CD146+ CD34− CD45− CD56−			CD146+ CD34+	
Corselli et al., 2013		CD146+ CD34− CD45− CD56−	CD34+ CD146+ CD31+	CD34+ CD31− CD146−		
Trakutev et al., 2008	CD34+ CD31− CD45− CD144−			CD34+ CD45− CD31−		
Eto et al., 2013						CD45+ CD14+ CD34+ CD206−

Hepatocyte growth factor-1 (HGF-1) is secreted in large amounts by MSCs. HGF-1 plays a role in angiogenesis and possesses the ability to promote cell growth and proliferation, and resist apoptosis. Indeed it has a neuroprotective effect, and in vitro studies illustrate that MSCs secrete HGF-1 which may have a protective effect on excitotoxicity-injured PC12 cells.[31] HGF-1 has demonstrated protective properties against autoimmune disease in vivo by activating regulatory T-cells, leading to the production of immunosuppressive cytokine IL-10.[32,33]

Matrix metalloproteinases (MMPs) are enzymes that are capable of degrading extracellular matrix proteins and can process a number of bioactive molecules. MMPs play a major role in neuroinflammation and pain through the division and suppression of extracellular matrix proteins, cytokines, and chemokines.[34] Nerve injury-induced changes in the dorsal root ganglion are responsible for neuropathic pain.[35] MMP-9, produced by injured dorsal root ganglions, provokes spinal microglia activation and neuropathic pain development due to MMP-9 pathophysiology, including IL-1 beta cleavage and microglia p38 activation in early-phase neuropathic pain. MMP-2 activation

TABLE 13.2

Differences between Bone Marrow and Adipose Tissue

	SVF	BM-MC	ASC	MSC
CD34	>30–70%	>2–30%	>2–30%	<2%
CD45	>30–70%	>70%	<2%	<2%
CD13	>2–30%	>70%	<2%	<2%
CD73	>2–30%	>2–30%	>70%	>70%
CD90	>2–30%	>2–30%	>70%	>70%
CD105	>2–30%	>2–30%	>70%	>70%
CD10			>70%	>30–70%
CD36			>30–70%	<2%
CD106			>2–30%	>30–70%
CFU-U	>1%	>0.001%	>5%	>5%

SVF = stromal vascular fraction
BM-MC = bone marrow mononucleated cells
ASC = adipose stem cells
MSC = mesenchymal stem cells

leads to late-phase neuropathic pain via IL-1 beta cleavage and astrocyte ERK activation.[35] Tissue inhibitor of metalloproteinases (TIMP) suppress neuropathic pain. TIMP-1 diminishes early-phase neuropathic pain, while TIMP-2 diminishes late-phase neuropathic pain.[35]

NEUROPATHIC PAIN

Neuropathic pain is one of the more difficult pain conditions to treat. Neuropathic pain is a progressive condition of the nervous system that is most often brought about by trauma, infection, or ischemia. Neuropathic pain symptoms include hyperalgesia and allodynia.[36] Diabetic neuropathy is one of the most common and serious complications of diabetes mellitus and metabolic syndrome.[37] Common treatments for neuropathic pain involve pharmaceutical intervention to mask or diminish symptoms with little effectiveness and many side effects.

MSCs have shown promise in the treatment of neuropathic pain in both animal and human studies. It is thought that this is due to the multipotency and paracrine effects of MSCs, in particular anti-inflammatory cytokines, proangiogenic factors, and neurotrophic factors.[38] Preclinical animal studies for trigeminal neuropathic pain, diabetic neuropathy, and hind paw neuropathic pain all suggest that MSCs are a promising method to treat various neuropathic pains.[26] For instance, a study conducted by Venturi et al.[39] used transperineal injections of autologous adipose tissue with stem cells to treat 15 female patients with pudendal neuralgia who were unresponsive to 3 months of medical treatments. Patients were examined clinically and evaluated using visual analog scale (VAS), validated SF-36 health survey, and pudendal nerve terminal motor latency (PNTML) before treatment, and 12 months following treatment. Twelve patients completed the protocol with no adverse events. Two patients reported no improvement in pain. The remainder of the patients showed significant improvement in VAS and SF-36 evaluation.

In another study, Vickers et al.[40] demonstrated the effects of SVF in ten subjects with neuropathic trigeminal pain who were unresponsive to traditional pharmacotherapy. The female patients underwent liposuction and the SVF was obtained via enzymatic digestion, centrifugation, and resuspension. The SVF was injected locally into the appropriate pain areas. Patients were examined clinically and evaluated using a ten-point pain intensity scale as well as the evaluation of the use of anti-neuropathic medication before and at 1 week, 1, 3, and 6 months after treatment. There were no systemic or local adverse effects as a result of treatment. Outcome results at 6 months showed that five out of nine subjects had both reduced pain intensity scores and reduced need for anti-neuropathic medication.

In a study using autologous bone marrow mononuclear cells, 168 patients with refractory diabetic neuropathy were evaluated. These patients underwent bone marrow aspiration, the mononuclear stem cells were separated using Ficoll-Hypaque density-gradient centrifugation, and then prepared for intramuscular injection. Patients were examined clinically and evaluated using the Toronto Clinical Scoring System (TCSS) and nerve conduction studies before and at 1, 3, 6, 12, 18, 24, and 36 months following treatment. Results of the study confirmed a decrease of the neuropathic signs and symptoms of neuropathy as evidenced by TCSS scores, motor nerve conduction velocity, sensory nerve conduction velocity, compound muscle action potential, and sensory nerve action potential. No adverse events or complications were observed.[41]

Indeed, many of these studies are small in size yet the collective results support the premise that patients can expect to see improvements from stem cell therapy for neuropathic pain. Most importantly, it was safe. More studies are needed to further evaluate dosage and length of effect.

DISCOGENIC PAIN

Low back pain is one of the leading causes of disability with a large social and economic impact. Disc degeneration occurs via hydration loss in the nucleus pulposus. The hydration loss manifests in instability, culminating in disc herniation, spondylolisthesis, facet joint dysfunction, and ultimately spinal stenosis.

It has been well-established that inflammatory cytokines secreted by the disc cells account for the pain experienced in disc degeneration.[42] This supports the notion that stem cell therapy maybe a viable option for discogenic pain. It is well-understood that MSCs have a paracrine effect which may address inflammation in the nucleus pulposus, as well as promoting the recruitment of other substances leading to the development of proteoglycans and type II collagen.[43] The use of MSCs is appropriate due to chondrogenic differentiation and immunomodulatory tendencies. Preclinical studies utilizing MSCs have demonstrated safety and efficacy in discogenic pain.[44]

Numerous human studies have shown favorable outcomes utilizing a variety of stem cell sources for discogenic pain. For instance, Mochida et al.[45] evaluated the use of autologous cultured nucleus pulposus chondrocytes that were co-cultured with MSCs in nine subjects with Pfirrman grade III disc degeneration and posterior lumbar intervertebral fusion. Patients were examined clinically and evaluated before and 3 years following treatment using the Japanese Orthopedic Association (JOA) scoring system for low back pain and MRI results. Clinical outcomes demonstrated significant improvement in JOA function and pain scores, as well as the safety of activated nucleus pulposus cell transplantation and the efficacy of the procedure to slow disc degeneration. Most importantly, there were no adverse events reported during the 3-year follow-up period.

In another study conducted by Orozco et al.,[46] the efficacy of autologous expanded bone marrow-derived MSCs was evaluated in ten patients with degenerative disc disease and persistent low back pain. The patients received injections directly into the nucleus pulposus. Patients were examined clinically and evaluated before and 1 year after treatment using visual analog scoring (VAS), Oswestry disability index (ODI), and MRI. Clinical outcomes illustrated that 71% of the patients had a decrease in pain and disability.

Pettine et al.[47–49] evaluated the use of nonexpanded autologous bone marrow concentration (BMAC) in 26 patients with moderate to severe discogenic low back pain. Patients were examined clinically before and at 3, 6, 12, 24, and 36 months following treatment utilizing ODI, VAS, and MRI. MRI results at 1-year post-procedure showed improvement of one modified Pfirrmann grade in 40% of the patients. After 36 months, 6 out of 26 patients moved forward to surgical intervention. The remaining subjects demonstrated evidence of safety and efficacy using bone marrow-derived MSCs as an intradiscal therapy.

A randomized study conducted by Noriega et al.[50] evaluated 24 patients with chronic low back pain with lumbar disc degeneration who were unresponsive to conservative treatments using allogeneic bone marrow MSCs via intradiscal injection. Subjects were examined clinically before treatment and after 12 months utilizing VAS, ODI, SF-12, and MRI. The MSC-treated patients showed a significant reduction in lumbar pain and disability at 3 months. The reduction was maintained at 6 and 12 months. Overall average reduction in disability was 28%, while 40% of those treated reported 100% improvement.

Coric et al.[51] evaluated the use of culture-expanded allogeneic juvenile chondrocyte cells in 15 patients with lumbar degenerative disc disease and low back pain. Patients were examined clinically before treatment and at 1, 3, 6, and 12 months following a single treatment utilizing MRI, ODI, Numerical Rating Scale (NRS), and the SF-36. Results from this study are very encouraging, with the average ODI, NRS, and SF-36 all showing significant improvement from baseline. Ten patients (77%) showed improvement in MRI. Only three subjects underwent surgical intervention by 12-month follow-up.

Centeno et al.[52] explored the use of culture-expanded autologous bone marrow-derived MSCs in 33 patients with lower back pain and degenerative disc disease. Patients were clinically evaluated before and after treatment and up to 72 months utilizing MRI, numeric pain score (NPS), modified single assessment numeric evaluation (SANE) rating, functional rating index (FRI), measurement of intervertebral disc dimension, and adverse events. Study results were very encouraging. NPS scores were significant relative to baseline at all evaluation intervals. SANE ratings showed an average improvement of 60% at 3 years post-treatment. Twenty patients underwent post-treatment MRI, and 85% demonstrated a reduction in disc bulge size of 23% post-procedure.

A phase I study conducted by Kumar et al.[53] evaluated the safety and efficacy of a combined treatment of autologous adipose-derived stem cells with hyaluronic acid derivative at two different doses in patients with chronic discogenic low back pain. Ten patients received either a dose of 2×10^7 cells/disc or 4×10^7 cells/disc. Safety and efficacy outcomes were determined utilizing VAS, ODI, SF-36, and MRI/X-ray at regular intervals for 1 year. Results demonstrated 60% significant improvement in VAS, ODI, and SF-36 in both dosage groups with no adverse events.

In summary, there are various studies suggesting MSCs may ameliorate the symptoms of discogenic pain. Most importantly, studies illustrate that the treatment is safe regardless of whether the cells were culture-expanded. These studies demonstrate that autologous MSCs from bone marrow would be a suitable in-office clinical application for discogenic pain with proper patient selection.

OSTEOARTHRITIS OR INFLAMMATORY PAIN

Osteoarthritis (OA) is considered to be the most common chronic joint disease in an increasingly growing elderly population. The Centers for Disease Control (CDC) estimate that OA affects over 30 million adults in the United States, with an associated cost of $185.5 billion per year.[54] While most consider OA an age-associated chronic degenerative disease, further research has revealed that cellular imbalance between catabolic/pro-inflammatory and anabolic pathways is behind the debilitating effects of OA.[55]

Conventional treatments for OA are designed to control symptoms rather than for disease modification. Most are pharmaceutical in nature and carry unwanted side effects with only limited benefit. The standard care for joint pain for those unresponsive to conventional therapy is joint replacement surgery, which is accompanied by significant complication risk, including pain or loss of function.[56]

OA treatments should have three objectives: relieve pain, control inflammation, and restore function and/or range of motion. MSCs are a suitable option for the treatment of OA due to their potential to regenerate cartilage tissue and control the inflammatory response. Cytokine and growth factor release convey immunomodulatory, anti-inflammatory, and analgesic effects.[57] Collectively this configuration of cells can help suppress cartilage destruction and its associated pain and inflammation. Moreover, preclinical OA models confirm MSCs' ability to differentiate into chondrocytes and repair damaged cartilage, as well as regulate local inflammatory environments and support a favorable healing environment via paracrine activities.

OA has been the most intensively investigated pain condition treated with MSCs. The majority of all OA studies using MSCs involve an intra-articular injection into the affected area. It is well-understood that intra-articular injections of MSCs are safe.[58] Moreover, there is an abundance of evidence demonstrating varying degrees of efficacy with a direct intra-articular injection of MSCs, particularly in the knee.

BONE MARROW-DERIVED STEM CELL STUDIES IN OA

Centeno et al. conducted a safety study of 339 patients with various joint conditions utilizing culture-expanded autologous bone marrow-derived MSCs which showed a greater than 75% improvement in 41% of patients treated, with greater than 50% improvement in 63% of those treated. The average reported pain relief improved throughout the 2-year study period. In terms of adverse events, only 2% reported self-limited increased pain and swelling at the injection site.[59]

In a smaller study of four patients, utilizing culture-expanded autologous bone marrow-derived MSCs showed improvement in VAS pain scores in all subjects from 24% to 50% at 6 months with no adverse events reported.[60] Although a small patient population, this study supports many other publications illustrating a decrease in pain.

Emadedin et al. investigated the safety of cultured autologous bone marrow-derived MSCs in 18 patients with OA of the hip, knee, or ankle. Each patient received one injection. Patients were clinically examined before treatments and at 2, 6, 12, and 30 months after treatment using MRI, VAS, and the Western Ontario and McMaster Universities Osteoarthritis Index (WOMAC). All patients improved in terms of increased walking distance, decreased VAS, and WOMAC scores, which were supported by MRI. No adverse events were reported.[61]

Orozco et al. conducted two prospective, observational studies to evaluate cartilage regeneration and clinical improvement in patients with OA. The first study involved an intra-articular injection of culture-expanded autologous bone marrow-derived MSCs in 12 patients with OA of the knee. Patients were evaluated clinically before and at 12 months after treatments using VAS, WOMAC scoring, and MRI. At 12 months, mean pain scores and WOMAC decreased significantly. MRI showed improvement in the quality of knee cartilage, and no adverse events were reported.[62]

One of the first to conduct a randomized controlled trial involving 50 patients with OA of the knee utilizing peripheral blood stem cells was Saw et al.[63] Patients were randomized into two groups. One group received a series of intra-articular hyaluronic acid injections, while the other group received peripheral blood stem cells following knee arthroscopy and chondroplasty. Patients were evaluated at baseline and 2 years post-treatment. Patients in both groups improved based on the International Knee Documentation Committee (IKDC) index score (reflecting pain, activity level) at 24 months. Patients receiving peripheral blood stem cells demonstrated increased cartilage quality at second-look arthroscopy.[63]

Wong et al. analyzed the results of a study performing intra-articular cultured autologous bone marrow-derived MSC injections combined with hyaluronic acid or hyaluronic acid alone in 56 subjects with arthroscopic microfracture and medial opening sedge high tibial osteotomy. Patients were divided evenly into two groups—a cell treatment group and a control group. The primary outcome measure was the IKDC score at baseline, 6 months, 1, and 2 years post-procedure. Secondary outcome measures included Tegner and Lysholm clinical scores as well as post-procedural Magnetic Resonance Observation of Cartilage Repair Tissue (MOCART) scores at 1 year. While both treatment arms demonstrated improvements in Tegner, Lysholm, and IKDC scores, the cell recipient group score showed statistically significant improvement.[64]

Kim et al. evaluated the efficacy of intra-articular injection of autologous bone marrow aspirate concentrate (BMAC) with adipose tissue in 41 patients with OA of the knee. Pain scores (VAS) and functional scales (SF-36, IKDC, Lysholm) were used for evaluation pre-procedure and 3, 6, and 12 months post-procedure. Results showed significant improvement in both knee pain and knee function scores.[65]

Soler et al. conducted a phase I-II prospective, open-label, single-dose, single-arm clinical trial assessing the feasibility, safety, and efficacy of ex-vivo expanded autologous MSCs infused intra-articular in patients with OA of the knee. Fifteen patients were clinically evaluated at baseline, 6, and 12 months using VAS, SF-36 questionnaire, Lequesne functional index, WOMAC, and MRI. Results showed significant improvements in VAS, WOMAC, and Lequesne scores. The treatment was well-tolerated with only a few reported mild adverse events (low back pain), while MRI showed signs of cartilage regeneration at 12 months.[66]

Most recently, Chahal et al. conducted a phase II non-randomized, open-label dose-escalation study in Canada to determine the safety and efficacy of culture-expanded autologous bone marrow-derived MSCs in 12 patients with late-stage knee OA. Patients were evaluated clinically at baseline and at 1, 2, and 6 weeks and 3, 6, and 12 months using the following patient outcome measures: KOOS, WOMAC, Whole Organ MRI Scores (WORMS), collagen content (T_2 scores), synovitis, and inflammation and cartilage biomarkers. Significant improvement was noted in KOOS pain and symptoms, and WOMAC overall. Interestingly, the high-dose cell group showed significantly lower anti-inflammatory biomarkers.[67]

A newly published study by Lamo-Espinosa et al. assessed the intra-articular injection of two doses of cultured autologous bone marrow-derived MSCs versus hyaluronic acid (control) in 30 patients with knee osteoarthritis. Patients were examined clinically at baseline, 12, and 48 months utilizing VAS and WOMAC scoring. No adverse events were reported. The cell-dose groups improved clinically according to VAS and WOMAC scores.[68]

Although all the studies are unique in their own way, they all demonstrate the safety of the use of bone marrow-derived MSCs. Indeed, there were varying degrees of efficacy, suggesting that bone marrow-derived MSCs may improve outcomes for patients suffering from OA.

ADIPOSE-DERIVED STEM CELL STUDIES IN OA

Similarly to the use of bone marrow-derived MSCs studies, many clinical research studies have been completed that demonstrate similar results. Here we will review several of them.

Jo et al. were the first to report results on dose-dependent direct intra-articular MSC injection for OA. This two-phase study consisted of 18 patients with OA of the knee. Phase I patients received either a low-, mid-, or high-dose injection of culture-expanded autologous adipose-derived MSCs. Phase II subjects all received the high-dose treatment. While all groups demonstrated improvement in pain and function as evidenced by WOMAC, VAS, and Knee Society Score (KSS, an index that measures pain, stability, and range of motion), the results were statistically significant in the high-dose group at 24 months.[69, 70]

Koh et al. conducted two studies utilizing autologous adipose-derived MSCs from the infrapatellar fat pad during arthroscopic debridement for the treatment of OA of the knee. The cells were injected intra-articular in a platelet-rich plasma suspension. Follow-up PRP treatments occurred on day 7 and day 14 post-treatment. Study results demonstrated a significant reduction of pain and improved quality of life via Lysholm score and KOOS 2 years post-treatment.[71, 72]

An open-label phase I study conducted in France and Germany by Pers et al.[73] evaluated the safety of a dose-escalation protocol of intra-articular injected cultured autologous adipose-derived MSCs in 18 patients with OA of the knee. Three groups received either a low, medium, or high dose of MSCs. Outcome parameters included adverse event reporting and WOMAC scores at baseline, 1 week, 3, and 6 months post-treatment. At 6 months, treatment was determined to be safe with no serious adverse events reported. The low-dose cell therapy group demonstrated significant improvement via WOMAC score.

Bansal et al.[74] evaluated the safety and preliminary effects of intra-articular injection of autologous adipose-derived SVF and platelet-rich plasma in ten patients with OA of the knee. Patients were evaluated at baseline, 3, 6, 12, 18, and 24 months utilizing WOMAC, 6-minute walk distance, and MRI. The results displayed a significant decrease in WOMAC scoring and significant improvement in walking distance.

In a phase II randomized placebo-controlled study by Lee et al.,[75] the safety and efficacy of a single intra-articular injection of autologous adipose-derived MSCs in 12 patients with OA of the knee were assessed. Patients were evaluated over a 6-month time frame. Outcome measures included WOMAC score, safety, and MRI. The results showed a significant improvement in WOMAC score at 6 months. There was no change in cartilage defect shown on MRI at 6 months. No serious adverse events were reported.

A newly published Australian randomized controlled study by Frietag et al.[76] evaluated the efficacy of autologous culture-expanded adipose-derived MSCs on pain, function, and disease modification in knee OA. Thirty patients were randomized into either a single-injection, two-injections (baseline and 6 months), or control group. Patients were evaluated at baseline, 1, 3, 6, and 12 months utilizing the following outcome measures: Numeric Pain Rating Scale (NPRS), KOOS, WOMAC, and MRI Osteoarthritis Knee Score (MOAKS). Results demonstrated significant pain reduction and functional improvement. Moreover, MOAKS demonstrated a modification of disease progression. No adverse events were reported.[76] Frietag et al.[77] also described the use of autologous culture-expanded adipose-derived MSCs for the treatment of acromioclavicular joint OA with positive findings. The patient received two injections, one at baseline and one at 5 months. Outcomes were evaluated utilizing NPRS, Quick Disability of Arm, Shoulder, Hand (QuickDASH), and MRI. The results showed pain reduction and functional improvement as well as structural improvement via MRI. This is the first reported use of MSCs therapy in upper limb OA.

Mautner and Bowers conducted a comparison study of autologous bone marrow aspirate concentrate (BMAC) versus autologous micro-fragmented adipose tissue MSCs in 76 patients with knee OA. Outcome measures included VAS, KOOS, and Emory Quality of Life (EQOL). The results demonstrated improved pain and function scores at 1 year for adipose and 1.5 years for BMAC with no significant differences between the two modalities. This is the first study to directly compare BMAC and adipose MSCs.[78]

In summary, although there are various different clinical study designs completed, they all illustrate that autologous adipose-derived stem cells are safe with varying amounts of efficacy. They all do demonstrate improvement in quality of life for patients suffering from OA.

ALLOGENEIC-DERIVED STEM CELLS

While the vast majority of clinical studies published utilize autologous stem cells for the treatment of OA, there is a growing body of evidence demonstrating that allogeneic sources are safe and effective. As the FDA compliance deadline for allogeneic product drug registration and approval approaches, more research will quickly emerge regarding safety and efficacy.

In a randomized study by Vega et al., culture-expanded allogeneic bone marrow-derived MSCs from 3 healthy donors were used in 30 patients with OA of the knee. The patients were randomized into two groups—allogeneic cell group and hyaluronic acid group. Patients were evaluated at baseline and followed for 1 year utilizing the following tests: VAS, Lequesne, WOMAC, and MRI. The results showed significant improvement in VAS, WOMAC, and Lequesne compared with hyaluronic acid at 6 and 12 months. Patient satisfaction in the cell-treated group was 77%, with no serious adverse events.[79]

Vangness et al. performed a randomized, double-blinded study to determine the safety of intra-articular injections of cultured allogeneic bone marrow-derived MSCs for knee OA, the ability of MSCs to promote meniscus regeneration, and the effects of MSCs on OA changes in the knee in 55 patients. The subjects underwent partial medial meniscectomy followed by an injection of either low-dose allogeneic MSC, high-dose allogeneic MSCs, or sodium hyaluronate vehicle control within 7 to 10 days post-procedure. Patients were evaluated at baseline and through 2 years to determine safety, meniscus regeneration, and pain. Results showed significantly increased meniscal volume in both cell groups. Those receiving cell treatment also experienced a significant reduction in pain according to VAS assessment at 12 months.[80]

Matas et al. assessed the safety and efficacy of either a single or repeated intra-articular injections of umbilical cord-derived allogeneic MSCs in OA of the knee. Twenty-eight patients were randomized to receive hyaluronic acid at baseline and 6 months, single-dose umbilical cord MSCs at baseline, or repeated doses at baseline and 6 months. Clinical outcomes were evaluated at 1, 4, 8, 12, 24, 36, and 52 weeks utilizing adverse event reporting, WOMAC, VAS, SF-36, and OARSI. Only patients in the cell-treated group experienced significant pain and function improvement from baseline. The umbilical MSCs group with repeated dose had the most improvement. No adverse events were reported, and no differences in MRI were detected.[81]

In summary, clinical studies utilizing MSCs for joint pain illustrate efficacy as well as safety, regardless of whether the cells were culture-expanded, or allogeneic. Patients' quality of life was improved, and they were satisfied with these treatments. However, correct dosing and standardized protocols have yet to be established. Most importantly, the overall results are very favorable compared to conventional treatment strategies. These studies suggest that allogeneic stem cells are a viable option for those suffering from inflammatory or OA pain.

CANCER PAIN

Pain resulting from cancer is a very common ailment. Cancer-related pain is experienced by 55% of patients undergoing treatments and by 66% of patients who have advanced, metastatic, or terminal disease.[82] Cancer pain is either a direct effect of the disease, such as nerve compression, or tumor extension into the tissue or bone, or the pain is related to treatment side effects such as chemotherapy-induced peripheral neuropathy, nerve injury, or lymphedema. The gold standard for cancer pain treatment is pharmaceutical intervention, in the form of opioids, steroids, antidepressants, and anticonvulsants. Many of these medications are accompanied by undesirable side effects.

The use of MSCs in treating cancer pain stems from the premise that chronic inflammation leads to cancer development.[83] A large amount of research has been devoted to the role of cytokines and chemokines in cancer. While the anti-inflammatory effect of MSCs is well-established, there is controversy surrounding the role of MSCs in tumor development. Numerous studies have shown that MSCs inhibit tumor growth, while just as many have suggested that MSCs possess protumor tendencies.[84] As a result of this controversy, there is little research regarding the use of MSCs for cancer pain. A preclinical study by Sun et al. evaluated the use of human bone marrow MSCs genetically engineered to express the human proenkephalin (hPPE) gene to treat bone cancer pain in a rat model.[85] Results demonstrated a decrease in pain threshold as well as a decrease in inflammatory cytokines interleukin-1 beta and interleukin-6. This demonstrates the possibility of using MSCs that may be genetically modified as a therapy for cancer pain, but more research is needed.

Author's note: the author recommends that, due to the even remote possibility of MSCs promoting tumor growth, any patients evaluated for stem cell treatment should not have had any active cancer within 5 years of treatment and should have a recent PAP smear, mammogram, CEA, and PSA testing before treatment.

MIGRAINE

Migraine is a complex episodic neurological disorder characterized by recurrent headaches, which may be accompanied by nausea, vomiting, and sensitivity to light and sound.[86] Visual aura is also experienced in approximately 30% of all migraine episodes, and migraines are three times more prevalent in females compared to males. Currently, there is no cure for migraine headaches. Conventional medical treatment consists of non-steroidal anti-inflammatory drugs (NSAIDs), triptans, anti-epileptics, beta-blockers, and calcium channel blockers, all of which vary in efficacy with significant side effects.[87]

The exact pathophysiology of migraine is not exactly known. There seems to be a hereditary component, as high as 50%. Most research points to the activation and sensitization of neurons in the trigeminal nerve as the trigger to migraine headaches. There are two possible theories as to how the nerve is aggravated—cortical spreading depression (CSD) and neurogenic inflammation. Cortical spreading depression is a wave of neural excitation activity followed by the depolarization of neurons. This may explain the aura some patients experience before the migraine episode. Neurogenic inflammation theory proposes that inflammatory neuropeptides lead to vasodilation and mast cell degranulation, followed by a release of various inflammatory compounds.[87]

Adult MSCs may help combat migraine due to their immunomodulatory effects. Studies using SVF have demonstrated efficacy in the treatment of trigeminal neuropathic pain. The activation of mast cells (which are derived from hematopoietic stem cells) triggers the release of inflammatory cytokines which result in many nervous system disorders, such as migraine.[88] Additionally, pericytes play a crucial role in neurological diseases. Used correctly, they may be used to increase blood flow, preserve blood–brain barrier function, and help repair glial scarring in areas of the central nervous system (CNS).[89] Moreover, MSCs studies have demonstrated that they are neuroprotective on dopaminergic neurons.[90]

There are only two published studies utilizing cells for the treatment of migraine. Bright et al. treated four females with long histories of migraine or tension-type headache systemically with autologous stromal vascular fraction isolated from lipoaspirate. Two of the four women ceased having migraines after 1 month; this lasted for a period of 12 to 18 months. A third patient had a significant reduction in the severity and frequency of migraine over 18 months. The fourth patient obtained a temporary decrease in symptoms for 1 month and was treated 18 months later. Most importantly, the dosage and types of pain medication were reduced in all patients.[91]

Mauksop and Rothaus investigated the intra-muscular injection of SVF in nine patients with severe migraine-related disability who failed botulinum toxin injections and three prophylactic drugs. The Migraine Disability Assessment Score (MIDAS) was used to assess the patients. Patients received injections in the pericranial, neck, and trapezius muscles and were evaluated at baseline and 3 months post-treatment. The mean MIDAS score decreased 34 points. Seven out of nine patients reported a decreased MIDAS score but only two experienced meaningful improvement.[92]

While these studies hold some promise for migraine treatment, the role of stem cells for migraines needs more research. Moreover, more studies with larger subject groups need to be completed to better evaluate the efficacy of stem cells for the treatment of migraine.

OPIOID TOLERANCE AND OPIOID-INDUCED HYPERALGESIA

Two of the most troublesome side effects of opioid use/abuse are the occurrence of opioid tolerance and opioid-induced hyperalgesia. Opioid tolerance occurs when an individual requires greater amounts of opioids over time to obtain the original degree of therapeutic effect. This does not necessarily involve addiction. Increased dosages however, can lead to overdose and death. Opioid-induced hyperalgesia describes a situation in which individuals taking opioids to treat pain paradoxically develop an increased sensitivity to noxious stimuli.[93] Currently, there are very few options in treating opioid tolerance or opioid-induced hyperalgesia other than medication rotation.

Molecular pathways and mechanisms tied to neuroinflammation appear to play similar, yet distinct roles in the development of both opioid tolerance and opioid-induced hyperalgesia. Opioids activate toll-like receptors on microglia, which leads to opioid tolerance. Opioid-induced hyperalgesia is mediated via μ-receptor dependent expression of P2X4 and the release of brain-derived neurotropic factor (BDNF) from microglia.[93] This pathway regulates microglia-to-neuron signaling, leading to the sensitization of spinal lamina I neurons and opioid-induced hyperalgesia. This suggests that mediating neuroinflammation would prove beneficial in treating opioid tolerance and opioid-induced hyperalgesia.

MSCs offer hope in the treatment of opioid tolerance and opioid-induced hyperalgesia, due mostly to their paracrine effects, mainly their immunomodulatory and anti-inflammatory effects. More specifically, MSCs impede opioid tolerance and opioid-induced hyperalgesia by hindering neuroinflammation. Repetitive opioid intake activates microglia and astrocytes in the spinal cord, as well as satellite cells in the dorsal root ganglion. Opioids also directly stimulate toll-like receptors (TLR-4), resulting in the manifestation of opioid tolerance. Additionally, opioids cause mu-opioid receptor (MOR)-mediated expression of punergic receptors P2X4R and the release of BDNF from microglia. Opioid-induced hyperalgesia occurs due to the sensitization of lamina I neurons modulated by microglia-to-neuron signaling via the P2X4-BDNF-TrkB pathway.

MSCs may prevent neuroinflammation by paracrine release of a number of exosomes, microvesicles, and growth factors including indoleamine 2,3-dioxygenase (IDO), prostaglandin-2 (PGE-2), IL-10, TGF-β, leukemia inhibiting factor (LIF), human leukocyte antigen-G5 (HLA-G5), and TSG-6. MSCs communicate with microglia, astrocytes, macrophages, and other immune cells via various signaling pathways to discourage the manufacture and release of interleukin-1-beta, IL-6, TNF-α, BDNF, NO, and other pro-inflammatory bioactives that contribute to the development of opioid tolerance and opioid-induced hyperalgesia.[94] Additionally, MSCs release growth factors that promote cell and tissue recovery via resident stem/progenitor cell stimulation, extracellular matrix remodeling, angiogenesis, and immune function modulation.[95]

Preclinical studies show promising results using MSCs to reverse opioid tolerance and opioid-induced hyperalgesia. Researchers at the Cleveland Clinic[93] conducted preclinical studies in rodents using MSCs harvested from rat bone marrow. Opioid tolerance was induced in rats using daily morphine injections for 3 to 4 weeks. MSCs were delivered by either intravenous or intrathecal administration 1 or 7 days before the administration of morphine to an opioid or control group. Outcome measures included paw withdrawal thresholds (PWT) to mechanical and thermal stimuli and tail flick tests. Intrathecal and intravenous MSCs did not cause any behavioral change in the control group. Both a single dose of intravenous or intrathecal administration in the opioid tolerance group significantly mitigated opioid tolerance for up to 26 days, regardless of the day of administration. The therapeutic effect took place as quickly as 2 days after treatment. In terms of opioid-induced hyperalgesia, both intravenous and intrathecal administration of MSCs produced similar degrees of anti-tolerance and anti-hyperalgesia effects. This is significant because intravenous injection is a much more easily tolerated route of administration with less risk. Immunohistochemistry illustrated that the treatments significantly reduced microglia and astrocyte activation in the spinal cord. These findings are significant as both opioid tolerance and opioid-induced hyperalgesia are the leading causes of overdose and death when increasing doses are necessary for pain relief. Human studies are currently under development to substantiate the preclinical findings. If successful, this will radically change the treatment approach to pain management.

In summary, MSCs may be promising for opioid tolerance and opioid-induced hyperalgesia assuming their main mechanisms of action are via paracrine effects. Indeed, preclinical data have illustrated a beneficial effect in animal models of addiction. More research and clinical work are needed to determine the efficacy of MSCs for opioid tolerance and opioid-induced hyperalgesia.

EXTRACELLULAR VESICLES

The use of extracellular vesicles is the next generation of possible therapies in the regenerative medicine sector. According to the International Society for Extracellular Vesicles (ISEV), extracellular vesicles (EV) is the generic term for particles naturally released from the cell that are delimited by a lipid bilayer and cannot replicate. EV subtypes should be defined by physical and biochemical characteristics and/or conditions/sources.[96] Another definition of EV is as a collective term for heterogeneous, small, double-layered lipid membrane vesicles typically 30–2000 nm, which serve as carriers for biologically active signaling molecules such as mRNA, microRNA, proteins, enzymes, lipids, and DNA fragments.[97] EV are nanoparticles secreted by virtually all cell types in the body. Their main function is intercellular communication. Included in the EV category are exosomes, microvesicles, and apoptotic bodies. Due to the lack of specific markers, as well as overlapping characteristics of size, composition, and density, it is challenging to pinpoint various subtypes of EV. Exosomes are EV that are released from a cell following the merging of a multivesicular body (MVB, or intermediate endocytic compartment) with the plasma membrane. This process frees the intraluminal vesicles into the extracellular space, releasing the exosomes.[98] Exosomes tend to range in size from 40 to 100 nanometers. Microvesicles range in size from 50 to 1000 nanometers and originate via outward budding of the cell membrane. Apoptotic bodies or apobodies are released by cells experiencing apoptosis and range in size from 1 to 5000 nanometers. EV can be isolated from most body fluids, as well as from the supernatant fluid of cell cultures. EV communication involves normal cellular processes as well as intercellular processes which are responsible for disease progression.[99]

Exosomes may prove an important vehicle for the treatment of pain management. They provide intracellular communication and transport macromolecules between cells. They contain a variety of bioactive materials including lipids (phosphatidylcholine, phosphatidylethanolamine, phosphatidylserine, lysophosphatidic acid, ceramide, cholesterol, sphingomyelin), and nucleic acids (miRNA, mRNA). Exosomes from MSCs work in the same fashion as stem cells but are smaller in size, possess lower immunogenicity tendencies, and are not subject to the restrictions of MSCs in terms of cell survival and unknown behavior over time. Other advantages of exosomes over stem cell therapy center around issues with direct cell transplantation, including risk of emboli due to intravenous infusion, tumorigenesis, and immune activation from allogeneic sources.[100]

Exosomes can be purified and stored for long time periods, and they can be evaluated more accurately than their MSCs counterparts for safety, dosage, potency, etc.[101] This translates into a more potent, standardized dosing regimen as well as a faster approval pipeline with the FDA.

There are some advantages of using MSCs-derived exosomes for joint pain over MSCs themselves. While they both may possess the same properties, exosomes can be cultured and secured at a certain growth or differentiation point under controlled conditions. Also, the removal of environmental properties and tendencies allows for their use in a pathological environment (i.e., the exosomes will not yield to the inflammatory environment common to degenerative disease states).[101] MSCs-derived EV have been shown to confer a number of favorable effects in preclinical models of OA, joint inflammation, and cartilage injury. EV enhanced cartilage metabolism and reduced inflammation in vitro, and preserved cartilage and prevented the advancement of OA in mice after joint injury.[102,103] EV demonstrated immunomodulatory and chondro-protective effects in vitro, as well as reducing cartilage degradation and anti-inflammatory tendencies in in vivo mice models of OA.[104–106] The use of EV in both rat and rabbit models of cartilage and osteochondral injury demonstrated significant defect repair as evidenced by the formation of hyaline-like collagen type II cartilage.[107–109]

Lui et al. studied the effects of exosome-mediated delivery of opioid receptor mu small-interfering RNA (siRNA) for the treatment of morphine relapse in vivo and in vitro and morphine relapse in mice. Results demonstrated that the exosomes delivered the opioid receptor mu (MOR) siRNA into the brain and successfully inhibited morphine relapse via the downregulation of opioid receptor mu expression levels. While more studies are needed, this could revolutionize the treatment of morphine, fentanyl, and methadone addiction.[110]

Exosomes hold promise for many degenerative conditions. Currently, human studies are underway using exosomes for conditions including cancer, diabetes, and wound healing. The current FDA position regarding exosomes is that due to their manipulation, they are considered a drug and are not permissible in clinical practice at this time. However, due to their standardization abilities and acellular nature, they may be the gateway to many FDA-approved products in the regenerative medicine sector.

In summary, the regenerative medicine sector will soon have an impact on pain management. There is an abundance of evidence that demonstrates both safety and efficacy with the use of stem cells for pain. Indeed, controlled studies are still needed, yet the evidence is relatively clear that stem cells help to decrease pain and improve quality of life for many. It remains to be seen if there will be large-scale controlled studies in the near future and what the FDA's position will be on the use of cells for pain management.

REFERENCES

1. Navani A. et al. Responsible, safe, and effective use of biologics in the management of low back pain: American Society of Interventional Pain Physicians (ASIPP) guidelines. *Pain Phys* 2019; 22(1S): S1–S74.
2. Caplan A.I., Sorrell J.M. The MSC curtain that stops the immune system. *Immunol Lett* 2015; 168(2): 136–9. http://dx.doi.10.1016/j.imlet.2015.06.005.
3. Caplan A.I., Hariri R. Body management: mesenchymal stem cells control the internal Regenerator. *Stem Cells Transl Med* 2015; 4(7): 695–701.
4. Murphy M.B., Moncivais K., Caplan A.I. Mesenchymal stem cells: environmentally responsive therapeutics for regenerative medicine. *Exp Mol Med* 2013; 45(11): e54.
5. Caplan A.I. MSCs: the sentinel and safe-guards of injury. *J Cell Physiol* 2016; 231(7): 1413–6. doi:10.1002/jcp.25255.
6. Dominici M. et al. Minimal criteria for defining multipotent mesenchymal stromal cells. The International Society for Cellular Therapy position statement. *Cytotherapy* 2006; 8(4): 315–17.
7. Pittenger M.E. et al. Multilineage potential of adult human mesenchymal stem cells. *Science* 1999; 284(5411): 143–7.
8. Watson L., Elliman S.J., Coleman C.M. From isolation to implantation: a concise review of mesenchymal stem cell therapy in bone fracture repair. *Cell Res Ther* 2014; 5(2): 51.
9. Sugaya H. et al. Comparative analysis of cellular and growth factor composition in bone marrow aspirate concentrate and platelet rich plasma. *Bone Marrow Res* 2018; 2018: 1549826. doi:10.1155/2018/1549826.
10. Schäfer R. et al. Quantitation of progenitor cell populations and growth factors after bone marrow aspirate concentration. *J Transl Med* 2019; 17(1): 115.
11. Friedlaender G.E., Lin S., Solchaga L.A., Snel L.B., Lynch S.E. The role of recombinant human platelet-derived growth factor-BB in orthopedic bone repair and regeneration. *Curr Pharm Des* 2013; 19(19): 3384–90.
12. Holmes K., Roberts O.L., Thomas A.M., Cross M.J. Vascular endothelial growth factor receptor-2 structure, function, intracellular signaling and therapeutic inhibition. *Cell Signal* 2007; 19(10): 2003–12.
13. Zuk P.A. et al. Multilineage cells from human adipose tissue: implications for cell-based therapies. *Tissue Eng* 2001; 7(2): 211–29.
14. Rodbell M., Jones A.B. Metabolism of isolated fat cells III: the similar inhibitory action of phospholipase C and of insulin on lipolysis stimulated by lipolytic hormones and theophylline. *J Biol Chem* 1996; 241(1): 140–2.
15. Zimmerlin L., Donnenberg V.S., Rubin J.P., Donnenberg A.D. Mesenchymal markers on human adipose stem/progenitor cells. *Cytom A* 2013; 83(1): 134–40.
16. Sumi M., Sata M., Toya N., Yanaga K., Ohki T., Nagai R. Transplantation of adipose stromal cells but not mature adipocytes, augments ischemia-induced angiogenesis. *Life Sci* 2007; 80(6): 559–65.
17. Tiemessen M.M., Jagger A.L., Evans H.G., van Herwijnen M.J., John S., Taams L.S. CD4+CD25+Foxp3+regulatory T cells induce alternative activation of human monocytes/macrophages. *Proc Natl Acad Sci USA* 2007; 104(49): 19446–51.
18. Eckes B., Nischt R., Krieg T. Cell-matrix interactions in dermal repair and scarring. *Fibrogenes Tiss Rep* 2010; 3: 4.
19. Guo J. et al. Stromal vascular fraction: a regenerative reality? Part 2: mechanisms of regenerative action. *J Plast Reconstr Surg* 2016; 69(2): 180–8. doi:10.1016/j.bjps.2015.10.014.
20. Bourin P. et al. Stromal cells from the adipose tissue-derived stromal vascular fraction and culture-expanded adipose tissue-derived stromal/stem cells: a joint statement of IFATS and ISCT. *Cytotherapy* 2013; 15(6): 641–8.
21. Hager G. et al. Three specific antigens to isolate endothelial progenitor cells from human liposuction material. *Cytotherapy* 2013; 15(11): 1426–35.

22. Bianchi F. et al. A new nonenzymatic method and device to obtain a fat tissue derivative highly enriched in pericyte-like elements by mild mechanical forces from human lipoaspirates. *Cell Transpl* 2013; 22(11): 2063–77.

23. Corselli M. et al. Identification of perivascular mesenchymal stromal/stem cells by flow cytometry. *Cytom A* 2013; 83(8): 714–20.

24. Traktuev D.O. et al. A population of multipotent CD34-positive adipose stromal cells share pericyte and mesenchymal surface markets, reside in periendothelial location, and stabilize endothelial netoworks. *Circ Res* 2008; 102(1): 77–85.

25. Eto H. et al. Characterization of human adipose tissue-resident hematopoietic cell populations reveals novel macrophage subpopulation with CD34 expression and mesenchymal multipotency. *Stem Cells Dev* 2013; 22(6): 985–97.

26. Echeverry S., Shi X.Q., Haw A., Liu H., Zhang Z.W., Zhang J. Transforming growth factor beta-1 impairs neuropathic pain through pleiotropic effects. *Mol Pain* 2009; 5: 16.

27. Chen N.F. et al. TGF-beta-1 attenuates spinal neuro-inflammation and the excitatory amino acid system in rates with neuropathic pain. *J Pain* 2013; 14: 671–85.

28. Lantero A., Tramullas M., Díaz A., Hurlé M.A. Transforming growth factor-beta in normal nociceptive processing and pathological pain models. *Mol Neurobiol* 2012; 45(1): 76–86.

29. Li J. et al. Interleukin-10 beta pretreated bone marrow stromal cells alleviate neuropathic pain through CCL7-mediated inhibition of microglial activation in the spinal cord. *Sci Rep* 2017; 7: 12260.

30. Sala E. et al. Mesenchymal stem cells reduce colitis in mice via release of TSG-6, independently of their localization to the intestine. *Gastroenterology* 2015; 149(1): 163–76.

31. Lu S. et al. Adipose-derived mesenchymal stem cells protect PC12 cells from glutamate excitotoxicity-induced apoptosis by upregulation of XIAP through P13-K/Akt activation. *Toxicology* 2011; 279(1–3): 189–95.

32. Okunishi K. et al. Hepatocyte growth factor significantly suppresses collagen-induced arthritis in mice. *J Immunol* 2007; 179(8): 5504–13.

33. Benkhoucha M. et al. Hepatocyte growth factor inhibits CNS autoimmunity by inducing tolerogenic dendritic cells and CD25+Foxp3+regulatory T cells. *Proc Natl Acad Sci USA* 2007; 107(14): 6424–9.

34. Rosenberg G.A. Matrix metalloproteinases in neuroinflammation. *Glia* 2002; 39(3): 279–91.

35. Kawasaki Y. et al. Distinct roles of matrix metalloproteases in the early- and late-phase development of neuropathic pain. *Nat Med* 2008; 14(3): 331–6.

36. Kerstman E., Ahn S., Battu S., Tariq S., Grabois M. Neuropathic pain. *Handb Clin Neurol* 2013; 110: 175–87.

37. Liu W. et al. Autologous bone marrow-derived stem cells for treating diabetic neuropathy in metabolic syndrome. *Hindawi Bio Med Res Int* 2017; 2017: 8945310. doi:10.1155/2017/8945310.

38. Kim H. et al. Bone marrow mononuclear cells have neurovascular tropism and improve diabetic neuropathy. *Stem Cells* 2009; 27(7): 1686–96.

39. Venturi M., Boccasanta P., Lombardi B., Brambilla M., Avesani E., Vergani C. Pudendaal Neuralgia: a new option for treatment? Preliminary results on feasibility and efficacy. *Pain Med* 2015; 16(8): 1475–81.

40. Vickers E.R., Karsten E., Flood J., Lilischkis R. A preliminary report on stem cell therapy for neuropathic pain in humans. *J Pain Res* 2014; 4(7): 255–63.

41. Mao H. et al. Efficacy of autologous bone marrow mononuclear cell transplantation therapy in patients with refractory diabetic peripheral neuropathy. *Chin Med J (Engl)* 2019; 132(1): 11–6.

42. Sanapati J. et al. Do regenerative medicine therapies provide long-term relief in chronic low back pain: a systematic review and metaanalysis. *Pain Phys* 2018; 21(6): 515–40.

43. Zhang J. et al. Molecular factors in intervertebral disc degeneration. *J Am Acad Reg Med* 2017; 1: 7203.

44. Oehme D., Goldschlager T., Ghosh P., Rosenfeld J., Jenkin G. Cell-based therapies used to treat lumbar degenerative disease a systematic review of animal studies and human clinical trials. *Stem Cells Int* 2015; 2015: 946031.

45. Mochida J., Sakai D., Nakamura Y., Watanabe T., Yamamoto Y., Kato S. Intervertebral disc repair with activated nucleus pulposus cell transplantation: a three-year, prospective clinical study of its safety. *Eur Cells Mater* 2015; 29: 202–12.

46. Orozco L., Soler R., Morera C., Alberca M., Sánchez A., García-Sancho J. Intervertebral disc repair by autologous mesenchymal bone marrow cells: a pilot study. *Transplantation* 2011; 92(7): 822–8.

47. Pettine K., Suzuki R., Sand T., Murphy M. Treatment of discogenic back pain with autologous bone marrow concentrate injections with minimum two-year follow-up. *Int Ortho* 2016; 40(1): 135–40.

48. Pettine K.A., Suzuki R.K., Sand T.T., Murphy M.B. Autologous bone- marrow concentrate intradiscal injection for the treatment of degenerative disc disease with three-year follow-up. *Int Ortho* 2017; 41(10): 2097–103.

49. Pettine K.A., Murphy M.B., Suzuki R.K., Sand T.T. Percutaneous injection of autologous bone marrow concentrate cells significantly reduces lumbar discogenic pain through twelve months. *Stem Cells* 2015; 33(1): 146–56.

50. Noriega D.C. et al. Intervertebral disc repair by allogeneic mesenchymal bone marrow cells: a randomized controlled trial. *Transplantation* 2017; 101(8): 1945–51.

51. Coric D., Pettine K., Sumich A., Boltes M.O. Prospective study of disc repair with allogeneic chondrocytes presented at the 2012 Joint Spine Section Meeting. *J Neurosurg Spine* 2013; 18(1): 85–95.

52. Centeno C. et al. Treatment of lumbar degenerative disc disease-associated radicular pain with culture-expanded autologous mesenchymal stem cells: a pilot study on safety and efficacy. *J Transl Med* 2017; 15(1): 197.

53. Kumar H. et al. Safety and tolerability of intradiscal implantation of combined autologous adipose-derived mesenchymal stem cells and hyaluronic acid in patients with chronic discogenic low back pain: one-year follow-up of a phase I study. *Stem Cell Res Ther* 2017; 8(1): 262.

54. https://www.cdc.gov/arthritis/basics/osteoarthritis.htm.

55. Goldring M.B. Osteoarthritis and cartilage: the role of cytokines. *Curr Rheumatol Rep* 2000; 2(6): 459–65.

56. Wylde V., Hewlett S., Learmonth I.D., Dieppe P. Persistent pain after joint replacement: prevalence, sensory qualities, and postoperative determinants. *Pain* 2011; 152(3): 566–72.

57. Dimarino A.M., Caplan A.I., Bonfield T.L. Mesenchymal stem cells in tissue repair. *Front Immunol* 2013; 4: 201.

58. Yubo M., Yanyan L., Li L., Tao S., Bo L., Lin C. Clinical efficacy and safety of mesenchymal stem cell transplantation for osteoarthritis treatment: a meta-analysis. *PLoS ONE* 2017; 12(4): e0175449.

59. Centeno C.J. et al. Safety and complications reporting update on the re-implantation of culture-expanded mesenchymal stem cells using autologous platelet lysate technique. *Curr Stem Cell Res Ther* 2011; 6(4): 368–78.

60. Davatchi F., Abdollahi B.S., Mohyeddin M., Shahram F., Nikbin B. Mesenchymal stem cell therapy for knee osteoarthritis. Preliminary report of four patients. *Int J Rheum Dis* 2011; 14(2): 211–15.

61. Emadedin M. et al. Long-term follow-up of intra-articular injection of autologous mesenchymal stem cells in patients with knee, ankle, or hip osteoarthritis. *Arch Iran Med* 2015; 18(6): 336–44.

62. Orozco L. et al. Treatment of knee osteoarthritis with autologous mesenchymal stem cells: a pilot study. *Transplantation* 2013; 95(12): 1535–41.

63. Saw K.Y. et al. Articular cartilage regeneration with autologous peripheral blood stem cells versus hyaluronic acid: a randomized controlled trial. *Arthroscopy* 2013; 29(4): 684.

64. Wong K.L., Lee K.B., Tai B.C., Law P., Lee E.H., Hui J.H. Injectable cultured bone marrow-derived mesenchymal stem cells in varus knees with cartilage defects undergoing high tibial osteotomy: a prospective, randomized controlled clinical trial with two years' follow-up. *Arthroscopy* 2013; 29(12): 2020–8.

65. Kim J.D. et al. Clinical outcome of autologous bone marrow aspirates concentrate (BMAC) injection in degenerative arthritis of the knee. *Eur J Orthop Surg Traumatol* 2014; 24(8): 1505–11.

66. Soler R. et al. Final results of a phase I–II trial using ex vivo expanded autologous mesenchymal stromal cells for the treatment of osteoarthritis of the knee confirming safety and suggesting cartilage regeneration. *Knee* 2016; 23(4): 647–54.

67. Chahal J. et al. Bone marrow mesenchymal stromal cells in patients with osteoarthritis results in overall improvement in pain and symptoms and reduces synovial inflammation. *Stem Cells Transl Med* 2019; 8(8): 746–757. doi:10.1002/sctm.18-0183.

68. Lamo-Espinosa J.M. et al. Intra-articular injection of two different doses of autologous bone marrow mesenchymal stem cells versus hyaluronic acid in the treatment of knee osteoarthritis: long-term follow-up of a multicenter randomized controlled clinical trial (phaseI/II). *J Transl Med* 2018; 16(1): 213.

69. Jo C.H. et al. Intra-articular injections of mesenchymal stem cells for the treatment of osteoarthritis of the knee: a proof-of-concept clinical trial. *Stem Cells* 2014; 32(5): 1254–66.

70. Jo C.H. et al. Intra-articular injection of mesenchymal stem cells for the treatment of osteoarthritis of the knee: a two-year follow-up study. *Am J Sports Med* 2017; 45(12): 2774–83.

71. Koh Y.G., Choi Y.J. Infrapatellar fat pad--derived mesenchymal stem cell therapy for knee osteoarthritis. *Knee* 2012; 19(6): 902–7.

72. Koh Y.G., Kwon O.R., Kim Y.S., Choi Y.J. Comparative outcomes of open-wedge high tibial osteotomy with platelet rich plasma alone or in combination with mesenchymal stem cell treatment: a prospective study. *Arthroscopy* 2014; 30(11): 1453–60.

73. Pers Y.M. et al. Adipose mesenchymal stromal cell-based therapy for severe osteoarthritis of the knee: a phase I dose-escalation trial. *Stem Cells Transl Med* 2016; 5(7): 847–56.

74. Bansal H. et al. Intra-articular injection in the knee of adipose derived stromal cells (stromal vascular fraction) and platelet rich plasma for osteoarthritis. *J Transl Med* 2017; 15(1): 141.

75. Lee W.S., Kim H.J., Kim K.I., Kim G.B., Jin W. Intra-articular injection of autologous adipose tissue-derived mesenchymal stem cells for the treatment of knee osteoarthritis: a phase IIb, randomized, placebo-controlled clinical trial. *Stem Cells Transl Med* 2019; 8(6): 504–11. doi:10.1002/sctm.18-0122. Epub ahead of print.

76. Freitag J. et al. Adipose-derived mesenchymal stem cell therapy in the treatment of knee osteoarthritis: a randomized controlled trial. *Regen Med* 2019; 14(3): 213–30 doi:10.2217//rme-2018-0161. Epub ahead of print.

77. Freitag J., Wickham J., Shah K., Tenen A. Effect of autologous adipose-derived mesenchymal stem cell therapy in the treatment of acromioclavicular joint osteoarthritis. *BMJ Case Rep* 2019; 12(2): e227865. doi:10.1136/bcr-2018-227865.

78. Bowers R.L. et al. Functional outcomes following micro-fragmented adipose tissue or bone marrow aspirate concentrate injections for symptomatic knee osteoarthritis. *Clin J Sports Med* 2018; 28: 235.

79. Vega A. et al. Treatment of knee osteoarthritis with allogeneic bone marrow mesenchymal stem cells: a randomized controlled trial. *Transplantation* 2015; 99(8): 1681–90.

80. Vangsness C.T., Farr J., Boyd J., Dellaero D.T., Mills C.R., LeRoux-Williams M. Adult human mesenchymal stem cells delivered via intra-articular injection to the knee following partial medial meniscectomy: a randomized, double-blind, controlled study. *J Bone Joint Surg Am* 2014; 96(2): 90–8.

81. Matas J. et al. Umbilical cord-derived mesenchymal stromal cells (MSCs) for knee osteoarthritis: repeated MSC dosing is superior to a single MSC dose and to hyaluronic acid in a controlled randomized phase I/II trial. *Stem Cells Transl Med* 2019; 8(3): 215–24.

82. Van den Beuken-van Everdingen M.H., Hochstenbach L.M., Joosten E.A., Tjan-Heijnen V.C., Janssen D.J. Update on prevalence of pain in patients with cancer: systemic review and meta-analysis. *J Pain Symptom Manag* 2016; 51(6): 1070–90.

83. Prakash M.D., Miller S., Randall-Demllo S., Nurgali K. Mesenchymal stem cell treatment of inflammation-induced cancer. *Inflamm Bowel Dis* 2016; 22(11): 2694–703.

84. Karroub A.E. et al. Mesenchymal stem cells within tumor stroma promote breast cancer metastasis. *Nature* 2007; 49: 557–63.

85. Sun Y., Tian Y., Haifeng L., Zhang D., Sun Q. Antinociceptive effect of intrathecal injection of genetically engineered human bone marrow stem cells expressing the human proenkephalin gene in rat model of bone cancer pain. *Pain Res Manag* 2017; 2017: 7346103.

86. Headache Classification Committee of International Headache Society, 2013. Available at: https://ichd-3.org/.

87. Samsam M. Central nervous system acting drugs in treatment of migraine headache. *Cent Nerv Syst Agents Med Chem* 2012; 12(3): 158–72.

88. Georgin-Lavialle S., Gaillard R., Moura D., Hermine O. Mastoytosis in adulthood and neuropsychiatric disorders. *Transl Res* 2016; 174: 77–85.

89. Cheng J., Korte N., Nortley R., Sethi H., Tang Y., Attwell D. Targeting pericytes for therapeutic approaches to neurological disorders. *Acta Neuropathol* 2018; 136(4): 507–23.

90. Bernstein C., Burstein R. Sensitization of the trigeminovascular pathway: perspective and implications to migraine pathophysiology. *J Clin Neurol* 2012; 8(2): 89–99.

91. Bright R., Bright M., Bright P., Hayne S., Thomas W. Migraine and tension-type headache treated with stromal vascular fraction: a case series. *J Med Case Rep* 2014; 7: 255–63.

92. Mauskop A., Rothaus K. Stem cells in the treatment of refractory chronic migraines. *Case Rep Neurol* 2017; 9(2): 149–55.

93. Hua Z. et al. Mesenchymal stem cells reversed morphine tolerance and opioid-induced hyperalgesia. *Sci Rep* 2016; 6: 32096. doi:10.1038/sreps32096.

94. Ferrini F. et al. Morphine hyperalgesia gated through microglia-mediated disruption of neuronal CI(-) homeostasis. *Nat Neurosci* 2013; 16(2): 183–92.

95. Li F., Liu L.P., Cheng K., Chen Z., Cheng J. The use of stem cell therapy to reverse opioid tolerance. *Clin Pharmacol Ther* 2018; 103(6): 971–4.

96. Théry C. et al. Minimal information for studies of extracellular vesicles 2018 (MISEV2018): a position statement of the International Society for extracellular Vesicles and update of the MISEV2014 guidelines. *J Extracell Vesicles* 2018; 7(1): 1535750.

97. Lamichhane T.N., Sokic S., Schardt J.S., Raiker R.S., Lin J.W., Jay S.M. Emerging roles for extracellular vesicles in tissue engineering and regenerative medicine. *Tissue Eng B* 2015; 21(1): 45–54.

98. Edgar J.R. Q&A: what are exosomes, exactly? *BMC Biol* 2016; 14: 46.

99. Rani S., Ryan A.E., Griffin M.D., Ritter T. Mesenchymal stem cell-derived extracellular vesicles: toward cell-free therapeutic applications. *Mol Ther* 2015; 23(5): 812–23.

100. Bjørge I.M., Kim S.Y., Mano J.F., Kalionis B., Chrzanowski W. Extracellular vesicles, exosomes, and shedding vesicles in regenerative medicine - a new paradigm for tissue repair. *Biomater Sci* 2017; 6(1): 60–78.

101. Li J.J., Hosseini-Beheshti E., Grau G.E., Zreiqat H., Little C.B. Stem cell-derived extracellular vesicles for treating joint injury and osteoarthritis. *Nanomaterials* 2019; 9(2): 261. doi:10.3390/nano9020261.

102. Tao S.C., Yuan T., Zhang Y.L., Yin W.J., Guo S.C., Zhang C.Q. Exosomes derived from the miR-140-5p-over-expressing human synovial mesenchymal stem cells enhance cartilage tissue regeneration and prevent osteoarthritis of the knee in a rat model. *Theranostics* 2017; 7(1): 180–95.

103. Vonk L.A. et al. Mesenchymal stromal/stem cell-derived extracellular vesicles promote human cartilage regeneration in vitro. *Theranostics* 2018; 8(4): 906–20.

104. Cosenza S. et al. Mesenchymal stem cells-derived exosomes are more immunosuppressive than microparticles in inflammatory arthritis. *Theranostics* 2018; 8(5): 1399–410.

105. Headland S.E. et al. Neutrophil-derived microvesicles enter cartilage and protect the joint in inflammatory arthritis. *Sci Transl Med* 2015; 7(315): 315ra190.

106. Lo Sicco C. et al. Mesenchymal stem cell-derived extracellular vesicles as mediators of anti-inflammatory effects: endorsement of macrophage polarization. *Stem Cells Transl Med* 2017; 6(3): 1018–28.

107. Lui X. et al. Integrations of stem cell-derived exosomes with in situ hydrogel glue as a promising tissue path for articular cartilage generation. *Nanoscale* 2017; 4: 4430–8.

108. Zhang S., Chu W.C., Lai R.C., Lim S.K., Hui J.H.P., Toh W.S. Exosomes derived from human embryonic mesenchymal stem cells promote osteochondral regeneration. *Osteoarthr Cartil* 2016; 24(12): 2135–40.

109. Zhang S., Chuah S.J., Lai R.C., Hui J.H.P., Lim S.K., Toh W.S. Mesenchymal stem cell exosomes mediate cartilage repair by enhancing proliferation, attenuating apoptosis, and modulating immune reactivity. *Biomaterials* 2018; 156: 16–27.

110. Yuchen L. et al. Targeted exosome-mediated delivery of opioid receptor Mu siRNA for the treatment of morphine relapse. *Sci Rep* 2015; 5: 17543. doi:10.1038/srep17543.

14 Adenine Dinucleotide
Past, Present, and Future

Richard F. Mestayer, III and Hyla Cass

CONTENTS

INTRODUCTION

The focus of this chapter will be on the use of intravenous nicotinamide adenine dinucleotide (NAD+), or DPN, as it was called in the older literature, and its clinical uses to date. Although there is additional, voluminous research being conducted on oral preparations of NAD+, these studies are excluded for the most part from this summary.

HISTORICAL PERSPECTIVE ON NAD+

In 2000, if someone did a search of the medical literature for information on nicotinamide adenine dinucleotide (NAD+), a particular coenzyme of niacin, they would have found maybe three or four articles. Conduct the same Medline search today, and you'd find literally hundreds. The explosion of interest in this particular molecule was highlighted in 2013, when David Sinclair published his work with mice showing a potential anti-aging effect using a precursor to NAD+ called NMN. But NAD+—or its more famous precursor, niacin—actually has a longer history in the annals of medicine, dating back to the pellagra epidemic of the early 1900s, which lasted for four decades in the United States.

According to Alfred J. Bollet, writing in the *Yale Medical Journal of Biology and Medicine*,[1] Pellagra was a new disease to American physicians when the first cases began to be reported. A single case in a Georgia farmer in 1902 was reported to the state Medical Association[2] and attributed to spoiled corn, but it attracted little interest. In 1906, Dr. George H. Searcy recognized pellagra at the Mount Vernon annex to the Bryce Hospital for Alabama Insane in Tuscaloosa. He described

88 cases, with a mortality rate of 64%, in the Alabama state medical journal in 1907[3] and in JAMA in 1907.[4]

The disease had first been described long before, however, in 1735 in Spain, where it was characterized by "the four Ds": dermatitis, especially a reddish-glossy rash on the dorsum of the hands and feet; diarrhea; dementia; and eventually, death.

Between 1906 and 1940, more than 3 million Americans—predominantly poor residents of the rural South—were affected by pellagra and more than 100,000 of its sufferers died. In 1915, an epidemiologist with the U.S. Public Health Service, Dr. Joseph Goldberger, discovered that the epidemic was linked to diet—and could be entirely remediated by adding fresh animal foods and a variety of green vegetables in place of the heavy reliance on corn by poor rural Americans.

The year following his study, only one of the original 172 patients met the criteria for diagnosis of pellagra. Dr. Goldberger was convinced diet played a major role, and additional studies showed that there was "a pellagra prevention" (PP) factor related to diet. Unfortunately, Dr. Goldberger died before the "PP" factor was identified by Conrad Elvehjem, an American agricultural chemist who identified two vitamins—nicotinic acid, also known as niacin, and nicotinamide—which were highly effective in curing black tongue in dogs,[5] a disease analogous to pellagra in humans. When clinical trials were conducted with humans, the elusive "PP" factor was identified as nicotinic acid.

The first report of NAD+'s use in treating addiction came in 1948, when Italian professor Paolo Ottenello published his findings in *Minerva Medica* that an intravenous injection of nicotinamide (1 g) and thiamine (25 mg) twice a day to morphine addicts and alcoholics enabled them to detox painlessly.[6]

A few years later, in 1954, Abram Hoffer, a Canadian biochemist and psychiatrist, became the first person to study the use of NAD+ (then called DPN, an acronym for diphosphopyridine nucleotide). Dr. Hoffer and his colleagues administered NAD+ and vitamin C to schizophrenics at the state hospital and reported that symptoms were reduced to the point that some no longer needed hospitalization. Moreover, those who were also alcoholics were able to quit drinking as a result of the treatment.[7] Apparently, patients who were unable to continue receiving the special NAD preparations experienced a relapse in symptoms, resulting in their return to the hospital.

Hoffer and his associates then published the first double-blind study of their treatment outcomes in the *American Journal of Psychiatry*, prompting additional studies and reports on niacin therapy for addiction by at least three other groups, including Russell Smith's work over 5 years with 500 alcoholic Catholic priests, 50% to 60% of whom had positive results.[8]

In the late 1950s, Dr. Paul O'Holleran, working at Seattle's Shick-Shadell Hospital, used an intravenous infusion of DPN (NAD+) to painlessly detox more than 11,000 alcoholics and more than 100 people addicted to various drugs with the exception of nicotine. Publishing his findings in the *Western Journal of Obstetrics and Gynecology* in 1961, he detailed to some degree his uses of intravenous DPN and thereafter obtained patents on the use of IV DPN in alcoholism, drug addiction, and schizophrenia. Several years later, an interesting monograph published in a United Nations periodical highlighted O'Holleran's work, and pointed out its parallels with the work of a compound discovered in Germany called methadone and its uses in treating drug addiction.[9] Thereafter, the use of oral methadone gained prominence and the use of intravenous detox treatments declined, never gaining traction in the United States or Europe.

However, in 1967 a South African researcher, Dr. J.P. Verster, wrote an article about the use of intravenous DPN in that country,[10] which was followed by a great deal of research as well as use of NAD+ in addiction treatment in South Africa. Verster's work was summarized by Dr. Theo Verwey in his book, *NAD+ Therapy: Too Good to be True?*[11] In his book, Verwey documented the use of intravenous NAD+ in some 20,000 patients treated for addiction and reported no significant side effects in that use. His only caution with the use of IV NAD+ was in those individuals with Gilbert's disease, a liver disease affecting bilirubin function. To this day intravenous NAD+ is used in South Africa to detox addiction patients.

In the 1980s, American physician William Hitt founded a clinic in Mexico to treat addiction, autoimmune disorders, allergies, and viruses with an intravenous delivery of various vitamins and amino acids prescribed for "neurotransmitter rebalancing." The active ingredient in this therapy was later identified as NAD+. The Hitt Center's detoxification protocol closely resembled the DPN therapy developed by Dr. Paul O'Halloren at Shick-Shadel Hospital and supported a rapid detox from alcohol, prescription, and illicit drugs. The treatment used no benzodiazepines or opiates to combat withdrawal symptoms and, over the years, boasted low rates of recidivism.

WHAT IS THE ROLE OF NAD+ IN THE BODY?

Figure 14.1 shows what we know of the many functions that NAD+ performs in healthy cells. NAD+ is essential in cell energy production—without which cells cannot do their work. It is involved in DNA repair and gene expression—the process by which genes are turned on and off. It is included in cell signaling, immune function, and the production of vital enzymes. It probably is involved in increasing the length of telomeres, which has anti-aging benefits. NAD+ is also thought to be a neurotransmitter. Any one of these functions would make NAD+ necessary, but the fact that NAD+ is involved in so many of them highlights the significance of this molecule and shows that prolonged depleted NAD+ levels can have profound health consequences. By the same token, as many of these functions consume NAD+, it is easy to see how, with accumulating stress, age, illness, and other factors, NAD+ levels can become depleted. Just how the body prioritizes which NAD+ functions it will carry out if levels are insufficient for them all is a fertile area for additional research.

CURRENT CLINICAL APPLICATIONS OF INTRAVENOUS NAD+

At Springfield Wellness Center, located in Springfield, Louisiana, psychotherapist Paula Norris Mestayer and Dr. Richard Mestayer developed the American protocols for intravenous use of NAD+ to treat addiction, alcoholism, depression, post-traumatic stress disorder (PTSD), and even neurodegenerative diseases such as Alzheimer's, Parkinson's, and CTE. However, because the preponderance of their experience with intravenous NAD+ in the treatment of addiction and alcoholism, we are confining our remarks to this application.

What is NAD+ Used for?

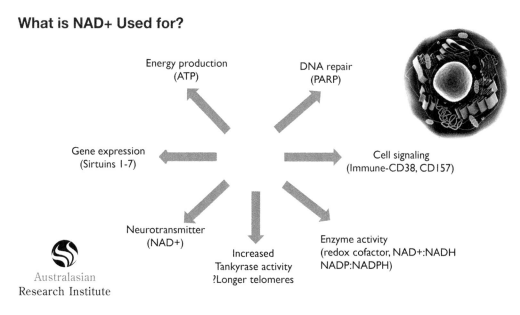

FIGURE 14.1   What is NAD+ used for?

NAD Reduces Cravings

Intravenous Administration of Nicotinamide Adenine Dinucleotide Significantly Reduces Self Report Craving Ratings Associated with Opiate and Alcohol Withdrawal

*S. L. BROOM[1], R. MESTAYER[2], E. STULLER[3], D. COOK[4], J. CARSON[2], K. SIMONE[2], P. NORRIS[2], P. HOTARD[2]
[1]Dept Psychol, William Carey Univ., Hattiesburg, MS; [2]Springfield Wellness Center, Springfield, LA; [3]Stullerresettings, LLC; [4] ABAM.SoberMD,LLC

INTRODUCTION

Introduction: Treatment of substance abuse disorders continues to challenge clinicians and "cravings" for the abused substance are often impediments to sobriety. Nicotinamide Adenine Dinucleotide (NAD) has been used in the past with claims of having anti-craving properties. Previous data from this clinic using a similar formulation of NAD support the use of NAD as a valid treatment for drug cravings. *This pilot study retrospectively examined the anti-craving properties of NAD in a group of 60 patients.* Additionally, patients were assessed on severity of cravings and relapse episodes at 12-20 months post treatment.

METHOD

The patients were adult males and females with addictions to primarily opiates or alcohol (N=60). Six patients were omitted due to incomplete data. The treatment, Brain Restoration Plus (BR+)™ comprised of IV infusions of NAD as well as vitamins, oral amino acids, NAC and variable PRN medications for an average of 10 consecutive days ranging from 5 to 10 hours daily at a dose range of 500mg-1500mg each day. Self-reported craving ratings (0-10 Scale) were collected on Day 1 (before starting treatment), Day 5, and on Day 10 (last day of treatment). Follow up phone surveys were conducted from 12-20 months post treatment (N= 27). Patients reported severity of cravings (1-5) and number of relapse episodes at the present time.

RESULTS

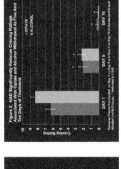

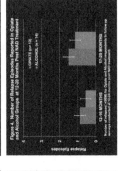

CONCLUSIONS

1) NAD is an effective detox treatment for alcohol and opiate addicts as evidenced by a significant reduction in craving ratings.

2) NAD was effective in reducing and maintaining the number of relapse episodes, as well as severity of drug cravings.

3) NAD shows potential as a long-term therapy in maintaining sobriety through minimizing drug cravings and preventing relapse.

ACKNOWLEDGMENTS

Thank you to Springfield Wellness Center for providing patient data. Thank you to William Carey University for providing a Professional Development Grant in support of this project.

FIGURE 14.2 NAD reduces cravings.

At the November 2014 Society of Neuroscience meeting in Washington, D.C., a group of Springfield Wellness colleagues presented the results of a study involving 60 adult patients (both male and female) detoxing from addiction (primarily to opiates and alcohol), who were treated over an average of 10 consecutive days with a proprietary formulation of BR+NAD™. This formulation was composed primarily of intravenous infusions of NAD+, along with oral amino acids and N-acetyl cysteine (NAC). The treatment was administered from 5 to 10 hours daily at a dose range of 500–1500 mg each day. Subjects reported that their cravings stopped or were significantly diminished by Day 2–Day 4 of treatment. Specifically, cravings dropped from an average rating of five or six (on a zero to ten scale) on Day 1 to a rating of two by Day 5 and an average of one or less by Day 10.[12]

In addition to significantly reduced cravings, study subjects also reported a dramatic reduction in withdrawal symptoms. These vary according to the addiction: for opiate withdrawal they typically include nausea, vomiting, and muscle spasms; for alcohol withdrawal tremors (DTs), and for crystal meth withdrawal the primary symptom is deep depression. They generalized from their experience with these and more than 1000 other patients that withdrawal symptoms are reduced by 60 to 75%. They have found this to be true no matter what patients have been addicted to—even methadone or Suboxone.

Intravenous NAD+ treatment for addiction also appears to be effective in reducing or eliminating post-acute withdrawal syndrome (PAWS), which, along with cravings, is a common reason for relapse. While PAWS can complicate opiate withdrawal for a year or more under conventional addiction treatment protocols, NAD+ detox treatment appears to *eliminate* PAWS initially and, if patients feel a return, they can be effectively re-treated for a day or two, after which PAWS again subside (Figure 14.2).

In addition to intravenous NAD treatment for addiction detox and PAWS remediation, we have utilized oral NAD supplements, nasal sprays, patches, and creams to extend the NAD boost provided intravenously. Moreover, although excellent research is now being done by David Sinclair and others on the role of NAD precursors such as NMN[13] in boosting cellular NAD levels, thus far intravenous NAD has given our patients the most robust clinical response.

Basic Research into the Mechanisms of NAD+ Effectiveness

Although the clinical results of intravenous NAD+ therapy for addiction detox are now well-established, the biochemical mechanisms for its effectiveness are still being studied.

Dr. James Watson is a well-respected surgeon on the clinical faculty of UCLA Medical School as well as the author of a website and blog on the molecular biology of aging.[14] As a result of his own research into NAD+, Dr. Watson was selected as one of the keynote speakers at the first 2015 Brain Restoration Summit, where he presented his analysis that the same processes that overwhelm the body's stress response systems and result in the degeneration associated with aging are also implicated in the disease of addiction.

In his summit presentation, Dr. Watson outlined three factors responsible for addiction: genetics (DNA), epigenetics (DNA regulation), and environment. Genes that have been identified as potential risk factors for addiction include those responsible for the brain's "reward" pathway, those responsible for ethanol (alcohol) stimulation or depression, those responsible for the "relief" pathway, and more.

Epigenetics (DNA regulation), though inherited, are also influenced by environmental factors such as stress, aging, disease, and drug use, that can turn gene expression off and on.

The third factor in addiction is environmental. A healthy diet plus regular exercise, for example, can confer positive epigenetic changes; whereas regular alcohol consumption, trauma, toxins, illness, or chronic stress adversely impacts a number of genetic switches.

Together, these three factors—genetics, epigenetics, and environment—could result in addiction due to the functioning of a single molecule: **NAD+.**

NAD+ plays a critical role in all three addiction risk factors, Watson explained. It repairs DNA, which can be damaged by oxidative stress, including drug use. It restores healthy epigenetic functioning—the turning off of epigenetic risk factors related to addiction—and it restores the brain to healthy functioning—including dopamine and endorphin production—so that the addict doesn't need a drug to get midbrain relief. Watson calls this the gene–environmental interaction (GEI or GXE). The environmental factor of oxidative stress triggers the epigenetic factor to turn on the expression of the genetic factor (DNA).

Watson notes that, although NAD+ is not the only epigenetic mechanism at the body's disposal, it *is* involved in several of the pathways implicated in addiction. His analysis also helps to explain how and why intravenous NAD+ given to detoxing patients confers such positive and immediate results: it starts to return the body to normal functioning, with positive genes turned on, negative genes turned off, oxidative stress better managed, mitochondrial energy production returned to normal, and DNA under repair.

Another research team, led by Corinne Lasmézas, has underscored the importance of NAD+ in DNA repair. Lasmézas and colleagues at the Scripps Research Institute showed that depletion of NAD+ drives neuronal death.[15]

Another research team, at the Linus Pauling Institute, Oregon State University, summarized some of the various implications of niacin—and its co-enzyme, NAD+—deficiency. Most notably, they wrote, "NAD+ is the sole substrate for PARP enzymes involved in DNA repair activity in response to DNA strand breaks; thus, NAD+ is critical for genome stability."[16]

Yet another researcher, Dr. Ross Grant of the University of New South Wales School of Medical Sciences, has published more than 50 papers on NAD+ metabolism—particularly NAD+'s role in aging and oxidative stress. His research shows that NAD+ levels in our bodies decline with age, triggering changes in certain genetic functions associated with maintaining cell health.[17]

Still other researchers are investigating the role of NAD+ in DNA repair—an ongoing process given the constant onslaught our bodies are subjected to via stress, environmental toxins, EMFs and RFs, poor diet, and more.

Human trials on NAD+ are underway around the world. These clinical trials are being led by Dr. Grant in Sydney, Australia; the staff at Springfield Wellness Center; Dr. David Lefer, Dr. David Polhemus, and Dr. Tom Sharp through NAD+ Research, Inc., and scientists at many other institutions.

For example, pilot studies conducted by NAD Research, Inc., in collaboration with Dr. Ross Grant, Dr. Jade Berg, and Nady Braidy, PhD, at the Australasian Research Institute, show that intravenous BR+NAD™ treatment reduces biomarkers reflective of inflammation in both alcohol and opiate detox patients, while increasing NAD+ levels and improving the NAD+/NADH ratio in plasma, which increases NAD+ effectiveness.

THE EFFECT OF ALCOHOL ON NAD+ LEVELS AND MARKERS FOR INFLAMMATION AND OXIDATIVE STRESS

Figure 14.3 shows that alcohol consumption greater than one drink/day decreases levels of NAD+ in the brain and increases inflammation as measured by readings of cerebrospinal fluid. With an intake greater than one alcoholic drink/day, average cerebrospinal NAD+ levels begin to drop, while cerebrospinal fluid levels of interleukin-6 (IL-6), which is a marker for inflammation, begin to rise. Alcohol's effect on both NAD+ levels and inflammation in the cerebrospinal fluid is likely reflective of NAD+ activity in the brain.

NAD+'S EFFECTIVENESS AT REDUCING INFLAMMATION AND OXIDATIVE STRESS LEVELS IN ADDICTION PATIENTS

Figure 14.4 shows the results of a pilot study that compared NAD+ plasma levels in 30 healthy participants with NAD+ plasma levels in 26 alcohol patients and 19 opiate patients, matched by age and gender. At the study's outset, levels of 8-isoprostane, a biomarker for oxidative stress, are higher in the addiction patients—both the alcohol and the opiate patients. After four days of intravenous BR+NAD™ therapy, another reading of plasma levels begins showing a dramatic reduction in the

Alcohol ↓ brain NAD⁺ & ↑ inflam.

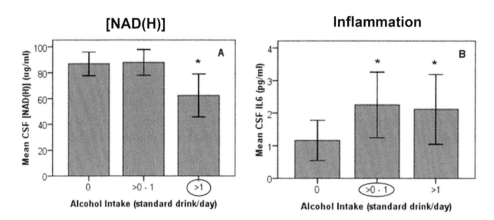

FIGURE 14.3 Alcohol consumption.

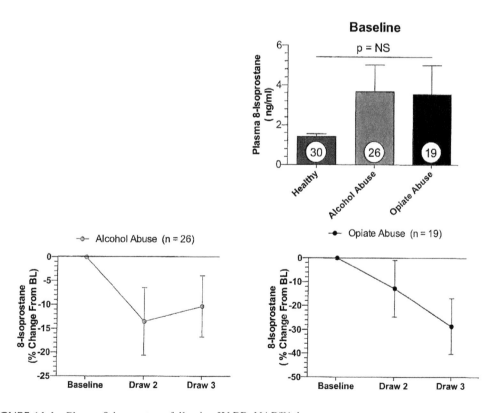

FIGURE 14.4 Plasma 8-isoprostane following IV BR+NAD™ therapy.

oxidative stress marker in both the alcohol patients and the opiate patients. For opiate patients, the levels of 8-isoprostane continue to drop all the way to the last day of treatment, while the decline of the oxidative stress marker tends to level off after Day 8, 9, or 10. This is a significant finding that warrants further research.

INTRAVENOUS NAD+ INFUSION REDUCES A SECOND MARKER FOR INFLAMMATION AND OXIDATIVE STRESS IN ADDICTION PATIENTS

The results from this pilot study show that levels of plasma TNF-alpha, a biomarker for inflammation and oxidative stress, are higher in alcohol and opiate patients than in healthy patients, and higher in alcohol patients than opiate patients (Figure 14.5).

It also shows that TNF-alpha levels respond positively following 4 days of intravenous BR+NAD™ therapy. The slide also indicates that for alcohol patients the drop in TNF-alpha tends to level off by the third draw, which is on Day 8, 9, or 10. In the opiate patients, however, we see a continued drop in TNF-alpha on the third draw, which is at the end of the BR+NAD™ treatment. It's interesting that, here again, we see two different patterns of reduction, which is seen in the 8-isoprostane level drops. In both cases, we've shown that intravenous NAD+ does help reduce markers of inflammation.

INTRAVENOUS BR+NAD™ INFUSIONS INCREASE THE NAD+/ NADH RATIO IN ALCOHOL ABUSE PATIENTS

Figure 14.6 again shows pilot data of the response to intravenous BR+NAD™ in 19 subjects treated for alcohol abuse. What's significant in this diagram, in addition to the rise in NAD+ plasma levels after 4 days of treatment, is a higher NAD+/NADH ratio, which suggests that better utilization of NAD+ will occur. Again, this warrants additional research to be followed up in clinical trials.

INTRAVENOUS BR+NAD™ INFUSIONS INCREASE THE NAD+/ NADH RATIO IN PATIENTS ADDICTED TO OPIATES

As in the previous diagram, Figure 14.7 shows pilot data of the response to intravenous BR+NAD™ for 17 subjects treated for opiate addiction. After 4 days of intravenous BR+NAD+™ treatment,

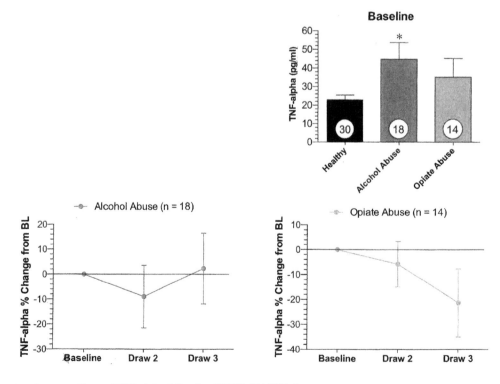

FIGURE 14.5   Plasma TNF-alpha following IV BR+NAD™ therapy.

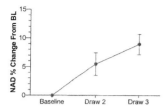
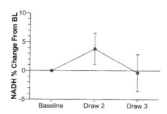
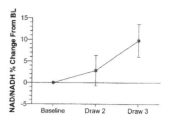

FIGURE 14.6 Response to intravenous BR+NAD™ therapy in subjects treated for alcohol abuse. (n=19 subjects.)

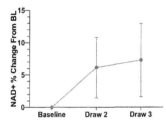
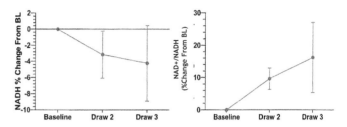

FIGURE 14.7 Response to intravenous BR+NAD™ therapy in subjects treated for opiate abuse. (n=17 subjects.)

NAD+ levels have risen in plasma; NADH levels have dropped; and the ratio of NAD+/NADH has increased, which we believe is significant. Again, this is unpublished pilot data, which could be used to design a more comprehensive study.

ESTABLISHING BASELINE NAD+ LEVELS

Yet another study undertaken at NAD Research Inc., in collaboration with the Australasian Research Institute, investigated the pharmacokinetic dynamics of intravenous NAD+ in 15 healthy males age 35–55.[18] This was an IRB-approved, double-blind, placebo-controlled pharmacokinetic study to establish baseline data on the metabolism of NAD+ in healthy individuals. This information will enable us to more readily determine when NAD+ levels are deficient in others. The study included 11 healthy males who were given intravenous NAD+ and 4 who were administered saline solution. Subjects' blood levels of NAD+ and its metabolites were monitored over time. The study's final conclusions were that:

- IV NAD+ does produce a significant increase in plasma NAD+ and its metabolites after 6 hours.
- There is only a modest rise (e.g., 35%) on RBC NAD+ 6 hours after infusion.
- A plateau effect of both plasma and urine levels of NAD+ was reached after 48 hours, with no apparent increase in RBC NAD+ after Day 1.
- It is probable that significant uptake or metabolism of NAD+ in tissue occurs early (e.g., in under 1 hour).
- The fate of most of the infused NAD+ is not yet determined.

ADDITIONAL NAD RESEARCH, INC., PARTNERSHIP STUDIES UNDERWAY OR PLANNED

A second study by NAD Research, Inc., led by Susan Broom, examined the response to IV NAD+ treatment in previous patients seeking treatment for alcohol addiction, opiate addiction, and neurodegenerative disease. Armed with baselines from the pharmacokinetic studies, we are examining whether the NAD+ treatment delivered the anticipated increase in plasma NAD+ and its metabolites. Preliminary findings are promising, and final results are expected in 2019.

We are also working to establish collaborative relationships with other researchers. A recent example involves a study by the Center of Magnetic Resonance Research at the University of Minnesota Medical School to measure NAD/NADH ratios in the brain utilizing a powerful MRI technique (In Vivo NAD+ Assay – Minn MRI Study). This study, which involved but a single individual, showed a dramatic increase in ATP production from a single dose of intravenous NAD+. We are currently designing an IRB-approved study to evaluate the cellular energy levels in the brains of additional healthy volunteers following a single dose of IV NAD+.

The implications of this study could be profound. In addition to validating the clinical results we see with intravenous NAD+ in detoxing addiction patients, a dramatic increase in brain cell energy levels could explain why Alzheimer's patients show improvement following intravenous NAD+ treatment and why we see such dramatic improvements in Parkinson's, CTE, and TBI patients following intravenous NAD+.

The next clinical studies in the queue include examining the response of alcohol-addicted patients to IV NAD+ versus standard of care and examining the response of PTSD patients to IV NAD+. These studies are in the design phase and currently seeking funding.

NAD Research, Inc., is guided by a highly qualified Board of Advisors. Led by co-chairs, Dr. Krishna Doniparthi and Dr. Susan Broom, members include Dr. Ross Grant, Dr. Jade Berg, Dr. Jim Watson, Dr. Elizabeth Stuller, Dr. Ken Starr, Dr. Walker Dixon, Dr. Halland Chen, Dr. David Lefer, Dr. Tom Sharp, and Dr. Richard Mestayer.

Many paths for research have developed, and it is our hope that clinical findings regarding the myriad uses and strategies for positively impacting health by way of NAD+ will emerge. We have no doubt that there will be more than three or four articles over the next 10 years.

REFERENCES

1. Bollet Alfred J., Politics and pellagra: the epidemic of pellagra in the US in the early twentieth century.*Yale Medical Journal of Biology and Medicine*, 65, 1992, pp. 211–221.
2. Harris H.F., A case of ankylostomiasis presenting the symptoms of pellagra. *Translational Medicine Association of Georgia*, 1902, pp. 220–227.
3. Searcy G.H., An epidemic of acute pellagra. *Translator Medicine* Association *State of Alabama*, 1907, pp. 387–392.
4. Searcy G.H., An epidemic of acute pellagra. *JAMA*, 37(1), 1907, p. 49.
5. Koehn C.J., Elvehjem C.A., Further studies on the concentration of the anti-pellagra factor. *Journal of Biological Chemistry*, 118(3), 1937, pp. 693–699.
6. Ottenello P., Il Complesso aneurina-vitamina PP nella cura del morfinismo e di altre intossi-cazioni voluttuaire/The use of thiamine and niacin in the detoxification of morphine addiction. *Minerva Medica*, 1948, pp. 213–215.
7. Hoffer A., Osmond H., Smythies J., Schizophrenia: a new approach II. Results of a year's research. *Journal of Mental Science*, 100(418), 1954, pp. 29–45.
8. Smith R.F., Status report concerning the use of megadose nicotinic acid in alcoholics. *Orthomolecular Psychiatry*, 3(4), 1974.
9. Harney Malachi L., *Current Provisions and Practices in the United States of America Relating to the Commitment of Opiate Addicts.* United Nations Office on Drugs and Crime, 1962, pp. 11–23.
10. Verster J.P., Alternative treatment of problem drinkers with DPN™: a brief overview. *The Journal of Modern Pharmacy*, 2003, p. 22.
11. Verwey T., *NAD+ Therapy: Too Good to Be True?* Alkogen e-book published on the internet in 2003 and available free from many online sources, or E-Mail alkogen@global.co.za.
12. Broom S.l., Carson J., Cook D., Hotard P., Mestayer R., Norris P., Simone K., Stuller E., Intravenous administration of nicotinamide adenine dinucleotide significantly reduces self-reported craving ratings associated with opiate and alcohol withdrawal. *Society of Neuroscience Poster Presentation*, 2014.
13. Wu L.E., Sinclair D., The elusive NMN transporter is found. *Nature Metabolism*, 1(1), 2019, pp. 8–9.

14. Giulano V., Watson J., www.Anti-agingFirewalls.com.
15. Zhou M., Ottenberg G., Sferrazza G.F., Hubbs C., Fallahi M., Rumbaugh G., Brantley A.F., Lasmézas C., Neuronal death induced by misfolded prion protein is due to NAD+ depletion and can be relieved *in vitro* and *in vivo* by NAD+ replenishment. *Brain*, 138(4), 2015, pp. 992–1008.
16. Higdon J., Drake V., Delage B., Meyer-Ficca M., *Niacin*. Linus Pauling Institute Micronutrient Information Center. http://lpi.oregonstate.edu/mic/vitamins/niacin.
17. Massudi H., Grant R., Braidy N., Guest J., Farnsworth B., Guillemin G.J., Age-associated changes in oxidative stress and NAD+ metabolism in human tissue. *PLOS ONE*, 2012. http://doi.org/10.1371/journal.pone.0042357.
18. Grant R., Berg J., Mestayer R.F., Braidy N., Bennett J., Broom S., Watson J., A pilot study investigating changes in the human plasma and urine NAD+ metabolome during a 6-hour intravenous infusion of NAD+. *Frontiers in Aging Neuroscience*, 2019. https://doi.org/10.3389/fnagi.2019.00257.

15 Ketamine Use in Pain Management

Sahar Swidan and Charles E. Schultz

CONTENTS

BACKGROUND

Ketamine is an N-methyl-D-aspartate (NMDA) non-competitive receptor antagonist that acts as an analgesic agent and has notable use in anesthesia, psychiatry, and pain management, among other disease states. N-methyl-D-aspartate amplifies pain signals, the development of central sensitization, and opioid tolerance.[1] The NMDA receptor is integral in learning, memory, and synaptic plasticity.

Ketamine, a phencyclidine derivative, was developed in the 1960s and was initially used as an anesthetic agent.[1] It has been shown to have antihyperalgesic effects, which can reduce or reverse opioid tolerance. Ketamine's role in pain management is centered on its NMDA receptor antagonism. Its analgesic action is effective at sub-anesthetic doses.[1] Moreover, its analgesic properties are augmented through ketamine's anti-inflammatory effects.

MECHANISM OF ACTION

Ketamine has multiple modalities of action, but most notably, it blocks the N-methyl-D-aspartate receptor (NMDAR). The excitatory glutamatergic NMDAR receptor is expressed throughout the brain and spinal cord and is integral in the chronification of pain.[2] Ketamine is also an agonist of AMPA, GABA, cholinergic, dopaminergic, and innate repair receptors, and an antagonist of HCN1, potassium, calcium, and sodium channels.[2]

While the NMDA receptor is the primary modality for ketamine's analgesic activity, its interaction with nicotinic and muscarinic acetylcholine receptors and voltage-sensitive sodium channels enhances its endogenous antinociceptive systems, which ultimately increase the descending inhibitory serotoninergic pathway.[1] The analgesic properties of ketamine for acute pain differ from its properties for chronic pain. For chronic pain, ketamine is purported to reverse central sensitization and enhance descending modulatory pathways, requiring higher cumulative dosages. Chronic pain management with ketamine is highly correlated to its psychomimetic effects. Acute pain management with ketamine is centered on the reversible antagonism of the NMDA receptor in addition to its various other modulated receptor activities.[3]

PHARMACOKINETICS

Ketamine is a lipophilic drug that crosses the blood–brain barrier and is available as a racemic mixture or as the S(+) enantiomer. The S(+) enantiomer is twice as potent as racemic ketamine and approximately four times as potent as the R(–) enantiomer.[4] Ketamine is N-demethylated via liver microsomes into its major metabolite norketamine. Norketamine is rapidly metabolized to ketamine's primary secondary metabolite, 6 hydroxynorketamine, and to a lesser extent 4-hydroxyketamine and 6-hydroxyketamine.[1] Ketamine's half-life in plasma is approximately 2.3 ± 0.5 hours, and it is primarily eliminated in the urine, mostly as hydroxylated or conjugated norketamine metabolites. Four percent is eliminated in the urine as unchanged ketamine. Less than 5% of ketamine is eliminated in the feces. The onset of action for intravenous ketamine is 1–5 minutes and approximately 30 minutes for intranasal ketamine. The duration of action is 10–15 minutes when parenterally administered and 1 hour when given intranasally.

PAIN MANAGEMENT WITH KETAMINE

With the impending opioid crisis, the use of ketamine is an attractive choice to help mitigate overusage of opioids. The American Society of Regional Anesthesia and Pain Medicine, the American Academy of Pain Medicine, and the American Society of Anesthesiologists issued consensus guidelines in 2018 for the management of acute and chronic pain with ketamine. The guidelines focus on the optimization of acute pain management while reducing exposure to chronic opioid use after acute opioid exposure.[3] Evidence supports the use of ketamine for acute pain in a variety of contexts, including as a stand-alone treatment, as an adjunct to opioids, and, to a lesser extent, as an intranasal formulation.[5] For acute pain management, ketamine use is indicated in severe postoperative pain management (i.e., abdominal, thoracic, orthopedic surgeries). Mild pain procedures such as tonsillectomy and head and neck surgery have not shown benefit from perioperative ketamine, and so it is not recommended.[3] In terms of duration of therapy with ketamine, there are variable recommendations and future studies are needed to optimize the safety and efficacy of ketamine intranasally and intravenously for pain management. Generally, intravenous infusions are limited to 48 hours, and, if extended past this time, will require slow tapers when stopping the medication. The duration of use for intranasal ketamine has not been defined in the literature and has suboptimal evidence-based recommendations.

Additionally, acute ketamine use is indicated in opioid-tolerant or opioid-dependent patients who present for surgery or acute exacerbations of chronic conditions manifesting with uncontrolled pain. Caution must be taken in this population as most of the literature supporting the use is limited to a few randomized controlled trials. A randomized controlled trial by Loftus et al.[5] in 102 opioid-dependent patients who had spinal surgery showed reduced opioid consumption by 48 hours as well as reduced opioid usage at 6 weeks in patients who received intraoperative ketamine only. Other studies have not shown benefit in this population. To date, many of the studies have been carried out in patients undergoing spine surgery. Other types of surgeries will need to be studied to see if the use of ketamine is applicable to the general population of opioid-tolerant patients who undergo surgery and require pain management. Additional studies are also needed to better establish efficacy in opioid-tolerant patients.

Non-surgical patients who have high opioid dependence and concomitant chronic conditions such as sickle cell disease have also been studied and may benefit from the use of ketamine in pain exacerbation. Ketamine has been found to improve analgesia in both adults and children, while reducing the need for opioids.[6,7] Additional studies are needed to establish efficacy in patients with chronic conditions, such as those who are high opioid users and require pain management in the setting of disease exacerbation.

Another niche of patients who may benefit from ketamine use are patients who are at an increased risk for opioid-related respiratory depression. These patients may include those who have obstructive sleep apnea. Opioids increase the severity of obstructive sleep apnea following surgery, and ketamine may have a role in limiting opioid consumption in this setting and improving outcomes of respiratory depression in these patients.[8–11]

Overall, ketamine has a place in therapy for pain management that includes the subset of patients with chronic pain not well-controlled with conventional pain management therapies. Ketamine can also be used as a third-line adjuvant agent for opioid-resistant pain in palliative care and intractable chronic noncancer pain.[1] Evidence among acute (non-surgical) pain, chronic pain, and noncancer pain is lacking, and further research is warranted for disease-state pain management with ketamine.

DOSAGES AND ROUTES OF ADMINISTRATION

Traditionally, ketamine is administered as intravenous or intramuscular. However, alternative routes have become more widespread including oral, nasal, transdermal, subcutaneous, and rectal administration.[2] The dosages and dose ranges provided below are based on published studies and consensus guidelines. Levels of evidence for dose ranges are per consensus guidelines and in accordance with the U.S. Preventive Services Task Force grading of evidence. Levels of evidence are based on the magnitude and certainty of benefit.

INTRANASAL

Acute Pain[12–14]
0.5 to 1 mg/kg/dose; may repeat in 10 to 15 minutes with 0.25 to 0.5 mg/kg/dose.

Chronic Pain[15]
10 mg every 90 seconds as needed until a maximum dose of 50 mg is reached or pain relieved.

INTRAVENOUS

Acute Pain[3]
- Bolus dose not to exceed 0.35 mg/kg (Grade C, moderate certainty)
- Infusions not to exceed 1 mg/kg per hour without intensive monitoring (Grade C, moderate certainty)
- Doses exceeding 1 mg/kg per hour only used in rare circumstances and on a case-by-case basis

Chronic Pain[16]
- Bolus dose: up to 0.35 mg/kg. (Grade C, low certainty.)
- Infusion: 0.5 to 2 mg/kg per hour, although dosages of up to 7 mg/kg per hour have been successfully used in refractory cases in ICU settings. (Grade C, low certainty.)
- There is evidence for a dose–response relationship, with higher dosages providing more benefit. Total dosages of at least 80 mg infused over a period of >2 h. (Grade C, low certainty.)

PARENTERAL KETAMINE

Parenteral ketamine can be used as a sole agent to manage acute pain or as a multimodal approach to pain management in combination with an opioid. However, most data support the use of parenteral ketamine to manage chronic pain.[16] There have been several double-blind randomized controlled trials that have found that the administration of intravenous ketamine was associated with a significantly greater reduction in pain compared with the control (often an opioid). The use of ketamine is an attractive choice to help mitigate over-usage of opioids to manage chronic pain, especially in opioid-tolerant patients who have opioid dependence.[16] In a randomized, double-blind, placebo-controlled trial in nine patients with central dysesthesia pain after a traumatic spinal cord injury, ketamine bolus IV of 60 mcg/kg followed by an infusion of 6 mcg/kg/min was associated with a marked reduction in both continuous and evoked pain.[17] Another randomized control trial by Amr et al.[18] found that patients who received IV ketamine 80 mg diluted in 500 cc of normal saline over 5 hours in conjunction with gabapentin had a 22-point reduction in the visual analog score compared with placebo plus gabapentin at the 2-week follow-up.

Aside from spinal cord injuries, parenteral ketamine has been shown to be beneficial in the management of chronic neuropathic pain. The effectiveness of IV ketamine was evaluated in a randomized, double-blind, cross-over study that also included lidocaine and placebo in 12 patients with chronic neuropathic pain due to accidental or surgical trauma or endogenous entrapment. The mean reduction in VAS scores was 55% for ketamine, 34% for lidocaine, and 22% for placebo. The response rate, defined as a 50% reduction in VAS-score during infusion, was highest for ketamine (7/12 patients), followed by lidocaine (4/12 patients), and placebo (2/12 patients).[19] In patients with fibromyalgia, two randomized controlled trials found a 20- to 25-point reduction in visual analog scale pain scores at 90 to 120 minutes following IV ketamine 0.3 mg/kg/dose compared with placebo.[20,21]

Many IV ketamine infusion protocols have been used for neuropathic pain; however, there is no consensus currently on an optimal protocol. Maher, Chen, and Mao[22] conducted a review of relevant, peer-reviewed articles that discussed ketamine infusion for the treatment of neuropathic pain to determine if there were any common components that could be associated with an increase in pain relief, duration of pain relief, and minimal side effects. A total of 26 qualifying studies were incorporated in the review. A formal meta-analysis was not possible due to the diversity of infusion protocols used. Study authors were able to identify some common trends in their review and suggest that a successful ketamine infusion protocol for neuropathic pain include the following components: (a) applying the longest possible ketamine infusion duration that is logistically feasible (rate of infusion does not appear to be a factor). Multi-hour outpatient treatments over the course of several days may provide more longer-lasting benefit than single or short-duration infusions; (b) using a dose of ketamine between 0.1 and 0.5 mg/kg/h to avoid excessive sedation in the majority of patients; (c) utilizing adjunct medications such as midazolam to decrease the incidence of psychomimetic side effects and potentially improve the degree of pain relief. Study authors note that additional clinical trials are needed to further optimize ketamine infusion protocols in the treatment of neuropathic pain, including comparative effectiveness trials of different ketamine infusion protocols and trials that identify optimal infusion protocols tailored to specific neuropathic pain conditions.

In patients with nociceptive pain, there have been mixed results in the literature. Ischemic pain attributed to severe peripheral disease had one randomized control trial that showed a 19% difference in pain relief between the ketamine infusion 0.6 mg/kg/dose plus regular opioid use over 4 hours compared to placebo infusion plus regular opioid use after 5 days.[23] A second cross-over, double-blind, randomized trial showed that there was no significant difference in pain scores between ketamine 0.15 to 0.45 mg/kg/dose over 5 minutes and morphine 10 mg.[24] This study was different because it compared ketamine to an opioid rather than strictly to placebo. This could contribute to the differences in findings and, thus, more studies are warranted to compare the effects of opioids and parenteral ketamine in the management of chronic pain. Another randomized, double-blind, placebo-controlled trial in patients with cancer pain refractory to opioids compared ketamine, dosed initially at 0.5 mg/kg/day followed by 1 mg/kg/day after 24 hours if the NPIS score remained ≥1 in combination with morphine, to placebo in combination with morphine. No significant differences were observed between the treatment groups during the 48-hour follow-up in terms of analgesic effects, tolerability, or patient satisfaction.[25] This particular study had a shorter follow-up time, and future studies may be needed to determine the significance of follow-up time for pain reduction.

Overall, the parenteral use of ketamine is highly effective in the management of chronic pain, especially as an alternative to an opioid or as a multimodal pain option. Additional studies are needed to further validate the results at longer follow-up intervals as well as head-to-head trials with opioids to assess the effectiveness of this class of medications. Patients with chronic pain are often high analgesic pain medication users and may be more susceptible to opioid use, so comparing the effectiveness of these agents in managing a variety of chronic pain disorders will be useful. Evidence is not as strong to support intravenous ketamine for acute pain, and further studies would be needed to confirm the use of parenteral ketamine in the acute pain setting.

INTRANASAL KETAMINE

Intranasal ketamine utilizes the nasal mucosa to bypass first-pass metabolism and the blood-brain barrier to ultimately be absorbed in the brain by olfactory sheets.[26] The large surface area, uniform temperature, and extensive vascularity of nasal mucosa make the intranasal route of administration able to easily facilitate rapid systemic absorption.[27] This method of administration may be of benefit in pain management to reduce the likelihood of dose-related dissociation and respiratory depression associated with ketamine. Low-dose ketamine with intranasal administration has been found to have a lower side effect and increased safety profile.[28–30]

A meta-analysis by Pakniyat et al.[31] explored the use of intranasal ketamine in the emergency department and demonstrated evidence to support the use of intranasal ketamine as an analgesic agent. The bioavailability of intranasal ketamine was reported to be 45–55%, and it is possible to be detect it in the blood 2 minutes after administration with a maximum concentration at 30 minutes post-administration. The duration of analgesia was documented as 1 hour. While the route of administration is easy and does not require venipuncture, ketamine for analgesic use in the emergency department may not be optimal due to its long onset of action. The dose of intranasal ketamine utilized among the studies ranged from 0.45 mg/kg/dose to 1.25 mg/kg/dose. Adverse events from the meta-analysis were mostly mild and related to bitter taste immediately after administration of the nasal spray, dizziness, and vomiting. The adverse events were transient and did not cause discontinuation of therapy. Also, systemic adverse events that are common with ketamine, such as hypertension, were not seen with the intranasal administration of ketamine. Overall, intranasal ketamine appears to be tolerated.

Shrestha et al.[32] studied intranasal ketamine administered at 0.7 mg/kg/dose. An additional dose of 0.3 mg/kg/dose could be given 15 minutes after the initial administration of intranasal ketamine. This study also looked at acute pain in the emergency department setting and analyzed the visual analog score and vital signs at 15, 30, and 60 minutes after initial administration. A total of 39 patients with various acute injuries participated in the study. At 15 minutes, 79% of patients achieved a >20 mm (VAS) reduction in pain and 100% had a reduction in pain by >20 mm at 30 and 60 minutes. An additional dose of ketamine was given to 17.6% of patients at 15 minutes. Adverse events were recorded and graded on a five-point scale using the Side Effect Rating Scale for Dissociative Anesthetics at 30 and 60 minutes and included fatigue, dizziness, nausea, headache, feeling of unreality, changes in hearing, mood change, general discomfort, and hallucinations.[32,33] The adverse events that were documented were mild and transient, resolving within 60 minutes after administration. There were no critical changes in vital signs noted in the study that required intervention or withdrawal from the drug. The results of this study concluded that there was significant pain relief with the administration of intranasal ketamine, showing its usefulness in the acute pain setting in the emergency department.[32]

Studies utilizing intranasal ketamine have been validated in both adults and pediatric patients. Miline K[34] wrote a case report looking specifically at intranasal fentanyl versus intranasal ketamine for pain relief in younger children who may present to the ER with an injury. Since children often present with oligoanalgesia, or poor pain management through the underuse of analgesics, pain can be difficult to manage in this patient population. Intranasal fentanyl has been utilized for pain reduction in the emergency department for children. This case report example states that a 0.5–1 mg/kg/ dose can provide rapid pain management for children who lack vascular access with the added benefit that intranasal ketamine has a sustained duration of action of 60 minutes compared to intranasal fentanyl's shorter duration of action of 30 minutes.

The use of intranasal ketamine in children was further explored in a noninferiority randomized clinical trial of 90 children presenting to the emergency department with a traumatic limb injury. The children received either intranasal ketamine 1.5 mg/kg/dose or intranasal fentanyl (2 mcg/kg/ dose). There was a mean reduction in the visual analog scale pain scores of 30.6 mm and 31.9 mm, respectively, at 30 minutes after administration. It was concluded that ketamine provides effective analgesia that is noninferior to intranasal fentanyl.[35]

Carr et al.[15] conducted a randomized, double-blind, placebo-controlled, crossover trial to evaluate the use of intranasal ketamine for breakthrough pain in adult patients with chronic pain. Prior to this study, few placebo-controlled trials investigating the use of intranasal ketamine in chronic pain existed. This study found that intranasal ketamine yielded a significant reduction in breakthrough pain following intranasal ketamine compared to placebo ($p < 0.0001$), with pain relief experienced within 10 minutes of dosing and lasting up to 60 minutes. Intranasal ketamine was well-tolerated with no serious adverse events, and the non-serious adverse events, including change in taste and rhinorrhea, were mostly transient. Overall, ketamine was recommended as a safe and effective option for breakthrough pain management in patients with chronic pain. More studies are needed to further validate these findings for the use of intranasal ketamine in the chronic pain setting.

Overall, it appears that the place in therapy for intranasal ketamine is for acute pain management. There have been a few studies exploring intranasal ketamine for the treatment of chronic pain, but more studies are needed to further validate its use in this patient population.

ADVERSE REACTIONS

The euphoric effects of ketamine can be a notable adverse reaction; however, in terms of its use as an anesthesia agent, it is also one of its therapeutic effects. Side effects such as hallucinations, paranoia, derealization/depersonalization, and panic attacks are common. Additionally, hypertension is a significant side effect that must be monitored and avoided in patients who have significant acute or chronic hypertension.[2] These side effects occur during administration and rapidly dissipate as the medication is eliminated from the body. Lower doses and concomitant use of a benzodiazepine help to increase tolerability in patients utilizing ketamine for indications requiring sustained use, such as chronic pain management.[2] Concomitant use of a benzodiazepine to prevent or reduce psychotomimetic effects and glycopyrrolate for excessive salvation or lacrimation may be considered to control side effects but this is not optimal.

Long-term side effects of ketamine include dependence and tolerance with prolonged use. A withdrawal syndrome with psychotic features has been described following discontinuation of long-term use. Moreover, ketamine is highly associated with the development of ulcerative cystitis, which is a painful bladder syndrome characterized by damage to the bladder's tissues leading to chronic,

TABLE 15.1
Ketamine Drug Interactions

Drug	Drug Interaction Severity Classification	Concomitant Use Documented Drug Interaction
St. John's Wort	Major	Increased risk of cardiovascular collapse
CNS depressants—loxapine, fentanyl, periciazine, nalbuphine, levorphanol, tramadol, dihydrocodeine, lofexidine, alfentanil, remifentanil, meperidine, metoclopramide, esketamine, flibanserin, bromazepam, clobazam, butorphanol, sufentanil, hydrocodone, methadone, buprenorphine, doxylamine, pentazocine, oxycodone, morphine, oxymorphone, cetirizine, codeine, cannabidiol, tapentadol, hydromorphone	Major	CNS depressants may result in potentiation of impaired cognitive function and motor skills and an increased risk of respiratory depression, hypotension, profound sedation, and syncope
Memantine	Major	May result in increased adverse events of N-methyl-D-aspartate antagonists
Seizure lowering agents—bupropion, donepezil, amifampridine	Major	May lower seizure threshold
Neuromuscular blockers—atracurium, tubocurarine	Moderate	May result in increased neuromuscular blockade
Metrizamide	Moderate	Increased risk of seizures
Theophylline	Moderate	May lower the seizure threshold

recurring pelvic pain with ulcers. About 33% of those who abuse ketamine develop reduced bladder volume and other kidney complications.[36]

DRUG INTERACTIONS

Ketamine has a few drug interactions that must be monitored, especially with concomitant drugs that cause respiratory depression and that lower seizure threshold. Drugs with similar indications and effects can have cumulative effects that result in the exacerbation of side effects if not monitored appropriately. Table 15.1 outlines documented ketamine drug interactions and their accompanying documented drug interaction.[37]

Ketamine is a substrate of CYP2B6 (major), CYP3A4 (major), and CYP2C9 (major), so CYP inhibitors of these enzymes can increase the serum concentrations and inducers can decrease the serum concentrations of these substrates (Table 15.2).

CONTRAINDICATIONS

Contraindications to ketamine include hypersensitivity to any component of ketamine as well as concomitant cardiovascular disease with uncontrolled blood pressure.

CONCLUSION

Both intravenous infusion and intranasal ketamine are effective routes of administration for analgesia; however, their appropriate places in therapy are different. Intravenous infusion ketamine is more appropriate for the management of chronic pain, while intranasal ketamine is most effective in the management of acute pain.

TABLE 15.2
Ketamine Cytochrome P450 Interactions

CYP2B6 Inducers	CYP2B6 Inhibitors	CYP3A4 Inducers	CYP3A4 Inhibitors	CYP2C9 Inducers	CYP2C9 Inhibitors
• Artemisinin • Carbamazepine • Efavirenz • Nevirapine • Phenobarbital • Phenytoin • Rifampin	Weak inhibitor 　• Crisaborole Other 　• Clopidogrel 　• Thiotepa 　• Ticlopidine 　• Voriconazole 　• Rucaparib	• Efavirenz • Nevirapine • Barbiturates • Carbamazepine • Glucocorticoids • Modafinil • Oxcarbazepine • Phenobarbital • Phenytoin • Pioglitazone • Rifabutin • Rifampin • St. John's Wort • Troglitazone • Brigatinib • Enzalutamide	Strong inhibitors 　• Indinavir 　• Nelfinivir 　• Ritonavir 　• Clarithromycin 　• Itraconazole 　• Ketoconazole 　• Nefazodone 　• Saquinavir 　• Telithromycin 　• Idelalisib 　• Ribociclib Moderate inhibitors 　• Aprepitant 　• Erythromycin 　• Fluconazole 　• Grapefruit juice 　• Verapamil 　• Diltiazem 　• Netupitant/ 　　palonosetron 　• Voriconazol Weak inhibitors 　• Cimetidine 　• Atomoxetine 　• Pantoprazole 　• Omeprazole 　• Lesinurad 　• Esomeprazole Other 　• Amiodarone 　• Ciprofloxacin 　• Fluvoxamine 　• Imatinib 　• Mifepristone 　• Nofloxacin 　• Norfluoxetine 　• Telaprevir 　• Boceprevir 　• Chloramphenicol 　• Delaviridine 　• Diethyl- 　　dithiocarbamate 　• Gestodene 　• Mibefradil 　• Azithromycin 　• Regorafenib 　• Starfruit	• Carbamazepine • Enzalutamide • Nevirapine • Phenobarbital • Rifampin • Secobarbital • St. John's Wort	Strong Inhibitors 　• Capecitabine Moderate Inhibitors 　• Amiodarone 　• Crisaborole 　• Voriconazole Other 　• Clopidogrel 　• Efavirenz 　• Fenofibrate 　• Fluconazole 　• Fluvastatin 　• Fluvoxamine 　• Isoniazid 　• Lovastatin 　• Metronidazole 　• Paroxetine 　• Phenylbutazone 　• Probenacid 　• Rucaparib 　• Sertraline 　• Sulfamethoxazole 　• Sulfaphenoazole 　• Teniposide 　• Zafilukast

REFERENCES

1. Bell R.F., Kalso E.A. Ketamine for pain management. *Pain Rep* 2018;3(5):e674.
2. Jonkman K., Dahan A., van de Donk T., et al. Ketamine for pain. *F1000Research* 2017;6(F1000 Faculty Rev):1711.
3. Schwenk E.S., Viscusi E.R., Buvanendran A., et al. Consensus guidelines on the use of intravenous ketamine infusions for acute pain management from the American society of regional anesthesia and pain medicine, the American academy of pain medicine, and the american society of anesthesiologists. *Reg Anesth Pain Med* 2018;43(5):456–466.
4. Mion G., Villevieille T. Ketamine pharmacology: an update (pharmacodynamics and molecular aspects, recent findings). *CNS Neurosci Ther* 2013;19(6):370–380.
5. Loftus R.W., Yeager M.P., Clark J.A., et al. Intraoperative ketamine reduces perioperative opiate consumption in opiate-dependent patients with chronic back pain undergoing back surgery. *Anesthesiology* 2010;113(3):639–646.
6. Tawfic Q.A., Faris A.S., Kausalya R. The role of a low-dose ketamine-midazolam regimen in the management of severe painful crisis in patients with sickle cell disease. *J Pain Symptom Manag* 2014;47(2):334–340.
7. Zempsky W.T., Loiselle K.A., Corsi J.M., Hagstrom J.N. Use of low-dose ketamine infusion for pediatric patients with sickle cell disease–related pain: a case series. *Clin J Pain* 2010;26(2):163–167.
8. Mulier J.P. Perioperative opioids aggravate obstructive breathing in sleep apnea syndrome: mechanisms and alternative anesthesia strategies. *Curr Opin Anaesthesiol* 2016;29(1):129–133.
9. Laskowski K., Stirling A., McKay W.P., Lim H.J. A systematic review of intravenous ketamine for postoperative analgesia. *Can J Anaesth* 2011;58(10):911–923.
10. Bell R.F., Dahl J.B., Moore R.A., Kalso E. Peri-operative ketamine for acute post-operative pain: a quantitative and qualitative systematic review (Cochrane review). *Acta Anaesthesiol Scand* 2005;49(10):1405–1428.
11. Elia N., Tramèr M.R. Ketamine and postoperative pain—A quantitative systematic review of randomised trials. *Pain* 2005;113(1–2):61–70.
12. Andolfatto G., Willman E., Joo D., et al. Intranasal ketamine for analgesia in the emergency department: a prospective observational series. *Acad Emerg Med* 2013;20(10):1050–1054.
13. Corrigan M., Wilson S.S., Hampton J. Safety and efficacy of intranasally administered medications in the emergency department and prehospital settings. *Am J Health Syst Pharm* 2015;72(18):1544–1554.
14. Yeaman F., Meek R., Egerton-Warburton D., Rosengarten P., Graudins A. Sub-dissociative-dose intranasal ketamine for moderate to severe pain in adult emergency department patients. *Emerg Med Australas* 2014;26(3):237–242.
15. Carr D.B., Goudas L.C., Denman W.T., et al. Safety and efficacy of intranasal ketamine for the treatment of breakthrough pain in patients with chronic pain: a randomized, double-blind, placebo-controlled, crossover study. *Pain* 2004;108(1–2):17–27.
16. Cohen S.P., Bhatia A., Buvandendran A., et al. Consensus guidelines on the use of intravenous ketamine infusion for chronic pain from the American society of regional anesthesia and pain medicine, the american academy of pain medicine, and the American society of anesthesiologists. *Reg Anesth Pain Med* 2018;43(5):521–546.
17. Eide P.K., Stubhaug A., Stenehjem A.E. Central dysesthesia pain after traumatic spinal cord injury is dependent on N-methyl-D-aspartate receptor activation. *Neurosurgery* 1995;37(6):1080–1087.
18. Amr Y.M. Multi-day low dose ketamine infusion as adjuvant to oral gabapentin in spinal cord injury related chronic pain: a prospective, randomized, double blind trial. *Pain Phys* 2010;13(3):245–249.
19. Kvarnström A., Karlsten R., Quiding H., Emanuelsson B.M., Gordh T. The effectiveness of intravenous ketamine and lidocaine on peripheral neuropathic pain. *Acta Anaesthesiol Scand* 2003;47(7):868–877.
20. Sörensen J., Bengtsson A., Bäckman E., Henriksson K.G., Bengtsson M. Pain analysis in patients with fibromyalgia. Effects of intravenous morphine, lidocaine, and ketamine. *Scand J Rheumatol* 1995;24(6):360–365.
21. Sörensen J., Bengtsson A., Ahlner J., Henriksson K.G., Ekselius L., Bengtsson M. Fibromyalgia—Are there different mechanisms in the processing of pain? A double blind crossover comparison of analgesic drugs. *J Rheumatol* 1997;24(8):1615–1621.
22. Maher D., Chen L., Mao J Intravenous ketamine infusions for neuropathic pain management: a promising therapy in need of optimization. *Anesth Analg* 2017;124(2):661–674.

23. Mitchell A.C., Fallon M.T. A single infusion of intravenous ketamine improves pain relief in patients with critical limb ischaemia: results of a double blind randomised controlled trial. *Pain* 2002;97(3):275–281.

24. Persson J., Hasselström J., Wiklund B., Heller A., Svensson J.O., Gustafsson L.L. The analgesic effect of racemic ketamine in patients with chronic ischemic pain due to lower extremity arteriosclerosis obliterans. *Acta Anaesthesiol Scand* 1998;42(7):750–758.

25. Salas S., Frasca M., Planchet-Barraud B., et al. Ketamine analgesic effect by continuous intravenous infusion in refractory cancer pain: considerations about the clinical research in palliative care. *J Palliat Med* 2012;15(3):287–293.

26. Westin U., Boström E., Gråsjö J., Hammarlund-Udenaes M., Björk E. Direct nose-to-brain transfer of morphine after nasal administration to rats. *Pharm Res* 2006;23(3):565–572.

27. Dale O., Hjortkjaer R., Kharasch E.D. Nasal administration of opioids for pain management in adults. *Acta Anaesthesiol Scand* 2002;46(7):759–770.

28. Galinski M., Dolveck F., Combes X., et al. Management of severe acute pain in emergency settings: ketamine reduces morphine consumption. *Am J Emerg Med* 2007;25(4):385–390.

29. Kennedy R., Porter F., Miller J., Jaffe D. Comparison of fentanyl/midazolam with ketamine/midazolam for pediatric orthopedic emergencies. *Pediatrics* 1998;102(4 Pt 1):956–963.

30. Gurnani A., Sharma P., Rautela R., Bhattacharya A. Analgesia for acute musculoskeletal trauma: low-dose subcutaneous infusion of ketamine. *Anaesth Intensive Care* 1996;24(1):32–36.

31. Pakniyat A., Qaribi M., Hezaveh D.R., Abdolrazaghnejad A. Intranasal ketamine as an analgesic agent for acute pain management in emergency department: a literature review. *J Acute Dis* 2018;7(6):241–246.

32. Shrestha R., Pant S., Shrestha A., Batajoo K.H., Thapa R., Vaidya S. Intranasal ketamine for the treatment of patients with acute pain in the emergency department. *World J Emerg Med* 2016;7(1):19–24.

33. Eide P., Jørum E., Stubhaug A., Bremnes J., Breivik H. Relief of post-herpetic neuralgia with the N-methyl-D-aspartic acid receptor antagonist ketamine: a double-blind, cross-over comparison with morphine and placebo. *Pain* 1994;58(3):347–354.

34. Miline K. Fentanyl versus intranasal for intranasal pain relief. *ACEP Now* 2019;38(3). https://www.acepnow.com/article/fentanyl-versus-ketamine-for-intranasal-pain-relief/. Accessed November 15, 2019.

35. Frey T.M., Florin T.A., Caruso M., Zhang N., Zhang Y., Mittiga M.R. Effect of intranasal ketamine vs fentanyl on pain reduction for extremity injuries in children: the PRIME randomized control trial. *JAMA Pediatr* 2019;173(2):140–146.

36. Kong Ho C.C., Pezhman H., Praveen S., et al. Ketamine-associated ulcerative cystitis: a case report and literature review. *Malays J Med Sci* 2010;17(2):61–65.

37. Drug interactions Flockhart Table™. Indiana University Department of Medicine Clinical Pharmacology. https://drug-interactions.medicine.iu.edu/Main-Table.aspx. Accessed December 2, 2019.

16 The Limbic System, Oxytocin, and Pain Management

Sahar Swidan and Charles E. Schultz

CONTENTS

THE LIMBIC SYSTEM

The limbic system is a complex set of structures in the midbrain that includes the hypothalamus, hippocampus, amygdala, and the cingulate cortex.[1] The components that make up the limbic system are responsible for "feeling and reacting" in the brain and are responsible for the formation of memories and assigning emotional significance to human senses. The limbic system is also closely integrated with the immune, endocrine, and autonomic nervous systems. Inflammation and physical trauma are two factors of many that can alter the functionality of the limbic system.[1] When the limbic system is not functioning appropriately due to injury or impairment, it becomes hypersensitive and begins to react to stimuli that are typically disregarded. This is a threat to the body and can result in inappropriate activation of the immune, endocrine, and autonomic nervous systems.[1] The over-firing of protection and threat mechanisms in the midbrain leads to distorted unconscious reactions, sensory perception, and protective responses. Over time, this state of hyperarousal can weaken the immune system, and affect systems associated in rest, digestion, detoxification, mood stability, and motor and cognitive function.[1]

The hypothalamus is the primary output node for the limbic system and is responsible for sexual function, endocrine function, behavioral function, and autonomic control. Notably, endocrine functions are controlled by either direct axonal connection to the posterior pituitary (vasopressin and oxytocin) or via secretion into the hypothalamic-hypophyseal portal system.

THE ROLE OF THE LIMBIC SYSTEM IN PAIN PERCEPTION

The limbic system, and more specifically the amygdala, is an important area of the brain for modulating the amount of pain experienced for a given noxious stimulus. The latero-capsular division of the central nucleus of the amygdala has been described as the "nociceptive amygdala" and appears to act at different levels of the pain neuraxis to both facilitate and inhibit pain modulation.[2] Since the limbic system is the center where emotions are processed, this component of the brain is heavily intertwined with pain recognition and management.[2] Pain is merely a "signal" that there is something wrong in the body; however, once this "signal" reaches the brain, the emotional center, hosted by the limbic system, transforms the "signal" into a response and pain is thus felt. The emotional response to pain involves the anterior cingulate gyrus and the right ventral prefrontal cortex.[3]

LIMBIC SYSTEM RETRAINING FOR PAIN MANAGEMENT

One school of thought is that limbic system retraining can be a useful non-pharmacologic modality for pain management to reverse hyperstimulation and depressed protective response. As with many disease states, non-pharmacological management is preferred as first-line therapy over medication-based treatments. Since chronic pain is often non-specific and widespread, pharmacologic-directed therapy is often difficult to utilize when there is not a clearly defined targeted source of pain.[4]

Limbic system retraining is a mechanism-targeted behavioral intervention that combines cognitive behavior therapy with emotional, behavioral, and cognitive restructuring along with neural linguistic reprogramming. The goal of limbic retraining is to reverse the maladaptive stress response and recover the necessary thoughts, emotions, and behavior patterns for the body to appropriately process stress and pain responses. Retraining the limbic system relies heavily on a psychological and neurophysiological approach to process pain signals that have been mismanaged by the emotional response.[5] This approach is patient-intensive, differing from traditional pharmacotherapy-directed therapies. For effective results, the patient must be compliant, as intermittent treatment is not as effective in redirecting the brain's maladaptive perception of painful stimuli.

Limbic system retraining is minimally documented in the literature, and more robust studies are needed to provide evidence-based recommendations on its effectiveness. Tinnitus retraining therapy has been shown to be successful in multiple published studies and relies heavily on limbic system retraining. Just as the limbic system and auditory systems are highly integrated, the limbic system and pain perception are directly related.[6] With tinnitus, it is not the auditory perception that is problematic but the presence of inappropriate associations between tinnitus-related neuronal activity and the reactions of the limbic and autonomic nervous systems. Therefore, in pain management, retraining the limbic system to recognize pain signals can lead to appropriate reactions of the limbic system and revive the protective mechanisms that can aid in the perception of pain.[6]

Limbic system retraining is a complex and labor-intensive psychological therapy. Its long-term utility requires more controlled studies. Pharmacological adjuvants may act synergistically to improve the process in terms of efficiency and effectiveness. Oxytocin may be one such compound that mechanistically is poised to fill this void.

OXYTOCIN AND THE LIMBIC SYSTEM

Oxytocin is the body's most potent natural pain modifier and a regulator of anxiety, stress-coping, and sociality. It is a highly abundant neurohypophysial peptide that has a prevalent expression localized to magnocellular neurons of the hypothalamic paraventricular and supraoptic nuclei.[7] Magnocellular oxytocin neurons of these nuclei innervate the forebrain and release the hormone into systemic circulation from the posterior pituitary in response to a variety of stimuli, including pain.[7,8] The parvocellular oxytocin neurons project to the brainstem and spinal cord where the oxytocin modulates inflammation and pain processing, thus modulating the limbic system.[7]

There is some speculative evidence that the oxytocin from the paraventricular nuclei of the hypothalamus can reach the central amygdala. Oxytocin has been known to reduce amygdala activity and is believed to have a neurocomputational mechanism underlying social-value representation, suggesting that oxytocin may promote pro-sociality by modulating the amygdala.[9,10] Administration of intranasal oxytocin has been shown to amplify the amygdala representation and increase prosocial behavior.

OXYTOCIN AND PAIN MANAGEMENT

With the continued rising concern surrounding the use of chronic opioids, oxytocin could prove to be an alternative pharmacotherapy, with the potential to modulate pain through both central and peripheral psychological and physiological processes (Figure 16.1).[8] Oxytocin receptors are located at multiple sites in the brain and throughout the spinal cord, and endogenous stimulation of oxytocin has been shown to decrease pain sensitivity.[11,12] The action of oxytocin's visceral nociceptive effects include the dorsal horn neuronal response to noxious visceral stimulation. Neuronal projections from the hypothalamus to the receptors in the dorsal horn of the spinal cord prevent pain signals from reaching the brain.[13] Oxytocin has been shown to indirectly reduce the activity of the spinal dorsal horn neurons following application of glutamate in rats.[14] In addition to decreasing sensitivity to pain, oxytocin has also been shown induce a state of calmness, and lower serum cortisol, stress, and anxiety.[15]

Oxytocin is commonly known for its use in labor and delivery, where it binds to G-protein coupled cell surface receptors that are highly expressed in mammary glands and the myometrium. It also causes dilation of vascular smooth muscle, thus increasing renal, coronary, and cerebral blood flow. While parturition has been the primary utilization for oxytocin in pain management, it has also shown evidence of effects on chronic pain and may be useful in other disease states such as headache, constipation, irritable colon, fibromyalgia, and other deep tissue disorders.[8,14,16–19]

The role of oxytocin in pain has mostly been studied in animal models, but oxytocin is increasingly being investigated for pain management in humans. While the majority of research suggests that oxytocin decreases sensitivity to pain in animals, data on the association between oxytocin and pain processing in humans are limited and mixed. Additionally, oxytocin studies have typically focused on acute pain with less of a focus on chronic pain.

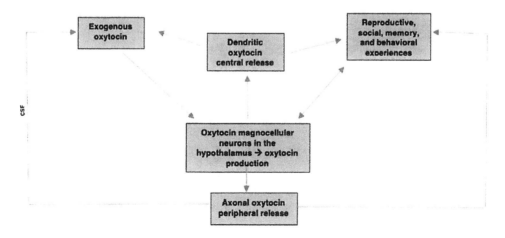

FIGURE 16.1 Oxytocin in pain modulation.

EFFECT OF OXYTOCIN ON PAIN VIA THE OPIOID AND CANNABINOID SYSTEMS

Animal data suggest that oxytocin, in addition to binding to its own receptors, also has effects on opioid and cannabinoid receptors, both of which are known to relieve pain. Oxytocin has been shown to bind to opioid receptors, stimulating endogenous opioid release in the brain.[20–22] In preclinical models, release of oxytocin from postsynaptic cells has been shown to increase intracellular calcium concentration, regulating the production of downstream endocannabinoids, which could be a plausible mechanism for its effects on cannabinoid receptors.[23]

Russo et al.[23] conducted a study in mice using a carrageenan-induced hyperalgesia pain model to investigate the effect of oxytocin on peripheral pain and the inflammatory process, and its potential involvement in the cannabinoid and opioid systems. Oxytocin was administered centrally via the intracerebroventricular (icv) route and peripherally via intraperitoneal and intraplantar routes. Peripheral pain was induced by carrageenan injection into the mouse paw and pain was measured during a carrageenan-only period and then again when carrageenan was administered post-oxytocin treatment. Oxytocin, administered icv at the highest dose (30 ng/mouse), produced significant antihyperalgesic effects at both 3 and 6 hours post-dose. The antihyperalgesic effects were not present at 24 hours post-dose. Another set of experiments demonstrated that the antihyperalgesic effects of oxytocin icv occurred in a dose-dependent manner. Oxytocin did not show any effect in reducing paw edema. Intraperitoneal and intraplantar injections did not reduce carrageenan-induced hyperalgesia.

Protein expression of inflammatory (COX-2, iNOS) and algesiogenic (nNOS) enzymes was evaluated in the spinal cord 3 hours post-carrageenan insult, and then again after the administration of icv oxytocin, to explore the effects of oxytocin on the inflammatory process. Carrageenan alone significantly increased the expression of COX-2, iNOS, and nNOS. Oxytocin administration significantly reduced nNOS expression but did not modify COX-2 or iNOS levels. Results were consistent with what was seen with the pain model, a reduction in pain but a lack of effect on edema. Direct involvement of the oxytocin receptor was confirmed using a specific receptor antagonist, which produced significant inhibition of oxytocin's antihyperalgesic effects.

The involvement of the cannabinoid system in oxytocin-induced antihyperalgesic effects was also explored with the use of specific CB_1 and CB_2 antagonists. Results showed that the antihyperalgesic effect of oxytocin was significantly reversed when used in conjunction with the CB_1 antagonist but not the CB_2 antagonist.

Naloxone was used to explore the effect of oxytocin on the opioid system. When administered alone, naloxone did not exert any significant effect on mechanical hyperalgesia. When used in conjunction with oxytocin, oxytocin's antihyperalgesic effects were significantly reversed at 3 hours but not 6 hours post-administration. Researchers were able to further elucidate the involvement specifically of the μ and κ receptors in oxytocin-induced antihyperalgesic effects through the use of opioid receptor subtype antagonists. The concomitant administration of oxytocin, naloxone, and the CB_1 antagonist produced the most significant reversion of oxytocin's antihyperalgesic effects, supporting the concept that both systems are involved with oxytocin's effects.[23]

HUMAN STUDIES OF OXYTOCIN FOR PAIN

A literature review by Rash et al.[16] identified nine qualifying studies that investigated the relationship between oxytocin and pain in humans. Multiple formulations of oxytocin were used in these studies, including the inhalation of oxytocin vapor, injection, and intranasal oxytocin. Four studies assessed endogenous oxytocin in blood plasma, four studies administered exogenous oxytocin relative to a placebo, and one study assessed the exogenous administration of oxytocin relative to a placebo as well as endogenous oxytocin concentrations in blood plasma. This review found that the effect of oxytocin on pain was generally consistent, suggesting that oxytocin may decrease pain sensitivity. Higher endogenous oxytocin concentrations were associated with lower pain sensitivity in four of five studies that assessed plasma oxytocin. Exogenous oxytocin was effective in reducing pain in three out of five studies. Each study is outlined below:

- Yang[24] studied intrathecal injection of oxytocin in 155 adult patients with acute and chronic lower back pain compared to 65 adult controls. Oxytocin was shown to relieve acute and chronic lower back pain, and both groups exhibited lower blood plasma oxytocin concentrations compared to pain-free controls.
- Alfven[25] studied the plasma oxytocin concentration of children with psychosomatic recurrent abdominal pain and children with organic abdominal disease producing pain. Plasma oxytocin (fasting morning sample) was measured by radioimmunoassay in 63 children with abdominal pain or inflammatory bowel disease and compared to a control group of 79 healthy children. Plasma oxytocin concentration was significantly lower in children with abdominal pain and inflammatory bowel disease compared to controls.
- Alfven, de la Torre, and Uvnas-Moberg[26] investigated the plasma concentrations of oxytocin, cortisol, and prolactin in 40 children with recurrent abdominal pain of non-organic origin compared to 34 controls. A blood sample (fasting morning sample) was collected and oxytocin, cortisol, and prolactin were measured by radioimmunoassay. Oxytocin and cortisol concentrations in the children with abdominal pain were found to be significantly reduced compared with those of the controls. The low oxytocin and cortisol levels persisted at a second examination 3 months later. No significant differences in the prolactin levels were observed between children with abdominal pain and controls.
- A double-blind, placebo-controlled pilot study was conducted by Ohlsson[27] et al. in 59 women with chronic constipation to examine the effects of long-term treatment with oxytocin. The study consisted of a 2-week baseline period followed by a 13-week treatment period of twice daily nasal oxytocin (40 IU twice daily) or placebo and a 2-week post-treatment follow-up period. Abdominal symptoms were rated daily. A total of 49 women were included in the analysis (23 women randomized to oxytocin, 26 women randomized to placebo). The oxytocin group demonstrated no significant advantage over placebo for constipation. Oxytocin seemed to have a positive effect on abdominal pain and discomfort and depressed mood.
- A study by Anderberg and Uvnäs-Moberg[28] assessed plasma oxytocin levels in 39 women with fibromyalgia with different hormonal status and in depressed and non-depressed patients and compared to 30 controls to relate oxytocin concentrations to adverse symptoms. Blood samples were drawn twice with an interval of 14 days during the 28-day period, and patients recorded symptoms daily. Oxytocin levels did not differ significantly between patients and controls or groups based on hormonal status compared to controls. Patients with high pain, stress, and depression had significantly lower levels of oxytocin when compared to patients who scored low in these symptoms. Low levels of oxytocin were also found in depressed patients with fibromyalgia compared to non-depressed patients.
- Uryvaev and Petrov[29] studied pain sensitivity after treatment with super low doses of oxytocin. Forty-eight healthy adults participated and received either oxytocin (n = 16), sub-threshold oxytocin (n = 16), or placebo (n = 16) by inhalation. A finger prick pain test was performed twice. Finger prick pain was reported as reduced when participants were infused with continuous inhalation of oxytocin (n = 16) relative to the continuous inhalation of placebo (n = 16). Subthreshold oxytocin resulted in no change.
- A study by Louvel et al.[30] studied the effects of oxytocin on colonic perception of intraluminal distension in 26 patients with irritable bowel syndrome (IBS), using a flaccid bag placed in the descending colon and connected to a computerized barostat. Symptomatic responses (first sensation and pain) were evaluated during isobaric distensions, performed automatically by the barostat, during a continuous infusion of oxytocin at various doses

or placebo. Continuous intravenous administration of oxytocin resulted in a dose response decrease in reports of pain.

- Singer et al.[31] measured the effects of oxytocin on pain processing in a double-blind placebo-controlled study of 20 male participants receiving painful electrical stimulation to their own hand (self-condition). The study consisted of two scheduled sessions approximately 10 days apart. Oxytocin nasal spray or placebo was administered to participants four times with a delay of 45 seconds between administrations at each session. Each administration of oxytocin contained approximately 4 IU, for a total of 32 IU. After each trial of painful stimulation, participants indicated how they felt about the stimulation by rating the degree of unpleasantness/pleasantness on an analogue rating scale. There was no significant difference between the oxytocin and placebo groups on the average unpleasantness ratings.

- A study by Grewen et al.[32] examined the relationship between plasma oxytocin and pain sensitivity and explored the relation of oxytocin to other factors known to influence pain perception. Forty-eight women (25 African American, 23 non-Hispanic white) participated in the study. Participants underwent three test pain procedures (ischemic, thermal heat, and cold pressor) to assess threshold, tolerance, and subjective intensity and unpleasantness of each type of pain stimulus. Measurements included plasma oxytocin levels measured by radioimmunoassay and depression and anxiety questionnaires. Greater oxytocin levels were correlated with greater tolerance to ischemic pain and cold pressor tolerance but not thermal heat tolerance. African American women demonstrated significantly lower pain tolerance across tasks compared with non-Hispanic Whites and also exhibited lower plasma oxytocin levels.[32] This study demonstrated that there may be an ethnic factor involved in oxytocin and pain modulation. More studies are needed to further explore this association.

OXYTOCIN FOR FIBROMYALGIA

In an effort to build upon the Anderberg and Uvnäs-Moberg et al.[28] study, which showed an inverse relationship between endogenous oxytocin plasma levels and severity of pain, anxiety, and depression in patients with fibromyalgia, Mameli[33] et al. conducted a double-blind, crossover, randomized study of intranasal oxytocin in fibromyalgia patients. The study included 14 females with fibromyalgia and comorbid disorders to receive oxytocin and placebo daily for 3 weeks of each treatment. Patients were randomly assigned to oxytocin-placebo or placebo-oxytocin. During the first week of oxytocin treatment, patients received 5 puffs twice daily (40 IU daily) of oxytocin, and then 10 puffs twice daily (80 IU daily) from the second week on. Medications for comorbid conditions were allowed to continue during the study if they had commenced at least 2 months prior to study start, and self-medications with nonsteroidal anti-inflammatories (NSAIDs) were also permitted and recorded both before and during the study. Thirteen of the 14 patients completed the study and were included in analyses. There were no differences between oxytocin and placebo in the number of doses of NSAIDs administered or in rating scales for pain, anxiety, depression, quality of sleep, or quality of life. There were also no significant differences in side effects between the two groups, with headache (53.8% oxytocin, 61.5% placebo), sleepiness (46.2% oxytocin, 38.5% placebo), dizziness (38.5% oxytocin, 30.8% placebo), and nausea/abdominal pain (46.2% oxytocin, 23.1% placebo) most common. Blood pressure, heart rate, body temperature, and laboratory tests were all within normal ranges. The study authors noted that several factors, including choice of dose, route of administration, and number of study patients, may have contributed to a lack of therapeutic effect. It was concluded in the original publication that higher doses or longer periods of time might further elucidate the analgesic effects of oxytocin. As a follow-up to the original study, the study authors noted that an ideal schedule may alternatively be more frequent daily administration with lower doses of oxytocin, for longer periods of time.[34] This conclusion was based on two additional studies, one that observed a stronger effect in cortical response to intense exercise with 24 IU of oxytocin as compared to 48 IU, and another that showed oxytocin as effective in reducing obesity if administered four times daily for 8 weeks.[35,36]

It was additionally noted that the lack of efficacy seen in the Mameli[33] et al. study could have also been due to concomitant use of NSAIDs.[37] This hypothesis is based on a study by Yeomans et al.,[38] which examined the effect of nasal oxytocin in chronic migraine patients. Nonsteroidal anti-inflammatory medications are known to block IL-6 production, a known driver of oxytocin receptor expression. Patients who had taken an NSAID within 24 hours of oxytocin dosing for migraine showed a strong decrease in the effect of oxytocin.

OXYTOCIN AND HEADACHE PAIN

Anecdotally, there are reports that women with chronic migraines have fewer attacks as they approach term in pregnancy, when oxytocin levels increase.[39] Preclinical studies have shown that intranasal oxytocin administration produces measurable oxytocin levels in all three branches of the trigeminal nerve, and reduced nociceptive responses to peripheral noxious stimulation.[40] Additionally, studies have found that oxytocin receptors located on the trigeminal nerve inhibit the nerve and block release of calcitonin gene-related peptide (CGRP) in vitro.[40] Calcitonin gene-related peptide is a protein that, when released around the brain, causes inflammation in the meninges and the resulting pain that is experienced during a migraine attack.

Tzabazis et al.[41] conducted a small placebo-controlled trial investigating the use of a single dose of intranasal oxytocin 32 IU at the outset of headache in 80 subjects with low-frequency, episodic migraines (42 in oxytocin group, 38 subjects in placebo group). Though not statistically significant, results trended strongly toward greater reductions in pain, photophobia, and phonophobia in the oxytocin group. The same researchers conducted a 28-day, open-label, multi-site study with 30 IU of intranasal oxytocin in 41 subjects (16 chronic and 25 high-frequency migraine sufferers), and found that mean migraine frequency decreased from 14.1 to 5.9 headache days, and mean severity decreased from 2.4 to 1.7 (0–3 scale). Lastly, the research group conducted an international study testing intranasal oxytocin 30 IU in 218 migraine sufferers (143 in oxytocin group, 75 in placebo group). The results showed a significant reduction in headache frequency, but an extremely large placebo phenomenon prevented statistical significance from being reached.

Wang et al.[19] assessed the effect of oxytocin on headache pain in a double-blind, placebo-controlled within-subject cross-over study. This study showed that patients with tension-type headache and migraine were relieved when using 400 ng of intranasal oxytocin (concentrations of 100 ng, 200 ng, or 400 ng of oxytocin were used in the study). Oxytocin relieved headaches in a dose-dependent manner. Oxytocin was most effective in the 400-ng group, consisting of 28 cases of headache patients. Complete remission in this group was achieved in 20 cases (71.4%) and partial remission in 8 cases (28.6%). Oxytocin concentrations in plasma and cerebrospinal fluid increased significantly in headache patients in relation with pain level, and there was positive relationship between plasma and cerebrospinal fluid oxytocin concentration in headache patients. Compared to healthy volunteers, plasma oxytocin concentrations were higher in patients with headache. It was concluded that intranasal oxytocin can be effective and safe in relieving human headaches in a dose-dependent manner.

DURATION OF OXYTOCIN TREATMENT

Oxytocin has been shown to be effective for a total of 7 days in mice for the management of pain. More than 7 days of treatment did not yield tolerance to use.[20] While some studies define duration of oxytocin use in their study methods, others such as Wang et al.[19] do not; however, Wang et al.[19] and others allude to a "short duration" of use. Ohlsson et al.[27] explored oxytocin twice daily for a total duration of 13 weeks in women with chronic constipation. Eleven (48%) of patients in the oxytocin group and 12 (47%) patients in the control group reported side effects. The most frequently reported side effects during the study were headache, nausea, abdominal pain, weight gain, and local irritation of the nasal mucosa. These side effects were distributed equally in the oxytocin and control groups. Overall, the duration of use of oxytocin in pain management is unclear, and further studies are warranted that focus on the optimal duration of use for effective pain management and the safety of extended use.

PHARMACOKINETICS

Although oxytocin has a short half-life of 1 to 6 minutes, administration of exogenous oxytocin crosses the blood–brain barrier, enters spinal fluid, and stimulates multiple receptors long after it is likely to be measurable in the serum.[42,43] The onset of action is 3 to 5 minutes when administered intramuscularly and approximately 1 minute when administered intravenously. The duration of action is 2 to 4 hours, but some patients have reported effects for as long as 6 to 8 hours.[44,45]

DOSAGE AND ADMINISTRATION

Although most of the literature suggests intranasal as the primary route of administration, oxytocin has also been shown to be effective when administered intranasal, sublingually as a liquid, dissolvable tablets, or as a troche. Dosages of 20 to 80 international units (IU) will result in pain relief within 15 minutes of administration.[16,45]

ADVERSE EFFECTS

The most common adverse effects associated with exogenous oxytocin are dizziness, nausea, and dysphoria, which are usually transient.[46] Since oxytocin causes the dilation of vascular smooth muscle, thus increasing renal, coronary, and cerebral blood flow, large doses or highly concentrated solutions of oxytocin can cause a transient increase in blood pressure. Blood pressure is unaffected by exogenous administration of oxytocin. Additionally, oxytocin has an antidiuretic effect, so severe and fatal that water intoxication has been reported with high doses (40–50 milliunits/minute) when infused over a long period. Since oxytocin is not typically administered as an IV formulation for chronic pain management, this adverse effect is less likely to be clinically significant.[47] There have been no reported drug interactions, but use is not recommended with ephedra or Ma Huang. More studies are needed to further assess the long-term analgesic efficacy and long-term safety and toxicity data.

CONCLUSION

Oxytocin has shown promising evidence of antihyperalgesic effects in animal models and in a limited number of human studies. Additional studies are needed to better understand how peripheral versus central oxytocin concentrations and route of administration affect pain conditions in humans. The optimal dose and duration of use of oxytocin for effective pain management will also need to be determined, as most experimental doses and treatment durations have been based on precedence. If proven therapeutic, oxytocin could provide a valuable and relatively inexpensive alternative to opioids, having a major advantage of low potential for addiction.

REFERENCES

1. Rajmohan V., Mohandas E.. The limbic system. *Indian J Psychiatry* 2007;49(2):132–139.
2. Neugebauer V., Li W., Bird G.C., Han J.S.. The amygdala and persistent pain. *Neuroscientist* 2004;10(3):221–234.
3. Hansen G.R., Streltzer J.. The psychology of pain. *Emerg Med Clin N Am* 2005;23(2):339–348.

4. Weisberg M.B., Clavel A.L. Jr. Why is chronic pain so difficult to treat? Psychological considerations from simple to complex care. *Postgrad Med* 1999;106(6):142–160.
5. Simons L., Elman I., Borsook D.. Psychological processing in chronic pain: a neural systems approach. *Neurosci Biobehav Rev* 2014;39:61–78.
6. Jastreboff P.J., Jastreboff M.M.. Tinnitus retraining therapy. *Semin Hear* 2001;22(1):51–64.
7. Nersesyan Y., Demirkhanyan L., Cabezas-Bratesco D., et al. Oxytocin modulates nociception as an agonist of pain-sensing TRPV1. *Cell Rep* 2017;21(6):1681–1691.
8. Tracy L.M., Georgiou-Karistanis N., Gibson S.J.. Oxytocin and the modulation of pain experience: implications in chronic pain management. *Neurosci Behav Rev* 2015;55:53–67.
9. Liu Y., Lin W., Li W., et al. Oxytocin modulates social value representations in the amygdala. *Nat Neurosci* 2019;22(4):633–641.
10. Sobota R., Mihara T., Forrest A., Featherstone R.E., Siegel J.J. Oxytocin reduces amygdala activity, increases social interactions and reduces anxiety-like behavior irrespective of NMDAR antagonism. *Behav Neurosci* 2015;129(4):369–398.
11. Barrett K.E., Boitano S., Barman S.M., Brooks H.L.. *Gangong's Review of Medical Physiology*, 24th ed. The McGraw-Hill Companies, Inc. 2012.
12. Jo Y.H., Stoeckel M.E., Freund-Mercier M.J., Schlichter R.. Oxytocin modulates glutamalergic synaptic transmission between cultured neonatal spinal cord dorsal horn neurons. *J Neurosci* 1998;18(7):2377–2386.
13. Reiter M.K., Kremarik P., Freund-Mercier M.J., Stoeckel M.E., Desaulles E., Feltz P.. Localization of oxytocin binding sites in the thoracic and upper lumbar spinal cord of the adult and postnatal rat: a histoautoradiographic study. *Eur J Neurosci* 1994;6(1):98–104.
14. Goodin B.R., Ness T.J., Robbins M.T.. Oxytocin— A multifunctional analgesic for chronic deep tissue pain. *Curr Pharm Des* 2015;21(7):906–913.
15. Windle R., Shanks N., Lightman S.L., Ingram C.D.. Central oxytocin administration reduces stress-induced corticosterone release and anxiety behavior in rats. *Endocrinology* 1997;138(7):2829–2834.
16. Rash J.A., Aguire-Camacho A., Campbell T.S.. Oxytocin and pain: a systematic review of synthesis and findings. *Clin J Pain* 2014;30(5):452–462.
17. Lee H.J., Macbeth A.H., Pagani J.H., Young W.S.. Oxytocin: the great facilitator of life. *Prog Neurobiol* 2009;88(2):127–151.
18. Douglas A.J., Neumann I., Meeren H.K.M., et al. Central endogenous opioid inhibition of supraoptic oxytocin neurons in pregnant rats. *J Neurosci* 1995;15(7):5049–5057.
19. Wang Y.L., Yuan Y., Yang Y., et al. The interaction between the oxytocin and pain modulation in headache patients. *Neuropeptides* 2013;47(2):93–97.
20. Reeta K.H., Mediratta P.K., Rathi N., Jain H., Chugh C., Sharma K.K.. Role of kappa-and delta opioid receptors in the antinociceptive effect of oxytocin in formalin-induced pain response in mice. *Regul Pept* 2006;135(1–2):85–90.
21. Breton J.D., Veinante P., Uhl-Bronner S., et al. Oxytocin-induced antinociception in the spinal cord is mediated by a subpopulation of glutamatergic neurons in lamina I–II which amplify GABAergic inhibition. *Mol Pain* 2008;4:19.
22. Gimpl G., Fahrenholz F.. The oxytocin receptor system: structure, function, and regulation. *Physiol Rev* 2001;81(2):629–683.
23. Russo R., D'Agostinoa G., Mattace Raso G., et al. Central administration of oxytocin reduces hyperalgesia in mice: implication for cannabinoid and opioid systems. *Peptides* 2012;38(1):81–88.
24. Yang J.. Intrathecal administration of oxytocin induces analgesia in low back pain involving the endogenous opiate peptide system. *Spine (Phila Pa 1976)* 1994;19(8):867–871.
25. Alfvén G.. Plasma oxytocin in children with recurrent abdominal pain. *J Pediatr Gastroenterol Nutr* 2004;38(5):513–517.
26. Alfvén G., de la Torre B., Uvnäs-Moberg K.. Depressed concentrations of oxytocin and cortisol in children with recurrent abdominal pain of non-organic origin. *Acta Paediatr* 1994;83(10):1076–1080.
27. Ohlsson B., Truedsson M., Bengtsson M., et al. Effects of long-term treatment with oxytocin in chronic constipation; a double blind, placebo-controlled pilot trial. *Neurogastroenterol Motil* 2005;17(5):697–704.
28. Anderberg U.M., Uvnäs-Moberg K.. Plasma oxytocin levels in female fibromyalgia syndrome patients. *Z Rheumatol* 2000;59(6):373–379.
29. Iu U., Petrov G.A.. Decreased pain sensitivity in man after treatment with superlow doses of oxytocin. *Biull Eksp Biol Med* 1996;122:487–489.
30. Louvel D., Delvaux M., Felez A., et al. Oxytocin increases thresholds of colonic visceral perception in patients with irritable bowel syndrome. *Gut* 1996;39(5):741–747.

31. Singer T., Snozzi R., Bird G., et al. Effects of oxytocin and prosocial behavior on brain responses to direct and vicariously experienced pain. *Emotion* 2008;8(6):781–791.

32. Grewen K.M., Light K.C., Mechlin B., Girdler S.S.. Ethnicity is associated with alterations in oxytocin relationships to pain sensitivity in women. *Ethn Health* 2008;13(3):219–241.

33. Mameli S., Pisanu G.M., Sardo S., et al. Oxytocin nasal spray in fibromyalgia patients. *Rheumatol Int* 2014;34(8):1047–1052.

34. Agabio R., Mameli S., Sardo S., Minerba L., melis M.R.. Oxytocin nasal spray in fibromyalgic patients: additional information: reply to the comment to the editor entitled 'future directions for the investigation of intranasal oxytocin and pain.' *Rheumatol Int* 2014;34(9):1335–1336.

35. Cardoso C., Ellenbogen M.A., Orlando M.A., Bacon S.L., Joober R.. Intranasal oxytocin attenuates the cortisol response to physical stress: a dose-response study. *Psychoneuroendocrinology* 2013;38(3):399–407.

36. Zhang H., Wu C., Chen Q., et al. Treatment of obesity and diabetes using oxytocin or analogs in patients and mouse models. *PLOS ONE* 2013;8(5):e61477.

37. Kwong K.K., Chan S.T.. Intranasal oxytocin and NSAIDs: comment on: oxytocin nasal spray in fibromyalgic patients (Rheumatol Int. 2014 Aug;34(8):1047-52.). *Rheumatol Int* 2015;35(5):941–942.

38. Yeomans D.C., Angst M., Mechanic J., Jacobs D.. Therapeutic effect of nasal oxytocin in chronic migraine:dependence on cytokines. *Cephalalgia* 2013;33(8):58, Abstract P59.

39. Goadsby P.J., Goldberg J., Silberstein S.D.. Migraine in pregnancy. *BMJ* 2008;336(7659):1502–1504.

40. Tzabazis A., Mechanic J., Miller J., et al. Oxytocin receptor: expression in the trigeminal nociceptive system and potential role in the treatment of headache disorders. *Cephalalgia* 2016;36(10):943–950.

41. Tzabazis A., Kori S., Mechanic J., et al. Oxytocin and migraine headache. *Headache* 2017;57(Suppl 2):64–75.

42. Striepens N., Kendrick K.M., Hanking V. *et al.* Elevated cerebrospinal fluid and blood concentrations of oxytocin following its intranasal administration in humans. *Sci Rep.* 2013;3:3440.

43. Modi M.E., Connor-Stroud F., Landgraf R., Young L.J., Parr L.A.. Aerosolized oxytocin increases cerebrospinal fluid oxytocin in rhesus macaques. *Psychoneuroendocrinology* 2014;45:49–57.

44. Tennant F.. *Oxytocin in Intractable Pain Patient Unresponsive to Standard Treatments.* Poster Presented at the 33rd Annual Meeting of the American Pain Society. April 30–May 3, 2014. Tampa, FL.

45. Tennant F., Pedersen C.. Sublingual Oxytocin and Ketamine for Pain Relief. Poster Presented at Pain week. September 5–9, 2017. Las Vegas, Nevada.

46. Kessner S., Sprenger C., Wrobel N., Young L.J., Parr L.A.. Effect of oxytocin on placebo analgesia: a randomized study. *JAMA* 2003;310(16):1733–1735.

47. *Pitocin (Oxytocin) Package Insert.* Rochester, MI: JHP Pharmaceuticals, LLC. September 2014.

17 Low-Dose Naltrexone
Immune and Inflammatory Mediator Extraordinaire

Sahar Swidan

CONTENTS

Naltrexone is an opiate antagonist approved by the Food and Drug Administration (FDA) for use in alcohol and opiate agonist dependence. It shows competitive inhibition at the mu (OP3), kappa (OP2), and delta (OP1) receptors with the ability to displace and prevent the binding of exogenous and endogenous opioids at FDA-approved doses. Naltrexone is commercially available as a tablet containing 50 mg of naltrexone hydrochloride and as long-acting 380 mg powder for injection. Orally, naltrexone is almost completely absorbed, but due to first-pass metabolism, only 5–40% reaches the bloodstream unchanged. It is metabolized in the liver to a less active metabolite called 6-beta-naltrexol, and then both the parent drug and metabolite are conjugated with glucuronate. The half-lives of naltrexone and 6-beta-natrexol are 4 hours and 14 hours, respectively, and both are excreted mainly by the kidneys.

Naltrexone, at normal doses of 50 mg to 150 mg daily, has traditionally been used for the treatment of alcohol and opiate agonist addiction. A Cochrane review investigating the effects of naltrexone therapy on alcohol dependence found that it reduced the risk of heavy drinking by 83% and decreased drinking days by 4% compared to placebo.[1] However, even at low or very low doses, naltrexone appears to improve positive outcomes for opioid- and alcohol-dependent patients. Two studies investigating the effects of very low-dose naltrexone (VLDN), at doses of 0.125 mg or 0.25 mg/day, on opioid-dependent patients with and without problem drinking showed promising results for opioid detoxification. They found that those patients who received VLDN with methadone experienced reduced withdrawal symptoms, reduced cravings, lower rates of treatment discontinuation, and fewer patients resuming alcohol following discharge.[2,3] Low-dose naltrexone (LDN) in combination with other medications, such as prazosin, has also been studied for alcohol addiction. Froehlich, Hausauer, and Rasmussen[4] discovered that combining LDN with prazosin was more effective at reducing alcohol intake compared to monotherapy. In addition to applications in alcohol and opioid addiction, LDN has been investigated as an adjunct therapy for cocaine addiction. The major effects of cocaine relate to the potent inhibition of dopamine and other monoamine neurotransmitters; however, there is also an important role of endogenous opioids in the pathophysiology of addiction. An animal study investigating LDN in combination with levo-tetrahydropalmatine (L-THP) showed reduced drug-seeking behavior compared to L-THP alone. Additionally, the study found an upregulatory effect on endogenous endorphins in the combination group.[5] It appears that LDN and VLDN have the potential to be effective as an adjunct therapy in multiple addictive disorders.

Low-dose naltrexone (1 mg to 5 mg), very low-dose naltrexone (0.001–1 mg), and ultra-low-dose naltrexone (ULDN) (<0.001 mg) have been investigated for their immune-modulatory and anti-inflammatory effects.[6] The most apparent effect at low doses is naltrexone's antagonism of toll-like receptor 4 (TLR4) within the microglia. Many studies have shown that TLR4 antagonism results in the downregulation of inflammatory cytokines and immune mediators such as interleukins (IL), interferons (IFN), tumor necrosis factors (TNF), and granulocyte colony-stimulating factor (G-CSF), among others. There has also been an observed compensatory release of endogenous opioids, such as opioid growth factor (OGF, [Met^5]-enkephalin) in response to low-dose naltrexone therapy, as well as a modulatory effect on the OGF–OGF receptor (OGFr) axis in cancer cell proliferation. The low concentration of naltrexone at the opioid receptors causes intermittent binding, which sends feedback to the central nervous system (CNS), mimicking opioid depletion and resulting in a compensatory release of endogenous opioids. Opioid growth factor is an inhibitory peptide in the human body exhibiting a role in cell proliferation as well as tissue organization in many biological and pathological conditions (e.g., cancer, wound healing, angiogenesis). The OGFr is an integral membrane protein that, when bound to OGF, modulates the signal transduction resulting in DNA activity.[7] It is important to note that to get the intermittent binding effect of LDN it must be prepared as an immediate-release formulation. According to Dr. Pradeep Chopra, using a sustained-release formulation would be detrimental because it is the "transient and reversible blockade of the opioid receptor" that is responsible for the upregulation of OGF. This effect is not seen with higher doses or sustained-release formulations of naltrexone (Yeazel D, e-mail communication, January 2018). Additionally, using fillers such as calcium carbonate during compounding can reduce absorption of naltrexone, thereby affecting the pharmacokinetic profile, and should be avoided.[8] Instead, inactive fillers such as Avicel®, sucrose, or lactose should be used in compounding.[9]

These immune, inflammatory, and opioid effects are key in managing the pathophysiology and progression of diseases such as multiple sclerosis (MS), Crohn's disease (CD), sarcoidosis, fibromyalgia (FM), complex regional pain syndrome (CRPS), painful diabetic neuropathy, autism, infections, and cancer.

MULTIPLE SCLEROSIS

Multiple sclerosis affects upwards of 400,000 people in the United States with approximately 10,000 new cases each year. The disease affects twice as many women as men, with women developing signs and symptoms earlier in life and ultimately more likely to develop progressive forms of MS. The primary signs and symptoms of MS are non-specific and may consist of complaints of altered visual acuity, gait problems, speech difficulty, fatigue, and tremor.

Central to the pathophysiology of MS is the migration of immune cells (e.g., T lymphocytes, B lymphocytes, macrophages) across the blood–brain barrier (BBB) into the CNS. Once they have crossed into the CNS, these immune cells cause the breakdown of the protective sheath covering the nerve fibers, which are made up of myelin cells. This demyelination can result in irreversible damage to the axons, which manifests as the symptoms of MS. Although T-cells contribute to the pathogenesis of MS, they also appear to have protective traits, which have led investigators to believe that T-cells have a level of plasticity in MS. Additional evidence suggests that a deficiency in T-regulatory (Treg) cells may play a role in active MS. Consequently, the autoimmune theory of MS elucidates that the initial destruction of myelin is due to CD4+ T-helper cells and that these cells may be activated following viral infection. The activated T-cells attach to the lining of the blood vessels composing the BBB and produce matrix metalloproteinases, which allows extravasation of T-cells into the CNS. These T-cells also produce proinflammatory cytokines (i.e., interleukins, interferons, tumor necrosis factors) contributing to the opening of the BBB, allowing B-cells, complement, macrophages, and antibodies into the CNS. Additionally, a recent study by Ludwig, Zagon, and McLaughlin[10] investigated serum [Met^5]-enkephalin levels as a biomarker for the onset of MS and response to therapy. The study found that serum [Met^5]-enkephalin levels are depressed prior to the clinical presentation of MS, and low doses of naltrexone restore [Met^5]-enkephalin to normal levels. This effect was not seen in normal subjects, thus making [Met^5]-enkephalin a possible future biomarker for MS, as well as showing a positive impact of LDN on endogenous opioids.

Traditionally, treatment options for MS include immunosuppressive and immune-modulatory therapies such as corticosteroids (e.g., methylprednisolone, prednisone) for the management of exacerbations and a variety of disease-modifying therapies (DMT) depending on the clinical symptoms (e.g., interferons, glatiramer acetate, natalizumab, fingolimod, mitoxantrone). Low-dose naltrexone can potentially provide multiple levels of therapeutic benefit in MS due to its immune-modulating and anti-inflammatory properties. Low-dose naltrexone may restore [Met^5]-enkephalin levels, which mediate the cell replication of T lymphocytes, astrocytes, and other glial cells associated with MS inflammation and degeneration. Studies on the effects of LDN on MS have resulted in a perceived decrease in fatigue, improvement or stabilization of the disease, and improved or stabilized quality of life for the participants at naltrexone doses of 3.5–4.5 mg once daily.[11] Two small pilot studies of 8 weeks and 6 months in duration found LDN to be safe and well-tolerated. One of these studies showed a significant reduction in spasticity in study participants, and the other demonstrated a significant improvement in mental health-related quality of life indices.[12,13] Another study reported no statistically meaningful differences in variables including presence of pain, energy, emotional well-being, social, cognitive, and sexual functions, role limitation due to physical and emotional problems, health distress, and overall QoL. A factor analysis showed a statistical difference in health perception scores between the groups before starting, in the middle, and at the end of the study.[14]

Raknes and Småbrekke looked at the effect of LDN prescribing on the prescribing of other mediations for MS using prescription data from the Norwegian prescription database. This pharmacoepidemiologic study was unable to associate the initiation of LDN therapy to a reduction in the dispensing of other MS medications. Opioid dispensing in the persistent LDN users group, defined as patients who collected four or more LDN prescriptions during the observation period, was significantly reduced. The persistent LDN users group showed a 42% decrease in cumulative opioid dose and a 9% decrease in number of users.[15]

Ludwig, Turel, Zagon, and McLaughlin[16] conducted a retrospective review over a 10-year period in patients with relapsing-remitting MS. Fifty-four patients were evaluated in the study: 23 who were initially prescribed LDN and not a DMT due to symptoms of fatigue or refusal to take a DMT at the time of first visit to the treatment center, and 31 patients who were treated with glatiramer acetate plus LDN as an adjunct to their DMT. Standard laboratory blood tests, timed walks, and changes in magnetic resonance imaging (MRI) reports were evaluated. There were no significant differences between the two groups in clinical assessments, and the study authors concluded that LDN alone did not result in an exacerbation of disease symptoms. This study suggests that LDN can be an inexpensive therapy for patients who are reluctant to take other, more costly DMTs.

CROHN'S DISEASE AND SARCOIDOSIS

There are between 18,000 to 45,000 new cases of Crohn's disease (CD), a subset of inflammatory bowel disease, each year in the United States. Crohn's disease has a dual peak incidence often occurring between the ages of 20–30 and 60–70, with females being 20–30% more likely to develop CD than males. The signs and symptoms of CD are highly variable, but patients typically present with diarrhea and abdominal pain. Additional symptoms can include hematochezia, perirectal lesions, and perianal lesions.

Crohn's disease is an inflammatory disease typically affecting the terminal ileum; however it may encompass any part of the gastrointestinal tract. The presence of TNFα, IL-2, and IL-10 leads to the inflammation of the gastrointestinal tract seen in CD. The inflammation of the gastrointestinal tract can cause edema, fibrosis, ulceration, mucosal thickening, narrowing of the intestinal lumen, and fistulas. Anemia and nutritional deficiencies due to bleeding in CD are common because of malabsorption, increased motility, and interactions between medications and nutrients. Additional complications include hepatobiliary, joint, ocular, dermatologic, coagulation, and metabolic disorders.

Treatment for CD focuses on inducing and maintaining remission, as well as improving the patients' quality of life. Pharmacologic therapy includes anti-inflammatory drugs to induce remission of the disease, such as aminosalicylates (ASAs), immunosuppressive drugs, biologic agents, and antimicrobials for infection prevention. Nutritional support is also extremely important in CD as there are elevated levels of IL-6 and TNFα, which can lead to increased protein loss and muscle wasting. Enteral nutrition might help reduce intestinal cytokine levels, thereby reducing inflammation and improving the possibility of remission.

Aminosalicylates are the mainstay of treatment for mild-moderate CD. The mechanism of action of ASAs is unclear, but may involve reducing oxidative stress, interfering with TNFα, suppressing IL-1 production, and inhibiting inflammatory pathways. The downfall of ASAs is that they can be expensive, difficult, or unpleasant to administer, and this can lead to decreased adherence. Low-dose naltrexone is inexpensive, easy to administer, and has shown promising results in studies on its effects on CD. In a study using 4.5 mg/day of naltrexone, 89% of patients with active CD showed a response to LDN therapy, 67% achieved remission, and there was a statistically significant improvement in the inflammatory bowel disease questionnaire (IBDQ) and SF-36 quality of life surveys.[17] Segal, MacDonald, and Chande[18] reported that LDN therapy resulted in a statistically significant clinical response in adults, exhibited as a decrease of greater than 70 on the Crohn's disease activity index (CDAI), as well as significant endoscopic response as evidenced by the greater than five-point drop in Crohn's disease endoscopic index of severity (CDEIS).

Lie et al.[19] conducted a study of LDN for the induction of remission in therapy-refractory inflammatory bowel disease (IBD) patients. This study also investigated if LDN has a direct modulatory effect on intestinal epithelial barrier function. A total of 47 IBD patients were enrolled (28 CD, 19 ulcerative colitis [UC]). All patients received 4.5 mg naltrexone daily, and self-assessed disease activity was recorded at 4, 8, and 12 weeks after initiation of LDN. Additionally, endoscopic evaluations, serum samples, and biopsies were collected. The effect of LDN on wound healing, cytokine production, and endoplasmic reticulum stress was also assessed. Thirty-five (74.5%) patients achieved a clinical response, defined as a decrease in disease activity within the first 4 weeks of LDN therapy lasting at least 4 weeks in total, with 25.5% of patients achieving a response of at least 3 months (8 CD, 4 UC). The remaining 48.9% of patients achieved short-lived improvements between 4 and 12 weeks (13 CD, 10 UC). Low-dose naltrexone improved epithelial barrier function by improving wound healing and decreasing endoplasmic reticulum stress levels. Cytokine levels were unaffected in the epithelial cells and serum collected from the IBD patients in this study. The authors concluded that naltrexone does not appear to positively impact inflammation through the modulation of intestinal epithelial cell cytokine production.

Raknes, Simonsen, and Småbrekke[20] conducted a pharmacoepidemiologic study using the Norwegian prescription database to determine the effect of initiating LDN on the prescribing patterns of other medications used specifically in the treatment of inflammatory bowel disease. Medication dispensing was compared 2 years before and after the first LDN prescription was given. This study showed a reduction in a number of different medications for the treatment of CD and UC following the dispensing of an LDN prescription. The study authors note that LDN may have the potential to reduce polypharmacy in IBD patients, resulting in a reduction of both cost and adverse effects.

Overall, the anti-inflammatory, immune-modulatory effects of LDN seem to be beneficial in CD severity and remission, making it ideal as an adjunct to traditional treatment or as a monotherapy.

The symptoms of CD can often be debilitating and interfere with normal daily functioning of the affected patients, making any treatment that improves functioning valuable.

Sarcoidosis is another inflammatory disease often presenting with gastrointestinal involvement. The usual treatment for sarcoidosis consists of the long-term use of prednisone, immunemodulators, or infliximab. These treatment options have many undesirable side effects including an increased risk of infection and malignancies. Because of the similarities between CD and sarcoidosis, LDN has been investigated as a therapeutic option for symptom management. In a case study by Weinstock, Myers, and Shetty,[21] LDN therapy improved fatigue, dyspnea, and parotitis when titrated from 1 mg up to 4.5 mg in a patient with a 39-year history of sarcoidosis.

FIBROMYALGIA

Approximately 2–5% of the world population has been diagnosed with fibromyalgia (FM) with more women than men affected. Fibromyalgia most commonly presents as a general pain-all-over, typically affecting the body bilaterally both above and below the waist. Pain on presentation is usually severe, poorly localized, and debilitating. Additionally, pain associated with FM exhibits increased sensitivity, or hyperalgesia.

Fibromyalgia is a conglomerate of many pain disorders, which makes diagnosis and treatment quite difficult. Inflammatory cytokines that are known to promote nociception, allodynia, and hyperalgesia in FM include TNFα and interleukins (1β, 2, 6, 15, 17). Parkinty and Younger[22] showed a reduction in serum concentrations of TNFα and interleukins during a 10-week, single-blinded, crossover trial investigating the effect of 4.5 mg naltrexone on serum markers of inflammation in eight women with fibromyalgia.

The most successful FDA-approved treatment options for FM have focused on afferent pain pathways. Drugs that affect the afferent pain pathways include antidepressants that modulate serotonin and/or norepinephrine (e.g., amitriptyline, duloxetine, milnacipran) and anticonvulsants acting as ligands of alpha-2-delta voltage-gated calcium channels in the CNS (e.g., gabapentin, pregabalin). It is important to note that FM is not effectively treated with opioid analgesics. Alternatively, opioids have been associated with opioid-induced hyperalgesia in the context of FM. Antidepressant and anticonvulsant medications manage the symptomatology of inflammation and immune dysfunction in FM, but do not directly affect the underlying pathology. As stated above, LDN has been shown to decrease the serum concentrations of immune and inflammatory cytokines, thus addressing FM pain from a more direct pathologic approach.[22]

A study in ten women with fibromyalgia who were administered 4.5 mg LDN daily for 8 weeks found that LDN reduced fibromyalgia symptoms for all study patients with a >30% improvement over placebo as measured by daily reports of symptom severity and tests. Twice monthly tests of mechanical, heat, and cold pain sensitivity demonstrated that mechanical and heat pain thresholds were improved with the drug. Patients with higher erythrocyte sedimentation rates had the greatest reduction in symptoms with LDN.[23]

A larger study in 31 women with fibromyalgia evaluated LDN 4.5 mg daily for a period of 12 weeks with 4 weeks of placebo taken either before or after the LDN treatment period depending on study arm assignment. This study also included a 2-week baseline period and a 4-week follow-up period for a total length of 22 weeks. All participants were told that they had the option to reduce their daily dosage to 3 mg if they experienced side effects. Self-assessed pain, fatigue, and other symptoms were recorded on a daily basis during the study and for 4 weeks after study medication was stopped. Twenty-eight women had sufficient data to be included in the analyses. Study patients experienced a significantly greater reduction in their pain scores while they were taking the LDN as compared with placebo (28.8% reduction versus 18.0% reduction; p=0.016). More participants met the criteria for response (defined as a significant reduction in pain plus a significant reduction in either fatigue or sleep problems) during LDN therapy compared to placebo (32% response during LDN versus 11% response during placebo; p=0.05). Participants also reported improved general satisfaction with life and improved mood while taking LDN. However, there was no improvement in fatigue or sleep. Four individuals (three while taking LDN and one while taking placebo) requested the 3 mg dosage due to side effects (headaches, heartburn, and irritability). These side effects were reduced by lowering the dosage to 3 mg/day.[24]

PAIN, COMPLEX REGIONAL PAIN SYNDROME, AND DIABETIC NEUROPATHY

According to the Centers for Disease Control and Prevention (2017), the sales of prescription opioids increased 400% between 1999 and 2014, but the incidence of pain in the U.S. did not change during that same period.[25] Notwithstanding, more than 100 million people in the U.S. live with chronic pain conditions. It is imperative, now more than ever, to find treatment options that are not only effective, but also safe for patients.

Pain is a very complex disease that is affected by both neural and immune systems in the peripheral nervous system (PNS) and CNS. It is categorized as either adaptive pain, immunologic pain, and/or maladaptive pain.

Adaptive pain is a result of tissue damage either from trauma or surgery and is propagated through the processes of transduction, conduction, transmission, perception, and modulation. Transduction involves the release of cytokines and chemokines from nociceptors in the somatic and visceral structures activated by mechanical, thermal, or chemical stimuli. Conduction involves the generation of action potentials by the depolarization of voltage-gated sodium channels. Transmission through afferent nerve fibers causes the release of glutamate and substance P acting as excitatory neurotransmitters, ultimately propagating the pain signal to the thalamus, where the signal is relayed to higher cortical structures. Perception is the result of the pain signals that reach the higher cortical structures becoming a conscious experience. Modulation is the result of many different neurotransmitters and receptor interactions that either strengthen or attenuate the pain signal. Excitatory neurotransmitters involved in pain include glutamate and substance P. Inhibitory neurotransmitters involved in pain include enkephalins, β-endorphins, GABA, norepinephrine, and serotonin. Additionally, NMDA receptors seem to influence opioid receptor responsiveness to exogenous and endogenous opioids.

The interaction between the immune system and pain has become an accepted theory in pain experience and management. It is believed that microglial cells in the CNS are activated following nerve injury, which is often seen in neuropathic pain conditions. Additionally, activation of microglia may play a role in tolerance to opioids as well as opioid-induced hyperalgesia.

Maladaptive pain is the result of damage or abnormal functioning of the PNS or CNS. It is manifested as ongoing nerve injury in either the PNS (e.g., postherpetic neuralgia, diabetic neuropathy) or the CNS (e.g., ischemic stroke, MS). Maladaptive pain may also be a result of disturbances in pain processing leading to hypersensitivity and spontaneous pain (e.g., FM, CD, tension headaches).

The treatment for pain should be individualized for each patient depending on the pathology and symptoms. The goals of pain management therapy are to improve the patient's level of functioning, decrease pain perception, reduce the use of medications when possible, and improve the quality of life. Traditional medication therapies for pain include the use of NSAIDs (e.g., ibuprofen, naproxen), non-opioid analgesics (e.g., acetaminophen), tricyclic antidepressants (e.g., amitriptyline, imipramine), and anticonvulsants (e.g., gabapentin). These treatment options focus on reducing the inflammatory response to pain stimuli as well as inhibiting afferent pain stimuli by acting as ligands of alpha-2-delta voltage-gated calcium channels in the CNS. Low-dose and ultra-low-dose naltrexone (ULDN) have been investigated for the management of pain, complex regional pain syndrome (CRPS), and painful diabetic neuropathy with encouraging results.

Ultra-low-dose naltrexone has been investigated as an adjunct to opioid agonist therapy for pain. The concept of using a low-dose naltrexone in combination with an opioid agonist is not new. In fact, there have been opioid agonist–antagonist combination drugs approved by the FDA, including Embeda® (morphine/naltrexone as 20 mg/0.8 mg, 30 mg/1.2 mg, 50 mg/2 mg, 60 mg/2.4 mg,

80 mg/3.2 mg, 100 mg/4 mg) and Troxyca ER® (oxycodone/naltrexone as 10 mg/1.2 mg, 20 mg/2.4 mg, 30 mg/3.6 mg, 40 mg/4.8 mg, 60 mg/7.2 mg, 80 mg/9.6 mg).[26,27]

In a review article by Leri,[28] opioid agonist and antagonist co-administration was investigated as a method to increase the desired effects of opioids and decrease the undesired effects. Leri stated that the effects of ULDN on, "analgesia, analgesic tolerance and opioid withdrawal have been consistently replicated." Similarly, Hay, La Vincente, Somogyi, Chapleo, and White[29] illustrated that ULDN significantly increased tolerance time to cold pressor pain compared to buprenorphine alone. These studies open the possibility of using ULDN as an adjunct to opioid pain management to increase the antinociceptive effects, ultimately reducing the dose needed for sufficient analgesia. This is likely due to the intermittent binding of ULDN to opioid receptors, resulting in the compensatory release of endogenous opioids. One of the more common side effects of opiate agonists is pruritus or itching. However, combination opiate agonist–antagonists have reduced the incidence of pruritus. Research into the effects of naltrexone cream and low-dose intravenous naltrexone has shown them to be significantly more effective at reducing pruritus associated with allergic dermatitis and liver disease, respectively.[30]

Firouzian et al.[31] conducted a randomized, double-blind, placebo-controlled study to evaluate the effects of a single ultra-low-dose infusion of naltrexone on pain intensity after lumbar discectomy in patients receiving patient-controlled anesthesia (PCA) with morphine. Eighty patients were randomized to receive naloxone, at a total dose of 0.25 mcg/kg/hr added to the normal saline infusion, or placebo post-surgery. All patients received a morphine PCA pump. Patients graded pain intensity, nausea, vomiting, and pruritus on a 0–10 VAS prior to being discharged from the anesthesia unit, and at 1, 6, 12, and 24 hours postoperatively. Infusion of ultra-low-dose naltrexone with morphine PCA resulted in a significant reduction in pain intensity, nausea, pruritus, and morphine consumption compared to the placebo group. The median (interquartile range) of morphine consumption after surgery was 26 (24.25 to 28) mg in the naloxone group compared to 34 (32–36) mg in the placebo group.

Xiao, Wu, Zhou et al.[32] conducted a randomized clinical study also looking at the effects of ultra-low-dose naltrexone infusion on postoperative opioid requirements and recovery in 72 patients undergoing open colorectal surgery. Patients were randomized to receive intraoperative remifentanil at either 0.1 mcg/kg/min, 0.30 mcg/kg/min, or 0.3 mcg/kg/min plus naltrexone at 0.25 mcg/kg/h after induction. Results showed that larger doses of remifentanil used intraoperatively triggered acute opioid tolerance postoperatively. Ultra-low-dose naltrexone improved opioid tolerance, improved functional recovery, and reduced the length of hospital stay.

A case report of a 35-year-old male with 2 years of chronic low back pain and a VAS score of 90–100 most of the time, interfering with daily activities, was initiated on 2 mg of LDN for 2 weeks, followed by an increase in dose to 4 mg daily at bedtime. At the time of presentation, his Modified Oswestry's Disability Questionnaire (MODQ) was 65–70%. Lumbar magnetic resonance imaging revealed diffuse posterior bulge and right posterolateral disc perfusion at L5-S1, causing bilateral compression of neural foramina. This patient reported no appreciable response in pain at the 2 mg dose. Two weeks after the 4 mg dose was initiated, the patient reported a 30–40% reduction in pain. After 4 weeks on the 4 mg dose, his VAS score was 35 and MODQ was 35.5%. Low-dose naltrexone was stopped after 6 weeks of administration. At the last follow-up (6 months post-LDN initiation), the patient reported minimal pain and was able to participate in all daily activities. No adverse events were noticed during or after LDN treatment in the patient.[33]

In a case report of a 48-year-old male with a history of diabetes mellitus II, hypertension, hyperlipidemia, coronary artery disease, and widespread complex regional pain syndrome (CRPS), 4.5 mg of LDN daily reduced pain on the Numeric Rating Scale (NRS) from an 8 to 10 prior to treatment to an NRS pain level of 5 to 6 after starting treatment. This patient was also receiving low-dose ketamine infusions prior to and during LDN treatment. After LDN treatment, this patient required lower doses of IV ketamine at decreased frequency (6-week intervals versus 3-week intervals with pain spikes not as high). The patient also recovered from CRPS flares more quickly, felt more energetic, tolerated pain better, and slept better within 2 months of treatment. His dystonic spasms stopped, and he was able to walk without a cane. It was noted that this patient's symptoms reduced in severity but not in distribution. Low-dose naltrexone was well-tolerated.[34] Therapy with LDN is thought to help reduce pain by antagonizing TLR4, which are upregulated in microglia cells in the CNS, thereby reducing inflammatory markers in the CNS.[35,36]

In a second case exploring the use of LDN therapy in CRPS, a 12-year-old female with a history of Ehlers–Danlos syndrome (EDS) hypermobility type 1, dysautonomia, non-epileptic seizures, chronic gastritis, mitochondrial dysfunction, asthma, vision loss, thyroid tumor, and anti-cardio-lipin antibodies was prescribed LDN 3 mg daily, in addition to ketamine troches (sublingual) 10 mg as needed. After 4 weeks, LDN was increased to 4.5 mg daily. After starting LDN, her pain scores dropped from an NRS of (7–10)/10 to an NRS of (3–5)/10. She also noted a decrease in allodynia and a decrease in sensitivity to touch and temperature change. There was no effect on dystonia. The patient was able to progressively reduce the use of ketamine troches 3 weeks after starting LDN and was taking them rarely after 8 weeks. Treatment with LDN was temporarily discontinued due to an ankle surgery and reinstated after 1 week postoperatively. The patient noticed a decrease in her postoperative pain 3 weeks after resuming LDN, with no spread of CRPS. The symptoms of CRPS resolved completely and LDN was well-tolerated. At the time of this case report, the patient had been maintained on LDN for 18 months.[34]

In a case report of a 76-year-old male with a 30-year history of type 2 diabetes and 7-year history of diabetic neuropathy, LDN therapy was associated with an improvement in VAS, short form McGill pain questionnaire, and 11-point Likert pain scale scores. The patient had previously tried amitriptyline, pregabalin, duloxetine, lamotrigine, NSAIDs, injectable vitamin B-complex, and injectable vitamin D in varying doses and combinations for 1–2 months with little to no relief. Naltrexone was administered at 1 mg for 2 weeks, 2 mg for 2 weeks, and finally 4 mg for 2 weeks. The patient did not show a response to the 1 mg dose; however he showed partial improvement in burning pain with the 2 mg dose. At 4 mg, the patient showed a reduction in VAS scores from 90% to 5%, the short form McGill pain questionnaire from 8 to 1, and the 11-point Likert scale from 8 to 2.[37]

CANCER

Cancer is the second leading cause of death in the U.S. and is a result of uncontrolled cellular growth, local tissue invasion, and distant metastases. Cancer is a complex disease caused by physical damage, chemical damage, biological damage, genetic alterations, and/or epigenetic alterations. Exposure or damage from a physical, chemical, or biological agent is believed to be the signal for cancer propagation. Additionally, genetic and epigenetic changes and predispositions play a role in the etiology of cancer.

The current body of literature on LDN and cancer explores the relationship between OGF and OGFr and their effect on cellular proliferation in ovarian, pancreatic, colorectal, and squamous cell carcinomas. Short-term LDN was observed to influence the OGF–OGFr axis, which is responsible for the regulation of cell proliferation.[38] Many other studies have investigated the use of LDN alone or in combination with standard therapies in ovarian cancer and renal carcinomas with promising results. Donahue, McLaughlin, and Zagon[39] observed that the combination of LDN and cisplatin in ovarian tumors enhanced the inhibition of tumorigenesis, depressed DNA synthesis, and reduced angiogenesis. Additionally, LDN seemed to reduce adverse events with cisplatin therapy. Another study confirmed that LDN upregulates OGF and OGFr, inhibiting tumorigenesis and cancer pro-liferation.[40] An alternative theory is that LDN prevents the prolonged cellular state of arrest in response to DNA damage, which places the cells in a state of cytostasis. This state of cytostasis reduces the sensitivity of the cell to treatment, preventing the cell from entering the apoptosis path-way. The intermittent binding of LDN does not block cells from entering this apoptosis pathway.[41]

Evidence seems to support LDN as an adjunct to current anticancer regimens, both by enhancing the drugs' anti-tumorigenesis effects and by decreasing the severity of side effects related to chemotherapy regimens.

A case study by Miskoff and Chaudhri[42] evaluated LDN in a 50-year-old male with prolonged survival and a history of prostate and lung cancer after a resection of adenocarcinoma in the right upper lobe of the lung. The patient began chemo-radiotherapy with cisplatin and pemetrexed post-surgery. Chemotherapy was stopped after the second treatment session due to intolerable side effects. After numerous additional health challenges, the patient was started on LDN 4.5 mg nightly. Imaging performed following the initiation of LDN has been unremarkable. At the time of publication by study authors, this patient had been on LDN for almost 4 years. More research is needed to assess the clinical efficacy of the use of LDN in these patients.

AUTISM SPECTRUM CONDITIONS

Autism spectrum conditions (ASC) are a heterogeneous collection of behavioral disorders with an estimated prevalence of 1 in 68 children in the U.S. One of the theories behind the pathophysiology of ASC is an imbalance of beta-endorphins resulting in behaviors such as decreased socialism, insensitivity to pain, and motor hyperactivity. Brown and Panksepp[43] discuss LDN's role in both immune and psychiatric regulation resulting in improved social bonding, emotional well-being, and relieving symptoms in autism and depression. Furthermore, Roy, Roy, Deb, Unwin, and Roy[44] investigated the effects of naltrexone on symptoms in patients with ASC. Participants were given 0.5–2 mg/kg of naltrexone with 77% showing improvement in irritability and hyperactivity compared to placebo. Naltrexone's effects on endorphins has clinically only been observed with low doses. Given the positive outcomes of the above-mentioned study using traditional dosing, it is logical to believe that LDN would have an equal or possibly more profound effect on ASC symptoms.

WOUND HEALING AND INFECTION

In their book *The Promise of Low Dose Naltrexone Therapy: Potential Benefits in Cancer, Autoimmune, Neurological and Infectious Disorders*, Moore et al.[45] discuss the difference between the effects of LDN and high-dose naltrexone (HDN). High-dose naltrexone has been observed to have a positive effect on cellular growth due to the selective blockade of the OGF–OGFr axis. The primary cell type in the granulation of cellular tissue is the fibroblast, the activity of which has been shown to be increased by HDN applied as a cream.[46] Additionally, in an animal study of wound healing in diabetic rats, topical 0.03% naltrexone cream applied to the wound accelerated DNA synthesis, increased mast cells, enhanced the expression of platelet-derived growth factor, and enhanced vascular endothelial growth factor.[47] The complete blockade of the OGF–OGFr axis by HDN appears to increase cellular growth and angiogenesis, both of which are important in wound healing. These are promising results for the use of naltrexone in wound healing, especially in patients with disease states with impaired wound healing, such as diabetes.

Alternatively, LDN has been studied in infection control due to its properties of inhibiting cellular growth through upregulating OGF levels. Tian, Jiao, and Wang et al.[48] showed that increased OGF exerted both a prophylactic and protective effect against the influenza A virus in mice. Additionally, LDN has been studied in HIV and hepatitis infections with similar protective results. It has been discussed above how LDN increases OGF levels, thereby explaining the relationship between LDN therapy and viral deterrence. Opioid growth factor receptors also appear to modulate the development of some bacterial species, activation of which seems to downregulate cellular growth. Low-dose naltrexone has been implicated in the prevention of *Staphylococcus aureus*, *Pseudomonas aeruginosa*, and *Streptococcus marcescens* growth, opening the possibility of using LDN in infection control.[45]

MYALGIC ENCEPHALOMYELITIS/CHRONIC FATIGUE SYNDROME (ME/CFS)

Myalgic encephalomyelitis/chronic fatigue syndrome is a complex, debilitating disease of unknown etiology. The prevalence varies widely. A systemic review and meta-analysis by Lim et al. estimates an overall prevalence of 0.89% according to the most commonly used CDC-1994 case definition criteria.[49] The peak age of onset is between 20 and 45 years, with a female to male ratio of 3:1.[50] Although the primary symptom is post-exertional fatigue, various neurologic, cardiovascular, respiratory, and gastrointestinal manifestations are commonly present. Currently, there are no known effective medical treatments, and diagnosis is primarily though the exclusion of other conditions. No controlled clinical trials of LDN use in this patient population have been reported in the literature. Case studies, retrospective chart reviews, and anecdotal reports have been published.

Bolton et al.[51] published three case reports of LDN administration for the treatment of chronic fatigue syndrome. The first case report is a 63-year-old female who developed profound weakness, fatigue, general malaise, light and sound sensitivity, repeated dizziness causing collapse, persistent anxiety, and widespread pain, all of which occurred after the development of viral meningitis. Pertinent history also includes an episode of gastroenteritis with subsequent multiple food intolerances. Multiple medications were tried with no improvement. In 2010, the patient was started on 1.5 mg of LDN daily, and the dose was increased slowly over the course of 2 years. Slight energy improvements and reduced intolerances to food were noticed at a dose of 4.5 mg/day, however, the dose was reduced to 3 mg due to headaches. The LDN dose was again slowly increased, and this patient has been maintained on 6 mg BID for the past 7 years at the time of publication. This patient reports a normal quality of life with symptoms such as poor sleep and excessive pain absent. Intellectual and cognitive functioning have returned. Energy levels were still noted to be reduced slightly during events such as infections, prolonged overexertion or excessive mental effort, with some reductions delayed up to 48 hours.

The second case report is of a 59-year-old female who was started on LDN 0.25 mg/day (at age 54) for a 25-year history of profound fatigue and weakness, flu-like symptoms, post-exertional malaise, cognitive impairment, nausea, widespread pain, and sleep disturbance. Possible precipitating factors that may have led to her diagnosis of ME/CFS include possible viral infection, early pregnancy, and exposure to ticks within 6 months of symptom onset. A very low dose of naltrexone was started due to known immune hypersensitivity (urticarial). Improved sleep and lower pain levels were noticed at a dose of 1 mg/day, approximately 6 months after LDN initiation. Pain and sleep issues continued, but at a lower level. Her functional level did not improve, and symptoms of post-exertional neuroimmune exhaustion, periodic muscle weakness, orthostatic intolerance, symptomatic sinus tachycardia, urticarial rashes, and susceptibility to bacterial infections are still present. This patient considered LDN to be beneficial long term, and she also takes ivabradine and certirizine to control these symptoms.

The third case report is a 39-year-old male who initiated LDN 1 mg/day (at age 37) for chronic fatigue syndrome that was diagnosed by his pediatrician during childhood. Pertinent medical history during childhood includes a head injury, glandular fever, severe tonsillitis, nasal polyps, sinusitis, and seasonal allergic rhinitis. The LDN dose was gradually increased to 4.5 mg/day. Improved sleep pattern and fewer colds, which are no longer associated with an energy dip or subsequent depression, were reported. Functional level improved from being mild/moderately limited on a daily basis (60–70% on functional activity scale) to mild limitations (80–90% on functional activity scale).

Polo et al.[52] investigated LDN in 218 ME/CFS patients through a retrospective chart review at a private sleep and breathing clinic. Typical ME/CFS patients at the clinic had been sick for several years and had undergone extensive tests at primary and secondary healthcare levels to rule out other diseases. The severity of symptoms ranged from mild to very severe. Patients were directed to start LDN 1.5 mg every morning for 1 week, followed by a dose increase to 3 mg (1.5 mg twice daily). The daily dose was allowed to be increased to 4.5 mg after 6 weeks on LDN therapy. Treatment was discontinued if no treatment effect was observed within the first 6 months. Treatment response and adverse effects were recorded during visits or upon renewal of prescription and were based on spontaneous reporting, without any structured questionnaire or rating scales. The magnitude of response was scored on a scale of 0–6 based on the number of symptom modalities for which any improvement was reported. Adverse effects were calculated with a similar scoring system. A large proportion of patients (73.9%) reported some degree of alleviation of ME/CFS symptoms after the initiation of LDN therapy, and approximately half of the patients experienced a response in at least two different ME/CFS symptoms. Improvement in vigilance/alertness was reported in 51.4% of patients, physical performance improvement in 23.9%, and cognitive dysfunction diminished in 21.1%. Adverse events were reported in 54.2% of patients, and 7.3% of patients discontinued treatment due to an adverse event. Most adverse symptoms were mild and temporary, with the most common being insomnia (15.3%) and nausea (15.3%). Adverse symptoms were more common than expected during the initial phase of treatment, including a wide spectrum of autonomic symptoms typically observed in ME/CFS. Study authors noted that an initial aggravation of symptoms followed by rapid alleviation suggests a possibility that LDN targets underlying nervous system dysfunction. While this retrospective study provides some preliminary information on the effectiveness and safety of LDN for ME/CFS, additional prospective, controlled clinical trials are needed.

DISCUSSION

Despite the negative connotations associated with naltrexone therapy, clinical evidence suggests that low doses of naltrexone provide benefits in multiple inflammatory and immune-modulatory disease states. Topics for future research should focus on other common inflammatory and immune-modulating diseases (e.g., asthma, chronic obstructive pulmonary disease, rheumatoid arthritis, diabetes). Previous studies on the effects of oral opiate antagonists on exercise-induced bronchospasms did not show a decrease in FEV1 following exercise.[53] However, we have only recently discovered the anti-inflammatory effects of low-dose opioid antagonists, and one of the previous studies investigated normal doses of nalmephene. To date, literature searches through PubMed have not produced any research on low-dose naltrexone in asthma, chronic obstructive pulmonary disease (COPD), or diabetes.

Only one study was found in PubMed for rheumatoid arthritis. This pharmacoepidemiologic study evaluated the effects of LDN on prescription medicine use in patients with rheumatoid arthritis (RA) and seropositive arthritis.[54] A total of 360 patients were identified from the Norwegian prescription database and stratified into three groups according to LDN exposure. Prescriptions were compared 1 year before and 1 year after starting LDN. Results showed that, in persistent users of LDN (four or more LDN prescriptions dispensed), there was a significant 13% relative reduction in the cumulative defined daily doses (DDDs) dispensed of all examined medicines at 1 year after the start of LDN when compared to 1 year prior. Persistent LDN users had significantly reduced DDDs of NSAID and opioids, and a lower proportion of users of DMARDs (–6.7 percentage points, 95% CI –12.3 to –1.0, p=0.028), TNF-α antagonists, and opioids. This study is unable to draw conclusions on the efficacy of LDN in RA/seropositive per se, but results suggest that persistent LDN use is associated with a reduced consumption of medications relevant to RA/seropositive arthritis.

The pathogenesis of rheumatoid arthritis (RA) involves both bone destruction and bone matrix degradation leading to the chronic inflammation of joint capsules and ultimately destruction of the joint. The autoimmune response seen in RA involves ILs, TNFs, and MMPs, all of which have been observed to be influenced by LDN therapy. Considering that 1% of the U.S. population has RA, research showing a positive impact with LDN would have modest application potential.

Asthma is characterized by outflow obstruction due to inflammation of the airways. The presence of CD4+ T-helper cells in asthma, along with other immune responders (e.g., eosinophils, basophils, macrophages) results in the release of proinflammatory cytokines. Interleukins, granulocyte-macrophage colony-stimulating factor, and leukotrienes, among other cytokines, further activate neutrophils, eosinophils, and macrophages in asthma, leading to acute and chronic inflammation. Low-dose naltrexone has been shown to mediate the replication of CD4+ T-helper cells in MS. Theoretically, the mediation of CD4+ T-helper cells in asthma may provide a preventative effect on asthma exacerbations. Given that more than 25 million people in the U.S. are affected by asthma, research into LDN's effect on exacerbations and quality of life has enormous potential.

Chronic obstructive pulmonary disease is a preventable and manageable disease that is not fully reversible due to destruction of the tissues in the airway. Major inflammatory cells involved in the pathology of COPD include TNFα, ILs, and leukotrienes. Bronchodilators are the mainstay of treatment for COPD and help reduce symptoms as well as improve quality of life. However, they may not slow the progression of the disease. Acute exacerbations of COPD increase disease progression and mortality. There is limited research on COPD exacerbations, but it is known that inflammatory mediators are present in sputum collected from patients who are experiencing an acute exacerbation. Low-dose naltrexone has shown to be effective at mediating inflammatory markers such as TNFα and ILs, so there may be a benefit to LDN therapy in either symptom management and/or prevention of acute exacerbations. COPD is the fourth leading cause of death in the U.S. and the only leading cause to increase in incidence over the past 30 years. Research into the impact of LDN on COPD mortality and morbidity would be invaluable.

Diabetes is typically characterized as a metabolic disorder due to either a deficiency of insulin secretion, sensitivity, or both. Type-1 diabetes mellitus (T1DM) is an autoimmune disease mediated by macrophage and T lymphocyte destruction of β-cells in the pancreas. Patients with type-2 diabetes mellitus (T2DM) often have high visceral adipose tissue, which produces several inflammatory and immune-modulatory cytokines (e.g., TNFα, IL-6, angiotensinogen). Low-dose naltrexone has been observed to have a modulating effect on macrophages and T-cells, as well as downregulating inflammatory and immune-modulatory cytokines. Additionally, Di Scala-Guenot and McIntosh[55] showed a relationship between OGF and pancreatic endocrine secretion of insulin. Naltrexone's ability to upregulate OGF and modulate the OGF–OGFr axis in low doses may play a role in the pancreatic secretion of insulin in diabetes. This theoretical and observed evidence may support the use of LDN as preventative or adjunct therapy in T1DM and T2DM patients.

Naltrexone overall appears to be safe and well-tolerated based on current studies and clinical experience. A systematic review and meta-analysis conducted by Bolton et al.[56] evaluated serious adverse events (SAEs) from randomized, placebo-controlled trials published with naloxone, at target doses of 3 mg to 250 mg, in a wide range of conditions (e.g., various addiction and psychiatric disorders, Crohn's disease, fibromyalgia, cancers) after January 1, 2001 through May of 2018. The analysis looked at 89 randomized controlled trials in 11,194 participants and found no evidence of an increased risk of SAEs occurring in the naltrexone group when compared to the placebo group. Data for reporting adverse events (AEs) in this study were poor, with fewer than 21 studies having AE data to contribute to analyses. A secondary analysis of 188 AEs indicated 6 AEs of statistical significance: decreased appetite, dizziness, nausea, sleepiness, sweating, and vomiting. These AEs were noted as mild in nature and common among all patients.

Dosing of LDN should be individualized with a "start low and go slow" approach. Patients may experience temporary and transient side effects upon initiation of LDN, including sleep disturbances and vivid dreams, nausea, and irritability. Side effects can be mitigated by decreasing the dose and titrating. A temporary addition of an H2 blocker, or administering LDN sublingual may be tried if nausea is experienced. Taking LDN in the morning instead of evening is recommended in cases of sleep disturbances. Low-dose naltrexone does not work immediately and can typically take anywhere from a few weeks to many months before patients begin to feel better due to LDN's immune-modulating effects.

Given the potential myriad of benefits of LDN, the question remains as to why it is not prescribed more frequently in the U.S. The answer most certainly is a result of lack of education in the healthcare field and minimal advertising to the public. In 2013, there was a surge in prescribing in Norway following a documentary about LDN therapy.[57] Prescriptions for LDN reached up to 0.3%

of the population of Norway following the documentary. To put that into perspective, 71% of general practitioners in Norway have acknowledged prescribing at least one LDN prescription between 2013 and 2014. If there were a similar influx of LDN prescriptions in the U.S., that would equate to nearly 1 million new patients. This may even be conservative given the almost universal potential for LDN in inflammatory and immune-modulatory diseases.

CONCLUSION

For those patients who have tried and failed other therapies for multiple sclerosis, Crohn's disease, sarcoidosis, fibromyalgia, and pain disorders, LDN is another potential therapy that may be helpful in disease management. Additionally, naltrexone may gain an increased acceptance as an adjunct therapy for autism spectrum conditions, wound healing, and antimicrobial stewardship. The wealth of research on the anti-inflammatory and immune-modulating effects of LDN has revealed promising results, and it should be a matter of time until LDN is recommended in the guidelines as adjunct therapy or monotherapy.

REFERENCES

1. Rösner S., Hackl-Herrwerth A., Leucht S., Vecchi S., Srisurapanont M., Soyka M. Opioid antagonists for alcohol dependence. *Cochrane Database Syst Rev* 2010;12(12):CD001867. doi:10.1002/14651858. CD001867.pub3.
2. Mannelli P., Patkar A.A., Peindl K., Gorelick D.A., Wu L.T., Gottheil E. Very low dose naltrexone addition in opioid detoxification: a randomized, controlled trial. *Addict Biol* 2009;14(2):204–213. doi:10.1111/j.1369-1600.2008.00119.x.
3. Mannelli P., Peindl K., Patkar A.A., Wu L., Tharwani H.M., Gorelick D.A. Problem drinking and low-dose naltrexone-assisted opioid detoxification. *J Stud Alcohol Drugs* 2011;72(3):507–513.
4. Froehlich J.C., Hausauer B.J., Rasmussen D.D. Combining naltrexone and prazosin in a single oral medication decreases alcohol drinking more effectively than does either drug alone. *Alcohol Clin Exp Res* 2013;37(10):1763–1770. doi:10.1111/acer.12148.
5. Sushchyk S., Xi Z., Wang J.B. Combination of levo-tetrahydropalmatine and low dose naltrexone: a promising treatment for prevention of cocaine relapse. *J Pharmacol Exp Ther* 2016;357(2):248–257. doi:10.1124/jpet.115.229542.
6. Toljan K., Vrooman B. Low-dose naltrexone (LDN)-review of therapeutic utilization. *Med Sci* (Besel) 2018;6(4):82.
7. Zagon I.S., Verderame M.F., McLaughlin P.J. The biology of the opioid growth factor receptor (OGFr). *Brain Res Brain Res Rev* 2002;38(3):351–376. doi:10.1016/s0165-0173(01)00160-6.
8. Leavitt S.B. Opioid antagonists in pain management. *Pract Pain Manag* 2011;9(3). www.practicalpain-management.com. Accessed February 7, 2020.
9. Behari B., Gluck D., Zagon I.S. Low dose naltrexone. www.lowdosenaltrexone.org. Accessed February 7, 2020.
10. Ludwig M.D., Zagon I.S., McLaughlin P.J. Featured article: serum [Met[5]]-enkephalin levels are reduced in multiple sclerosis and restored by low-dose naltrexone. *Exp Biol Med (Maywood)* 2017;242(15):1524–1533. doi:10.1177/153570217724791.
11. Turel A.P., Oh K.H., Zagon I.S., McLaughlin P.J. Low dose naltrexone for treatment of multiple sclerosis: a retrospective chart review of safety and tolerability. *J Clin Psychopharmacol* 2015;35(5):609–611. doi:10.1097/jcp.0000000000000373.
12. Gironi M., Martinelli-Boneschi F., Sacerdote P., Solaro C., Zaffaroni M., et al. A pilot trial of low-dose naltrexone in primary progressive multiple sclerosis. *Mult Scler* 2008;14(8):1076–1083.
13. Cree B.A.C., Kornyeyeva E., Goodin D.S. Pilot trial of low-dose naltrexone and quality of life in multiple sclerosis. *Ann Neurol* 2010;68(2):145–150.
14. Sharafaddinzadeh N., Moghtaderi A., Kashipazha D., Majdinasab N., Shalbafan B. The effect of low-dose naltrexone on quality of life of patients with multiple sclerosis: a randomized placebo-controlled trial. *Mult Scler* 2010;16(8):964–969.
15. Raknes G., Småbrekke L. Low dose naltrexone in multiple sclerosis: effects on medication use: a quasi-experimental study. *PLOS ONE* 2017;12(11):e0187423.

16. Ludwig M.D., Turel A.P., Zagon I.S., McLaughlin P.J. Long-term treatment with low dose naltrexone maintains stable health in patients with multiple sclerosis. *Mult Scler J Exp Transl Clin* 2016;2:2055217316672242.

17. Smith J.P., Stock H., Bingaman S., Mauger D., Rogosnitzky M., Zagon I.S. Low-dose naltrexone therapy improves active Crohn's disease. *Am J Gastroenterol* 2007;102(4):820–828. doi:10.1111/j.1572-0241.2007.01045.x.

18. Segal D., MacDonald J.K., Chande N. Low dose naltrexone for induction of remission in Crohn's disease. *Cochrane Database Syst Rev* 2014;21(2):cd010410. doi:10.1002/14651858.cd010410.

19. Lie M.R.K.L., van der Giessen J., Fuhler G.M., de Lima A., Peppelenbosch M.P., et al. Low dose naltrexone for induction of remission in inflammatory bowel disease patients. *J Transl Med* 2018;16(1):55.

20. Raknes G., Simonsen P., Småbrekke L. Corrigendum: the effect of low-dose naltrexone on medication in inflammatory bowel disease: a quasi experimental before-and-after prescription database study. *J Crohns Colitis* 2019;13(12):1588–1589.

21. Weinstock L.B., Myers T.L., Shetty A. Low-dose naltrexone for the treatment of sarcoidosis. *Sarcoidosis Vasc Dif* 2017;34(2):184–187.

22. Parkitny L., Younger J. Reduced pro-inflammatory cytokines after eight weeks of low-dose naltrexone for fibromyalgia. *Biomedicines* 2017;5(2):16. doi:10.3390/biomedicines5020016.

23. Younger J., Mackey S. Fibromyalgia symptoms are reduced by low-dose naltrexone: a pilot study. *Pain Med* 2009;10(4):663–672.

24. Younger J., Noor N., McCue R., Mackey S. Low-dose naltrexone for the treatment of fibromyalgia: findings of a small, randomized, double-blind, placebo-controlled, counterbalanced, crossover trial assessing daily pain levels. *Arthritis Rheum* 2013;65(2):529–538. doi:10.1002/art.37734.

25. Centers for Disease Control and Prevention. Opioid prescribing. https://www.cdc.gov/features/opiod-prescribing-guide/index. Accessed February 7, 2020.

26. Embeda [package insert]. Bristol, TN: King Pharmaceuticals, Inc. 2009.

27. Troxyca E.R. [package insert]. New York: Pfizer, Inc. 2016.

28. Leri F. Co-administration of opioid agonists and antagonists in addiction and pain medicine. *Expert Opin Pharmacother* 2008;9(8):1387–1396. doi:10.1517/14656566.9.8.1387.

29. Hay J.L., La Vincente S.F., Somogyi A.A., Chapleo C.B., White J.M. Potentiation of buprenorphine antinociception with ultra-low dose naltrexone in healthy subjects. *Eur J Pain* 2011;15(3):293–298. doi:10.1016/j.ejpain.2010.07.009.

30. Moore E.A., Wilkinson S. *The Promise of Low Dose Naltrexone Therapy: Potential Benefits in Cancer, Autoimmune, Neurological and Infectious Disorders.* Jefferson, NC: Mcfarland & Company, 2009.

31. Firouzian A., Gholipour Baradari A., Alipour A., Emami Zeydi A., Zamani Kiasari A., et al. Ultra-low-dose naloxone as an adjuvant to patient controlled analgesia (PCA) with morphine for postoperative pain relief following lumber discectomy: a double-blind, randomized, placebo-controlled trial. *J Neurosurg Anesthesiol* 2018;30(1):26–31.

32. Xiao Y., Wu L., Zhou Q., Xiong W., Duan X, Huang X. A randomized clinical trial of the effects of ultra-low-dose naloxone infusion on postoperative opioid requirements and recovery. *Acta Anaesthesiol Scand* 2015;59(9):1194–1203.

33. Ghai B., Bansal D., Hota D., Shah C.S., Pharm M. Off-label, low-dose naltrexone for refractory chronic low back pain. *Pain Med* 2014;15(5):883–884.

34. Chopra P., Cooper M.S. Treatment of complex regional pain syndrome (CRPS) using low dose naltrexone (LDN). *J Neuroimmune Pharmacol* 2013;8(3):470–476. doi:10.1007/s11481-013-9451-y.

35. Younger J., Parkitny L., McLain D. The use of low-dose naltrexone (LDN) as a novel anti-inflammatory treatment for chronic pain. *Clin Rheumatol* 2014;33(4):451–459. doi:10.1007/s10067-014-2517-2.

36. Sturm K.M., Collin M. Low-dose naltrexone: a new therapy option for complex regional pain syndrome type I patients. *Int J Pharml Compd.* 2016;20(3):197–201.

37. Hota D., Srinivasan A., Dutta P., Bhansali A., Chakrabarti A. Off-label, low-dose naltrexone for refractory painful diabetic neuropathy. *Pain Med* 2016;17(4):790–791. doi:10.1093/pm/pnv009.

38. Donahue R.N., McLaughlin P.J., Zagon I.S. Low-dose naltrexone targets the opioid growth factor-opioid growth factor receptor pathway to inhibit cell proliferation: mechanistic evidence from a tissue culture model. *Exp Biol Med (Maywood)* 2011;236(9):1036–1050. doi:10.1258/ebm.2011.011121.

39. Donahue R.N., McLaughlin P.J., Zagon I.S. Low-dose naltrexone suppresses ovarian cancer and exhibits enhanced inhibition in combination with cisplatin. *Exp Biol Med (Maywood)* 2011;236(7):883–895. doi:10.1258/ebm.2011.011096.

40. Zagon I.S., Donahue R., McLaughlin P.J. Targeting the opioid growth factor: opioid growth factor receptor axis for treatment of human ovarian cancer. *Exp Biol Med (Maywood)* 2013;238(5):579–587. doi:10.1177/1535370213488483.

41. Liu W.M., Scott K.A., Dennis J.L., Kaminska E., Levett A.J., Dalgleish A.G. Naltrexone at low doses upregulates a unique gene expression not seen with normal doses: implications for its use in cancer therapy. *Int J Oncol* 2016;49(2):793–802. doi:10.3892/ijo.2016.3567.

42. Miskoff J.A., Chaudhri M. Low dose naltrexone and lung cancer: a case report and discussion. *Cureus* 2018;10(7):e2924.

43. Brown N., Panksepp J. Low-dose naltrexone for disease prevention and quality of life. *Med Hypotheses* 2009;72(3):333–337. doi:10.1016/j.mehy.2008.06.048.

44. Roy A., Roy M., Deb S., Unwin G., Roy A. Are opioid antagonists effective in attenuating the core symptoms of autism spectrum conditions in children: a systematic review. *J Intellect Disabil Res* 2015;59(4):293–306. doi:10.1111/jir.12122.

45. Moore E.A., Wilkinson S. *The Promise of Low Dose Naltrexone Therapy.* Jefferson, NC: Mcfarland & Company, Inc. 2009.

46. Immonen J.A., Zagon I.S., McLaughlin P.J. Selective blockade of the OGF-OGFr pathway by naltrexone accelerates fibroblast proliferation and wound healing. *Exp Biol Med (Maywood)* 2014;239(10):1300–1309. doi:10.1177/1535370214543061.

47. McLaughlin P.J., Cain J.D., Titunick M.B., Sassani J.W., Zagon I.S. Topical naltrexone is a safe and effective alternative to standard treatment of diabetic wounds. *Adv Wound Care* 2017;6(9):279–288. doi:10.1089/wound.2016.0725.

48. Tian J., Jiao X., Wang X., Geng J., Wang R., et al. Novel effect of methionine enkephalin against influenza a virus infection through inhibiting TLR7-MyD88-TRAF6-NF-kB p65 signaling pathway. *Int Immunopharmacol* 2017;55:38–48. doi:10.1016/j.intimp.2017.12.001.

49. Lim E.-J., Ahn Y.-C., Jang E.-S., Lee S.-W., Lee S.-H., Son C.-G. Systmatic review and meta-analysis of the prevalence of chronic fatigue syndrome/myalgic encephalomyelitis (CFS/ME). *J Trans Med* 2020;18(1):100. doi:10.1186/s12967-020-02269-0.

50. Cortes Rivera M., Mastronardi C., Silva-Aldana C.T., Arcos-Burgos M., Lidbury B.A. Myalgic encephalomyelitis/chronic fatigue syndrome: a comprehensive review. *Diagnostics* 2019;9(3):E91. doi:10.3390/diagnostics9030091.

51. Bolton M.J., Chapman B.P., Van Marwijk H. Low-dose naltrexone as a treatment for chronic fatigue syndrome. *BMJ Case Rep* 2020;13(1):e232502. doi:10.1136/bcr-2019-232502.

52. Polo O., Pesonen P., Tuominen E. Low-dose naltrexone in the treatment of myalgic encephalomyelitis/chronic fatigue syndrome (ME/CFS). *Fatigue Biomed Health Behav* 2019;7(4):207–217. doi:10.1080/21641846.2019.1692770.

53. Christopher M.A., Wyzan D., Harman E., Hendeles L. The effects of nalmephene, a potent oral opiate antagonist, on exercise-induced bronchospasm. *J Allergy Clin Immunol* 1988;82(6):1037–1041. doi:10.1016/0091-6749(88)90141-8.

54. Raknes G., Småbrekke L. Low dose naltrexone: effects on medication in rheumatoid and seropositive arthritis. A nationwide register-based controlled quasi-experimental before-after study. *PLoS ONE* 2019;14(2):e0212460.

55. Di Scala-Guénot D., McIntosh C.H. The effect of met-enkephalin and naloxone on somatostatin and insulin secretion from the isolated, perfused rat pancreas. *Diabetes* 1985;34(12):1283–1287. doi:10.2337/diab.34.12.1283.

56. Bolton M., Hodkinson A., Boda S., Mould A., Panagioti M., et al. Serious adverse events reported in placebo randomised controlled trials of oral naltrexone: a systematic review and meta-analysis. *BMC Med* 2019;17(1):10.

57. Raknes G., Småbrekke L. A sudden and unprecedented increase in low dose naltrexone (LDN) prescribing in Norway. Patient and prescriber characteristics, and dispense patterns: a drug utilization cohort study. *Pharmacoepidemiol Drug Saf* 2017;26(2):136–142. doi:10.1002/pds.4110.

18 Topical Pain Medications and Their Role in Pain Management

Sahar Swidan and Mara Rubin

CONTENTS

The goal of this chapter is to review topical pain medications and their place in therapy. The ability to bypass first-pass metabolism and minimize systemic side effects allows for safer options, especially for patients on multiple medications. There is a growing interest in utilizing compounded preparations to improve adherence and efficacy.

Topical pain medications have applications in many different disease states. They can be utilized to help manage pain symptoms or combined to offer synergistic effects. Neuropathic pain (NP) is a debilitating condition that impairs patient quality of life. The international association for the study of pain defines NP as "pain caused by a lesion or disease of the somatosensory nervous system."[1] Patients will often present with burning, tingling, and the description of needles poking their skin. Due to variability in subjective response to analgesia, oftentimes patients will try multiple different therapies to try and manage pain.

CAPSAICIN

- Capsaicin is a lipophilic compound that diffuses poorly into aqueous solutions in the body, making it ideal for topical, localized delivery. It functions by acting as a vanilloid receptor agonist, binding at the transient potential vanilloid receptor 1 (TRPV1). It acts by depleting substance P from sensory nerve endings to modulate neuropathic pain. Chronic exposure to capsaicin can produce a persistent local effect on cutaneous nociceptors, which is best described as "defunctionalization" and is constituted by reduced spontaneous activity and a loss of responsiveness to a wide range of sensory stimuli.[2,3]
- A literature review by Pickering et al.[4] was performed to evaluate local treatments for localized neuropathic pain. Results showed that both topical 8% capsaicin and topical 5% lidocaine were efficacious for localized neuropathic pain. Both were well-tolerated and safe when used long term and should be considered for first-line use, especially in elderly patients, patients with multiple comorbidities, and polypharmacy.

- A Cochrane review was done to explore high-dose topical capsaicin for neuropathic pain in adults. Randomized controlled trials studying capsaicin 8% patches were included. Four studies featuring 1272 patients treated for postherpetic neuralgia showed significantly improved efficacy outcomes over controls. At both 8 and 12 weeks of therapy, more patients reported feeling much or very much better using high-concentration capsaicin than controls. Two studies involved 801 participants treated for HIV neuropathy. Both studies showed an average reduction in pain intensity by 30% with high-concentration capsaicin. Local adverse reactions were common, such as pruritus, erythema, and burning at the application site.[5]
- A systematic review was done to evaluate the evidence of both oral and topically applied medications in the treatment of osteoarthritis. Capsaicin gel was effective in the management of osteoarthritis. Five randomized controlled trials (RCTs) were evaluated and showed treatment efficacy. In three of the trials, patients applied 0.025% capsaicin four times daily for 4–12 weeks. In the fourth study, 0.015% capsaicin was applied once daily for 6 weeks. The fifth study utilized 0.075% capsaicin four times daily for 4 weeks. In all trials, capsaicin showed a significant improvement in pain compared to placebo. All trials also showed a significant improvement in pain upon movement. Adverse effects included redness and burning sensation.[6]
- A randomized, double-blind, crossover, placebo-controlled clinical study conducted by Kulkantrakorn et al.[7] investigated the efficacy and safety of a 0.075% topical capsaicin lotion on painful diabetic neuropathy. The study included patients with both types 1 and 2 diabetes mellitus who had suffered from painful diabetic neuropathy for at least 1 month. Treatment intervention was studied for 8 weeks followed by a 4-week washout period before crossing over to the other treatment. Participants were instructed to apply the capsaicin lotion to the painful area three times a day. The primary outcome of this study was a reduction in mean pain score from baseline, which was assessed using the visual analog scale (VAS). The secondary endpoints included score changes in neuropathic pain scale, assessing pain with the short form McGill Pain Questionnaire, and the proportion of patients with pain score reductions of 30% to 50%. Safety was also investigated at each visit during the study. There were no significant improvements in pain control compared to placebo for any of the pain measures or for the proportion of patients with pain score reductions of 30% to 50%. There were some adverse effects seen from the group using capsaicin including burning, edema, and erythema. This study failed to show that there was a benefit from using a capsaicin lotion with a concentration of 0.075%.
- Casanueva et al.[8] conducted a two-armed randomized clinical trial testing the effectiveness of Sensedol®, a 0.075% capsaicin topical treatment, in patients with severe fibromyalgia. The primary outcome of this study was a change in the overall score of pain. The secondary outcomes included other fibromyalgia-related variables. A total of 130 patients were treated for 6 weeks and evaluated both at the beginning and end of the 6-week treatment period and again at 6 weeks post-treatment. Participants were instructed to apply the cream three times a day to the affected area. The researchers found that at the end of the 6-week treatment period, patients had shown significant improvements in myalgic score. Six weeks after treatment, patients showed significant improvement in several clinical outcomes, including myalgic score and pressure pain threshold, but the VAS score for pain did not show statistically significant improvement. The overall conclusion from this study was that 0.075% capsaicin cream can provide short-term improvement. The researchers acknowledged that the treatment duration was short and recognize that further studies are needed.

LIDOCAINE

- Baron et al.[9] conducted an open-label, non-inferiority study comparing a 5% lidocaine patch versus pregabalin capsules in post-herpetic neuralgia and diabetic peripheral neuropathy. The primary outcome was response rate after 4 weeks. Secondary outcomes included 30% and 50% reductions in 11-point Numerical Rating Scale (NRS-3), a change in allodynia severity, quality of life (QoL), and patient satisfaction with therapy. Ninety-six patients with post-herpetic neuralgia and 204 with painful diabetic peripheral neuropathy were analyzed. In post-herpetic neuralgia, lidocaine 5% had a 62.2% response while pregabalin had a 46.5% response. Both treatments reduced allodynia severity, and 30–50% reductions in NRS-3 scores and QoL scores were greater with 5% lidocaine. The response to both treatments was comparable in painful diabetic neuropathy. Patients on lidocaine experienced fewer adverse events than those taking pregabalin. This study supports 5% lidocaine as a potential first-line therapy for patients with localized neuropathic pain.

AMITRIPTYLINE

- Oral amitriptyline is currently used for neuropathic pain; however, it can be limited by dose-related anticholinergic effects.
- Chemotherapy-induced peripheral neuropathy (CIPN) is extremely debilitating, and patients have limited options for relief. Dose reduction or the discontinuation of chemotherapy regimens may result from severe CIPN. A pilot study done by Rossignol et al.[10] investigated the application of amitriptyline 10% cream on neuropathic pain. Patients who had hematological or solid tumors with CIPN of the hands and feet were given amitriptyline 10% cream twice a day. Pain intensity scores were assessed by the VAS at 1, 2, and 4 weeks, followed by monthly for up to 1 year. A total of 44 patients were enrolled in the study. The median pain score was 7 at baseline which decreased to a median of 2 after 4 weeks of topical treatment. This led to 11/44 patients with reduced initial chemotherapy doses, as well as 5 patients who discontinued chemotherapy, to resume chemotherapy after treatment with topical amitriptyline 10%.
- A double-blind, randomized, placebo-controlled crossover study compared the effectiveness of 5% lidocaine, 5% amitriptyline, and placebo gel with neuropathic pain. Thirty-five patients with postsurgical neuropathic pain, postherpetic neuralgia, or diabetic neuropathy with allodynia or hyperalgesia were instructed to apply 3–5 mL of the study drug twice a day for a week. There was a washout period of 1 week following each treatment. After the washout periods, patients would be presented with a different study drug. The primary outcome of this study was to determine if either 5% lidocaine or 5% amitriptyline was effective in alleviating symptoms of neuropathic pain. The researchers found that there was a significant reduction in pain intensity in the patients treated with the lidocaine, but this result was not surprising as lidocaine has been shown to be effective as a patch in previous studies. The researchers found that there was no significant change in pain intensity score for both the placebo and amitriptyline. When comparing the treatments, the researchers found topical lidocaine and placebo reduced pain more than amitriptyline.[11]

GABAPENTIN

- Boardman et al.[12] investigated the use of topical gabapentin 2% to 6% in the treatment of localized and generalized vulvodynia. A retrospective study based off a 10-point VAS was done comparing pain scores pre- and post-treatment. Between January 2001 and December 2006, 51 women with vulvodynia received topical gabapentin anywhere from 2% to 6%. After 8 weeks, the mean pain score was significantly reduced from 7.26 to 2.49 among the 35 evaluable participants. Eighty percent of evaluable women showed at least a 50% improvement in pain scores. Sexual function also improved in 17 out of 20 evaluable women. Fourteen percent of the women treated discontinued therapy. Topical gabapentin seems to offer significant pain relief in women with vulvodynia.

BACLOFEN

- Topical baclofen acts as an agonist at the GABA-B receptor. By the activation of tetraethylammonium-sensitive K+ channels on GABA-B, peripheral antinociceptive effects are observed. The intracellular increase in K+ is accompanied by a decrease in calcium ions, which alter membrane permeability, leading to a slow and prolonged inhibitory transmission.[13] Baclofen is used mostly in combination with other topical formulations for combined analgesia, as efficacy has not been established for monotherapy.
- Keppel Hesselink et al.[14] investigated the use of baclofen 5% and palmitoylethanolamide 400 mg TID for the treatment of idiopathic vulvodynia and proctodynia. This case consisted of a 33-year-old woman with intractable chronic vulvar and anal pain, resulting in abstinence from sexual intercourse and the inability to cycle or sit for more than 5 minutes. After 3 months of topical baclofen 5% and palmitoylethanolamide 400 mg TID, her symptoms decreased by more than 50% and she was able to have pain-free sexual intercourse. This case suggests that this formulation should be a viable treatment in patients with chronic vulvodynia and proctodynia.
- A study was performed by Ala et al.[15] that investigated the effects of topical 5% baclofen in patients after a hemorrhoidectomy. They conducted a randomized, double-blind, placebo-controlled clinical trial with 60 participants. Participants received either baclofen (5%) cream or placebo immediately after surgery and then every 12 hours for 14 days. Pain was assessed using the VAS, and analgesic requirement was measured by analgesic consumption. Pain ratings did not differ significantly between the baclofen and placebo groups at both 24 and 48 hours after the surgical procedure. The baclofen group showed a significantly lower pain score on weeks 1 and 2 post-surgery compared to the placebo group. The baclofen group also reported less concomitant use of oral systemic analgesics compared to placebo on week 1 and 2. There were reports of slight itching and bleeding from both groups, but there was no discontinuation of treatment due to adverse effects.

KETAMINE

- Ketamine is an anesthetic that exerts its analgesic properties at lower doses. Mechanistically, it works via non-competitive NMDA receptor blockade. This leads to the blocking of glutamate production, and thus ameliorating analgesic effects.
- Finch et al.[16] studied the use of topical ketamine 10% cream on 20 patients with complex regional pain syndrome (CRPS). Sensory tests on both symptomatic and non-symptomatic limbs were performed, both before and 30 minutes after ketamine cream was applied, to evaluate pain response. Ketamine inhibited allodynia to light brushing and hyperalgesia to punctate stimulation when applied to the symptomatic limb. Systemic ketamine levels were below detectable limits. Topical ketamine can be used to reduce allodynia in patients with CRPS.
- Rabi et al.[17] looked at the use of topical ketamine 10% for neuropathic pain in spinal cord injury. An open-label trial was conducted in five subjects at an outpatient rehabilitation hospital with spinal cord injury. Ketamine 10% was applied three times a day for 2 weeks. Numerical pain scores (NPS) were recorded from 0 to 10. At the end of 2 weeks, all five subjects had a decrease in their NPS ranging from 14 to 63%. The duration of effect varied, ranging from 1 hour in one subject to the next application in other subjects with no adverse effects. Four of the five patients reported satisfaction with their treatment. Topical ketamine 10% should be considered for patients with neuropathic pain in spinal cord injury.
- A retrospective review was conducted in patients from a specialty pain clinic suffering from complex regional pain syndrome. Sixteen patients were included in the review and were treated from May of 2006 to April of 2013. The patients were prescribed one of nine different ketamine combination topical formulations containing ketamine in either 6%

or 10%. Eight of the patients reported a reduction in pain, seven reported a worsening of pain, and one reported no benefit. The researchers concluded that the use of topical ketamine should be considered as it shows promise and there are limited treatment options for CRPS. They highlighted that additional efficacy trials with topical ketamine are needed before it can be implemented as a first-line therapy.[18]

CLONIDINE

- Clonidine is an alpha 2 adrenergic receptor agonist. Topical use targets alpha 2 receptors located in the brain, spinal cord, the dorsal root ganglia on sensory neurons, and nociceptors. When these G protein-coupled receptors are activated, downregulation of adenylate cyclase and other secondary messengers that support abnormal excitability of nociceptors occurs.
- Campbell et al.[19] conducted a randomized, double-blind, placebo-controlled, parallel-group, multicenter trial of topical clonidine 0.1% gel for the treatment of painful diabetic neuropathy. A total of 179 subjects applied clonidine 0.1% gel three times daily or placebo for 12 weeks on their feet. Outcomes were measured using a 0–10 NPS. The clonidine-treated group had decreased foot pain by an average of 2.6 points compared to 1.4 for placebo. This study showed that topical clonidine significantly reduced foot pain in patients with diabetic neuropathy.
- Kiani et al.[20] compared the safety and efficacy of topical clonidine gel and capsaicin cream in the treatment of painful diabetic neuropathy. A 12-week randomized double-blind and parallel-group trial of 139 patients with type 2 DM and a VAS of at least 4 were treated for up to 3 months. Outcomes were assessed via the VAS to measure a reduction in the median pain score from baseline. Both drugs proved to be efficacious, with an average of a 4-point reduction in VAS scores. There was no difference in efficacy between the two drugs; however capsaicin had a higher discontinuation rate due to dermatologic side effects. This study shows that both topical preparations may be used to treat diabetic neuropathies, and selection should be done on a patient-specific basis to minimize side effects.

PHENYTOIN

- Phenytoin acts by blocking voltage gated sodium channels. Kopsky and Keppel-Hesselink[21] examined the usefulness of topical phenytoin in patients suffering from refractory neuropathic pain. Three patients were given a topical cream based on phenytoin 5% or 10% after experiencing no analgesia from gabapentin 10% cream. Case 1 was a 69-year-old male with diabetic neuropathy who first received phenytoin 5% cream for allodynia at night. Phenytoin 5% cream reduced the allodynia and other pain symptoms to 3 on the NRS with an onset of action of 5 minutes and duration of effect of 8 hours. After increasing to phenytoin 10% cream twice daily for 3 months, the patient did not experience any allodynia symptoms at night (0 on NRS). Pain reduction appeared within 5 minutes after application and was maintained for at least 12 hours. Case 2 was a 71-year-old male suffering from combined chronic idiopathic axonal polyneuropathy (CIAP) and chemotherapy-induced polyneuropathy (CIPN). He was given phenytoin 5% cream, leading to a reduction in tingling, pins and needles, and burning pain within 20 minutes. His pain score reduced from 8 to 3 on the NRS and the duration of effect was at least 5 hours. His sleep quality also improved. The patient applied the cream three times daily during a period of 2 months. Case 3 was a 53-year-old female who suffered from CIPN in both hands. She was given phenytoin 5% cream and asked to compare it to baclofen 5% cream (previous use reduced her pain to 3 on the NRS, although allodynia was still present). Before application of both creams, her pain was 7 on the NRS. The patient's pain was reduced with baclofen 5% cream from 7 to 3 with a time of onset of 20 minutes. With phenytoin 5% cream, her pain went from 7 to 0 on the NRS with a time of onset of 30 minutes. The duration of effect of phenytoin 5% cream was 4 hours. With phenytoin 10% cream, the time of onset for analgesia decreased, and within 10–15 minutes she experienced a reduction in pain from 7 to 0 on the NRS. The duration of effect was increased to 6 hours.

- Kopsky et al.[22] looked at a cohort of 70 patients who were treated with either 5% or 10% phenytoin cream for neuropathic pain. The onset of pain relief, duration of effect, and reduction in pain intensity were measured on the 11-point NRS. Nine patients applied phenytoin 5%, and 61 patients applied phenytoin 10%. After grouping the effects of all of the patients, the mean onset of pain relief was 16.3 minutes and the mean duration of effect was 8.1 hours. The mean pain reduction on the NRS was 61.2%, which was statistically significant. No systemic phenytoin side effects were reported. Phenytoin cream reduced neuropathic pain considerably, while providing a quick onset of relief.

NON-STEROIDAL ANTI-INFLAMMATORY DRUGS (NSAIDs)

- Topical NSAIDs work by inhibiting the enzyme cyclooxygenase. Cyclooxygenase has two isoforms, COX-1 and COX-2, where inhibition mediates the production of prostaglandins and thromboxane A2. Prostaglandins play a role in inflammatory and nociceptive processes, so targeting local areas of effect can provide symptom relief that is musculoskeletal in nature.[23]
- Derry et al.[24] reviewed topical NSAIDs for chronic musculoskeletal pain in adults. Randomized, double-blind, controlled trials on the efficacy and safety of topical NSAIDs were filtered through databases and reviewed. All studies selected examined topical NSAIDs for osteoarthritis treatment. In studies lasting 6–12 weeks, topical diclofenac and topical ketoprofen were significantly more effective in reducing pain with 60% of participants having much reduced pain. There were infrequent serious adverse effects reported, making this a more attractive option for patients with comorbid conditions.
- Derry et al.[25] reviewed topical NSAIDs for acute musculoskeletal pain resulting from strains, sprains, or sports or overuse type injuries. Randomized, double-blind, active or placebo (inert carrier)-controlled trials on the efficacy and safety of topical NSAIDs were filtered through databases and reviewed. Results showed that formulations of diclofenac, ibuprofen, ketoprofen, piroxicam, and indomethacin demonstrated significantly higher rates of clinical success defined by at least a 50% reduction in pain intensity. Adverse effects were minimal, suggesting that patient tolerability and adherence are improved with topical NSAID use.

COMBINATION THERAPY

- Tam and Furlan[26] investigated a transdermal combination of lidocaine and ketamine cream in neuropathic pain for effectiveness and tolerability. A retrospective chart review of 854 patients was studied. Twenty-one patients with neuropathic pain signs/symptoms/diagnosis were given a transdermal prescription containing lidocaine and ketamine. Results showed that 8 out of 11 patients experienced analgesia from the combination cream. Two patients discontinued treatment due to skin reactions. This combination shows promise as an alternative to oral medications for neuropathic pain.
- An open-label study done by Lynch et al.[27] looked at a combination of topical amitriptyline 2%/ketamine 1% cream administered over 6–12 months in the setting of moderate to severe peripheral neuropathy. Outcomes measured included perceived analgesic effect, patient satisfaction, and safety over a 6–12-month period. Twenty-eight subjects participated in the study, and 21 completed the study. At 6 months, results showed that there was an average 34% reduction in pain, minimal systemic absorption, and no serious medication-related adverse events with the combination. At 12 months the average reduction in

pain was 37%. We can conclude that this combination is a potential option for long-term analgesia. The analgesic effects can be attributed to NMDA receptor blockade, and local anesthetic properties, as well as interactions with the adenosine system.

- A multicenter phase III, double-blind, randomized, placebo-controlled trial was conducted by Gewandter et al.[28] to investigate the effectiveness of a 2% ketamine and 4% amitriptyline combination cream on chemotherapy-induced neuropathy (CIPN). There were 458 patients who participated in the trial. Patients were required to keep a diary of their pain based on a numerical rating scale from 0 to 10 (10 being the worst pain) 1 week prior to treatment, 3 weeks, and 6 weeks post-treatment. The primary outcome of this study was to assess the change in pain score at week 6 of treatment. There was no statistically significant change in pain symptoms in the patients who used the topical ketamine/amitriptyline cream. The researchers concluded that amitriptyline and ketamine in combination does not decrease symptoms of CIPN, and that further research should be geared toward novel medications for pain management in this population.

- Barton et al.[29] performed a double-blind, placebo-controlled trial of a combination topical pain gel to investigate its effect on chemotherapy-induced neuropathic pain. The compounded cream contained 10 mg baclofen/40 mg amitriptyline HCl/20 mg ketamine. The researchers measured outcomes based on three components of sensory neuropathy: sensory (i.e., numbness, tingling, burning sensation in the hands and feet), motor (i.e., ability to hold a pen, opening jars, and cramping), and autonomic (i.e., erectile dysfunction, dizziness, vision). This study confirmed that the combination gel trended toward more improvement in sensory neuropathy. Higher doses of the combination gel (30 mg baclofen/60 mg amitriptyline/30 mg ketamine formulation) were initially proposed, but due to a lack of data on the systemic absorption of the triple combination, the FDA approved an investigational new drug application for this combination with the lower dose cream that was used in this trial. The researchers point out that the lower doses may have been associated with less effectiveness.

- Complex regional pain syndrome (CRPS) is a condition that develops in the limbs following surgery or trauma. This syndrome involves multiple pathological mechanisms including vasoconstriction, free radical generation, and the production of inflammatory cytokines. There is limited documentation for treatment for this syndrome, but it has been found that a multimodal treatment approach is effective at combatting this condition. A retrospective review of patients who were prescribed a compounded cream containing ketamine 10%/pentoxifylline 6%/clonidine 0.2%/dimethyl sulfoxide 6% to 10% was conducted to assess the effectiveness of this topical formulation on CRPS. Thirteen patients in total were included in the study. Nine patients reported pain reduction following treatment. Seven of those reported a major benefit and two reported complete resolution; however, all patients were on additional medications. Six of them were taking an additional opioid analgesic and one was taking prednisone. The average change in numerical pain score was 3.4 for the patients who reported benefit. The overall conclusion from this study was that compounded analgesic creams have the potential to be an effective adjunctive treatment for pain in patients suffering from CPRS.[30]

- A retrospective analysis of patient data obtained from prescribing physicians was performed by Somberg and Molnar[31] to compare the effectiveness of two compounded creams and diclofenac gel in chronic noncancer pain. The primary outcome of this analysis was to obtain a quantitative measure of efficacy from pre- to post-treatment using the Visual Numeric Pain Intensity Scale. Pain types included chronic extremity, joint, musculoskeletal, neuropathic, and other chronic pain conditions. This analysis included 2177 patients. Cream I contained flurbiprofen (20%), tramadol (5%), clonidine (0.2%), cyclobenzaprine (4%), and bupivacaine (3%). Cream II contained flurbiprofen (20%), baclofen (2%), clonidine (0.2%), gabapentin (10%), and lidocaine (5%). The diclofenac gel contained 1% diclofenac sodium. The researchers found that pain intensity scores dropped 37% and 35% from pre- to post-treatment for cream I and cream II, respectively. There was a 19% decrease in pain from pre- to post-treatment for the diclofenac gel. While this is valuable data suggesting that these two creams could be effective for treatment of a number of various chronic pain conditions, the researchers pointed out that treating physicians may have had prescribing bias. This could mean that the patients who had more severe pain were prescribed one of the two compounded creams as opposed to those with less severe pain, making it appear that the compounded creams are more efficacious than the diclofenac gel. Despite this potential bias, the compounded creams did show a statistically significant decrease in pain for those who used them in comparison to the diclofenac gel. Further study may be required in order to ascertain their efficacy.

- A study conducted by Brutcher et al.[32] investigated the effects of three separate compounded topical creams to treat localized chronic pain. This trial was a double-blind, randomized, parallel study that compared the effectiveness of three separate topical compounded creams to placebo. The primary outcome for this study was the average pain score on a 0–10 numerical rating scale. Included in the secondary outcomes were reductions in analgesic use, mean worst pain score, and treatment adherence. Participants did a follow-up at 1 month and 3 months if they had a positive outcome at the first follow-up. The study population consisted of individuals experiencing localized pain in the face, back or buttocks, neck, abdomen, chest, groin, or up to two extremities. Participants had to have experienced symptoms for longer than 6 weeks and have an average pain score of at least 4 during the week preceding the beginning of the trial. Patients were diagnosed with one of three separate pain conditions: neuropathic, nociceptive, or mixed pain. They were then separated into three different groups accordingly. The three creams that were compounded for neuropathic, nociceptive, and mixed pain contained 10% ketamine/6% gabapentin/0.2% clonidine/2% lidocaine; 10% ketoprofen/2% baclofen/2% cyclobenzaprine/2% lidocaine; and 10% ketamine/6% gabapentin/3% diclofenac/2% baclofen/2% cyclobenzaprine/2% lidocaine, respectively. The creams were formulated using a lipophilic-based carrier (transdermal pain base [Medisca]). The researchers found that, although there were slight differences among the three groups, the change in pain score did not differ significantly between the placebo and drug groups for any of the three pain classifications. Worst pain score and analgesic medication reduction at both 1 and 3 months did not differ between the drug and placebo groups. Seventy-seven percent of patients reported full adherence at both the 1- and 3-month follow-ups.

The authors of this paper noted that study participants in both the treatment and placebo groups did show improvement in pain throughout the study, but that those changes were not statistically significant. Despite the known analgesic effects of NSAIDs and lidocaine, the lack of efficacy seen with these compounded formulations was attributed to poor diffusion into the skin. Study limitations included a study population that had failed previous pain treatment options, lack of exclusion of capsaicin as an ingredient in the creams, and a younger demographic that may not have been representative of what older individuals experience in regard to pain. This study did not provide enough evidence to substantially demonstrate the effectiveness of topical combination pain creams.

Various pain syndromes often have multiple relevant pathway malfunctions, further complicating therapy considerations. In the case of the rare orphan disease Charcot–Marie–Tooth type 1A (CMT1A), neuropathy results from an autosomal dominant duplication of a gene encoding for the structural myelin protein PMP22. Patients suffer from abnormal Schwann cell differentiation and demyelination, leading to axonal suffering, then loss and muscle wasting. Attarian et al.[33] conducted a study looking at a low-dose compounded combination of PTX3003, which consists of baclofen, naltrexone, and sorbitol. Eighty patients with mild-moderate CMT1A received placebo or one of three increasing doses of PXT3003 for 1 year to assess safety and tolerability. Both safety and tolerability were confirmed for PXT3003. The highest dose showed the best improvement beyond stabilization.

Currently, other agents are being investigated for pain relief that seem promising but have not yet shown enough evidence to warrant a clinical recommendation. Further studies are needed before incorporating these agents into treatment algorithms.

Ambroxol is an agent that is most commonly used to treat respiratory diseases to combat excessive mucus production. Mechanistically, it acts as a voltage gated sodium channel blocker, blocking subtype Na_v 1.8 expressed on nociceptive C fiber neurons.[34]

An initial clinical observation through retrospective chart review was done by Kern and Weiser.[34] Seven patients with severe neuropathic pain were treated in this study with ambroxol 20% cream, which was repeatedly applied in the area of neuropathic pain. Individual mean pain intensity reported was between 4 and 6 on a 10-point NRS. The pain reduction following treatment with ambroxol was between 2 and 8 points within 30 mins with a duration of 3–8 hours. Four patients refractory to lidocaine relief and one patient refractory to capsaicin 8% all experienced analgesia with ambroxol 20% cream. No patient has reported any side effects or skin changes during treatment that has been continued for up to 4 years. While the analgesic effects seem very promising, the small sample size in this study indicates that more research is needed.

CONCLUSION

Various pain syndromes are multi-factorial and difficult to treat. Often, a multimodal treatment approach is needed to best help the patients with these severe and refractory conditions. The evidence for the efficacy of topical pain gels is conflicting depending on the various studies cited here; however, some do show great efficacy and warrant a trial in patients who are not responding to the various modalities. In general, they are easy to apply, and many have lower side effect profiles as compared to oral medications.

REFERENCES

1. Murnion B.P. Neuropathic pain: current definition and review of drug treatment. *Aust Prescr* 2018;41(3):60–63.
2. Anand P., Bley K. Topical capsaicin for pain management: potential mechanisms of action of the new high-concentration capsaicin 8% patch. *Br J Anesth* 2001;107(4):490–502. doi:10.1093/bja/aer260.
3. Casale R., Symeonidou Z., Bartolo M. Topical treatments for localized neuropathic pain. *Curr Pain Headache Rep* 2017;21(3):15. doi:10.1007/s11916-017-0615-y.
4. Pickering G., Elodie M., Tiberghien F., Delorme C., Mick G. Localized neuropathic pain: an expert consensus on local treatments. *Drug Des Devel Ther* 2017;11:2709–2718.
5. Derry S., Sven-Rice A., Cole P., Tan T., Moore R.A. Topical capsaicin (high concentration) for chronic neuropathic pain in adults. *Cochrane Database Syst Rev* 2013;2(2):CD007393. doi:10.1002/14651858. CD007393.pub3.
6. Silva V., El-Metwallya E.E., Lewith G., Macfarlane G.J. Arthritis Research UK Working Group on Complementary and Alternative Medicines. Evidence for the efficacy of complementary and alternative medicines in the management of osteoarthritis: a systematic review. *Rheumatology* 2011;50(5):911–920. doi:10.1093/rheumatology/keq379.
7. Kulkantrakorn K., Chomijit A., Sithinamsuwan P., Tharavanij T., Suwankanoknark J., Napunnaphat P. 0.075% capsaicin lotion for the treatment of painful diabetic neuropathy: a randomized, double-blind, crossover, placebo-controlled trial. *J Clin Neurosci* 2019;62:174–179.
8. Casanueva B., Rodero B., Quintial C., Llorca J., González-Gay M.A. Short-term efficacy of topical capsaicin therapy in severely affected fibromyalgia patients. *Rheumatol Int* 2013;33(10):2665–2670.
9. Baron R., Mayoral V., Leijon G., Binder A., Steigerwald I., Serpell M. 5% lidocaine medicated plaster versus pregabalin in post-herpetic neuralgia and diabetic polyneuropathy: an open-label, non-Inferiority two-stage RCT study. *Curr Med Res Opin* 2009;25(7):1663–1676. doi:10.1185/03007990903047880.
10. Rossignol J., Cozzi B., Liebaert F. et al. High concentration of topical amitriptyline for treating chemotherapy induced neuropathies. *Support Care Cancer* 2019;27(8):3053–3059. doi:10.1007/s00520-018-4618-y.
11. Ho K.Y., Huh B.K., White W.D., Yeh C.C., Miller E.J. Topical amitriptyline versus lidocaine in the treatment of neuropathic pain. *Clin J Pain* 2008;24(1):51–55. doi:10.1097/AJP.0b013e318156db26.

12. Boardman L., Cooper A.S., Blais L.R., Raker C.A. Topical gabapentin in the treatment of localized and generalized vulvodynia. *Obstet Gynecol* 2008;112(3):579–585. doi:10.1097/AOG.0b013e3181827c77.

13. Reis G.M., Duarte I.D. Baclofen, an agonist at peripheral GABAB receptors, induces antinociception via activation of TEA-sensitive potassium channels. *Br J Pharmacol* 2006;149(6):733–739. doi:10.1038/sj.bjp.0706898.

14. Keppel Hesselink J.M., Kopsky D.J., Sajben N.L. Vulvodynia and proctodynia treated with topical baclofen 5 % and palmitoylethanolamide. *Arch Gynecol Obstet* 2014;290(2):389–393. doi:10.1007/s00404-014-3218-4.

15. Ala S., Alvandipour M., Saeedi M., Mansourifar M., Monajati M., Shiva A. Effect of topical baclofen 5% on post-hemorrhoidectomy pain: randomized double blind placebo-controlled clinical trial. *J Gastrointest Surg* 2020;24(2):405–410. doi:10.1007/s11605-019-04147-7.

16. Finch P., Knudsen L., Drummond P.D. Reduction of allodynia in patients with complex regional pain syndrome: a double-blind placebo-controlled trial of topical ketamine. *Pain* 2009;146(1–2):18–25.

17. Rabi J., Minori J., Abad H., Lee R., Gittler M. Topical ketamine 10% for neuropathic pain in spinal cord injury patients: an open-label trial. *Int J Pharm Compd* 2016;20(6):517–520.

18. Durham M.J., Mekhjian H.S., Goad J.A., Lou M., Ding M., Richeimer S.H. Topical ketamine in the treatment of complex regional pain syndrome. *Int J Pharm Compd* 2018;22(2):172–175.

19. Campbell C.M., Mark K., Bruce S. et al. Randomized control trial of topical clonidine for treatment of painful diabetic neuropathy. *Pain* 2012;153(9):1815–1823. doi:10.1016/j.pain.2012.04.014.

20. Kiani J., Sajedi F., Nasrollahi S.A., Esna-Ashari F. A randomized clinical trial of efficacy and safety of the topical clonidine and capsaicin in the treatment of painful diabetic neuropathy. *J Res Med Sci* 2015;20(4):359–363.

21. Kopsky D.J., Keppel Hesselink J.M. Topical phenytoin for the treatment of neuropathic pain. *J Pain Res* 2017;10:469–473. doi:10.2147/JPR.S129749.

22. Kopsky D.J., Keppel Hesselink J.M. Phenytoin cream for the treatment for neuropathic pain: case series. *Pharmaceuticals (Basel, Switzerland)* 2018;11(2):53. doi:10.3390/ph11020053.

23. Derry S., Wiffen P.J., Kalso E.A. et al. Topical analgesics for acute and chronic pain in adults - an overview of cochrane reviews. *Cochrane Database Syst Rev* 2017;5:CD008609. doi:10.1002/14651858.CD008609.pub2.

24. Derry S., Conaghan P., Da Silva J.A., Wiffen P., Moore R.A. Topical NSAIDs for chronic musculo-skeletal pain in adults. *Cochrane Database Syst Rev* 2016;2016(4):CD007400. doi:10.1002/14651858.CD007400.pub3.

25. Derry S., Moore R.A., Gaskell H., McIntyre M., Wiffen P. Topical NSAIDs for acute musculoskeletal pain in adults. *Cochrane Database Syst Rev* 2015;2015(6):CD007402. doi:10.1002/14651858.CD007402.pub3.

26. Tam E., Furlan A.D. Transdermal lidocaine and ketamine for neuropathic pain: a study of effectiveness and tolerability. *Open Neurol J* 2012;6:58–64. doi:10.2174/1874205X01206010058.

27. Lynch M.E., Clark A.J., Sawynok J., Sullivan M.J. Topical amitriptyline and ketamine in neuropathic pain syndromes: an open-label study. *J Pain* 2005;6(10):644–649.

28. Gewandter J.S., Mohile S.G., Heckler C.E. et al. A phase-III randomized, placebo-controlled study of topical amitriptyline and ketamine for chemotherapy-induced peripheral neuropathy (CIPN): a university of rochester CCOP study of 462 cancer survivors. *Support Care Cancer* 2014;22(7):1807–1814.

29. Barton D.L., Wos E.J., Qin R. et al. A double-blind, placebo-controlled trial of a topical treatment for chemotherapy-induced neuropathy: NCCTG trial N06CA. Support Care Center 2011;19(6):833–841.

30. Russo M.A., Santarelli D.M. A novel compound analgesic cream (ketamine, pentoxifylline, clonidine, DMSO) for complex regional pain syndrome patients. *Pain Pract* 2016;16(1):E14–20. doi:10.1111/papr.12404.

31. Somberg J.C., Molnar J. Retrospective evaluation on the analgesic activities of 2 compounded topical creams and voltaren gel in chronic noncancer pain. *Am J Ther* 2015;22(5):342–349.

32. Brutcher R.E., Kurihara C., Bicket M.C. et al. Compounded topical pain creams to treat localized chronic pain: a randomized controlled trial. *Ann Intern Med* 2019;170(5):309–318. doi:10.7326/M18-2736.

33. Attarian S., Vallat J.M., Magy L. et al. An exploratory randomised double-blind and placebo-controlled phase 2 study of a combination of baclofen, naltrexone and sorbitol (PXT3003) in patients with charcot-marie-tooth disease type 1A. *Orphanet J Rare Dis* 2014;9:199. doi:10.1186/s13023-014-0199-0.

34. Kern K.-U., Weiser T. Topical ambroxol for the treatment of neuropathic pain: an initial clinical observation. *Schmerz Berl Germany* 2015;29(Suppl 3):S89–96. doi:10.1007/s00482-015-0060-y.

19 Herbal and Supplement Use in Pain Management

Sahar Swidan and Mara Rubin

CONTENTS

CAPSICUM

- *Class*: analgesic and anti-inflammatory agent.
- *Mechanism of action*: repeated use of capsaicin depletes substance p, which decreases the neuronal transmission of pain.[1]
- *Use*: osteoarthritis, fibromyalgia.
- *Dosing*:
  - *Fibromyalgia*:
    - Topical: apply 0.025% or 0.075% capsaicin cream three or four times daily for 4–6 weeks modestly to reduce pain at tender points.[2] Long-term benefits are not

known, and more studies are needed in order to further assess capsaicin as a long-term therapy in the symptom management of fibromyalgia.[1]

- *Adverse effects*: gastrointestinal, burning of mucosal membranes if rubbed on by mistake.
- *Drug interactions*: moderate theoretical risk with anticoagulants/antiplatelet warfarin, antidiabetic, antihypertensive, cefazolin, aspirin.
- Fifty-two minor interactions (e.g., ACE-inhibitor induced cough may be induced or exacerbated).
- *Cautions*: none known.

CAT'S CLAW

- *Class*: analgesic and anti-inflammatory agent.
- *Mechanism of action*: according to in vitro and clinical research, the anti-inflammatory properties of *Uncaria guianensis* and *Uncaria tomentosa* may result from their ability to inhibit TNF-alpha and, to a lesser extent, prostaglandin E2 (PGE2) production. In vitro, cat's claw was a potent inhibitor of TNF-alpha production.[3]
- *Use*: osteoarthritis, rheumatoid arthritis.
- *Dosing*:
  - Osteoarthritis: 100 mg by mouth once daily.[4]
  - Rheumatoid arthritis: 20 mg three times daily.[5]
- *Adverse effects*: generally, well-tolerated.
- *Contraindications*: hypersensitivity to cat's claw or its components.
- *Drug interactions*:
  - *Anticoagulant/antiplatelet drugs*: cat's claw contains rhynchophylline and isorhyncho-phylline. Research suggests that concurrent use of cat's claw and anticoagulant/anti-platelet drugs can reduce platelet aggregation and cause an increased risk of bleeding in some patients.[6]
  - *Antihypertensive drugs*: cat's claw contains rhynchophylline and isorhynchophyl-line. Concurrent use of cat's claw and antihypertensive drugs may increase the risk of hypotension.[7]
  - *Calcium channel blockers "moderate risk"*: animal research suggests that the vari-ous alkaloids in cat's claw can lower blood pressure by acting as a calcium channel blocker—(TRC Natural Medicines).
  - *CYP P450 3A4 substrates*: cat's claw inhibits 3A4 and may increase levels of drugs metab-olized by CYP3A4, including ketoconazole, itraconzole, fexofenadine, and triazolam.[8]
  - *Immunosuppressants*: cat's claw may interfere with immunosuppressants due to the immunostimulating activity of cat's claw. It stimulates phagocytosis and increases respiratory cellular activity and the mobility of leukocytes.[3]
  - *Protease Inhibitors*: cat's claw may increase levels of protease inhibitors because cat's claw inhibits CYP 3A4. Use with caution.[9]
- *Cautions*:
  - Do not use in pregnancy. There is concern that it may be unsafe due to its traditional use as a contraceptive.[10]
  - Do not use in lactation due to insufficient evidence of safety.[10]

DEVIL'S CLAW

- *Class*: analgesic and anti-inflammatory agent.
- *Mechanism of action*: the iridoid glycoside constituents of devil's claw seem to have an anti-inflammatory effect. Some preliminary research suggests that harpagoside inhibits both the cyclooxygenase (COX) and lipoxygenase inflammatory pathways.[11]
- *Use*: osteoarthritis, back pain, rheumatoid arthritis.

- *Dosing*:
  - *Back pain*:
    - (Doloteffin, ardeypharm) 2400 mg taken in three divided doses daily for up to 1 year has been used.[12]
  - (WS 1531) 600–1200mg of harpagophytum extract twice daily for 4 weeks.[13]
  - *Osteoarthritis*:
    - 670–800 mg three times daily up to 2 months.
    - (Doloteffin, ardeypharm) 2400 mg taken in three divided doses daily for up to 1 year has been used.[12]
- *Adverse effects*: gastrointestinal pain, allergic skin reactions, dysmenorrhea, throbbing frontal headache, tinnitus, anorexia, loss of taste, anxiety, somnolence, and insomnia, but most of these are rare and overall devil's claw is well-tolerated.[12]
- *Contraindications*: hypersensitivity to devil's claw and its components.
- *Drug Interactions*:
  - *CYP 2C19, 2C9, 3A4 substrates*: devil's claw inhibits these CYP enzymes and can increase levels of these substrates.[14]
  - *H2 blockers and proton pump inhibitors*: minor interaction that devil's claw may increase stomach acid and decrease the effectiveness of H2 blockers and PPIs.[15,16]
  - *Warfarin*: concurrent use of warfarin and devil's claw may increase risk of bleeding and warfarin—dose adjustments may be necessary.[17]
- *Cautions*:
  - Do not use in pregnancy. Data suggest that devil's claw has oxytocic effects and can induce contractions of uterine muscle.[18]
  - Insufficient evidence for lactation. Do not use when breastfeeding.[18]

GINGER

- *Class*: analgesic and anti-inflammatory agent.
- *Mechanism of action*: anti-inflammatory effects through the inhibition of arachidonic acid and inhibition of prostaglandin and leukotriene synthesis.
- *Use*: osteoarthritis, dysmenorrhea, migraine headache, rheumatoid arthritis (further studies needed to evaluate effectiveness and dosing), post-operative recovery (further studies needed to evaluate effectiveness and dosing).
- *Dosing*:
  - *Osteoarthritis*:
    - *Orally*: 1000 mg daily for 4 weeks or 170 mg three times daily for 3 weeks has been used.[19]
    - *Topically*: ginger and plai 4% by weight—4 grams/day in four divided doses for 6 weeks has been applied.[20]
  - *Dysmenorrhea*: 250 mg four times daily orally for 3 days from the start of the menstrual period or until pain relief.[21]
  - *Migraine headache*: 250 mg orally as a single dose at the onset of the migraine.[22]
- *Adverse effects*: generally-well tolerated, but in doses higher than 5 g per day may have side effects such as abdominal discomfort, heartburn. Encapsulated ginger opposed to ginger powder yields less abdominal discomfort.[23]
- *Contraindications*: hypersensitivity to ginger and its components.
- *Drug interactions*:
  - *Anticoagulant/antiplatelet drugs*: moderate interaction due to inhibition of thromboxane synthetase and decreased platelet aggregation leading to an increased risk of bleeding.[24]
  - *Diabetic drugs*: ginger may increase insulin levels and/or decrease blood glucose levels, leading to an additive effect with blood glucose-lowering drugs and a higher risk of hypoglycemia.[25]

- ◦ *Antihypertensive drugs*: ginger may have hypotensive effects leading to an additive effect with calcium channel blocker and other antihypertensive medications.[26]
- ◦ *Cyclosporine*: ginger may reduce the maximum concentration and AUC of cyclosporine by 51.4% and 40.3%, respectively, as found in a study. A decrease in the effectiveness of cyclosporine has been observed when ginger is taken before cyclosporine and this should be avoided.[27]
- ◦ *Metronidazole*: ginger may increase the absorption and plasma half-life of metronidazole. Also, the elimination rate of metronidazole may be reduced with co-administration with ginger.[28]
- • *Cautions*: none reported.

INDIAN FRANKINCENSE (*BOSWELLIA*)

- • *Class*: analgesic and anti-inflammatory agent.
- • *Mechanism of action*: boswellic acids, especially AKBA, inhibit 5-lipoxygenase and reduce leukotriene synthesis and inhibit leukocyte elastase, which are the likely mechanisms for its anti-inflammatory and analgesic properties.[29]
- • *Use*: osteoarthritis, rheumatoid arthritis.
- • *Dosing*: (5-Loxin) 100–250 mg daily for 90 days has been used.[30]
- • *Adverse effects*: diarrhea, nausea, abdominal pain, heartburn, itching, skin rash, headache, edema.[31]
- • *Contraindications*: hypersensitivity to *Boswellia* or any of its components.
- • *Drug interactions*:
  - ◦ *CYP1A2, 2C19, 2C9, 2D6, and 3A4 substrates*: *Boswellia* inhibits cytochrome P450 enzymes, increasing drug levels of these substrates.[32]
  - ◦ *Immunosuppressants*: *Boswellia* has immunostimulant properties that may decrease the effectiveness of immunosuppressive drugs.[33]
- • *Cautions*: insufficient reliable information available about safety during pregnancy and lactation, so avoid use.

LIMBREL (FLAVOCOXID)

- • *Class*: analgesic and anti-inflammatory medical food.
- • *Mechanism of action*: Limbrel decreases COX-2 and lipoxygenase.
- • *Use*: osteoarthritis.
- • *Dosing*: 250–500 mg BID[34] (with or without food).
- • *Adverse effects*: jaundice, pruritus, abdominal pain, fever, rash.
  - ◦ More severe adverse reactions include increases in AST and ALT, which were found to resolve completely within 3 months of discontinuation. Liver damage can occur with Limbrel, and caution should be taken.
  - ◦ Primus announced a voluntary product recall on January 26, 2018, due to sustained pressure from the FDA.
- • *Contraindications*: patients with liver dysfunction at baseline.[34]
- • *Drug interactions*: none known.
- • *Cautions*: report any signs of liver toxicity such as jaundice, fatigue, or abdominal pain.[34]

TURMERIC

- • *Class*: analgesic and anti-inflammatory agent.
- • *Mechanism of action*: turmeric has anti-inflammatory properties that affect the production of cyclooxygenase-2, prostaglandins, and leukotrienes.[35]

- *Use*: osteoarthritis, rheumatoid arthritis.
- *Dosing*:
  - *Osteoarthritis*: 500 mg twice daily for 6 weeks.[36]
  - *Rheumatoid arthritis*:
    - 250–500 mg twice daily for 8 weeks to 3 months.
    - 400 mg three times daily for 2 weeks.
    - 400–600 mg up to three times/day for inflammation relief (Arthritis Foundation).
- *Adverse effects*: constipation, dyspepsia, diarrhea, distention, GERD, nausea, vomiting.[37]
- *Drug interactions*:
  - *Anticoagulant/antiplatelet drugs*: turmeric has antiplatelet effects and may increase the INR.[38]
  - *Antidiabetic drugs*: turmeric and its constituent curcumin can reduce levels of blood glucose and HbA1C and potentiate the effects of antidiabetic drugs leading to an increased risk of hypoglycemia.[39]
  - *Camptothecin*: curcumin inhibits camptothecin-induced apoptosis of breast cancer cells by up to 71%.[40]
  - *Cyclophosphamide*: in an animal model, curcumin 25 g/kg appears to inhibit cyclophosphamide-induced tumor regression.[40]
  - *CYP P450 1A1, 1A2, 3A4 substrates*: turmeric and its constituent curcumin inhibit some cytochrome P450 enzymes and can increase drug levels of substrates metabolized by these enzymes.[41]
  - *Docetaxel/paclitaxel*: turmeric's constituent curcumin can enhance the bioavailability of docetaxel and increase the blood levels. Monitor concurrent use.[42]
  - *Doxorubicin*: curcumin has been shown to inhibit doxorubicin-induced apoptosis of breast cancer cells by up to 65%.[40]
  - *Estrogen*: curcumin may displace the binding of estrogen to its receptors.[43]
  - *Glyburide*: pharmacokinetic research shows that curcumin 475 mg for 10 days prior to taking glyburide 5 mg increases blood levels of glyburide by 12% at 2 hours after the dose in patients with type 2 DM.[44]
  - *Mechlorethamine*: curcumin may inhibit mechlorethamine-induced apoptosis of breast cancer cells by up to 70%.[40]
  - *Norfloxacin*: curcumin can increase blood levels of orally administered norfloxacin, increasing the effects and adverse effects of the medication.[45]
  - *P-glycoprotein*: curcuminoids and other constituents in turmeric can inhibit P-glycoprotein expression and activity, causing an increase in absorption of p-glycoprotein substrates.[46]
  - *Sulfasalazine*: curcumin can cause an increase in blood levels of sulfasalazine by 3.2-fold and increase the effects and adverse effects of sulfasalazine.[47]
  - *Tacrolimus*: turmeric and its constituent curcumin inhibit CYP3A4. Avoid large doses of turmeric with tacrolimus.[48]
- *Cautions*: use with caution in patients with gallstones or gallbladder disease, and patients with iron deficiency due to a risk of reduced iron absorption with turmeric administration.

WILLOW BARK

- *Class*: analgesic and anti-inflammatory agent.
- *Use*: osteoarthritis.
- *Dosing*: salicin 120–240 mg daily for 2–6 weeks.[49]
- *Adverse effects*: gastrointestinal adverse effects, itching, rash.[50]
- *Contraindications*: allergy to aspirin since willow bark contains salicylates, allergy to salicylates.

- *Drug interactions*:
  - *Acetazolamide*: willow bark contains salicin and can lead to an increase in plasma levels of acetazolamide.[51]
  - *Anticoagulant/antiplatelet*: concomitant use of willow bark and anticoagulant/antiplatelet drugs can increase the risk of bleeding due to decreased platelet aggregation. Willow bark has less severe antiplatelet effects compared to warfarin.[52]
  - *Salicylate-containing drugs*: willow bark contains salicin, a plant salicylate. Willow bark may have an additive effect with other salicylate-containing drugs.[53]
- *Cautions*: willow bark contains salicylates which are excreted in breast milk and have been linked to adverse effects in breast-fed infants.[51]

SUPEROXIDE DISMUTASE

- *Class*: antioxidant.
- *Mechanism of action*: superoxide dismutase catalyzes the conversion of superoxide to oxygen and hydrogen peroxide, reducing damage from radical oxygen species.
- *Use*: osteoarthritis, rheumatoid arthritis.
- *Dosing*:
  - *Osteoarthritis*: 16 mg as an intra-articular injection every two weeks.[54]
  - *Rheumatoid arthritis*: 4 mg intra-articular injection once weekly for up to 6 weeks.[55]
- *Adverse effects*: pain or allergic reaction at the injection site.[56]
- *Contraindications*: hypersensitivity to superoxide dismutase or any of its components.
- *Drug interactions*: none known.
- *Cautions*: insufficient reliable information available regarding pregnancy and lactation; avoid using.

VITAMIN C

- *Class*: water-soluble vitamin, antioxidant.
- *Mechanism of action*: mechanism of action related to pain is unknown and further research is needed to understand how vitamin C helps to alleviate pain in osteoarthritis and post-operative pain.
- *Use*: osteoarthritis, post-operative pain.
- *Dosing*:
  - *Osteoarthritis*: vitamin C in the form of calcium ascorbate 1 gram daily for 2 weeks has been used.[57]
  - *Postoperative pain*: a single prophylactic dose of 2 grams of vitamin C by mouth, 1 hour prior to anesthesia has been used in patients (tested in patients receiving cholecystectomy).[58]
- *Adverse effects*: dose-related adverse effects, most common including nausea, vomiting, esophagitis, heartburn, abdominal cramps, gastrointestinal obstruction, fatigue, flushing, headache, insomnia, sleepiness, and diarrhea.[59]
  - Doses greater than the tolerable upper limit of 2 g per day can increase the risk of severe adverse effects such as osmotic diarrhea.
- *Contraindications*: hypersensitivity to vitamin C and any of its components.
- *Drug interactions*:
  - *Acetaminophen*: high doses of vitamin C (3 grams) competitively inhibit the sulfate conjugation of acetaminophen, resulting in an increase in the fractions of the dose of acetaminophen excreted as acetaminophen glucuronide and a decrease in the fraction excreted as acetaminophen sulfate. May not be clinically significant.[60]
  - *Alkylating agents*: use of vitamin C during chemotherapy may reduce the activity of chemotherapy and generate free radicals.[61]

- ○ *Aluminum*: vitamin C can increase the amount of aluminum absorbed from aluminum compounds.[62]
- ○ *Aspirin/salicylates*: acidification of the urine by vitamin C could increase reabsorption of salicylates by the renal tubules and increase plasma salicylate levels.[63]
- ○ *Estrogen*: vitamin C may increase plasma estrogen levels up to 47% when vitamin C is taken with oral contraceptives or hormone replacement therapy, including topical products.[64]
- ○ *Fluphenazine*: vitamin C may decrease fluphenazine levels when used concurrently with vitamin C 500 mg twice daily.[65]
- ○ *Protease inhibitors*: taking vitamin C orally along with indinavir may modestly reduce indinavir levels.[66] Vitamin C may modestly reduce levels of other protease inhibitors as well.
- ○ *Dihydropyridine calcium channel blockers*: these medications (e.g., nicardipine) inhibit uptake of vitamin C by intestinal cells. It is unknown if this is clinically significant.[67]
- ○ *Warfarin*: high doses of vitamin C may reduce the response to warfarin, possibly causing diarrhea and reduced warfarin absorption, and it was concluded that it was not clinically significant.[68]
- *Cautions*: do not exceed tolerable upper limit of 2g per day.

VITAMIN E

- *Class*: antioxidant.
- *Mechanism of action*: mechanism in relation to pain reduction is not known and further research is needed.
- *Use*: osteoarthritis, rheumatoid arthritis.
- *Dosing*:
  - ○ *Rheumatoid arthritis/osteoarthritis*: 600 mg orally twice daily.[69]
- *Adverse effects*: nausea, diarrhea, intestinal cramps, weakness, headache, blurred vision, rash, gonadal dysfunction, and creatinuria.[70]
- *Contraindications*: none known.
- *Drug interactions*:
  - ○ *Alkylating agents*: the use of antioxidants such as vitamin E during chemotherapy can interfere with chemotherapy activity and may generate free radicals.[61]
  - ○ *Anticoagulant/antiplatelet drugs*: concomitant use of vitamin E and anticoagulant or antiplatelet drugs might increase the risk of bleeding by inhibition of platelet aggregation and antagonization of the effects of vitamin K-dependent clotting factors.[71]
  - ○ *Cytochrome P450 3A4 substrates*: vitamin E may increase the metabolism of drugs metabolized by CYP3A4. Vitamin E appears to bind with the nuclear receptor (pregnane X receptor [PXR]), which may result in increased expression of CYP4A4.[72]
- *Warfarin*: greater than 400 IU of vitamin E per day may prolong prothrombin time, INR, and increase the risk of bleeding due to interference with vitamin K-dependent clotting factors.[73]
- *Cautions*: none reported.

CHONDROITIN SULFATE

- *Class*: structure-modifying agent.
- *Mechanism of action*: in chondrocytes, chondroitin sulfate has been suggested to reduce the interleukin-1 (IL-1) beta-induced increase in p38 mitogen-activated protein kinase (p38MAPK) and signal-regulated kinase ½ (Erk1/2) phosphorylation, resulting in a decrease in the nuclear translocation of nuclear factor-kappaB (NF-kappaB) and the reduction of proinflammatory cytokine and enzyme production.[74]
- *Use*: osteoarthritis, exercise-induced muscle soreness.
- *Dosing*: 800 to 2000 mg daily as a single dose or in two or three divided doses for up to 3 years.[75]

- *Adverse effects*: well-tolerated.
- *Contraindications*: allergy to shark and bovine.
- *Drug interactions*:
  - ◦ *Warfarin*: taking chondroitin in combination with glucosamine might increase the anticoagulation effects of warfarin and increase risk of bruising and bleeding. May increase INR.[76]
- *Cautions*: allergy to shark and bovine.

GLUCOSAMINE SULFATE

- *Class*: structure-modifying agent.
- *Mechanism of action*: as sulfate is required for articular cartilage glycosaminoglycan synthesis, some researchers think the sulfate moiety in glucosamine sulfate might be responsible for its effect on osteoarthritis and the additional glucosamine might increase the absorption of sulfate. It has been shown that glucosamine sulfate increases serum and synovial sulfate levels.[77]
- *Use*: osteoarthritis, exercise-induced muscle soreness.
- *Dosing*: 1500 mg daily as a single dose or three divided doses for up to 3 years.[78]
- *Adverse effects*: well-tolerated.
- *Contraindications*: allergy to shellfish.
- *Drug interactions*:
  - ◦ *Acetaminophen*: adding glucosamine to acetaminophen may decrease pain in patients with osteoarthritis. Some research suggests that the sulfate portion of glucosamine sulfate might contribute to its effect in osteoarthritis.[79]
  - ◦ *Anti-diabetic drugs*: glucosamine might increase insulin resistance or decrease insulin production leading to worsened diabetes and a decrease in effectiveness of diabetic drugs.[80]
  - ◦ *Topoisomerase II inhibitors*: glucosamine might induce resistance to etoposide and doxorubicin by reducing the drug's inhibition of topoisomerase II. Other drugs such as mitoxantrone and anthracyclines may also be affected.[81]
  - ◦ *Warfarin*: taking chondroitin in combination with glucosamine might increase the anticoagulant effects of warfarin and increase risk of bruising and bleeding. May increase INR.[76]
- *Cautions*: allergy to shellfish.

METHYLSULFONYLMETHANE (MSM)

- *Class*: antiarthritic, free radical scavenger.
- *Mechanism of action*: MSM is primarily used for osteoarthritis. Preliminary research suggests MSM might inhibit degenerative changes in joints in animal models of osteoarthritis.[82] It might also stabilize cell membrane, slow or stop leakage from injured cells, and scavenge hydroxyl free radicals which trigger inflammation.[83]
- *Use*: osteoarthritis, joint pain.
- *Dosing*: 1.5 to 6 grams daily in three divided doses for up to 12 weeks.[84]
- *Adverse effects*: nausea, diarrhea, bloating, headache, fatigue, insomnia, and difficulty concentrating.
- *Contraindications*: none known.
- *Drug interactions*: none known.
- *Cautions*: insufficient reliable evidence for use during pregnancy and lactation; avoid use.

S-ADENOSYLMETHIONINE (SAME)

- *Class*: analgesic, anti-inflammatory, primary methyl group donor.
- *Mechanism of action*: SAMe is a molecule that is naturally formed in the body from homo-cysteine and 5-methylene tetrahydrofolate. It is important for the synthesis, activation, and metabolism of many different reactions throughout the body.
- *Use*: osteoarthritis, fibromyalgia.
- *Dose*:
  - *Osteoarthritis*: 600–1200 mg daily in up to three divided doses for up to 84 days has been tested.[85]
  - *Fibromyalgia*
    - Clinical trials have shown a modest improvement as compared to placebo or compared to TENS therapy.[86]
    - *Oral*: SAMe 800 mg daily in two divided doses for 6 weeks has been used.[87]
    - *IV*: there is conflicting evidence on the use of SAMe for fibromyalgia.
    - 600 mg IV SAMe once daily for 10 days does not seem to help improve symptoms. Other research suggests that 400 mg IV once daily for 15 days significantly reduces pain, the number of tender points, and depression compared to baseline.[88,89]
- *Adverse effects*: flatulence, nausea, vomiting, diarrhea, constipation, dry mouth, headache, mild insomnia, anorexia, sweating, dizziness, and nervousness.
- *Contraindications*: hypersensitivity to SAMe or any of its components.
- *Drug interactions*:
  - *Anti-depressants, meperidine, MAOIs, pentazocine, tramadol*: concurrent use might cause additive serotonergic effect and increase the risk of serotonin syndrome.[90]
  - *Dextromethorphan*: concurrent use may cause additive serotonergic effects and increase the risk of serotonin syndrome.[90]
  - *Levodopa*: SAMe methylates levodopa and may lead to worsening of Parkinsonian syndrome. SAMe administration may lead to a decreased effect of levodopa.[91]
- *Cautions*: none known.

5-HYDROXYTRYPTOPHAN (5-HTP)

- *Class*: produced in the body from the essential amino acid L-tryptophan.
- *Mechanism of action*: it is converted to the neurotransmitter serotonin. 5-HTP increases the production of serotonin in the central nervous system.
- *Use*: fibromyalgia, tension headache.
- *Dose*:
  - *Fibromyalgia*: 100 mg orally three times daily for 30 days to 90 days can help to improve pain, tenderness, sleep, anxiety, fatigue, and morning stiffness in those with fibromyalgia.[92,93]
- *Adverse effects*: nausea, vomiting, abdominal, or epigastric pain, diarrhea, and anorexia.
- *Contraindications*: hypersensitivity to 5-HTP or any of its components.
- *Drug interactions*:
  - *Anti-depressant drugs, carbidopa, meperidine, MAOIs, pentazocine, tramadol*: concurrent use might cause additive serotonergic effect and increase the risk of serotonin syndrome.[94]
  - *Dextromethorphan*: concurrent use may cause additive serotonergic effects and increase the risk of serotonin syndrome.[94]
- *Cautions*: insufficient reliable information available for pregnancy and lactation; avoid use.

MAGNESIUM

- *Class*: chemical element.
- *Mechanism of action*: magnesium is a chemical element that is important to normal bone structure. It also plays a role in more than 300 cellular reactions.[95]
- *Use*: fibromyalgia, cancer-associated neuropathic pain, cluster headache, postoperative pain, migraine headache.
- *Dose*:
  ○ *Fibromyalgia*: magnesium citrate 300 mg daily for 8 weeks improved symptoms of fibromyalgia such as number of tender points and comorbidities such as depression as compared to baseline.[96]
  ○ *Cancer-associated neuropathic pain*: 500 mg to 1 g IV magnesium sulfate can relieve pain.[97]
  ○ *Postoperative pain*: 25 to 100 mg intrathecally increases time until onset by up to 23 minutes following surgery compared to local anesthetics alone or lipophilic opioid.[98]
  ○ *Migraine headache*: magnesium sulfate 400 mg by mouth daily.[99]
- *Adverse effects*: gastrointestinal irritation, nausea, vomiting, and diarrhea.
- *Contraindications*: hypersensitivity to magnesium or any of its constituents, heart block, kidney dysfunction.
- *Drug interactions*:
  ○ *Aminoglycosides*: concurrent use can lead to neuromuscular weakness because both reduce presynaptic acetylcholine release, leading to neuromuscular blockade. More likely to occur with IV magnesium.[100]
  ○ *Antacids*: the use of antacids may reduce the laxative effect of magnesium oxide.[101]
  ○ *Anticoagulant/antiplatelet*: magnesium sulfate inhibits platelet aggregation at concentrations as low as 0.5–1 mM.[102]
  ○ *Bisphosphonates*: magnesium may decrease bisphosphonate absorption. Separate doses of magnesium from bisphosphonates by at least 2 hours.[103]
  ○ *Calcium channel blockers*: magnesium inhibits calcium entry into smooth muscle cells and may interfere and have additive effects leading to an increased risk of hypotension.[63]
  ○ *Digoxin*: clinical evidence suggests that treatment with oral magnesium hydroxide may reduce absorption from the intestines and decrease its therapeutic effect.[104]
  ○ *Gabapentin*: magnesium used concurrently with gabapentin may lead to decreased gabapentin maximum concentration by 33%, time to maximum concentration by 36%, and AUC by 43%.[105]
  ○ *Potassium-sparing diuretics*: potassium-sparing diuretics also have magnesium-sparing properties, which can counteract the magnesium loss associated with loop and thiazide diuretics, and increased magnesium levels could result.[106]
  ○ *Quinolone antibiotics*: magnesium can form insoluble complexes with quinolones and decrease their absorption.[63]
  ○ *Skeletal muscle relaxants*: parenteral magnesium can potentiate the effects of skeletal muscle relaxants by decreasing acetylcholine release from motor nerve terminals.[63]
  ○ *Sulfonylureas*: concomitant administration of magnesium hydroxide and sulfonylureas may increase the absorption and increase the risk of hypoglycemia by up to 35%.[107]
  ○ *Tetracyclines*: magnesium can form insoluble complexes with tetracyclines and decrease their absorption and antibacterial activity. Separate by 2 hours before, or 4 to 6 hours after tetracycline administration.[108]
- *Cautions*: none known.

COENZYME Q10

- *Class*: fat-soluble compound and anti-oxidant.
- *Mechanism of action*: coenzyme Q10 is involved in many biochemical processes throughout the human body. It is found endogenously, mostly in the heart, liver, kidney, and pancreas.[109]
- *Use*: fibromyalgia, diabetic neuropathy, migraine headache.
- *Dose*:
  - *Diabetic neuropathy*: 400 mg orally for 12 weeks.[110]
  - *Fibromyalgia*:
    - *Oral*: 300 mg daily orally for 40 days reduced fibromyalgia pain by 52% to 56%. Fatigue was also reduced by 47%, morning tiredness by 56%, and tender points 44% compared to baseline.[111] It has also been shown that coenzyme Q10 200 mg in combination with ginkgo biloba 200 mg daily by mouth for 12 weeks improves quality of life measures including physical fitness, emotional feelings, social activities, overall health, and pain.[112]
  - *Migraine headache*: 100 mg daily for 3 months.[113]
- *Adverse effects*: nausea, vomiting, diarrhea, appetite suppression, heartburn, and epigastric discomfort.
- *Contraindications*: hypersensitivity to co-enzyme Q10 and its components.
- *Drug interactions*:
  - *Alkylating agents*: antioxidants might protect tumor cells from chemotherapeutic agents that work by inducing oxidative stress and may reduce effectiveness.[114]
  - *Antihypertensive drugs*: CoQ10 may decrease blood pressure and might have additive blood pressure-lowering effects when used with antihypertensive drugs, leading to an increased risk of hypotension when used concurrently.[115]
  - *Warfarin*: concomitant use might reduce the anticoagulation effects of warfarin leading to decreased warfarin efficacy. CoQ10 has vitamin K-like procoagulant effects.[116]
- *Cautions*: insufficient reliable evidence for use during pregnancy and lactation; avoid use.

MELATONIN

- *Class*: indole neurohormone compound produced in the brain by the pineal gland.[117]
- *Mechanism of action*: the synthesis and release of melatonin in the body are stimulated by darkness and suppressed by light, suggesting the involvement of melatonin in circadian rhythm.
- *Use*: fibromyalgia.
- *Dose*:
  - *Fibromyalgia*: melatonin is thought to decrease the severity of pain and synthesis as well as the number of painful joints in people with fibromyalgia.[118]
    - *Oral*: melatonin 3 mg to 5 mg for up to 60 days.[118]
- *Adverse effects*: drowsiness, hypothermia (may decrease body temperature by about 0.5–1.5°F).
- *Contraindications*: hypersensitivity to melatonin or other components in the supplement product.
- *Drug interactions*:
  - *Anticoagulant drugs*: minor bleeding and decreased prothrombin activity.
  - *Antihypertensive drugs*: decrease blood pressure in healthy adults and lower both systolic and diastolic blood pressure in those with high blood pressure at night. Additive effect with antihypertensive drugs.

- ○ *Anticonvulsants*: lower seizure threshold and may increase seizure frequency in patients, particularly children with neurological defects.
- ○ *Immunosuppressant drugs*: melatonin can stimulate immune function and might interfere with therapy. Avoid administering both during the same regimen time.
- ○ *Amphetamine-containing drugs*: exacerbate adverse effects including decreased levels in tryptophan hydroxylase, tyrosine hydroxylase, and dopamine.
- ○ *CNS depressants*: additive sedation.
- ○ *Anti-diabetic drugs*: melatonin may impair glucose utilization and increase insulin resistance. However, some research also shows that melatonin can improve glycemic control and decrease HbA1c and has no effect on glucose levels.
- ○ *Benzodiazepines*: may decrease endogenous levels of melatonin.
- ○ *Contraceptive drugs*: may increase the levels of melatonin and exacerbate adverse reactions.
- ○ *Fluvoxamine*: significantly increases melatonin levels and may increase bioavailability of exogenously administered melatonin up to 20 times.
- ○ *Verapamil*: increased excretion of melatonin through CYP interactions.
- *Cautions*:
  - ○ Avoid melatonin with lactose in patients who have hereditary galactose intolerance, glucose-galactose malabsorption, or LAPP lactase deficiency.
  - ○ Do not use in patients with hepatic impairment or autoimmune disease.
  - ○ Caution use in patients with renal impairment.
  - ○ Melatonin may worsen restless leg syndrome.

RIBOSE

- *Class*: ribose is an aldopentose, monosaccharide that contains five carbon atoms.
- *Mechanism of action*: ribose is a building block of RNA, which is one of the two backbone chains in nucleic acids.
- *Use*: fibromyalgia.
- *Dose*:
  - ○ *Fibromyalgia*:
    - – *Oral*: 5 grams three times a day can improve energy, sense of well-being, and decrease pain in patients with fibromyalgia.[119] A duration of therapy has not been specified in preliminary clinical trials for the indication of fibromyalgia.
- *Adverse effects*: hypoglycemia, diarrhea, nausea, and headache.
- *Contraindications*: hypersensitivity to ribose and any of its components.
- *Drug interactions*:
  - ○ *Alcohol*: ribose may increase the hypoglycemic effect of ethanol.[120]
  - ○ *Anti-diabetic drugs*: ribose may increase the hypoglycemic effect of oral antihyperglycemic agents.[120]
  - ○ *Salicylate drugs*: ribose may enhance the hypoglycemic effect of salicylate drugs.[120]
- *Cautions*: insufficient reliable information available for use during pregnancy and lactation; avoid using.

VITAMIN D

- *Class*: vitamin D is a fat-soluble vitamin.
- *Use*: fibromyalgia.
- *Dose*:

- ○ *Fibromyalgia*: preliminary clinical research suggests that taking cholecalciferol reduces the pain that fibromyalgia patients experience.[121] The greatest effects were in patients who also had low serum levels of vitamin D compared with that of placebo. Quality of life was not affected.[121] The dose depended on the patient's plasma vitamin D status, with patients taking 2400 IU daily if calcifediol levels were <60 nmol/L or 1200 IU daily if serum calcifediol were 60–80 nmol/L at baseline. Supplementation was conducted to achieve and maintain blood levels between 32 and 48 ng/mL for 20 weeks.[121]
- *Adverse effects*: well-tolerated when taken in appropriate doses. Symptoms of vitamin D toxicity include hypercalcemia, azotemia, and anemia.
- *Contraindications*: hypersensitivity to vitamin D or any of its components.
- *Drug interactions*:
  - ○ *Aluminum*: the protein that transports calcium across the intestinal wall can also bind and transport aluminum. This protein is stimulated by vitamin D, which may therefore increase aluminum absorption.[122]
  - ○ *Atorvastatin/CYP 3A4 substrates*: atorvastatin is metabolized in the gut by CYP 3A4 and vitamin D is thought to induce this enzyme, resulting in reduced bioavailability of atorvastatin and other CYP3A4 substrates.[123]
  - ○ *Calcipotriene*: a vitamin D analog used topically for psoriasis that can be absorbed in sufficient amounts to cause systemic effects, including hypercalcemia. Tell patients not to take vitamin D supplements if they are taking calcipotriene.[124]
  - ○ *Cimetidine*: inhibits an enzyme involved in the conversion of vitamin D to its active form in the liver. It does not affect the formation of active vitamin D metabolites in the kidneys.[125]
  - ○ *Digoxin*: high doses of vitamin D can cause hypercalcemia, and hypercalcemia increases the risk of fatal cardiac arrhythmias with digoxin. Avoid vitamin D above the tolerable upper intake level of 2000 units/day, and monitor serum calcium levels in people taking vitamin D and digoxin concurrently.[124]
  - ○ *Non-dihydropyridine calcium channel blockers*: high doses of vitamin D can cause hypercalcemia. Hypercalcemia can reduce the effectiveness of calcium channel blockers in atrial fibrillation.[124]
  - ○ *Heparin and LMWH*: unfractionated heparin is associated with reduced bone density and osteoporotic fractures, especially when doses of 15,000 units/day or more are used for 3 months or longer. Heparin can increase bone resorption and reduce bone formation.[126]
  - ○ *Thiazide diuretics*: thiazide diuretics decrease urinary calcium excretion, which could lead to hypercalcemia if vitamin D supplements are taken concurrently.[127]
- *Cautions*: none known.

ACETYL L-CARNITINE

- *Class*: L-carnitine is a non-protein amino acid naturally found in the body.[128] Acetyl L-carnitine is the derivative of the amino acid L-carnitine.
- *Mechanism of action*: the body converts L-carnitine into acetyl-L-carnitine. The main function of L-carnitine is to transfer long-chain fatty acids in the form of their acyl-carnitine esters across the inner mitochondrial membrane before beta-oxidation.[129]
- *Use*: fibromyalgia.
- *Dose*:
  - ○ *Fibromyalgia*: one clinical study suggests that taking acetyl L-carnitine 1000 mg per day orally plus acetyl-L-carnitine 500 mg/day IM for 2 weeks, followed by acetyl-L-carnitine 1500 mg/day orally for 8 weeks can reduce muscle pain and improve mood,

general health, and quality of life compared to placebo in patients with fibromyalgia.[129] Another study showed that 1500 mg/day of acetyl-L-carnitine orally in three divided doses for 12 weeks improved depression symptoms, but not pain, quality of life, or anxiety, compared to baseline in patients with fibromyalgia.[130]

- *Adverse effects*: nausea, vomiting, gastrointestinal upset, dry mouth, anorexia, agitation, headache, insomnia
- *Contraindications*: hypersensitivity to acetyl L-carnitine or any of its constituents.
- *Drug interactions*:
  - *Acenocoumarol*: taking L-carnitine 1 gram/day seems to significantly increase the anticoagulant effect, similar to warfarin but shorter-acting. Use of acetyl-L-carnitine concurrently with warfarin can lead to increases in INR.[131]
  - *Warfarin*: use cautiously with warfarin because acetyl L-carnitine can significantly increase the anticoagulant effect.[130]
- *Cautions*: insufficient reliable information available regarding use during pregnancy and lactation; avoid use.

VITAMIN B1 (THIAMINE)

- *Class*: water-soluble B-complex vitamin.
- *Use*: diabetic neuropathy.
- *Dosing*:
  - *Diabetic neuropathy*: 100 mg orally three times daily for 3 months.[132]
- *Adverse effects*: generally well-tolerated.
- *Drug interactions*:
  - *Diuretic drugs*: diuretic drugs increase urinary thiamine excretion and evidence of this vitamin deficiency may occur. Depletion of this supplement can worsen heart failure.
- *Contraindications*: hypersensitivity to thiamine products.
- *Cautions*: none known.

VITAMIN B12

- *Class*: essential, water-soluble vitamin.
- *Use*: diabetic neuropathy, postherpetic neuralgia, peripheral neuropathy.
- *Dosing*:
  - *Diabetic neuropathy*:
    - Cyanocobalamin 0.25 mg three times daily for 9 weeks, methylcobalamin 1500 mcg daily for 3–4 months.[133]
  - *Postherpetic neuralgia*: methylcobalamin 100 mcg SC six times weekly for 4 weeks.[134]
  - *Peripheral neuropathy*: preliminary clinical research shows that taking a specific product containing 3 mcg vitamin B12, folic acid 400 mcg, and uridine monophosphate 50 mg (Keltican) daily for 60 days reduced pain by 44% and decreased concomitant analgesic requirements by over 75% compared to baseline in patients with peripheral neuropathy, including those with lumbar/lumbosacral radiculopathy, sciatic pain, and cervical radiculopathy.[135]
- *Adverse effects*: none noted, generally well-tolerated.
- *Contraindications*: hypersensitivity to cobalt, B12 products, or any component of the supplement product.
- *Drug interactions*:
  - *Chloramphenicol*: limited case reports suggest that chloramphenicol can delay or interrupt the reticulocyte response to supplemental vitamin B12 in some patients. Monitor blood counts closely if this combination is needed and cannot be avoided.[130]

- *Cautions*: not recommended in those with Leber's disease as it may increase the risk of sudden and severe optic atrophy; patients with severe megaloblastic anemia may have increased risk of hypokalemia, thrombocytosis, and sudden death with administration of B12.

BIOTIN

- *Class*: water-soluble B vitamin also known as B7.
- *Mechanism of action*: biotin modulates gene expression and alters pro-astrocyte glucose utilization that can improve symptoms associated with diabetic neuropathy by activating the Krebs cycle in demyelinating nerve cells and activating fatty acid synthesis that is required for myelin synthesis.[136]
- *Use*: diabetic neuropathy.
- *Dosing*:
  - *Diabetic neuropathy*: 5 mg orally for 130 weeks preceded by 12 weeks of IM injections.[137]
- *Adverse effects*: gastrointestinal upset.
- *Contraindications*: hypersensitivity to biotin or any of its constituents.
- *Drug interactions*:
  - *CYP1B1 inducer*: interaction with CYP1B1 substrates can decrease levels of these drugs metabolized by this enzyme.[138]
  - *Anticonvulsants*: can impair biotin absorption.
- *Lab interactions*:
  - High-dose biotin has been shown to interfere with many lab tests and yield false positive or negative results. Most of the published research on biotin interference covers hormone tests, such as parathyroid hormone (PTH), thyroid-stimulating hormone (TSH), and T4 and T3 tests, as well as tests for troponin. However, because biotin is used in so many immunoassays, scientists say it could interfere with many others.

EVENING PRIMROSE

- *Class*: biennial plant.
- *Mechanism of action*: rich in omega 6 fatty acids and has direct action on immune cells.
- *Use*: diabetic neuropathy, relapsing-remitting MS, rheumatoid arthritis.
- *Dosing*:
  - *Relapsing-remitting MS*: 0.6–0.7 g three times daily in combination with hemp seed oil for a period of 6 months.[139]
  - *Diabetic neuropathy*: 360–480 mg daily for 6 months to a year.[140]
- *Adverse effects*: gastrointestinal pain, distention and fullness, diarrhea, vomiting, flatulence, and dyspepsia.
- *Contraindications*: hypersensitivity to evening primrose or any of its components.
- *Drug interactions*:
  - *Anesthetic medications*: reports of seizures. Unclear in studies if due to evening primrose.
  - *Anticoagulant and antiplatelet drugs*: reduces platelet aggregation and prolongs bleeding time.
  - *Protease inhibitor drugs*: may increase the levels of lopinavir and ritonavir when used in combination.
  - *Phenothiazines*: may lower seizure threshold. Unclear whether primrose has epileptogenic effects with the drug as there is no evidence that evening primrose alone causes seizures.
- *Cautions*: N/A.

MILK THISTLE (SILYMARIN)

- *Class*: silybin or silibinin is thought to be the most active component of silymarin.
- *Mechanism of Action*: there is interest in using silymarin for complications of diabetes, such as diabetic nephropathy, which is thought to be caused by oxidative stress and inflammation.[141] Silymarin also possesses anti-fibrotic properties via downregulation of transforming growth factor-beta (TGF-beta). TGF-beta plays a role in diabetic nephropathy as it causes hardening of the glomerulus in the kidney as well as interstitial fibrosis.
- *Use*: multiple sclerosis, diabetic neuropathy.
- *Dosing*:
  - *Diabetic neuropathy*: 140 mg orally three times daily for 3 months, in combination with conventional treatment.[142]
- *Adverse effects*: nausea, vomiting, abdominal pain, sweating, and weakness.
- *Contraindications*: hypersensitivity to milk thistle or any of its components.
- *Drug interactions*:
  - *Anti-diabetic drugs*: can have additive effects of lowering blood glucose, HbA1c levels, and insulin resistance.
  - *CYP 2C9, 2D6, and 3A4*: silymarin is a CYP inhibitor and can increase the levels of CYP substrates of these enzymes.
  - *Glucuronidated drugs*: may affect the clearance of drugs undergoing glucuronidation and can inhibit uridine diphospho-glucuronosyl transferase, which is necessary for the glucuronidation process.
  - *Raloxifene*: milk thistle contains silibinin constituents and silymarin.
  - that, when in combination with raloxifene, inhibit the glucuronidation of raloxifene.
  - *Sirolimus*: silymarin also interacts with sirolimus. The combination decreases sirolimus clearance and is found in hepatically and renally impaired patients.
  - *P-glycoprotein substrates*: Milk thistle inhibits P-glycoprotein substrates and increases drug levels of these medications.
  - *Tamoxifen*: The constituent silibinin in milk thistle may increase plasma levels of tamoxifen, and later conversion into the active metabolite.
- *Cautions*: insufficient reliable information available for use in pregnancy and lactation; avoid use.

FEVERFEW

- *Class*: anti-inflammatory, anti-histamine, analgesic.
- *Mechanism of action*: it's not yet clear how feverfew works in the prevention of migraine.
- *Use*: migraine headache.
- *Dosing*: 50 to 150 mg once daily.[143]
- *Adverse effects*: generally well-tolerated.
- *Contraindications*: hypersensitivity to feverfew or any of its components.
- *Drug interactions*:
  - *Anticoagulant/antiplatelet drugs*: feverfew may inhibit platelet aggregation and may have additional effects and increase the risk of bleeding with these drugs.[144]
  - *Cytochrome P450 1A2, 2C19, 2C8, 2C9, 2D6, 3A4*: feverfew may inhibit CYP 1A2, 2C19.[14]
- *Cautions*: insufficient reliable information for pregnancy and lactation; avoid use.

REFERENCES

1. Natural Medicines. Natural medicines in the clinical management of fibromyalgia. http://naturaldataba se.therapeuticresearch.com.pitt.idm.oclc.org/ce/CECourse.aspx?cs=naturalstandard&s=ND&pm=5 &pc=17-108 (accessed 27 December 2017).

2. McCarty D.J., Csuka M., McCarthy G., Trotter D. Treatment of pain due to fibromyalgia with topical capsaicin: a pilot study. *Semin Arthritis Rheum* 1994;23(6):41–7.
3. Sandoval M., Charbonnet R.M., Okuhama N.N., et al. Cat's claw inhibits TNFalpha production and scavenges free radicals: role in cytoprotection. *Free Radic Biol Med* 2000;29(1):71–8.
4. Piscoya J., Rodriguez Z., Bustamante S.A., et al. Efficacy and safety of freeze-dried cat's claw in osteoarthritis of the knee: mechanisms of action of the species Uncaria guianensis. *Inflamm Res* 2001;50(9):442–8.
5. Mur E., Hartig F., Eibl G., Schirmer M. Randomized double blind trial of an extract from the pentacyclic alkaloid-chemotype of Uncaria tomentosa for the treatment of rheumatoid arthritis. *J Rheumatol* 2002;29(4):678–81.
6. Chen C.X., Jin R.M., Li Y.K., et al. Inhibitory effect of rhynchophylline on platelet aggregation and thrombosis. *Zhongguo Yao Li Xue Bao* 1992;13(2):126–30.
7. Zhou J., Zhou S. Antihypertensive and neuroprotective activities of rhynchophylline: the role of rhynchophylline in neurotransmission and ion channel activity. *Jethnopharmacol* 2010;132(1):15–27.
8. Budzinski J.W., Foster B.C., Vandenhoek S., Arnason J.T. An in vitro evaluation of human cytochrome P450 3A4 inhibition by selected commercial herbal extracts and tinctures. *Phytomedicine* 2000;7(4):273–82.
9. Müller A.C., Kanfer I. Potential pharmacokinetic interactions between antiretrovirals and medicinal plants used as complementary and African traditional medicines. *Biopharm Drug Dispos* 2011;32(8):458–70.
10. McGuffin M., Hobbs C., Upton R., Goldberg A., eds. *American Herbal Products Association's Botanical Safety Handbook*. Boca Raton, FL: CRC Press, LLC, 1997.
11. Chantre P., Cappelaere A., Leblan D., et al. Efficacy and tolerance or Harpagophytum procumbens versus diacerhein in treatment of osteoarthritis. *Phytomedicine* 2000;7(3):177–83.
12. Chrubasik S., Thanner J., Künzel O., et al. Comparison of outcome measures during treatment with the proprietary Harpagophytum extract doloteffin in patients with pain in the lower back, knee or hip. *Phytomedicine* 2002;9(3):181–94.
13. Chrubasik S., Junck H., Breitschwerdt H., Conradt C., Zappe H. Effectiveness of Harpagophytum extract WS 1531 in the treatment of exacerbation of low back pain: a randomized, placebo-controlled, double- blind study. *Eurj Anaesthesiol* 1999;16(2):118–29.
14. Unger M., Frank A. Simultaneous determination of the inhibitory potency of herbal extracts on the activity of six major cytochrome P450 enzymes using liquid chromatography/mass spectrometry and automated online extraction. *Rapid Commun Mass Spectrom* 2004;18(19):2273–81.
15. Romiti N., Tramonti G., Corti A., Chieli E. Effects of devil's claw (Harpagophytum procumbens) on the multidrug transporter transporter ABCB1/P-glycoprotein. *Phytomedicine* 2009;16(12):1095–100.
16. Brinker F. *Herb Contraindications and Drug Interactions*, 2nd ed. Sandy, OR: Eclectic Medical Publications, 1998.
17. Shaw D., Leon C., Kolev S., Murray V. Traditional remedies and food supplements: a 5-year toxicological study (1991–1995). *Drug Saf* 1997;17(5):342–56.
18. Mahomed I.M., Ojewole J.A.O. Oxytocin-like effect of Harpagophytum procumbens [Pedaliacae] secondary root aqueous extract on rat isolated uterus. *Afr J Trad CAM* 2006;3(1):82–9.
19. Haghighi M., Khalva A., Toliat T., Jallaei S. Comparing the effects of ginger (Zingiber officinale) extract and ibuprofen on patients with osteoarthritis. *Arch Iran Med* 2005;8:267–71.
20. Niempoog S., Siriarchavatana P., Kajsongkram T. The efficacy of Plygersic gel for use in the treatment of osteoarthritis of the knee. *J Med Assoc Thai* 2012;95(Suppl 10):S113–9.
21. Ozgoli G., Goli M., Moattar F. Comparison of effects of ginger, mefenamic acid, and ibuprofen on pain in women with primary dysmenorrhea. *J Altern Complement Med* 2009;15(2):129–32.
22. Maghbooli M., Golipour F., Moghimi Esfandabadi A., Yousefi M. Comparison between the efficacy of ginger and sumatriptan in the ablative treatment of the common migraine. *Phytother Res* 2014;28(3):412–5.
23. Grøntved A., Brask T., Kambskard J., Hentzer E. Ginger root against seasickness: a controlled trial on the open sea. *Acta Otolaryngol* 1988;105(1–2):45–9.
24. Srivastava K.C. Effect of onion and ginger consumption on platelet thromboxane production in humans. *Prostaglandins Leukot Essent Fatty Acids* 1989;35(3):183–5.
25. Akhani S.P., Vishwakarma S.L., Goyal R.K. Anti-diabetic activity of zingiber officinale in streptozotocin-induced type I diabetic rats. *J Pharm Pharmacol* 2004;56(1):101–5.
26. Ghayur M.N., Gilani A.H. Ginger lowers blood pressure through blockade of voltage-dependent calcium channels. *J Cardiovasc Pharmacol* 2005;45(1):74–80.

27. Chiang H.M., Chao P.D., Hsiu S.L., et al. Ginger significantly decreased the oral bioavailability of cyclo-sporine in rats. *Am J Chin Med* 2006;34(5):845–55.
28. Okonta J.M., Uboh M., Obonga W.O. Herb-drug interaction: a case study of effect of ginger on the pharmacokinetic of metronidazole in rabbit. *Indian J Pharm Sci (India)* 2008;70(230):232.
29. Safayhi H., Mack T., Sabieraj J., et al. Boswellic acids: novel, specific, nonredox inhibitors of 5-lipoxy-genase. *J Pharmacolexpther* 1992;261(3):1143–6.
30. Sengupta K., Alluri K.V., Satish A.R., et al. A double blind, randomized, placebo controlled study of the efficacy and safety of 5-Loxin for the treatment of osteoarthritis of the knee. *Arthritis Res Ther* 2008;10(4):R85.
31. Holtmeier W., Zeuzem S., Preiss J., et al. Randomized, placebo-controlled, double-blind trial of Bosewellia Serrata in maintaining remission of Crohn's disease: good safety profile but lack of efficacy. *Inflamm Bowel Dis* 2011;17(2):573–82.
32. Frank A., Unger M. Analysis of frankincense from various Boswellia species with inhibitory activity on human drug metabolising cytochrome P450 enzymes using liquid chromatography mass spectrometry after automated on-line extraction. *J Chromatogr A* 2006;1112(1–2):255–62.
33. Mikhaeil B.R., Maatooq G.T., Badria F.A., Amer M.M. Chemistry and immunomodulatory activity of frankincense oil. *Z Naturforsch C J Biosci* 2003;58(3–4):230–8.
34. Chalasani N., Vuppalanchi R., Navarro V., et al. Acute liver injury due to flavocoxid (Limbrel), a medi-cal food for osteoarthritis: a case series. *Ann Intern Med* 2012;156(12):857–60.
35. Zhang F., Altorki N.K., Mestre J.R., Subbaramaiah K., Dannenberg A.J. Curcumin inhibits cyclooxy-genase-2 transcription in bile acid- and phorbol ester-treated human gastrointestinal epithelial cells. *Carcinogenesis* 1999;20(3):445–51.
36. Madhu K., Chanda K., Saji M.J. Safety and efficacy of curcuma longa extract in the treatment of painful knee osteoarthritis: a randomized placebo-controlled trial. *Inflammopharmacology* 2013;21(2):129–36.
37. Sharma R.A., McLelland H.R., Hill K.A., et al. Pharmacodynamic and pharmacokinetic study of oral curcuma extract in patients with colorectal cancer. *Clin Cancer Res* 2001;7(7):1894–900.
38. Shah B.H., Nawaz Z., Pertani S.A., et al. Inhibitory effect of curcumin, a food spice from turmeric, on platelet-activating factor- and arachidonic acid-mediated platelet aggregation through inhibition of thromboxane formation and Ca2+ signaling. *Biochem Pharmacol* 1999;58(7):1167–72.
39. Arun N., Nalini N. Efficacy of turmeric on blood sugar and polyol pathway in diabetic albino rats. *Plant Foods Humnutr* 2002;57(1):41–52.
40. Somasundaram S., Edmund N.A., Moore D.T., et al. Dietary curcumin inhibits chemotherapy-induced apoptosis in models of human breast cancer. *Cancer Res* 2002;62(13):3868–75.
41. Price R.J., Scott M.P., Giddings A.M., et al. Effect of butylated hydroxytoluene, curcumin, propyl gallate and thiabendazole on cytochrome P450 forms in cultured human hepatocytes. *Xenobiotica* 2008;38(6):574–86.
42. Yan Y.D., Kim D.H., Sung J.H., Yong C.S., Choi H.G. Enhanced oral bioavailability of docetaxel in rats by four consecutive days of pre-treatment with curcumin. *Int J Pharm* 2010;399(1–2):116–20.
43. Shenouda N.S., Zhou C., Browning J.D., et al. Phytoestrogens in common herbs regulate prostate cancer cell growth in vitro. *Nutrcancer* 2004;49(2):200–8.
44. Neerati P., Devde R., Gangi A.K. Evaluation of the effect of curcumin capsules on glyburide therapy in patients with type-2 diabetes mellitus. *Phytother Res* 2014;28(12):1796–800.
45. Pavithra B.H., Prakash N., Jayakumar K. Modification of pharmacokinetics of norfloxacin following oral administration of curcumin in rabbits. *J Vet Sci* 2009;10(4):293–7.
46. Junyaprasert V.B., Soonthornchareonnon N., Thongpraditchote S., Murakami T., Takano M. Inhibitory effect of thai plant extracts on P-glycoprotein mediated efflux. *Phytotherres* 2006;20(1):79–81.
47. Kusuhara H., Furuie H., Inano A., et al. Pharmacokinetic interaction study of sulphasalazine in healthy subjects and the impact of curcumin as an in vivo inhibitor of BCRP. *Br J Pharmacol* 2012;166(6):1793–803.
48. Nayeri A., Wu S., Adams E., et al. Acute calcineurin inhibitor nephrotoxicity secondary to turmeric intake: a case report. *Transplant Proc* 2017;49(1):198–200.
49. Unsworth J., d'Assis-Fonseca A., Beswick D.T., Blake D.R. Serum salicylate levels in a breast fed infant. *Ann Rheum Dis* 1987;46(8):638–9.
50. Schmid B., Lüdtke R., Selbmann H.K., et al. Efficacy and tolerability of a standardized willow bark extract in patients with osteoarthritis: randomized placebo-controlled, double blind clinical trial. *Phytother Res* 2001;15(4):344–50.
51. Sweeney K.R., Chapron D.J., Brandt J.L., et al. Toxic interaction between acetazolamide and salicylate: case reports and a pharmacokinetic explanation. *Clin Pharmacol Ther* 1986;40(5):518–24.

52. Krivoy N., Pavlotzky E., Chrubasik S., Eisenberg E., Brook G. Effect of salicis cortex extract on human platelet aggregation. *Planta Med* 2001;67(3):209–12.
53. Schmid B., Kötter I., Heide L. Pharmacokinetics of salicin after oral administration of a standardized willow bark extract. *Eur J Clin Pharmacol* 2001;57(5):387–91.
54. McIlwain H., Silverfield J.C., Cheatum D.E., et al. Intra-articular orgotein in osteoarthritis of the knee: a placebo-controlled efficacy, safety, and dosage comparison. *Am J Med* 1989;87(3):295–300.
55. Goebel K.M., Storck U., Neurath F. Intrasynovial orgotein therapy in rheumatoid arthritis. *Lancet* 1981;1(8228):1015–7.
56. Nielsen O.S., Overgaard J., Overgaard M., et al. Orgotein in radiation treatment of bladder cancer. A report on allergic reactions and lack of radioprotective effect. *Acta Oncol* 1987;26(2):101–4.
57. Jensen N.H. Reduced pain from osteoarthritis in hip joint or knee joint during treatment with calcium ascorbate. A randomized, placebo-controlled cross-over trial in general practice. *Ugeskr Laeger* 2003;165(25):2563–6.
58. Kanazi G.E., El-Khatib M.F., Yazbeck-Karam V.G., et al. Effect of vitamin C on morphine use after laparoscopic cholecystectomy: a randomized controlled trial. *Can J Anaesth* 2012;59(6):538–43.
59. Levine M., Rumsey S.C., Daruwala R., Park J.B., Wang Y. Criteria and recommendations for vitamin C intake. *JAMA* 1999;281(15):1415–23.
60. Houston J.B., Levy G. Drug biotransformation interactions in man VI: acetaminophen and ascorbic acid. *J Pharm Sci* 1976;65(8):1218–21.
61. Labriola D., Livingston R. Possible interactions between dietary antioxidants and chemotherapy. *Oncology (Williston Park)* 1999;13(7):1003–8.
62. Fairweather-Tait S., Hickson K., McGaw B., Reid M. Orange juice enhances aluminium absorption from antacid preparation. *Eur J Clin Nutr* 1994;48(1):71–3.
63. Hansten P.D., Horn J.R. *Drug Interactions Analysis and Management.* Vancouver, WA: Applied Therapeutics Inc., 1997.
64. Back D.J., Breckenridge A.M., MacIver M., et al. Interaction of ethinyloestradiol with ascorbic acid in man. *Br Med J (Clin Res Ed)* 1981;282(6275):1516.
65. Dysken M.W., Cumming R.J., Channon R.A., Davis J.M. Drug interaction between ascorbic acid and fluphenazine. *JAMA* 1979;241:2008.
66. Slain D., Amsden J.R., Khakoo R.A., et al. Effect of high-dose vitamin C on the steady-state pharmacokinetics of the protease inhibitor indinavir in healthy volunteers. *Pharmacotherapy* 2005;25(2):165–70.
67. Kuo S.M., Lin C.P., Morehouse H.F. Jr. Dihydropyridine calcium channel blockers inhibit ascorbic acid accumulation in human intestinal Caco-2 cells. *Life Sci* 2001;68(15):1751–60.
68. Feetam C.L., Leach R.H., Meynell M.J. Lack of a clinically important interaction between warfarin and ascorbic acid. *Toxicol Appl Pharmacol* 1975;31(3):544–7.
69. Edmonds S.E., Winyard P.G., Guo R., et al. Putative analgesic activity of repeated oral doses of vitamin E in the treatment of rheumatoid arthritis. Results of a prospective placebo controlled double blind trial. *Ann Rheum Dis* 1997;56(11):649–55.
70. Anon. Dietary supplementation with n-3 polyunsaturated fatty acids and vitamin E after myocardial infarction: results of the GISSI-Prevenzione trial. Gruppo Italiano per lo Studio della Sopravivenza nell'Infarto miocardico. *Lancet* 1999;354(9177):447–55.
71. Liede K.E., Haukka J.K., Saxén L.M., Heinonen O.P. Increased tendency towards gingival bleeding caused by joint effect of alpha-tocopherol supplementation and acetylsalicylic acid. *Ann Med* 1998;30(6):542–6.
72. Landes N., Pfluger P., Kluth D., et al. Vitamin E activates gene expression via the pregnane X receptor. *Biochem Pharmacol* 2003;65(2):269–73.
73. Steiner M. Vitamin E, a modifier of platelet function: rationale and use in cardiovascular and cerebrovascular disease. *Nutr Rev* 1999;57(10):306–9.
74. du Souich P., García A.G., Vergés J., Montell E. Immunomodulatory and anti-inflammatory effects of chondroitin sulphate. *J Cell Mol Med* 2009;13(8A):1451–63.
75. Morreale P., Manopulo R., Galati M., et al. Comparison of the anti-inflammatory efficacy of chondroitin sulfate and diclofenac sodium in patients with knee osteoarthritis. *J Rheumatol* 1996;23(8):1385–91.
76. Rozenfeld V., Crain J.L., Callahan A.K. Possible augmentation of warfarin effect by glucosamine-chondroitin. *Am J Health Syst Pharm* 2004;61(3):306–7.
77. Hoffer L.J., Kaplan L.N., Hamadeh M.J., Grigoriu A.C., Baron M. Sulfate could mediate the therapeutic effect of glucosamine sulfate. *Metabolism* 2001;50(7):767–70.
78. Rindone J.P., Hiller D., Collacott E., Nordhaugen N., Arriola G. Randomized, controlled trial of glucosamine for treating osteoarthritis of the knee. *West J Med* 2000;172(2):91–4.

79. Bush T.M., Rayburn K.S., Holloway S.W., et al. Adverse interactions between herbal and dietary substances and prescription medications: a clinical survey. *Altern Ther Health Med* 2007;13(2):30–5.

80. Balkan B., Dunning B.E. Glucosamine inhibits glucokinase in vitro and produces a glucose-specific impairment of in vivo insulin secretion in rats. *Diabetes* 1994;43(10):1173–9.

81. Yun J., Tomida A., Nagata K., Tsuruo T. Glucose-regulated stresses confer resistance to vp-16 in human cancer cells through a decreased expression of DNA topoisomerase II. *Oncol Res* 1995;7(12):583–90.

82. Murav'ev I.u.V., Venikova M.S., Pleskovskaia G.N., Riazantseva T.A, Sigidin I.a.A. Effect of dimethyl sulfoxide and dimethyl sulfone on a destructive process in the joints of mice with spontaneous arthritis. Patol Fiziol Eksp Ter 1991;2:37–9.

83. Brien S., Prescott P., Lewith G. Meta-analysis of the related nutritional supplements dimethyl sulfoxide and methylsulfonylmethane in the treatment of osteoarthritis of the knee. *Evid Based Complement Alternat Med* 2011;2011:528403.

84. Usha P.R., Naidu M.U. Randomised, double-blind, parallel, placebo-controlled study of oral glucosamine, methylsulfonylmethane and their combination in osteoarthritis. *Clin Drug Investig* 2004; 24(6):353–63.

85. Domljan Z., Vrhovac B., Dürrigl T., Pucar I. A double-blind trial of ademetionine vs naproxen in activated gonarthrosis. *Int J Clin Pharmacol Ther Toxicol* 1989;27(7):329–33.

86. Tavoni A., Vitali C., Bombardieri S., Pasero G. Evaluation of S-adenosylmethionine in primary fibromyalgia. A double-blind crossover study. *Am J Med* 1987;83(5A):107–10.

87. Jacobsen S., Danneskiold-Samsøe B., Andersen R.B. Oral S-adenosylmethionine in primary fibromyalgia. Double-blind clinical evaluation. *Scand J Rheumatol* 1991;20(4):294–302.

88. Volkmann H., Nørregaard J., Jacobsen S., et al. Double-blind, placebo-controlled cross-over study of intravenous S-adenosyl-L-methionine in patients with fibromyalgia. *Scand J Rheumatol* 1997;26(3):206–11.

89. Tavoni A., Jeracitano G., Cirigliano G. Evaluation of S-adenosylmethionine in secondary fibromyalgia: a double-blind study. *Clin Exp Rheumatol* 1998;16(1):106–7.

90. Iruela L.M., Minguez L., Merino J., Monedero G. Toxic interaction of S-adenosylmethionine and clomipramine. *Am J Psychiatry* 1993;150(3):522.

91. Charlton C.G., Crowell B. Jr. Parkinson's disease-like effects of S-adenosyl-L-methionine: effects of L-dopa. *Pharmacol Biochem Behav* 1992;43(2):423–31.

92. Sarzi Puttini P., Caruso I. Primary fibromyalgia syndrome and 5-hydroxy-l-tryptophan: a 90-day open study. *J Int Med Res* 1992;20(2):182–9.

93. Caruso I., Sarzi Puttini P., Cazzola M., Azzolini V. Double-blind study of 5-hydroxytryptophan versus placebo in the treatment of primary fibromyalgia syndrome. *J Int Med Res* 1990;18(3):201–9.

94. Singhal A.B., Caviness V.S., Begleiter A.F., et al. Cerebral vasoconstriction and stroke after use of serotonergic drugs. *Neurology* 2002;58(1):130–3.

95. Shils M., Olson A., Shike M. *Modern Nutrition in Health and Disease*, 8th ed. Philadelphia, PA: Lea and Febiger, 1994.

96. Bagis S., Karabiber M., As I., Tamer L., Erdogan C., Atalay A. Is magnesium citrate treatment effective on pain, clinical parameters and functional status in patients with fibromyalgia? Rheumatol Int 2013;33(1):167–72.

97. Crosby V., Wilcock A., Corcoran R. The safety and efficacy of a single dose (500 mg or 1 g) of intravenous magnesium sulfate in neuropathic pain poorly responsive to strong opioid analgesics in patients with cancer. *J Pain Symptom Manag* 2000;19(1):35–9.

98. Albrecht E., Kirkham K.R., Liu S.S., Brull R. The analgesic efficacy and safety of neuraxial magnesium sulphate: a quantitative review. *Anaesthesia* 2013;68(2):190–202.

99. Gallelli L., Avenoso T., Falcone D., et al. Effects of acetaminophen and ibuprofen in children with migraine receiving preventive treatment with magnesium. *Headache* 2014;54(2):313–24.

100. L'Hommedieu C.S., Nicholas D., Armes D.A., et al. Potentiation of magnesium sulfate--Induced neuromuscular weakness by gentamicin, tobramycin, and amikacin. *J Pediatr* 1983;102(4):629–31.

101. Yamasaki M., Funakoshi S., Matsuda S., et al. Interaction of magnesium oxide with gastric acid secretion inhibitors in clinical pharmacotherapy. *Eur J Clin Pharmacol* 2014;70(8):921–4.

102. Ravn H.B., Vissinger H., Kristensen S.D., Husted S.E. Magnesium inhibits platelet activity–An in vitro study. *Thromb Haemost* 1996;76(1):88–93.

103. Dunn C.J., Goa K.L. Risedronate: a review of its pharmacological properties and clinical use in resorptive bone disease. *Drugs* 2001;61(5):685–712.

104. Rodin S.M., Johnson B.F. Pharmacokinetic interactions with digoxin. *Clin Pharmacokinet* 1988; 15(4):227–44.

105. Yagi T., Naito T., Mino Y., Umemura K., Kawakami J. Impact of concomitant antacid administration on gabapentin plasma exposure and oral bioavailability in healthy adult subjects. *Drug Metab Pharmacokinet* 2012;27(2):248–54.

106. Ryan M.P. Diuretics and potassium/magnesium depletion. Directions for treatment. *Am J Med* 1987;82(3A):38–47.

107. Kivistö K.T., Neuvonen P.J. Enhancement of absorption and effect of glipizide by magnesium hydroxide. *Clin Pharmacol Ther* 1991;49(1):39–43.

108. Sompolinsky D., Samra Z. Influence of magnesium and manganese on some biological and physical properties of tetracycline. *J Bacteriol* 1972;110(2):468–76.

109. Greenberg S., Frishman W.H. Co-enzyme Q10: a new drug for cardiovascular disease. *J Clin Pharmacol* 1990;30(7):596–608.

110. Hernández-Ojeda J., Cardona-Muñoz E.G., Román-Pintos L.M., et al. The effect of ubiquinone in diabetic polyneuropathy: a randomized double-blind placebo-controlled study. *J Diabetes Complications* 2012;26(4):352–8.

111. Cordero M.D., Alcocer-Gómez E., de Miguel M., et al. Can coenzyme Q10 improve clinical and molecular parameters in fibromyalgia? *Antioxid Redox Signal* 2013;19(12):1356–61.

112. Lister R.E. An open, pilot study to evaluate the potential benefits of coenzyme Q10 combined with Ginkgo biloba extract in fibromyalgia syndrome. *J Int Med Res* 2002;30(2):195–9.

113. Shoeibi A., Olfati N., Soltani Sabi M., et al. Effectiveness of coenzyme Q10 in prophylactic treatment of migraine headache: an open-label, add-on, controlled trial. *Acta Neurol Belg* 2017;117(1):103–9.

114. Portakal O., Ozkaya O., Erden Inal M., et al. Coenzyme Q10 concentrations and antioxidant status in tissues of breast cancer patients. *Clin Biochem* 2000;33(4):279–84.

115. Langsjoen P., Willis P., Folkers R., Folkers K.. Treatment of essential hypertension with coenzyme Q10. *Mol Aspects Med* 1994;15(Suppl 1):S265–72.

116. Spigset O. Reduced effect of warfarin caused by ubidecarenone. *Lancet* 1994;344(8933):1372–3.

117. Brzezinski A. Melatonin in humans. *N Engl J Med* 1997;336(3):186–95.

118. Citera G., Arias M.A., Maldonado-Cocco J.A., et al. The effect of melatonin in patients with fibromyalgia: a pilot study. *Clin Rheumatol* 2000;19(1):9–13.

119. Teitelbaum J.E., Johnson C., St Cyr J. The use of D-ribose in chronic fatigue syndrome and fibromyalgia: a pilot study. *J Altern Complement Med* 2006;12(9):857–62.

120. Burke E.R. *D-Ribose What You Need to Know.* Garden City Park, NY: Avery Publishing Group, 1999: 1–43.

121. Wepner F., Scheuer R., Schuetz-Wieser B., et al. Effects of vitamin D on patients with fibromyalgia syndrome: a randomized placebo-controlled trial. *Pain* 2014;155(2):261–8.

122. Moon J. The role of vitamin D in toxic metal absorption: a review. *J Am Coll Nutr* 1994;13(6):559–64.

123. Schwartz J.B. Effects of vitamin D supplementation in atorvastatin-treated patients: a new drug interaction with an unexpected consequence. *Clin Pharmacol Ther* 2009;85(2):198–203.

124. McEvoy G.K., Drug A.H.F.S. *Information.* Bethesda, MD: American Society of Health-System Pharmacists, 1998.

125. Odes H.S., Fraser G.M., Krugliak P., Lamprecht S.A., Shany S. Effect of cimetidine on hepatic vitamin D metabolism in humans. *Digestion* 1990;46(2):61–4.

126. Tannirandorn P., Epstein S. Drug-induced bone loss. *Osteoporos Int* 2000;11(8):637–59.

127. Tatro D.S., ed. *Drug Interactions Facts.* St. Louis, MO: Facts and Comparisons Inc., 1999.

128. Vidal-Casariego A., Burgos-Peláez R., Martínez-Faedo C., et al. Metabolic effects of L-carnitine on type 2 diabetes mellitus: systematic review and meta-analysis. *Exp Clin Endocrinol Diabetes* 2013;121(4):234–8.

129. Rossini M., Di Munno O., Valentini G., et al. Double-blind, multicenter trial comparing acetyl l-carnitine with placebo in the treatment of fibromyalgia patients. *Clin Exp Rheumatol* 2007;25(2):182–8.

130. Leombruni P., Miniotti M., Colonna F., et al. A randomised controlled trial comparing duloxetine and acetyl L-carnitine in fibromyalgic patients: preliminary data. *Clin Exp Rheumatol* 2015;33(1 Suppl 88):S82–5.

131. Martinez E., Domingo P., Roca-Cusachs A. Potentiation of acenocoumarol action by L-carnitine. *J Intern Med* 1993;233(1):94.

132. Rabbani N., Alam S.S., Riaz S., et al. High-dose thiamine therapy for patients with type 2 diabetes and microalbuminuria: a randomized, double-blind placebo-controlled pilot study. *Diabetologia* 2009;52(2):208–12.

133. Devathasan G., Teo W.L., Mylvaganam A. Methylcobalamin in chronic diabetic neuropathy. A double-blind clinical and electrophysiological study. *Clin Trials J* 1986;23:130–40.

134. Xu G., Lv Z.W., Feng Y., Tang W.Z., Xu G.X. A single-center randomized controlled trial of local methylcobalamin injection for subacute herpetic neuralgia. *Pain Med* 2013;14(6):884–94.

135. Negrão L., Almeida P., Alcino S., et al. Effect of the combination of uridine, folic acid and vitamin B12 on the clinical expression of peripheral neuropathies. *Pain Manag* 2014;4(3):191–6.

136. Sedel F., Papeix C., Bellanger A., et al. High doses of biotin in chronic progressive multiple sclerosis: a pilot study. *Mult Scler Relat Disord* 2015;4(2):159–69. doi:10.1016/j.msard.2015.01.005.

137. Koutsikos D., Agroyannis B., Tzanatos-Exarchou H. Biotin for diabetic peripheral neuropathy. *Biomed Pharmacother* 1990;44(10):511–4.

138. Rodriguez-Melendez R., Griffin J.B., Zempleni J. Biotin supplementation increases expression of the cytochrome P450 1B1 gene in Jurkat cells, increasing the occurrence of single-stranded DNA breaks. *J Nutr* 2004;134(9):2222–8.

139. Rezapour-Firouzi S., Arefhosseini S.R., Mehdi F., et al. Immunomodulatory and therapeutic effects of hot-natured diet and co-supplemented hemp seed, evening primrose oils intervention in multiple sclerosis patients. Complement Ther Med 2013;21(5):473–80.

140. Keen H., Payan J., Allawi J., et al. Treatment of diabetic neuropathy with gamma-linolenic acid: the gamma-linolenic acid multicenter trial group. *Diabetes Care* 1993;16(1):8–15.

141. Voroneanu L., Nistor I., Dumea R., Apetrii M., Covic A. Silymarin in type 2 diabetes mellitus: a systematic review and meta-analysis of randomized controlled trials. *J Diabetes Res* 2016;2016:5147468.

142. Fallahzadeh M.K., Dormanesh B., Sagheb M.M., et al. Effect of addition of silymarin to renin-angiotensin system inhibitors on proteinuria in type 2 diabetic patients with overt nephropathy: a randomized, double-blind, placebo-controlled trial. *Am J Kidney Dis* 2012;60(6):896–903.

143. Johnson E.S., Kadam N.P., Hylands D.M., Hylands P.J. Efficacy of feverfew as prophylactic treatment of migraine. *Br Med J (Clin Res Ed)* 1985;291(6495):569–73.

144. Awang D.V.C. Prescribing therapeutic feverfew (Tancetum pathrnium (L.) Schultz Bip., syn. Chrysanthemumparthenium (L.) Bernh). *Int Med* 1998;1(1):11–3.

20 PEA
A Novel Fatty Acid in the Treatment of Pain

Sahar Swidan

CONTENTS

The topic of peroxisome proliferator-activated receptor (PPAR) ligands typically involves a discussion of the lipid-lowering effects of fibrates and the blood sugar-lowering effects of thiazolidinediones. However, more recent research has investigated the role of the endogenous PPAR-α ligand, palmitoylethanolamide (PEA) on inflammation, pain, neurodegenerative diseases, stroke, spinal cord injury, and neuropsychiatric disorders.[1] Palmitoylethanolamide is a naturally occurring fatty acid belonging to the *N*-acylethanolamine (NAE) class of signaling molecules and can be isolated from egg yolks, peanut meal, and lecithin. It is rapidly metabolized in the human body via fatty acid amide hydrolase (FAAH) and *N*-acylethanolamine-hydrolyzing acid amidase (NAAA) to inactive metabolites palmitic acid and ethanolamine.[2,3] Initial pharmacokinetic research by Lambert et al.[2] assumed a ligand-binding relationship between PEA and the endogenous cannabinoid 2 (CB2) receptor. However, these initial claims proved to be incorrect and were explained as the entourage effect, where PEA competes with the endocannabinoid anandamide (AEA) for FAAH, resulting in higher concentrations of AEA.[4] Although it does have a structural relationship to AEA and other endocannabinoids, PEA was found to have pharmacologic activity at PPAR-α, PPAR-γ, PPAR-δ, G protein-coupled receptor (GPR) 55, GPR119, transient receptor potential channel type (TRP) V1, ATP-sensitive potassium channels, and calcium-activated potassium channels. Additionally, PEA appears to inhibit ceramidases, and potassium channels Kv4.3 and Kv1.5, as well as interacting with NF-κB, cyclooxygenase (COX), TNFα, interleukin (IL)-4, IL-6, IL-8, nitric oxide (NO), and substance P mast cell activation. This variety of interactions has afforded PEA the title of being "promiscuous."[4,5]

Many of the receptors, channels, and cytokines that PEA interacts with are involved in inflammatory pain signaling (e.g., PPAR-α), immune systems (e.g., GPR55), and endocrine systems (e.g., GPR119). As discussed by Skaper et al.,[1] inflammation is a protective response in the human body that is initiated during the cellular healing process. However, when inflammation is prolonged it can cause damage and lead to pain, neurologic diseases, and other inflammatory disorders. Palmitoylethanolamide accomplishes its anti-inflammatory and anti-nociceptive effects by binding to and modulating PPAR-α, which is a regulator of the gene networks controlling pain and inflammation. This gene network switches NF-κB off, which is involved in the pathology of peripheral neuropathies, carpal tunnel syndrome, sciatic pain, osteoarthritis, low-back pain, dental pain, multiple sclerosis, chronic pelvic pain, postherpetic neuralgia, and vaginal pain.[5] The cannabinoid-like receptors GPR55 and GPR119 have been linked to inflammation in the gut related to immune system modulation and GLP-1 secretion from entero-endocrine cells, respectively.[6] Additionally, PEA influences potassium channels involved in pain perception and desensitizes the TRPV1 channel on sensory neurons. These pharmacodynamic relationships are what gives PEA its anti-inflammatory, immune-modulatory, and anti-nociceptive properties.

PAIN, ENDOMETRIAL PAIN, FIBROMYALGIA, AND IBS-RELATED PAIN

The interaction between PEA and PPAR-α has been demonstrated by comparing the observed effects of PEA on normal mice to those that have been genetically altered without PPAR-α. When exposed to PEA, the PPAR-α null mice did not experience the anti-nociceptive effects of PEA.[7,8] Based on animal studies, the hypothesis that PPAR-α has anti-nociceptive and anti-inflammatory effects is supported by showing reduced edema and macrophage infiltration, and increased myelin sheath, axonal diameter, and number of fibers. PEA was also associated with a reduction of inflammatory markers (e.g., COX-2, inducible NO synthase, malondialdehyde). Consequently, it was determined that PEA not only exerts anti-inflammatory and anti-nociceptive effects, but also prevents neurotoxicity and neurodegeneration.[1,7]

PEA has been shown to be effective in a number of chronic pain conditions both as an adjunct therapy to other pain medication and as a monotherapy. Gatti et al.[9] performed a prospective observational study on the effects of PEA in several chronic pain conditions including diabetic neuropathy, post-herpetic neuralgia, and osteoarthritis. This study consisted of 564 patients suffering from various pathological conditions who were either undergoing standard therapy with unsatisfactory results or who had discontinued therapy because of side effects. Adult patients greater than 18 years old, with chronic pain for more than 6 months, and a Numerical Rating Scale (NRS) score of 4 or greater were included in the study. Study participants were instructed to take 600 mg of PEA (Normast®) twice daily for 3 weeks followed by once daily dosing for 1 week. The NRS was used to evaluate changes in pain before and after the treatment period. Participants were separated into two groups based on whether they were taking concomitant medication with PEA or PEA alone. The researchers reported that the PEA treatment markedly decreased the mean score pain intensity from a baseline value of 6.4 to 2.5 for all study participants. Their analysis of the data using a mixed model repeated measure ruled out any other factors beside the PEA treatment for the improvement of pain. The study also highlighted the value of having a group that was taking the PEA as a monotherapy for pain by stating that there was a similar reduction in pain seen with this group as compared to the other group.

Human studies on the effects of PEA on endometrial pain have shown promising results. Keppel Hesselink[10] observed a therapeutic response with the combination of PEA and trans-polydatin, as measured by the visual analogue scale (VAS) score within 1–4 weeks of treatment, of at least 50% when compared to baseline in patients with chronic pelvic pain related to endometriosis. Mast cells have been associated with endometrial pain, and PEA has been shown to be effective in reducing mast cell activation.[1,5,6]

Another study was conducted in 2015 on the effects of PEA and trans-polydatin as a treatment for primary dysmenorrhea. This randomized placebo-controlled study investigated the effects of a PEA + trans-polydatin combination on 220 adolescent and young women (mean age 19 years) who experienced primary dysmenorrhea. The researchers found that an improvement in pelvic pain was seen in 98.18% of the cases in the group treated with the combination medication versus 56.36% in the placebo group. The average improvement in pain in the treatment group was 4 points based on the VAS as compared to only 1 point in the placebo group. While this was a small sample size, the researchers noted that this therapy would, at the very least, be a good adjunct treatment to the traditional use of NSAIDs or oral contraceptives for the relief of primary dysmenorrhea. Using this combination would lead to a decrease in side effects seen from the use of these traditional treatments.[11]

Cobellis et al.[12] investigated the effectiveness of a PEA+ trans-polydatin combination in endometriosis through a randomized, double-blind, parallel-group, placebo-controlled clinical study. The 61 participants in this study were female between the ages of 24 and 41 who had a confirmed diagnosis of endometriosis. The participants were separated into three separate groups and were given the PEA + trans-polydatin combination (400 mg + 40 mg twice daily for 3 months), placebo, or celecoxib (200 mg twice daily for 7 consecutive days). Study participants completed a questionnaire for pelvic pain assessment and rated their pelvic pain using the VAS both before and after treatment. The researchers reported that there was a larger reduction in pain with the PEA + trans-polydatin compared to placebo reported by the patients. Additionally, there was a reduction in pain seen in the celecoxib group. While NSAIDs are an effective symptomatic therapy for endometriosis, they have a number of side effects that can make them dangerous for long-term use. This study highlighted that the PEA + trans-polydatin combination would be a good option for patients suffering from endometriosis if they have absolute contraindications for NSAIDs. While this study was promising, more research needs to be done to establish the effectiveness of PEA on endometriosis.

Giugliano et al.[13] performed a study investigating the effects of a PEA + trans-polydatin combination on endometriosis pain. This was a prospective cohort clinical study with 47 participants. They were separated into two groups based on where the endometriosis was located; group A had endometriosis located at the recto-vaginal septum and group B at the ovary. All patients were treated with estrogen-progestin therapy and anti-inflammatory therapy for at least 6 months prior to the start of the trial and continued that therapy for the duration of the trial. Every patient received the same treatment (PEA + trans-polydatin, 400 mg + 40 mg twice daily) for 90 days. Patients rated the severity of dysmenorrhea, chronic pelvic pain, dyspareunia, and dyschezia using the VAS prior to the start of treatment and at 30 (T1), 60 (T2), and 90 (T3) days after treatment. At the beginning of the trial the average mean scores for chronic pelvic pain, dysmenorrhea, dyspareunia, and dyschezia were 5.11, 6.7, 3.85, and 2.57, respectively. Except for dyschezia, there was a significant reduction in pain observed among the two groups over the period of 90 days. Specifically, reductions in chronic pelvic pain in the patients with recto-vaginal endometriosis and dysmenorrhea in patients with ovarian endometriosis were observed. This study demonstrated the efficacy of a PEA + trans-polydatin combination as an adjunct therapy in the treatment of endometriotic pain. The authors of this paper noted that the patients who participated in this study started out with moderate endometriotic pain; therefore, they cannot attest to the efficacy of PEA + trans-polydatin in patients with severe endometriotic pain.

Fibromyalgia is a complex disease state that encompasses many different pain disorders, making diagnosis and treatment difficult. The presence of inflammatory cytokines is key to the nociception, allodynia, and hyperalgesia seen in fibromyalgia patients. Del Giorno et al.[14] investigated the efficacy of a combination therapy consisting of duloxetine, pregabalin, and PEA. The results of the study showed a significant reduction of painful tender points and global pain with the addition of PEA. This provides evidence for the PEA as an adjunct to pain management in fibromyalgia.

Irritable bowel syndrome (IBS) is a gastrointestinal disorder that typically presents with pain associated with the alteration of bowel function. Recent evidence has shown a link between endogenous cannabinoid receptors (e.g., CB_1, CB_2), cannabinoid-like receptors (e.g., TRPV1, GPR55), and endogenous ligands (e.g., AEA, PEA) with attenuation of IBS-related pain.[15] Irritable bowel syndrome can be divided into two main categories based on symptomatology. Type-D patients present with diarrhea, whereas type-C patients present with constipation. Fichna et al.[15] found that patients with IBS-D have lower plasma levels of PEA, correlating with cramping pain, and patients with IBS-C have higher levels of endogenous cannabinoids combined with lower levels of FAAH. Russo et al.[16] reported that PEA has been well-established as an effective anti-inflammatory, analgesic in inflammatory bowel disease (IBD), and their work in animal models showed a reduction in inflammation and pain in IBD pain animal models. Depending on the type and presentation, a

PEA agonist and/or antagonist may prove to be an effective treatment option for patients with IBS and IBD.

A study performed by Cremon et al.[17] investigated the analgesic properties of a PEA/polydatin (200 mg/20 mg) combination and its effect on patients with IBS. This was a pilot, phase IIb, randomized, double-blind, placebo-controlled, parallel-arm, multicenter trial that lasted for 12 weeks and included 54 patients. Irritable bowel syndrome can lead to alteration of the intestinal mucosal barrier that allows for the passage of immune mediators, including the recruitment of mast cells and their activation. This study reported the effects of the PEA/polydatin combination on mast cell count, mast cell/immune cell activation, and the effect of treatment on immune activation, the effect of treatment on the endocannabinoid system, and the effect of treatment on digestive symptoms associated with IBS. Based on tissue samples taken from the colon, those with IBS had a higher area occupied by mast cells than the tissue samples from healthy patients. The researchers found that the treatment and placebo groups did not have statistically significant differences in the area taken up by mast cells. Immune factor parameters did not differ significantly between the healthy patients and those with IBS, and there was no significant difference between the placebo and treatment groups over time. The researchers did observe a decrease in the severity of abdominal pain and discomfort over time with the treatment group compared to the placebo. They showed that 62.1% of the patients on the PEA/polydatin treatment responded versus 40% in the placebo group. Other symptoms of IBS, including bloating severity and frequency, bowel habits, and dyspeptic and gastro-esophageal reflux symptoms, were found to be unaffected by the interaction between treatment and duration of treatment. The lack of effect seen on the endocannabinoid receptors and endocannabinoid-like mediators suggests that, with respect to IBS, PEA acts through a different pathway to exert its effects. This study suggested that PEA/polydatin was markedly effective in reducing the severity of abdominal pain and discomfort in IBS, and that it may act through an alternate pathway besides the endocannabinoid system. This study set a path for further study on this supplement and its use in the treatment of IBS symptoms.

PARKINSON DISEASE, ALZHEIMER DISEASE, AND BRAIN ISCHEMIA

The disabling motor disturbances seen in Parkinson disease (PD) are a result of the neurodegeneration of dopaminergic nigrostriatal neurons. The cause of this neurodegeneration is thought to be related to the activation of glial cells leading to inflammation. In an animal model by Esposito et al.,[18] MPTP was administered to mice to induce PD, followed 24 hours later by the administration of PEA. Treatment with PEA resulted in reduced glial cell activation and reversed the MPTP-associated motor deficits. Palmitoylethanolamine-induced neuroprotection was observed to be partially dependent on PPAR-α as evidenced by the MPTP toxicity in PPAR-α null mice. Brotini et al.[19] showed that the use of an ultra-micronized form of PEA in addition to conventional levodopa therapy significantly improved motor and non-motor symptoms in PD patients. This poses a possible new therapeutic approach for patients with Parkinson disease as well as other neurodegenerative diseases caused by glial cell-activated inflammation.

Alzheimer disease (AD) is characterized by beta amyloid plaques, gliosis, and tau protein hyperphosphorylation leading to cognitive deficits in those affected. In an animal study by Scuderi et al.,[20] beta amyloid was administered to the hippocampus of rats followed by PEA and the PPAR-α antagonist GW6471. The investigators found that PEA administration was correlated with a reduction in amnestic and cognitive deficits in the AD model rats. These results show a possible therapeutic option for AD patients for the improvement in cognitive deficits as well as disease progression.

Brain ischemia can result from a variety of disease states including trauma, hypoxia, toxicity, cytokines, etc. Mast cells are the human body's defense against pathogens as well as inflammation. In brain ischemia, mast cells relocate to the site of damage and degranulate, causing the release of inflammatory mediators. Parrella et al.[21] found that PEA, in addition to the flavonoid luteolin, exerts a mast cell modulatory effect in the context of brain ischemia cellular models. The addition of

PEA-luteolin prevented the degranulation of mast cells in response to oxygen and glucose deprivation and provided a direct synergistic neuroprotective effect. This research provides a basis for the potential use of PEA in the treatment and management of brain ischemia.

TRAUMATIC BRAIN INJURY AND SPINAL CORD INJURY

Traumatic brain injury (TBI) has a high mortality rate and is associated with behavioral dysfunction, chronic pain syndromes, anxiety, memory, and/or learning deficits. Palmitoylethanolamide was investigated in a mouse model of TBI, where mice exhibited anxiety, aggressiveness, and reckless behavior.[22] Depressive behavior also impaired the social interactions of the mice with TBI. Guida et al.[22] showed that the altered behavior was associated with changes in IL-1β expression, as well as changes in neuronal firing in the cortices of these mice. Administration of PEA restored the behavioral, biochemical, and functional changes in the TBI mice compared to placebo.

Another approach to combating neuroinflammation is by inhibiting NAAA responsible for metabolizing PEA. Impellizzeri et al.[23] investigated the use of the oxazoline derivative of PEA (PEA-OXA) as an inhibitor of NAAA. Mice with spinal and traumatic brain injuries were treated with PEA-OXA showing reduced histological alterations, behavioral deficits, and improved motor function. The investigators also observed a reduction in glial cell activation, NF-κB, COX-2, TNF-α, inducible NO synthase, and IL-1β. It appears that inhibiting the metabolism of endogenous PEA could be an effective therapeutic choice for patients with TBI and spinal cord injuries.

A large percentage of individuals with a spinal cord injury (SCI) also experience neuropathic pain and spasticity. Andresen et al.[24] conducted a randomized, double-blind, placebo-controlled, parallel, multicenter clinical trial investigating the effects of sublingual ultra-micronized PEA (um-PEA) as an adjunct treatment for neuropathic pain in this patient population. The strength of um-PEA used was 600 mg sublingually twice daily for 12 weeks. Seventy-three patients participated in this study and were responsible for keeping a daily pain diary that documented average pain, spasticity, sleep disturbances, and use of rescue medication for pain. The primary outcome of this study was to observe the average change in pain from baseline to the last week of treatment using the Numerical Rating Scale. In order to be included in this study, patients had to be older than 18 years of age with an SCI that was older than 6 months and experiencing neuropathic pain for more than 3 months. After the treatment period, the researchers found that the um-PEA as an adjunct therapy failed to make improvements in neuropathic pain. Additionally, there was no effect on spasticity or other secondary outcomes (i.e., sleep disturbances, muscle stiffness intensity, use of rescue medication). Seven of the patients in this study reported adverse events, including a urinary tract infection, paralytic ileus, cholecystolithiasis, and erysipelas. Study results indicated that the patients using the um-PEA did show a statistically significant decline in the use of rescue medication compared to the placebo group. Limitations of this study include incorrect dosing (a higher dose may have been required to show effects), and limited pharmacokinetic data highlighting um-PEA's ability to penetrate into the cerebrospinal fluid. Additionally, the variation in concomitant medication use among the study population varied, which could have affected the effectiveness of the um-PEA. This was the first trial of its kind investigating um-PEA as an adjunct therapy in central pain. Further study with a larger sample size and a more homogenous study population should be conducted in order to draw a more substantial conclusion regarding um-PEA's efficacy in neuropathic pain in SCI patients.

GLAUCOMA, DIABETIC RETINOPATHY, AND DIABETIC NEUROPATHY

Glaucoma is the second most common cause of blindness, and diabetic retinopathy is the most common microvascular complication in diabetes. Both ophthalmic disorders share a common pathology: inflammation. Hesselink et al.[25] report that PEA levels are often decreased in the eyes of patients who have glaucoma. Multiple studies comparing PEA to standard treatment or placebo showed a significant decrease in intraocular pressure, the major risk factor for the development of glaucoma.[25]

Costagliola et al.[26] performed an open-label 6-month study on the effects of PEA on visual field damage progression in patients with normal tension glaucoma (NTG). This is a form of glaucoma that is characterized by optic nerve damage and vision loss despite normal intra-ocular pressure levels. Thirty-two patients were split equally between a treatment group with PEA and a control group that received no treatment. All of the patients who participated in the study had been treated with once-daily latanoprost for at least 3 months. The participants in the treatment group were instructed to take one tablet after breakfast and dinner for 6 months. Best corrected visual acuity (BCVA), intraocular pressure (IOP) with the patient in a sitting position, central corneal thickness, and blood pressure were measured at baseline. The researchers reported that IOP dropped from a mean value of 14.4 to 11.1 in patients treated with PEA. There were no statistically significant changes in the BCVA. The mean deviation and pattern standard deviation visual field parameters diminished in the PEA group compared to the control. The findings of this study show that PEA can be helpful in reducing IOP and recovering mean deviation and pattern standard deviation in glaucoma patients suffering from normal tension glaucoma.

Diabetes is starting to become accepted as an inflammatory disease. This is supported by the elevation of inflammatory markers in diabetic patients, such as C-reactive protein (CRP), IL-6, and TNFα. Hyperglycemia associated with diabetes can lead to increased production of inflammatory markers from the Müller cells. Müller cells are the major source of inflammatory cytokines in the retina, but microglia and astrocytes also seem to have a role in the immune response to advanced glycation end products.[25] Palmitoylethanolamide has an inhibitory effect on inflammatory cytokines as well as toll-like receptors (TLR). In patients with diabetes, TLR-4 is upregulated, resulting in damage due to reactive oxygen species and inflammation. It appears that PEA may have a place in the prevention and treatment of both glaucoma and diabetic retinopathy.

Patients with chronic diabetes often experience diabetic neuropathy characterized by hyperalgesia and allodynia that can result in decreased quality of life. In an open-label study investigating micronized PEA in diabetic neuropathy, 300 mg of PEA-micronized (Normast) twice daily significantly reduced pain severity and related symptoms.[25] Thirty patients suffering from diabetic neuropathic pain were included in this study. All patients in the trial had been previously diagnosed with type II diabetes. The researchers assessed the symptoms of the study participants using the Michigan Neuropathy Screening Instrument (MNSI); the total symptom score (TSS) was used to assess the intensity and frequency of symptoms (i.e., burning, paresthesia, numbness/lack of sensitivity). The researchers also used the Neuropathic Pain Symptom Inventory (NPSI) to assess the diverse manifestations of neuropathic pain (i.e., paresthesia/dysesthesia, burning pain, deep pain, paroxysmal pain, evoked pain). Evaluations were performed at baseline, 30 days, 60 days, and 90 days. The researchers showed that MNSI, TSS, and NPSI test scores decreased significantly over the course of the 60-day treatment period. The TSS specifically showed improvement in all four symptom areas over the course of the 60-day study. The same trend was seen with the NPSI scores in all the subcategories listed above. There were no reports of adverse effects from the PEA. The limitations of this study include an open-label trial design and the small sample size. The researchers noted that this study demonstrating efficacy of PEA warrants further placebo-controlled trials with PEA and neuropathic pain.[27]

Another study was done on 27 human subjects to assess the short-term efficacy of PEA on uncontrolled neuropathic pain in patients with diabetes or traumatic chronic neuropathic pain. All of the study participants had been taking pregabalin, or gabapentin/tramadol, but failed to achieve pain relief. The VAS (range 2–10), NPSI, and the health questionnaire five dimension for quality of life (EQ-5D) were used to assess the effectiveness of PEA in the study participants. Ultra-micronized PEA was administered at 1200 mg/day sublingually for 10 days and then as a tablet between the 10th and 40th day of the study. Patients continued concomitant therapy for pain during the study. At 10 days patients were evaluated using only the VAS. Researchers reported that patients showed an improvement in pain score reduction from a mean score of 8.20 to 6.40. At the end of the study this score further decreased to 5.80. The overall NPSI score decreased from 5.2 to 3.8 and the EQ-5D score increased from –0.30 to 0.5, indicating a higher quality of life based on the parameters tested in the questionnaire. The researchers concluded that PEA may be an efficacious add-on therapy for the management of peripheral neuropathic pain.[28]

These studies show a possible therapeutic benefit of PEA in diabetic neuropathy as either adjunct therapy or monotherapy.

INFLUENZA AND COMMON COLD

Many early studies investigating the prophylaxis and treatment of influenza and common cold infections explored the link between the consumption of eggs and improved outcomes. We now know that PEA is abundant in egg yolks, and the anti-inflammatory and immune-modulating effects seen in these studies were most likely due to the ingestion of PEA. Several studies in the 1960s and 1970s explored the use of PEA as a prophylaxis and treatment of influenza and the common cold. The results of these trials showed that patients treated with PEA had fewer episodes of fever, headache, sore throat, and incidence of disease compared to placebo.[6] Given that there is still no absolute treatment for the common cold and the varied successes of recent influenza vaccines, PEA provides a valid option for treatment and prevention.

CONCLUSION

Palmitoylethanolamide appears to have many applications in inflammatory and immune-modulatory diseases. The profound effects on PPAR-α, NF-κB, inflammatory cytokines, COX, and substance P mast cell activation support the use of PEA in the treatment of pain, neurodegenerative diseases, neural injury, ophthalmic disorders, and viral infections, among a multitude of other diseases. With such a phenomenal safety profile as well as no documented drug or disease interactions, it is a wonder that PEA is not utilized more often.

REFERENCES

1. Skaper S.D., Facci L., Barbierato M. et al. *N*-palmitoylethanolamine and neuroinflammation: a novel therapeutic strategy of resolution. *Mol Neurobiol* 2015;52(2):1034–1042. doi:10.1007/s12035-015-9253-8.
2. Lambert D.M., Vandevoorde S., Jonsson K., Fowler C.J. The palmitoylethanolamide family: a new class of anti-inflammatory agents? *Curr Med Chem* 2002;9(6):663–674.
3. Alhouayek M., Muccioli G.G. Harnessing the anti-inflammatory potential of palmitoylethanolamide. *Drug Discov Today* 2014;19(10):1632–1639. doi:10.1016/j.drudis.2014.06.007.
4. Keppel Hesselink J.M., Kopsky D.J., Witkamp R.F. Palmitoylethanolamide (PEA)-'promiscuous' anti-inflammatory and analgesic molecule at the interface between nutrition and pharma. *PharmaNutrition* 2014;2(1):19–25. doi:10.1016/j.phanu.2013.11.127.
5. Keppel Hesselink J.M., Hekker T.A.M. Therapeutic utility of palmitoylethanolamide in the treatment of neuropathic pain associated with various pathological conditions: a case series. *J Pain Res* 2012;5:437–442. doi:10.2147/JPR.S32143.
6. Keppel Hesselink J.M.K., de Boer T., Witkamp R.F. Palmitoylethanolamide: a natural body-own anti-inflammatory agent, effective and safe against influenza and common cold. *Int J Inflam* 2013;2013:1–8. doi:10.1155/2013/151028.
7. Mannelli L.D.C., D'Agostino G., Pacini A. et al. Palmitoylethanolamide is a disease-modifying agent in peripheral neuropathy: pain relief and neuroprotection share a PPAR-alpha-mediated mechanism. *Mediators Inflam* 2013;2013:1–12. doi:10.1155/2013/328797.
8. Sasso O., Russo R., Vitiello S. et al. Implication of allopregnanolone in the antinociceptive effect of *N*-palmitoylethanolamide in acute or persistent pain. *Pain* 2012;153(1):33–41. doi:10.1016/j.pain.2011.08.010.
9. Gatti A., Lazzari M., Gianfelice V., Di Paolo A., Fabrizio Sabato A., Sabato A.F. Palmitoylethanolamide in the treatment of chronic pain caused by different etiopethogenesis. *Pain Med* 2012;13(9):1121–1130. doi:10.1111/j.1526-4637.2012.01432.x.

10. Keppel Hesselink J.M. Effectiveness of the association micronized N-palitoylethamolamine (PEA)-tranpolydatin in the treatment of chronic pelvic pain. *Eur J Obstet Gynecol Reprod Biol* 2011;159(2):488–489. doi:10.1016/j.ejogrb.2011.06.005.

11. Tartaglia E., Armentano M., Giugliano B. et al. Effectiveness of the association *N*-palmitoylethanolamine and transpolydatin in the treatment of primary dysmenorrhea. *J Ped Adolesc Gynecol* 2015;28(6):447–450. doi:10.1016/j.jpag.2014.12.011.

12. Cobellis L., Castaldi M.A., Giordano V. et al. Effectiveness of the association micronized *N*-Palmitoylethanoleamine (PEA) – transpolydatin in the treatment of chronic pain related to endometriosis after laproscopic assessment: a pilot study. *Eur J Obstet Gynecol Reprod Biolo* 2011;158(1):82–86. doi:10.1016/j.ejogrb.2011.04.011.

13. Giugliano E., Cagnazzo E., Soave I., Lo Monte G., Wenger J.M., Marci R. The adjuvant use of N-palmitoylethanolamine and transpolydatin in the treatment of endometriotic pain. *Eur J Obstet Gynecol Reprod Biolo* 2013;168(2):209–213. doi:10.1016/j.ejogrb.2013.01.009.

14. Del Giorno R., Skaper S., Paladini A., Varrassi G., Coaccioli S. Palmitoylethanolamide in fibromyalgia: results from prospective and retrospective observational studies. *Pain Ther* 2015;4(2):169–178. doi:10.1007/s40122-015-0038-6.

15. Fichna J., Wood J.T., Papanastasiou M. et al. Endocannabinoid and cannabinoid-like fatty acid amide levels correlate with pain-related symptoms in patients with IBS-D and IBS-C: a pilot study. *PLOS ONE* 2013;8(12):1–8. doi:10.1371/journal.pone.0085073.

16. Russo R., Cristiano C., Avagliano C. et al. Gut-brain axis: role of lipids in the regulation of inflammation, pain and CNS diseases. *Curr Med Chem* 2018;25(32):3930–3952. doi:10.2174/09298673246661702 16113756.

17. Cremon C., Stanghellini V., Barbaro M.R. et al. Randomised clinical trial: the analgesic properties of dietary supplementation with palmitoylethanolamide and polydatin in irritable bowel syndrome. *Aliment Pharmacol Ther* 2017;45(7):909–922. doi:10.1111/apt.13958.

18. Esposito E., Impellizzeri D., Mazzon E. , Paterniti I., Cuzzocrea S. Neuroprotective activities of palmitoylethanolamide in an animal model of Parkinson's disease. *PLOS ONE* 2012;7(8):1–14. doi:10.1371/journal.pone.0041880.

19. Brotini S., Schievano C., Guidi L. Ultra-micronized palmitoylethanolamide: an efficacious adjuvant therapy for Parkinson's disease. *CNS Neurol Disord Drug Targets* 2017;16(6):705–713. doi:10.2174/187 1527316666170321124949.

20. Scuderi C., Stecca C., Valenza M. et al. Palmitoylethanolamide controls reactive gliosis and exerts neuroprotective functions in a rat model of Alzheimer's disease. *Cell Death Dis* 2014;5:e1419. doi:10.1038/cddis.2014.376.

21. Parrella E., Porrini V., Iorio R. et al. PEA and luteolin synergistically reduce mast cell-mediated toxicity and elicit neuroprotection in cell-based models of brain ischemia. *Brain Res* 2016;1648(A):409–417. doi:10.1016/j.brainres.2016.07.014.

22. Guida F., Boccella S., Iannotta M. et al. Palitoylethanolamide reduces neuropsychiatric behaviors by restoring cortical electrophysiological activity in a mouse model of mild traumatic brain injury. *Front Pharmacol* 2017;8(95):1–14. doi:10.3389/fphar.2017.00095.

23. Impellizzeri D., Cordaro M., Bruschetta G. et al. *N*-palmitoylethanolamine-oxazoline as a new therapeutic strategy to control neuroinflammation: neuroprotective effects in experimental models of spinal cord and brain injury. *J Neurotrauma* 2017;34(18):2609–2623. doi:10.1089/neu.2016.4808.

24. Andresen S.R., Bing J., Hansen R.M. et al. Ultramicronized palmitoylethanolamide in spinal cord injury neuropathic pain: a randomized, double-blind, placebo-controlled trial. *Pain* 2016;157(9):2097–2103. doi:10.1097/j.pain.0000000000000623.

25. Keppel Hesselink J.M., Costagliola C., Fakhry J., Kopsky D.J. Palmitoylethanolamide, a natural retinoprotectant: its putative relevance for the treatment of glaucoma and diabetic retinopathy. *J Ophthalmol* 2015;2015:1–9. doi:10.1155/2015/430596.

26. Costagliola C., Romano M.R., dell'Omo R., Russo A., Mastropasqua R., Semeraro F. Effect of palmitoylethanolamide on visual field damage progression in normal tension glaucoma patients: results of an open-label six-month follow-up. *J Medl Food* 2014;17(9):949–954. doi:10.1089/jmf.2013.0165.

27. Schifilliti C., Cucinotta L., Fedele V., Ingegnosi C.,Luca S., Leotta C. Micronized palmitoylethanolamide reduces the symptoms of neuropathic pain in diabetic patients. *Pain Res Treat* 2014:1–5. doi:10.1155/2014/849623.

28. Cocito D., Peci E., Ciaramitaro P., Merola A., Lopiano L. Short-term efficacy of ultramicronized palmitoylethnaolamide in peripheral neuropathic pain. *Pain Res Treat* 2014;2014:1–4. doi:10.1155/2014/854560.

21 Lifestyle and Its Relationship to Pain

Hal S. Blatman

CONTENTS

INTRODUCTION

Lifestyle is expressed in the behavior patterns of individuals and groups. It encompasses opinions, values, interests, and goals, as well as particular activities. A good part of patient care involves lifestyle coaching for improvement in health issues. While many practitioners realize the importance of life practices, the time constraints of medical practice and personal conviction are likely to affect their efforts in persuading patients toward change. With the surge of trained health coaches, more emphasis is being given to helping patients make lifestyle changes that can result in decreased pain.

There are many aspects of lifestyle that affect pain, and it is not possible here to be totally inclusive in the specifics. A thorough discussion would at least have to include:

- Sleep
- Diet
- Smoking
- Exercise
- Recreation
- Stress
- Work/occupation
- Body work

It is easy to agree that each of these will have some effect on a person's experience of pain. In 30 years of practice and teaching, it has become evident that some of this list is more important and should be described here and emphasized in practice. A discussion of partial credit is also warranted, because some issues of pain, at least from dietary exposure, seem to be more absolute than expected.

Years of practice have also shown me some techniques of persuasion that have resulted in wonderful and rewarding changes in the lives of many of my patients. Where this sharing may add to the efficacy of a reader's communication skills, it is also meant to trigger a response and collaboration among students.

WHAT MATTERS MOST?

With the myriad of things on the list during any patient encounter, how do you decide what to discuss? And after the problem list, the patient's chief concerns, and the required monitoring of medication, there may be little time for anything else. In the limited time remaining, how do you decide which issues are most important, and of those, which are possible or perhaps easiest for the patient to discuss and understand? Healing and reducing pain have a specific hit list in lifestyle behaviors that can be promoting or detrimental. Our biology is very good at healing, but chronic pain and dysfunction follow from some degree of failure in the recovery system. The basics of requirements for healing on one side include the avoidance of activities that hamper healing, and on the other providing the resources needed for biologic restoration.

Coaching a patient to get out of the way of their body's efforts and ability to heal involves education and finding their keys to motivation. This can make the treatment of pain very personal, and much more so than procedures and prescription medication. Action steps can be taken to reduce inflammatory pain and also reduce the compromise of tissue oxygenation. These steps may lead to reduced pain in most chronic pain patients. Augmenting healing involves providing needed nutrients that facilitate the biochemistry of repair.

There are many lifestyle issues and changes from which to choose and propose to any particular patient. When it comes to reducing pain, diet and nutrition seem to matter most. Every practitioner has their own lifestyle bias in patient coaching and has to determine what is sensible and reasonable and tailor their specific patient recommendations. What is generally considered a sensible effort at change, however, is clearly not enough to effect the changes in inflammatory and healing biology for the average pain patient to realize the dramatic improvement that comes with absolute adherence. This becomes a question of *partial credit* and is discussed later. To add more confusion, some substances that are inflammatory and pain-inducing for one person may not affect another. Fortunately, there is a short list of substances that seem to be most universally important. For every patient, an understanding of which behavior patterns are most counterproductive, together with a feeling of general receptivity to change, allow more effective prioritization of discussion during an office visit. This may also help with making better referrals to those outside a practitioner's expertise.

In my experience patients are rarely exposed to the idea that food choices can make a tremendous difference in how much they suffer from pain. A pharmaceutical and procedure-based education and pain practice rarely give time for discussion about nutrition. Moreover, there is much conflicting education among the various practitioners who teach our patients. Evidence is accumulating that suggests dietary ingredients may modulate chronic pain through the modulation of inflammation and oxidative stress.[1] This may include inflammatory foods on the causative side as well as nutritional supplements on the treatment side.

Medical practice has taught me that there are a few things that make a more significant difference in clinical outcome than our training has led us to believe. Simply thinking that food has something to do with pain does not compare with the significance of knowing that these changes can reduce pain by more than 40%. The clinical efficacy of reducing pain by lifestyle changes is reliable, especially when pain is more severe, and the changes are more dramatic. Often the extent to which proposed changes matter is severely under appreciated.

While everyone knows that smoking is bad, its influence on healing and pain is underestimated. Elective surgeries and procedures are still performed on smokers when they are at a disadvantage for complications and healing issues. The consequences of smoking and inflammatory food are also grossly underappreciated. The inflammatory effect of starch (sugar) and hydrogenated oil is certainly enough to cause increased inflammation in injured fascia and thereby increased pain. A review by Frances Bell et al. further outlines and emphasizes how different foods can contribute to allodynia, hyperalgesia, and also pain relief.[2] While it is easy to suggest cutting down on French fries and white bread, very few practitioners feel confident to speak with the conviction necessary to propose that a single French fry can increase back pain for 2–4 days. In my vast clinical experience, I've consistently seen many such examples of how small amounts and even cross-contamination by inflammatory food induces dramatic exacerbations of pain.

In my opinion, the single most important lifestyle issues affecting pain involve food and nutrition. Even if the pathology is permanent and diet is all that can be changed, it is possible for more than 40% of most patients' chronic pain to disappear within 6 weeks of the last even minuscule exposure to a highly inflammatory constituent. With such relief as a strong possibility, many can be persuaded to *give it a try*. Most might see enough improvement to help them make the leap to correlating stricter change with even better results. On the other hand, make sure also to call attention to exacerbations of pain and look to correlate the ingestion of inflammatory food the day before onset. As inflammatory foods come out of the diet, relapse with a now unusual dose can bring on a significant increase in pain and stiffness as the inflamed fascia "glues" together. This may be especially identifiable in people with low back pain and headache.

In my experience, the smoking of tobacco should always be a priority of discussion. Next should be the understanding that a patient's first monetary resources should be spent on good food and clean water. Food has to be considered medicine if we are going to help patients heal from their old injuries and get off drugs.

The average person thinks little of *why* we eat. It is not about hunger or taste since these issues more help determine when and what we eat. The *why* requires some thought, and people will stop and reflect. Most people will readily agree that primary reasons for eating include:

- Providing fuel to burn for energy.
- Providing raw materials from which to build new and spare parts.

Where people can understand this about appliances and automobiles, they can make the connection to helping their body heal or continuing to watch it wear out more quickly than need be.

An example to understand quality of fuel parallels the level of octane in gasoline. For many cars the manufacturer advises 87 octane. High-performance automobiles however may require 93 octane and racing fuel may be higher than 100 octane. Help the patient compare the octane of their chosen food fuels with their level of pain and fatigue. It can be easy to see a relationship between energy level, fatigue, and high-sugar/low-octane fuels. Octane here refers to the level of nutrition, not the number of calories. Deteriorating health can also be correlated with a body *falling apart* from being maintained and built from *inferior* parts. Manufactured and prepared food may not carry the nutritive value of organically grown fresh food.

In considering change, many aspects of a person's life may be part of an office visit discussion. With regard to food changes, there may be barriers to progress that are insurmountable. Spousal and family support can be essential, as well as funding for more costly ingredients. Simple food changes may require significant preparation in addition to the involvement of family members and friends. What if the patient needs to be gluten-free and housemates do not understand cross-contamination? In some cases, it may even be necessary to change relationships. This level of coaching and support requires something different than what is provided by the average pain practice.

Through all of this, what a patient sees first and last is the behavior and lifestyle of the practitioner. A smoker cannot easily persuade a client to quit smoking except by getting sick and passing away. A can of soda on the desk will send a different message than a cup of tea or glass of clean water. Patients notice everything, and might be likely to ask: "what did you eat for breakfast doc?"

PARTIAL CREDIT

Throughout our lives we are taught the value of partial credit. From honorable mention to answering a question on a test, some credit is better than none. And certainly, there is a lot of good to be said for the concept. Cutting down from two packs to six cigarettes per day is a valuable lifestyle change. Eating less French fries, sugar, and white flour are healthy changes that require praise and reinforcement.

When it comes to pain, some lifestyle changes will result in the partial credit of feeling better. Feeling really good and getting out of pain require a different attitude and level of attention to detail. Partial credit with hammers is the example that being hit hard will hurt a lot more than being hit softly. With bees it can be agreed that 20 bee stings will likely hurt more than 1. But with regard to pain it is the immune system that has to settle, and if your system is sensitive to bees it only takes one to kill you. So, while there is likely to be some improvement in pain levels with appropriate dietary restriction, the best results may come from total abstinence from even the tiniest morsel of a particular substance for more than 4–6 weeks. Partially or almost gluten-free may be as meaningful as a little pregnant.

In this fashion, there are some foods and food products that often seem to require black and white abstinence for getting out of pain. For these items, the slightest amount can cause severe pain lasting for several weeks, and these likely need to be totally avoided. Classically trained physicians may initially think it extreme and unlikely for food triggers to be characterized in this fashion. Recall however the severity of reaction in someone sensitive to bee stings to the sting of even one bee. And then consider how many days or weeks it can take to settle immune sensitivity and allergy reactions. For certain people specific foods and even ingredients can upregulate the immune system and provoke the upregulation of inflammatory and pain-increasing mediators. In these circumstances, a trace of dairy can cause the onset of head and neck pain within hours, and a trace of gluten can cause the onset of lower back pain by the next morning. As I paid more attention to this in my practice, I began to realize these phenomena were much more widespread among my patients than I ever imagined. Indeed, it is a rare chronic pain patient who is not affected to this degree.

On the other hand, there are many foods that are necessary for providing important nutrients for healing and should be deliberately ingested. The patient who will not eat any vegetables and lives on fast food is at a disadvantage for healing. In considering food choices, and in addition to micro- and macronutrients, attention must also be given to the microbiome.[3] And while every patient is different, there is a general commonality and order for where to start that is applicable to most situations.

New information related to the microbiome and pain is even more impressive and further relates pain and food. While the microbiome has been related to digestive issues and visceral pain, there is new correlation to inflammatory pain, neuropathic pain, headache, and even opioid tolerance. Almost every one of my patients who radically decreases sugar, wheat, and potato notices a dramatic increase in the efficacy of their opiates. To go along with these experiences, we are learning more about mechanisms for the clinical observance of the relationship of inflammatory food to pain. One such discovery is that microbiota in the gut produce mediators that modulate and induce peripheral sensitization.[4] This relates food choices to allodynia.

A microbiome effect may also lead to a better understanding of the observation that it may not be enough to just be gluten-free. Many people have told me gluten-free provided no improvement until they were also sugar-, dairy-, and potato-free.

Becoming more important in our lives will be the awareness of the effects of long-term low-level exposures to toxic metals, pesticides, herbicides, and more. Low-level constant exposures may steadily increase body burden, and many of these substances have half-lives of many years. It is possible to test for levels of heavy metals and herbicides, and then treat to accelerate detoxification. One of the mechanisms of their adverse effects on our biology is an increase in oxidative stress. More and more it is being recognized that oxidative stress is a common denominator for many health issues.[5] These efforts at diagnosis and treatment can help patients with chronic pain and also fatigue.

EXAMPLE SIDE BAR

In a brief discussion, an acquaintance admitted he had experience with a low-carb diet, and had lost weight and felt great. I asked, and he revealed that of course it was past tense. I further asked why, and couldn't he stand feeling that good? His reply speaks volumes, in that it was about life-style and he wanted to eat the bread. It later occurred to me that this was not lifestyle at all. Among other things, lifestyle is about spending time with those who matter, participating in activities of recreation, and meditating in nature. Eating bread is more about disease style than lifestyle. What chronic illnesses is one signing up for, and what complications and health issues that otherwise might never happen are now more likely to occur sooner?

As I observed the painful and inflammatory consequences of bread flour on myself and my patients, I was still not convinced that these issues were important for those with no pain. That was until several years ago when I learned about zonulin proteins. Zonulin proteins are secreted by our own cells to enhance the absorption of needed nutrients across membrane barriers. Gluten inges-tion is associated with increased zonulin proteins, and thereby also associated with changes in the permeability characteristics of our intestinal barriers, lung barriers, and blood–brain barrier.[6] When a substance can compromise the integrity of a protective barrier, it should be recognized as univer-sally detrimental by a multitude of effects. This phenomenon seems to be universal to our species and therefore may make the ingestion of bread more disease style than lifestyle.

SMOKING AND TOBACCO

It is not disputed that smoking tobacco is harmful to health. Helping a person through this kind of lifestyle change can be challenging. Most patients know that smoking is not to their advantage, but comparatively few are successful in quitting. A significant success rate in effecting change occurs when coaching educates and brings people along, as opposed to trying to more impress them with the threat of severe and dire consequences. Helpful suggestions that provide a way out can be much more effective than reminders of cancer risk.

At some point in a patient's encounter must come the realization that there has been an injury that their body could not heal well enough for them to be living without the remnant of chronic pain. Sometimes it is a tendon injury, other times it might be a joint or spine injury. Explaining that the body has a very difficult time healing bone, ligament, and tendon with nicotine and tobacco exhaust in the blood may provide a different motivation for cutting down or quitting. Patients need to realize that providing opiate medication to make inflammation-producing behaviors more comfortable has quite gone out of style, since high levels of these medicines have been shown to be dangerous and even counterproductive.

Rather than discussing lung cancer, there is a different impact to discussing how cigarette smoke closes blood vessels and decreases blood supply to injured tissue.[7] And in the absence of nicotine, even a tobacco extract adversely affects healing.[8] There may be a more significant impact to hear-ing that one's tender and injured tendon or ligament cannot heal as well with nicotine in the blood than a discussion about lung cancer. At a later visit further discussion can include encouraging the patient to look up the health effects of cadmium poisoning, and later keep asking why they continue to sign up for this exposure.

In the meantime, it is imperative that the patient see decreasing smoking as easier and less threatening than expected. Suggesting the same old path they've tried before, or some therapy like acupuncture or hypnosis that requires a prohibitive expenditure does not help break down their difficult barriers to success. In considering the use of tobacco, I refer to three main addictions:

- Nicotine
- Social (purchase, friends, breaks, ritual of lighting, etc.)
- Chemicals in the tobacco smoke, planted by manufacturers to maintain addiction

Of these, the most significant is the addictive effect from what is added to the tobacco in process of making cigarettes.[9] This realization can have a profound effect on the psychology of quitting. Learning that the tobacco companies *deliberately did this to you* needs to come at the same time as providing an easy solution for getting out of this circle. All that one has to do to make this first change in behavior is to self-roll all cigarettes from organic or other pipe tobacco. Now without quitting or even the anxiety of setting a quit date, it is possible to detox from these chemicals over the next 2 months, and the most difficult next steps of cutting down are likely to be easier.

Encouraging change and providing a path and choice with little downside increases the likelihood of success. Admit that rolling requires effort and will taste different. Getting over these differences is important, and a certain amount of "sucking it up" will be necessary. Suggest that immediate cost savings could be better than 50% and why not check it out. At the next visit the not yet motivated person might be reminded about why they haven't yet looked into saving all that money. Also suggest shopping carefully for a cigarette rolling machine. The process of self-rolling needs to be as easy as possible, and available devices have different degrees of difficulty for deployment. With this philosophy of discussion, you are now on your patient's side against a problem with which they have struggled for perhaps many years. The balance of motivation and fear just needs a little tilting, and making it easier to change encourages people to flex their power of self-control.

Another and gentler step toward quitting is to only smoke cigarettes out of doors. Just this step may decrease exposure by more than 75% without even changing the number of cigarettes smoked. Smoking inside a closed environment dramatically increases toxic exposures to many chemicals.[10] For patients who live with smokers, this can be a therapeutically powerful negotiation in gaining health and self-respect.

Suggest not smoking in the car, especially on the way to their office visit. No one in your office needs to be exposed to the high level of toxicity that comes off the clothes of someone who was just in a smoke-filled closed space. Perhaps set a day aside for "stinky people" delegated to patients who are the worst offenders of your office environment. You might also start leaving the worst offenders in the exam room with a HEPA filter for 30–40 minutes before going in to see them. Making their disrespecting behavior inconvenience them can reduce your exposure *and* provide motivation for change, especially if someone else drove them.

A good next step is the progression to vaporizer technology that avoids fire and resultant cadmium exposure while maintaining the social structure of the habit. Odor disappears, toxicity of clothing decreases, and possibilities for quitting concomitantly increase. Suggesting using vaporizer technology indoors and all fire and flame outside can be a helpful step, especially for situations where other family members smoke. While vaporizing is not without toxicity, chemical exposures for oneself and one's contacts are dramatically lower, and for many this step can be very helpful progress.[11]

Along with sharing the effect tobacco smoking has on healing, comes the practitioners' advice to delay elective surgery or elective dental work until enough changes can be made in these lifestyle parameters for an improved chance of success. People can understand not wanting to sign up for an elective procedure when conditions for healing are significantly compromised, especially when they can see good possibilities for lifestyle change. These surgeries may include elective dental work of tooth pulling and implants, joint fusions, tendon repair, and joint replacement surgery.

INFLAMMATORY FOOD AND PAIN

One of the most significant deficiencies in medical education is nutrition and the effect of food choices on inflammatory pain.[12] Dietary ingredients have been increasingly recognized to play a role in the balance of oxidative stress, inflammation, and resultant pain. Rondanelli et al. looked at 172 studies and proposed a food pyramid for subjects with chronic pain.[13] Recommendations take into account providing better raw materials for the body to utilize and limiting inflammatory triggers. There are recommendations to limit high-glycemic foods and also to ingest some nutritional supplements.

Clinical experience during the past 25 years has continued to demonstrate a list of foods and ingredients that aggravate chronic pain from all causes in most patients. While there are exceptions, they are rarer than ever suspected. Expectations for real improvement through experimentation of dietary elimination can really only come with total black and white adherence to avoidance of the particular substance.

These include:

- Wheat
- Most sugar
- Potato
- Fruit juice
- Fake fat and hydrogenated oil
- Artificial sweeteners

Each of these inflammatory and toxic instigators should be discussed with pain patients. Learning what each does and its effect on pain can provide powerful motivation for change. A big help for the practitioner working with skeptical patients are two widely sold books that motivate change and are relatively easy for many people to understand. These are *Wheat Belly* by William Davis and *Grain Brain* by David Perlmutter. Each provides an independent source of information with a consistent and important message for people in pain.

One common factor among the foods on this list is the induction of insulin and increase in visceral fat. Another is the increase in zonulin proteins that regulate intestinal permeability. This has been linked to inflammation, autoimmunity, and cancer.[14]

Wheat, especially that grown in the U.S., and bread flour have a unique and perhaps multifactorial influence on chronic pain. Clinically we consistently observe lower back pain, joint stiffness, and pain related to barometric change to be often dramatically increased by even a very small amount of flour. This effect seems independent of celiac disease.

Sucrose has been linked to many chronic illnesses. It also affects the intestinal microbiome. These changes may have far-reaching consequences in how people function and behave. Mice fed a simulated Western diet showed reduced cognitive flexibility.[15] Changing how patients respond and even think about pain and healing may be negatively influenced by their choices of food.

Sugar also increases the likelihood of intestinal overgrowth of yeast. One of the easiest to spot physical signs of yeast overgrowth is a coating on the tongue. In general, the thicker the coating, the worse the problem. The pictures in Figure 21.1 are the same man, before and 3 months after taking sugar out of his diet.

Sugar has also been shown to significantly augment the nociceptive properties of morphine in the rat.[16] Rats given sucrose exhibited augmented antinociceptive effects of morphine to the hot-plate test when heated to 51 and 53°C. This may help explain some of the observed clinical response to opiates. Where sugar potentiates opiate pain relief, the effect wears off in a couple of hours, perhaps leaving the person with only their opioid medicine "on board." To that effect, we hear our patients report that their pain medication only lasts 2 or 3 hours.

Sugar-sweetened beverages are known to have adverse effects on glucose and lipid metabolism, especially if consumed in high quantities and by overweight people. A study published in 2011

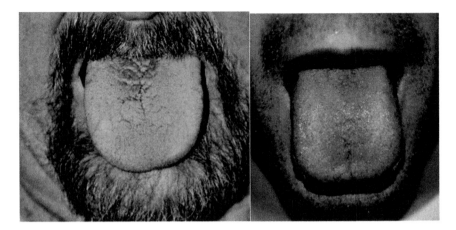

FIGURE 21.1   Tongue on left with white coating and brown stains; same tongue on right, 3 months after sugar-free diet.

studied the effect of these drinks on normal-weight subjects. The data showed elevated cardiac risk markers and hs-CRP after low to moderate consumption within just 3 weeks.[17]

Whether the mechanism relates to nociceptive properties or the induction of inflammation, our clinical experience is that opiates provide longer and more consistent relief when sugar and insulin-raising, or inflammatory foods are totally avoided.

The power of this in practice is that an office visit changes from negotiating for more opiate medication to a patient needing to learn what to do or not to do so that the medication you are willing to prescribe can work more to their satisfaction. To pull this off, it is best that the practitioner set an example, and is firm in their belief that this inflammatory food avoidance will be helpful.

Stevia is not an artificial sweetener and does not seem to instigate an insulin or inflammatory response and resultant or consequential pain. While it may prove to be one of the best alternatives for sweet taste, safety may be overestimated.

POTATO

Many of my patients have noted that white, red, and blue potatoes cause exacerbation of lower back pain starting the next day and lasting 2–4 days. There are glycoalkaloids in potato that increase intestinal permeability and aggravate inflammatory bowel disease.[18,19] Moreover, frying concentrates these glycoalkaloids and makes them even more dangerous.[20] The prevalence of irritable bowel disease is highest in countries where fried potato consumption is highest.[11] It is perhaps this relationship that helps define the origin of increased lower back pain with even a teaspoon of white potato.

Conversely, it is interesting to note that, when an ethanolic extract from potato tubers is administered orally to mice, there is evidence of decreased inflammation and pain.[21]

FRUIT JUICE

Fruit juice is on the inflammatory food list for the same reasons as sugar. Certainly, it can be argued that fruit juice is just natural sugar. In this fashion fruit juices have been promoted to be among the healthier drinks. Just as easily however, it can also be argued that much of the fruit's beneficial nutrition is removed in the juicing process. One study shows the average sugar content of a 100% fruit juice category was 10.7 g/100 ml.[22] A dental pH/plaque study investigated the potential cariogenicity of fruit juices. Testing orange and apple juice preparations with and without added sugar, it was demonstrated that all carried "substantial quantities of sugar" and were equally cariogenic.[23] While fruit juices contain some nutrition from the fruit, there are untoward effects like those from sucrose. In our clinical experience fruit juices contribute to the body-wide inflammatory issues that adversely affect pain. Regarding the exacerbation of chronic pain, a glass of orange juice may be no different than a can of soda.

HYDROGENATED OIL

Hydrogenation changes natural oils and makes them resistant to spoilage. It allows popular brands of peanut butter to be opened and not spoil or grow mold when stored in a cabinet at room temperature for long periods of time. Other effects flow through from fatty acid metabolism pathways, the incorporation of these materials into cell membranes, and other effects on metabolism. Perhaps the biologic antithesis of these substances is the effect of omega-3 polyunsaturated fatty acid supplementation. As the ingestion of hydrogenated fats may increase pain, omega-3 supplementation decreases inflammatory joint pain in rheumatoid arthritis, inflammatory bowel disease, and dysmenorrhea.[24] Patients can understand that if food won't grow mold, then it won't grow them either. While there are exceptions, this demonstrates a negative biologic effect of hydrogenated oil in food.

ARTIFICIAL SWEETENERS

Aspartame has been noted to increase pain symptoms and even simulate fibromyalgia and total body pain. More than 20 years ago I gave a presentation at a pain conference that prompted an attendee to write me a few months later to say that 2 months after no diet soda, her fibromyalgia pain was gone. Aspartame has been shown to have an effect on NMDA receptors, and perhaps from this line of research will come a better understanding of a relationship to pain.[25]

Perhaps the pain effect of aspartame is related to increased oxidative stress. Serum methanol concentrations are elevated after the ingestion of a single dose of aspartame,[26] and other measurements after aspartame administration demonstrate increased oxidative stress.[27] In addition, aspartame is linked to an increased formation of formaldehyde adducts.[28] When formaldehyde binds to DNA it forms formaldehyde–DNA adducts. This process may lead to inaccurate DNA replication and resultant mutations and cancerous tumors. One analysis indicated that aspartame is a multipotential carcinogenic agent, even at a daily dose of 20 mg/kg body weight, much less than current daily acceptable intake.[29] Aspartame has also been implicated in worsening depression in those with a history of mood disorders.[30]

Sucralose is derived from sucrose by substituting three atoms of chlorine for three hydrogen-oxygen groups of the sucrose molecule. A study in male rats demonstrated altered gut microflora and other effects after a 12-week exposure.[31] In 2006 there was a case report of sucralose causing migraine.[32]

Saccharin (ortho-sulfobenzoic acid imide) has also shown to alter intestinal bacteria and change the microbiome. A mice study reported in 2017 showed the induction of liver inflammation, perhaps associated with the perturbation of the gut microbiota.[33] Newer technology is allowing study of the microbiome and a relationship to pain conditions. One such relationship has been shown with chronic prostatitis and chronic pelvic pain syndrome.[34]

DRINKING WATER AND CHLORINATION BYPRODUCTS

The importance of clean water is not commonly discussed with the average pain patient. Our body is more than 70% water, and water is required for detoxification and the elimination of waste. It may be challenging enough to coach the elimination of soda and fruit juices from the diet, much less have a discussion of prescribed number of glasses of water/day. Fortunately, as we become more aware of the relationship between inflammatory pain and oxidative stress, it is convenient that water filters are more popular as well as easily and inexpensively available. Jiang-Hua Li et al. showed negative rat health effects from swimming training in chlorinated pools and hypothesized a relationship to increased metabolic stress, especially to the liver.[35] Chlorinated drinking water is also associated with bladder cancer, and consideration should also be given regarding exposure to the associated disinfection byproducts that include trihalomethanes.[36] Increased oxidative stress from toxic exposures would lead to decreased physical capacity, and arguably increased pain, especially in a patient whose symptoms are aggravated by physical activity.

STAGES OF LEARNING

Guiding patients starts with presumed credibility and them listening to you. The best goal is for the patient to learn to listen to their own body. Ultimately our body can be our best teacher if we can only hear the message. In learning the language, realize our body's job is to make us feel good all the time. When we are physically hurting, our body is telling us it does not like something we have done. Again, both my personal and clinical experience has led to the firm understanding that exacerbations of pain are rarely unprovoked. Most of the time, carefully questioning the patient will bring out the truth of these four rules:

1. Pain does not fall down from the sky.
2. If you wake up in the morning with pain you did not have the night before, and you did not fall out of a tree or out of bed overnight, the pain is inflammatory and comes from last night's dinner or after dinner food.
3. If you go to bed with pain you did not have in the morning and did not do anything big enough to make this pain, it most likely comes from breakfast or lunch.
4. If you feel more pain when the barometer changes, you have eaten something inflammatory to your body in the past 6 weeks.

With this information, exacerbations of pain become a joint search for the offending food or injury instead of a negotiation for increased medication. Now the office visit can turn into a teaching and learning experience.

Another consistency is the analogy that the body will not teach you 11th grade lessons until you graduate from 10th grade. So, you might not be able to feel a reaction to potato, perhaps, until you have learned to totally avoid bread flour. The reaction from flour may overpower the effect of potato. And you might not feel either if you are more affected by dairy or sugar.

Another consistency is that you will get smacked harder when the body thinks you should have already learned a particular lesson.

1. In 9th grade you learned that if you ate the whole pizza, you got sent to see the principal.
2. In 10th grade you learned that if you ate a piece of the pizza, you had to stay after school.
3. In 11th grade you learned that if you ate a bite of the pizza, you had detention for a week.
4. In 12th grade you learned that if you ate a crumb of the pizza, you were suspended.
5. First year of college you learned about cross-contamination…and…

And so on…

Teach your patients how and what to look for in the search: from where did the increased pain come?

1. Start with what is obvious and visible…bread, wheat, potato, soda, etc.
2. If nothing obvious, then check the ingredients on every label of whatever was opened and put into the food.
3. If nothing is noted, write down everything that can be remembered during the past 48–72 hours and put it in a drawer.
4. Go through this process every time there is unexplained pain and start to notice the common denominators.

EXERCISE

Exercise has been shown to be generally helpful for many issues from heart disease to cancer. There are also many studies showing various benefits for people in chronic pain. Hoffman and Hoffman in 2007 showed improvement in mood and perception of pain, and that exercise may also offer some protection from depression.[37] Smith and Grimmer-Somers reported a review of 15 studies and concluded in favor of the efficacy of exercise programs for chronic low back pain for up to 6 months after cessation of treatment.[38] Many patients will do better with regular exercise and varying intensity by having respect for physical tolerance and medical issues.

REST/SLEEP

Sleep and rest are of paramount importance in treating a person with chronic pain. There is a strong clinical relationship between pain symptoms and disordered sleep. This is true in both pain patients and healthy subjects. In addition, the effect goes both ways, in that pain may worsen sleep, and sleep deprivation increases pain. In summarizing this, Hajak proposed that psychotherapy needed to support both pain management and sleep.[39]

Numerous studies have shown the importance of treating sleep apnea for its co-morbidity with several conditions. Aytekin et al. investigated the presence of chronic widespread musculoskeletal pain in patients with obstructive sleep apnea and showed a 55.4% prevalence.[40]

Fortunately, there is a long list of possibly helpful treatment options for assisting pain patients who have difficulty falling asleep and staying asleep. These include herbal medicine, homeopathic remedies, sleep hygiene, investigation and treatment for apnea, not eating sugar in the evening, various medications, medical marijuana, CBD oil, and more. Evening food choices are not generally considered and probably should be. An insulin-raising snack at 9 pm may induce a hypoglycemic event several hours later with a resultant cortisol release causing awakening at about 3 am. Another common oversight involves the use of herbal agents as sleep aids. In general, they are not as potent as benzodiazepines but allow the maintenance of sleep architecture. Their strength is to mute an adrenalin response to stress and may be best taken at 5 pm and again at 10 pm for an 11 pm bedtime.

MEDITATION

Mindfulness meditation has also been studied for its effects on pain relief. This technique has long been utilized as part of integrative medicine pain treatment. A study in 2015 shows mindfulness meditation-related pain relief was associated with stimulation of the orbitofrontal, subgenual anterior cingulate, and anterior insular cortex of the brain.[41] The insular cortex is the focus of interoception, and greatly affects how a person "feels" and thinks about their pain.

Meditation can also help regenerate the distraction pathway and reduce perceived pain.[41] Daily exercise of these techniques can become part of a lifestyle.

BODY WORK

Body work can be considered as only important for specific therapy, and it can also be considered as a lifestyle. All kinds of touch and energy therapies are considered here under the heading of body work. In the 11-2018 issue of Townsend Letter, Blatman discusses a new paradigm for understanding pain and the sensations promoted by kinks in the fascia that compress unmyelinated nerve endings in the ropey bands and trigger points resultant from injury. In addition, many therapies have an effect on fascia as a common denominator. These include:

- Myofascial release
- Chiropractic

- Acupuncture
- Dry needling
- Myotherapy
- Alexander work
- Trigger point injection
- Massage therapy
- Osteopathic manipulation
- Healing touch
- Homeopathy
- And more…

Incorporating some of these on a regular basis can be part of a healthy and preventive lifestyle. It is easy to understand the importance of their incorporation into the lifestyle of those who suffer from chronic pain.

SUMMARY

Pain care has long been focused on helping the hopeless cope with an unfortunate situation. The assumption of intractability provides justification for ablative procedures and high doses of medication for the purpose of providing what is often not enough relief.

A different discussion centers healing and reducing inflammation as opposed to ablation procedures and medication. Successfully reducing inflammation has to start with food, or medication and procedure efficacy will be correspondingly limited.

Finding and healing the injuries of a lifetime that culminate to result in chronic pain require a focus on fascia. Many of these injuries are under the radar of the person in pain who is understandably much more aware of only their more severe injuries. It is the inflammation from food and environmental toxicity that *lights* their more severe and impactful injuries up like a *Christmas tree*. Increased pain from weather change (rain pain) is also due primarily to this inflammatory response to food that ignites the injuries of a lifetime.

When lifestyle changes decrease inflammation and toxicity, the *electricity* and *lights* get turned down, and the brain will ignore all but the most severe issues. As this happens, more pain will disappear than the patient ever thought possible—almost like it was never there.

In any person, there are many more tender areas than those associated with the predominant pain complaints. We are usually only aware of our most significant injuries and then only the ones causing pain at this moment. Patients do not need their injuries to be "all better," they only need to be 99% ignorable—all over their body.

All parts of life can be directed toward the goal of healing and becoming pain-free. Much like training for Olympic competition, the life of pain can be approached from many directions to effect change. Lifestyle choices can "make or break" the potential for successful treatment.

Medical studies often focus on changing only a few variables at a time. Successful integrative treatment often involves doing everything at once and not knowing which intervention makes the most difference. The body has to put itself back together. Limiting therapeutic directions and options is self-defeating, because any one sub-optimal link can prevent progress.

Encourage patient learning as a lifestyle. Teach and encourage reading and expanding on the basics of what can be given within the model of provided medical care. Starting the work of change often brings more change and also self-reinforcing development.

And lastly, consider *your* lifestyle. What example do you set for your patients and their healing? Do you enjoy your practice? What would it take for you to enjoy it more? I have found my pain practice to be fun and rewarding. Patients learn to take responsibility for how they feel, learn to do their own body work, stop smoking, and change their food. Then body work directed toward unkinking trigger points, fascia healing, and regenerative medicine can provide up to 90% relief for many of our patients in chronic pain. Almost none ever again opt for epidural steroids, radiofrequency ablation, or high-dose medication.

For many of us, job satisfaction is related to knowing we made a difference in people's lives. When you influence people to make lifestyle changes for their health and watch their pain go away, your influence is self-reinforcing and most people will continue the growth you started. This will bring you joy at night, excitement in the morning for your day, and professional satisfaction.

REFERENCES

1. Rondanelli M. et al., Food pyramid for subjects with chronic pain: foods and dietary constituents as anti-inflammatory and antioxidant agents. *Nutrition Research Reviews* **31**(1):131–151 (2018).
2. Bell, R.F., Borzan, J., Kalso, E. & Simonnet, G. Food, pain, and drugs: does it matter what pain patients eat? *Pain* **153**(10), 1993–1996 (2012).
3. Tick, H. Nutrition and pain. *Physical Medicine and Rehabilitation Clinics* **26**(2):309–320 (2015).
4. Guo, R., Chen, L.-H., Xing, C. & Liu, T. Pain regulation by gut microbiota: molecular mechanisms and therapeutic potential. *British Journal of Anaesthesia* **123**(5), 637–654 (2019).
5. Marchev, A.S. et al. Oxidative stress and chronic inflammation in osteoarthritis: can NRF2 counteract these partners in crime? *Annals of the New York Academy of Sciences* **1401**(1), 114–135 (2017).
6. Rittirsch, D. et al. Zonulin as prehaptoglobin2 regulates lung permeability and activates the complement system. *American Journal of Physiology Lung Cellular Molecular Physiology* **304**, L863–L872 (2013).
7. Silverstein, P. Smoking and wound healing. *The American Journal of Medicine* **93**(1A), S22–S24 (1992).
8. Skott, M. et al. Tobacco extract but not nicotine impairs the mechanical strength of fracture healing in rats. *Journal of Orthopaedic Research* **24**(7), 1472–1479 (2006).
9. Gonseth, S. & Cornuz, J. Chemicals added to cigarettes and their effects on tobacco dependence. *Revue Médicale Suisse* **5**(210), 1468–1471 (2009).
10. Licht, A.S., Hyland, A., Travers, M.J. & Chapman, S. Secondhand smoke exposure levels in outdoor hospitality venues: a qualitative and quantitative review of the research literature. *Tobacco Control* **22**(3), 172–179 (2013).
11. Jensen, R.P., Luo, W., Pankow, J.F., Strongin, R. & Peyton, D.H.M. Hidden formaldehyde in e-cigarette aerosols. *The New England Journal of Medicine* **372**(4), 392–394 (2015).
12. Mogre, V., Stevens F.C.J., Aryee P.A., Amalba A., Scherpbier A.J.J.A. Why nutrition education is inadequate in the medical curriculum: a qualitative study of students' perspectives on barriers and strategies. *BMC Med Educ.* **18**(1),26 (2018).
13. Rondanelli, M. et al. Food pyramid for subjects with chronic pain: foods and dietary constituents as anti-inflammatory and antioxidant agents. *Nutrition Research Reviews* **31**(1), 1–21 (2018). doi:10.1017/S0954422417000270.
14. Fasano, A. Zonulin and its regulation of intestinal barrier function: the biological door to inflammation, autoimmunity, and cancer. *Physiological Reviews* **91**(1), 151–175 (2011).
15. Magnusson, K.R. et al. Relationships between diet-related changes in the gut microbiome and cognitive flexibility. *Neuroscience* **300**, 128–140 (2015).
16. Kanarek, R.B. & Homoleski, B. Modulation of morphine-induced antinociception by palatable solutions in male and female rats. *Pharmacology Biochemistry and Behavior* **66**(3), 653–659 (2000).
17. Aeberli, I. et al. Low to moderate sugar-sweetened beverage consumption impairs glucose and lipid metabolism and promotes inflammation in healthy young men: a randomized controlled trial. *The American Journal of Clinical Nutrition* **94**(2), 479–485 (2011).
18. Iablokov, V. et al. Naturally occurring glycoalkaloids in potatoes aggravate intestinal inflammation in two mouse models of inflammatory bowel disease. *Digestive Diseases and Sciences* **55**(11), 3078–3085 (2010).
19. Patel, B. et al. Potato glycoalkaloids adversely affect intestinal permeability and aggravate inflammatory bowel disease. *Inflammatory Bowel Diseases* **8**(5), 340 (2002).
20. Tajner-Czopek, A., Rytel, E., Kita, A., Pęksa, A. & Hamouz, K. The influence of thermal process of coloured potatoes on the content of glycoalkaloids in the potato products. *Food Chemistry* **133**(4), 1117–1122 (2012).
21. Choi, E. & Koo, S. Anti-nociceptive and anti-inflammatory effects of the ethanolic extract of potato (Solanum tuberlosum). *Food and Agricultural Immunology* **16**(1), 29–39 (2010).
22. Boulton, J. et al. OP52 how much sugar is hidden in drinks marketed to children? *Journal of Epidemiology and Community Health* **69**(Suppl 1), A31–A32 (2015).

23. Mahajan, N. et al. Effect of commonly consumed sugar containing and sugar free fruit drinks on the hydrogen ion modulation of human dental plaque. *Journal of Indian Society of Pedodontics and Preventive Dentistry* **32**(1), 26–32 (2014).

24. Goldberg, R.J. & Katz, J. A meta-analysis of the analgesic effects of omega-3 polyunsaturated fatty acid supplementation for inflammatory joint pain. *Pain* **129**(1–2), 210–223 (2007).

25. Pan-Hou, H., Suda, Y., Ohe, Y., Sumi, M. & Yoshioka, M. Effect of aspartame on N-methyl-d-aspartate-sensitive l-[3H]glutamate binding sites in rat brain synaptic membranes. *Brain Research* **520**(1–2), 351–353 (1990).

26. Davoli, E., Cappellini, L., Airoldi, L. & Fanelli, R. Serum methanol concentrations in rats and in men after a single dose of aspartame. *Food and Chemical Toxicology* **24**(3), 187–189 (1986).

27. Choudhary, A. & Devi, R. Serum biochemical responses under oxidative stress of aspartame in wistar albino rats. *Asian Pacific Journal of Tropical Disease* **4**, S403–S410 (2014).

28. Trocho, C. et al. Formaldehyde derived from dietary aspartame binds to tissue components in vivo. *Life Sciences* **63**(5), 337–349 (1998).

29. Soffritti, M. et al. First experimental demonstration of the multipotential carcinogenic effects of aspartame administered in the feed to Sprague-dawley rats. *Environmental Health Perspectives* **114**(3), 379–385 (2006).

30. Walton, R.G., Hudak, R. & Green-Waite, R.J. Adverse reactions to aspartame: double-blind challenge in patients from a vulnerable population. *Biological Psychiatry* **34**(1–2), 13–17 (1993).

31. Abou-Donia, M.B., El-Masry, E.M., Abdel-Rahman, A.A., McLendon, R.E. & Schiffman, S.S. Splenda alters gut microflora and increases intestinal P-glycoprotein and cytochrome P-450 in male rats. *Journal of Toxicology and Environmental Health, Part A* **71**(21), 1415–1429 (2008).

32. Bigal, M.E. & Krymchantowski, A.V. Migraine triggered by sucralose—A case report. *Headache: The Journal of Head and Face Pain* **46**(3), 515–517 (2006).

33. Bian, X. et al. Saccharin induced liver inflammation in mice by altering the gut microbiota and its metabolic functions. *Food and Chemical Toxicology* **107**(B), 530–539 (2017).

34. Arora, H.C., Eng, C. & Shoskes, D.A. Gut microbiome and chronic prostatitis/chronic pelvic pain syndrome. *Annals of Translational Medicine* **5**(2), 30 (2017).

35. Li, J.-H. et al. Health effects from swimming training in chlorinated pools and the corresponding metabolic stress pathways. *PLOS ONE* **10**(3), e0119241 (2015).

36. Li, X.-F. & Mitch, W.A. Drinking water disinfection byproducts (DBPs) and human health effects: multidisciplinary challenges and opportunities. *Environmental Science and Technology* **52**(4), 1681–1689 (2018).

37. Hoffman, M.D. & Hoffman, D.R. Does aerobic exercise improve pain perception and mood? A review of the evidence related to healthy and chronic pain subjects. *Current Pain and Headache Reports* **11**(2), 93–97 (2007).

38. Smith, C. & Grimmer-Somers, K. The treatment effect of exercise programmes for chronic low back pain. *Journal of Evaluation in Clinical Practice* **16**(3), 484–491 (2010).

39. Hajak, G. CS03-02 - sleep and chronic pain. *European Psychiatry* **26**(S2), 1775 (2011).

40. Aytekin, E. et al. Chronic widespread musculoskeletal pain in patients with obstructive sleep apnea syndrome and the relationship between sleep disorder and pain level, quality of life, and disability. *Journal of Physical Therapy Science* **27**(9), 2951–2954 (2015).

41. Zeidan, F. et al. Mindfulness meditation-based pain relief employs different neural mechanisms than placebo and sham mindfulness meditation-induced analgesia. *The Journal of Neuroscience* **35**(46), 15307–15325 (2015).

22 Developing Education and Treatment Protocols for Substance Use Disorders That Are Socially Responsible, Accountable, and Integrated

Recovery Engagement— Recognize and Treat

Brian Spitsbergen

CONTENTS

OVERVIEW

Educating medical professionals regarding opioid use disorders and the process of developing an increased knowledge base to improve decision-making regarding patients continues to be an important topic in the area of treating *substance use disorders* (SUD). Increased knowledge and improved processes for dealing with a patient in crisis struggling with an SUD will assist medical professionals dealing with this population toward making better and, in some cases, lifesaving decisions. There appears to be a persistent gap between the medical professionals and addiction professionals regarding the importance of sharing knowledge and experiences in the effective treatment of SUD that could significantly improve the outlook and prognosis and treatment outcomes. This chapter will discuss the scope of the problem, recognition of common SUD symptoms, basic information regarding the diagnosis and treatment of SUD, basic information about diagnosis and addiction severity, understanding motivation for the patient struggling with an SUD, and promising approaches or best practices for the treatment of SUD with this population.

SCOPE OF THE PROBLEM

Volkow et al.[1] (2014) estimated that over 2 million people in the United States suffer from substance use disorders related to prescription opioid pain relievers. The Institute of Addiction Medicine (2008) reported that Americans, who represent less than 5% of the world's population, are by far the largest group of opioid users; 80% of the world's supply of opioids (99% of the hydrocodone available globally) are used by people in the United States, and nearly 31% started with the nonmedical use of prescription drugs. Despite this knowledge regarding the effect on the general population, only recently has there been training and information provided to medical professionals about how to recognize symptoms of an SUD. Even then, there seems to be minimal resources dedicated to providing education to medical professionals regarding addiction severity, the role of treatment, and finally misunderstanding about the purpose and goals of treatment and recovery.

RECOGNITION OF SUD SYMPTOMS AND PATIENT MOTIVATION

Recognition of an SUD necessitates that any medical professional faced with a patient in medical crisis must first have some level of awareness that any patient in front of them could be struggling with an active SUD while experiencing other medical conditions that require immediate attention. Patients struggling with an SUD in "active" use often will have a history of other mental health or medical conditions that are, according to them, urgent and in need of immediate attention. *A patient struggling with an SUD will often NOT be motivated to see their SUD as a problem, but rather be motivated to find a solution to their discomfort that will include continued use.* Addiction will manifest itself in a variety of forms and substance preferences, but the culture surrounding their addictive thoughts and behaviors will have some universality.

For example, let's take a patient with active SUD whose drugs of choice are prescribed medications such as an opioid or benzodiazepine. In spite of observable symptoms—restlessness, disturbed sleeping patterns, confused thinking, or exaggerated physical aches and pains—this patient will maintain that their prescribed medications are necessary and helpful. There will be no overt or noticeable motivation by the patient to consider ceasing any or all substance use. It is also doubtful that ceasing use will be their first thought or choice. It is realistic to expect that many will become defensive about a previous diagnosis that precipitated the necessity of prescription(s) and will attempt to explain and defend the importance of maintaining these prescriptions. *It is common, regardless of the substance of preference, for these types of observable behaviors to be present when a patient is dealing with any acute or chronic medical condition and an SUD.* Now, let's explore specific symptoms and their impact on motivation.

PROGRESSION

There are various explanations of why some patients escalate into an SUD. Some will point to a biological cause, such as having a family history of drug or alcohol abuse. Others will suggest abusing drugs can lead to affiliation with using peers, which, in turn, exposes the individual to progressive use. For example, Hawkins et al.[2] (1992) studied youth risk and protective factors and found that those individuals who rapidly escalated into an SUD tend to have higher risk factors and lower levels of protective factors. Gender, race, and geographic location have also been found to play a role. One critical factor to consider is age—*the earlier people are exposed to substance use the more likely they are to experience a change in brain state.* There are several qualitative studies that suggest that patients who end up addicted and struggling with an SUD described their initial exposure to a mood-altering substance at extraordinarily young ages, which likely exposed a developing brain to the increased risks associated with SUD.

A practical conceptual framework of progression is best described as a patient's increased use of any mood-altering substances over the course of time. A practical definition of progression is a patient's need *to self-regulate through the use of mood-altering chemicals to alleviate any perceived discomfort, perceived pain, or emotions that appear disruptive despite the increased risk.*

The precise relationship between self-regulation and substance use disorders is still not fully explained through research. Several researchers have investigated the role that self-regulatory temperament (e.g., relatively stable individual differences in self-regulatory ability) may play in promoting vulnerability to or resilience relevant to other contextual risk factors for substance use,[3–5] but there is not a conclusive answer as to the reasons why people use substances to self-regulate. However, we can look at examples of responses in a variety of external stressors—for example medical problems—that over time start to appear irrational, exaggerated, or self-justified.

When people have progressed into a state of active addiction, they have progressed into a chronic, often relapsing, but treatable brain disease. One characteristic of addiction is cravings. Essentially, cravings tell a patient's brain that continued use is critical to survival. *Cravings are what drive the addicted patient to continue to use and progress to increased amounts*, despite the damage that it creates in their life and in the lives of those around them. Patients struggling with an SUD will often attempt to *minimize their levels of progression* and the damage this progression has caused.

TOLERANCE

Renaldi et al.[6] (1988) described tolerance occurring when the person no longer responds to the drug in the way that person initially responded. Stated another way, it will take a higher dose of the drug to achieve the same level of response achieved initially. For the patient struggling with an SUD, tolerance often develops quickly, and therefore the amount required for relief increases over time to meet their level of tolerance. In some cases, *tolerance can be identified at first exposure to substance use*, particularly as described earlier, when first exposure to substances occurs during early adolescence. Patients with a likely predisposition to SUD ordinarily report having different kinds of experiences than their non-SUD peers including using more than intended on their first exposure, limited physical consequences (e.g., no hangover), and a quick recovery post-initial exposure. This type of information can be extremely valuable and can quickly assist the medical professional in recognizing some of the initial warning signs or indicators. Recognizing the development of tolerance at the beginning of their using career can help medical professionals clarify their decision-making because symptoms of tolerance early in their substance use will likely include some of the following consequences: reduced academic success and increased medical and legal histories. It also can provide guidance toward determining if this patient took additional significant risks to health, education, and legal freedoms in order to obtain and recreate that initial experience.

CHRONICITY AND WITHDRAWAL

Baldacchino et al.[7] (2012) indicated that chronic opioid use and withdrawal experiences have been reported to be associated with a number of neuropsychological impairments during both active use and after a period of abstinence. As drugs produce less and less of the desired effect, risk-taking will become extensive. When the inability to sustain current levels of use is paired with the inability to manage use or afford the consequences of this maintenance, there will be a noticeable increase in anxiety as the patient begins to realize that their current level of substance use is not sustainable. Due to the increase in required substance use to avoid withdrawal, fear will begin to motivate and take over most aspects of this patient's behavior. For example, in the mind of the patient struggling to find the maintenance solution to their SUD, fear of withdrawal becomes the most important issue that requires resolution with the resolution being more use. It is likely that this patient will display behaviors that are aggressive, irrational, and suggest that any and all measures will be taken to continue using. *The brain and the body are "dysregulated" to the point where the patient struggling with SUD will continue seeking use of substances for relief and regulation at all costs.*

When fear, increased dosages, and reduced options in obtaining drugs lead to further increases in reckless use, the result will be yet even more examples of extreme negative consequences and cycles of depression partnered with intense mood swings. The downward trajectory of this patient is even quicker when the onset of use occurs at a younger age. Normally, a patient struggling with an SUD has likely considered suicide. Many will not follow through on these thoughts but due to the chronicity of use, consequences, and intense fear of withdrawal it should be expected that there is always potential for suicidal ideations. Some will report multiple suicide attempts. Using an extensive amount of substances on a single occasion just to see "what might happen" should also be considered a suicide attempt.

Even when attempts are made to limit or stop using—most often under external pressure from the legal system/medical professionals, or even family and other social supports—the combination of emotional pain and physical discomfort that goes with withdrawal often becomes too intense. It is common for the outcome in this case to be to see a patient frequently, with periods of sobriety being brief. Remember, for the user substances are now the *solution* to their problem as long as they can maintain use. For many with an SUD, years have passed with little to no progress toward the expansion of emotional, intellectual, and spiritual maturation. In short, a patient with an SUD has chronologically grown up, but their other aspects of development have likely been inhibited. Interestingly, they are often unaware that they have fallen behind non-addicted peers regardless of their age or developmental stage.

Withdrawal experiences are experienced as extreme negative events, and the emotions (dysregulation) associated with the negative events are intense. Patients with SUD often drift toward isolation. Isolation further exacerbates fears and insecurities which further diminishes the ability to receive support from family and friends. Episodes of depression and extreme moods become so intense that the inability to understand or control emotions becomes normalized.

RECOGNIZING LEVELS OF IMPAIRMENT

One important aspect of classifying and finding appropriate services for an SUD is recognizing levels of impairment. *Impairment for a patient struggling with SUD refers to reductions in functioning due to ineffective coping strategies.* The activation of the brain's reward system is central to problems arising from an SUD; the rewarding feeling that people experience as a result of taking drugs may be so profound that they neglect other normal activities in favor of taking the drug. This is the place where impairment begins.

Not all impairments will be the same from patient to patient—perhaps a better way to process impairment is through identification of addiction severity. Addiction is best intervened in with clear recognition of severity levels and risk of relapse potential. Frequently, the level of severity creates cognitive and emotional deficiencies that for short periods might be difficult to detect but will result in re-engagement in active use if severity is not understood, thus directing professionals toward making decisions toward an appropriate level of care.

Previous research on addiction severity began with the *Addiction Severity Index (ASI)* developed by McLellan, Luborsky, Woody, and O'Brien (1980).[8] The ASI is a structured clinical interview tool developed to fill the need for a reliable, valid, and standardized diagnostic and evaluative instrument in the field of alcohol and drug abuse. The ASI focuses on producing 10-point problem severity ratings in each of the six areas commonly affected by addiction. Several factors contribute to this: potency of desired drug(s) of choice; age and frequency of onset; developmental maturity; and experiences surrounding trauma of all socioeconomic, physical, and emotional types.

Indicators of severity will vary at different points in time, but will generally follow a specific path consistent with progression and will show signs/symptoms that advance over time. There is no one single impairment indicator that will automatically define severity for a substance use disorder, but rather a collection of clinical symptoms that trigger decisions. *It is important to note that symptoms of severity and level of impairment do not automatically change immediately with the removal of the substance use.*

Tice et al.[9] (2001) described identifying impairments and the associated severity of an SUD to the extreme risks taken and high emotional stress present paired with loss of control over impulses with the inability to inhibit inappropriate behaviors or to delay gratification.

Campbell's[10] (2003) research discussed the common etiology of substance and behavioral addictions including faulty volitions instigated by cognitive impairments. These impairments and subsequent level of severity are likely to continue beyond the cessation of substance use. Cognitive impairment minimizes the recall of the negative effects of the addictive behavior which is viewed as necessary and causal to all addictions. Campbell suggested that a patient's impairment and subsequent level of severity can occur for several months or longer, with cognitive and emotional impairments accounting for a substantial proportion of patients in early recovery having trouble achieving and maintaining sobriety.

Spitsbergen[11] (2017) also discussed the severity and impairment stemming from withdrawal symptoms where there was a consistent theme of overwhelming fear of withdrawal (referred to as dope sickness) in the study of barriers to successful recovery for opioid users aged 18–25, where users almost universally reported impaired decision-making processes and high levels of addiction severity often to the point where their value systems became compromised and systems so dysregulated that they feared withdrawal more than they feared death.

IDENTIFYING EMOTIONAL DYSREGULATION

Patients with SUD in an emergency or critical care situation will almost certainly be experiencing emotional dysregulation. In this scenario, it should be expected that a patient will display some common symptoms: extreme anxiety or fear, symptoms of trauma, depression, near-death experiences, and suicidal ideations. Emotional dysregulation likely will drive a patient in crisis to look for an immediate solution to these intense emotions. Let's look at some of the common indicators of dysregulation.

DEPRESSIVE EPISODES

Depressive episodes are extraordinarily common for SUD patients. Davis et al.[12] (2005) reported in their analysis that nearly one-third of patients with major depressive disorder also have substance use disorders, and the comorbidity yields a higher risk of suicide and greater social and personal impairment as well as other psychiatric conditions. Viewed in this light, mental health issues affecting patients with an acute SUD precipitate a higher degree of risk factors. Patients with a pattern of acute and chronic SUD issues may describe depressive-related issues as frequent and which have become a normalized experience for them. For medical professionals it should be anticipated that dealing with active SUD means the severe depressive episodes will be cumulative in terms of frequency and impact. Depression will most likely be one of the most troublesome intense moods experienced when attempting to recover from an SUD. Spitsbergen[11] (2017) noted that depression mixed with other mental health concerns was acknowledged as an issue affecting patients during the transition to recovery.

DEPRESSION ASSOCIATED WITH DETOXIFICATION

Many patients struggling with SUD are going to experience intense negative moods associated with depression when faced with detoxification. Depression, paired with negative experiences associated with active use or severe medical consequences, can produce intense short-term episodes of depression and anxiety. *The most important risk here is that, when these depressed moods mixed with anxiety are at the point of highest intensity at detoxification, there is increased vulnerability to suicidal ideations.*

Dreissen et al.[13] (2002) concluded that severe trait anxiety persisting after 3 weeks of abstinence, comorbid depressive and/or anxiety disorders, and combinations of these with moderate or severe current anxiety and depressive states represent the greatest risks of relapse and therefore may indicate a treatment need. In other words, when a patient with an SUD experiences depression during detoxification, these increased intense feelings of depression post-detoxification will likely get "worse" upon full detoxification. This increases the possibility of being subjected to increased anxiety or even panic in regard to any post-detoxification depression. *This post-detoxification process is often familiar to a patient with SUD and can influence decisions to follow medical advice at the point of detoxification.*

SUICIDAL IDEATION

It is not uncommon for patients with SUD to experience pervasive suicidal thoughts. In fact this can often be viewed as progressive, beginning during adolescence and increasing in frequency over the course of their lifetime. Spitsbergen[11] (2017), for example, reported that younger users of opioids described their suicidal ideations as progressive from a very young age while recognizing the emotional costs of not addressing suicidal thoughts prior to an extreme medical crisis because they felt they could manage their thoughts with more substance use.

TRAUMA

Previous studies have established the association of childhood trauma exposure with the development and progression of drug use and dependence in adolescence and early adulthood.[14–19] Research has also begun to delineate the short- and long-term sequelae associated with exposure to trauma, substance abuse, and the combination of these experiences. These problems include PTSD, depression, behavioral problems, disruptions in development, attachment and interpatiental difficulties, somatic complaints, and cognitive impairments.[20] Many of these problems will persist well into adulthood and are linked with increased risk for morbidity and mortality.[21–23]

It is common for those struggling with an SUD to have experienced physical, emotional, or sexual consequences within their environment. *Examples of traumas include: car accidents, fights, accidents involving physical injury, mourning the death of a loved one, physical pain, mental instability, physical and emotional abuse, grief and loss, and sexual assault.* Additionally, there is a possibility of some undiagnosed concussion or brain trauma either unreported or untreated.

NEAR-DEATH EXPERIENCES

Patients with an SUD commonly will be familiar with near-death experiences during their active use. In many cases, repeated exposure to near-death experiences may condition them to not even recognize some near-death experiences as being critical ones. Many of these "experiences" may include witnessing or being connected to life events that result in trauma. Experiences could include harm from weapons, physical altercation requiring medical attention, car accidents, witnessing accidental death, and death and revival. Additionally, many will suffer from physical health issues—overdosing, contracting a sexually transmitted infection, or contracting hepatitis C, or a patient revival from death.

DIAGNOSIS OF SUD—DSM-5

Diagnosis of SUD is performed using the *Diagnostic Statistical Manual – DSM-5*.[24] The DSM is the standard psychiatric system of classification for mental disorders used for clinical, research, policy, and reimbursement purposes in the United States. It has widespread importance and influence on how disorders are diagnosed, treated, and investigated. Since its first publication in 1952, DSM has been reviewed and revised five times; the new version, DSM-5, was published in 2013. The Diagnostic and Statistical Manual of Mental Disorders (DSM) is the handbook used by healthcare professionals in the United States and much of the world as the authoritative guide toward the diagnosis of mental disorders.

The DSM-5 recognizes substance-related disorders resulting from the use of ten separate classes of drugs: alcohol; caffeine; cannabis; hallucinogens (phencyclidine or similarly acting arylcyclohexylamines, and other hallucinogens, such as LSD); inhalants; opioids; sedatives, hypnotics, or anxiolytics; stimulants (including amphetamine-type substances, cocaine, and other stimulants); tobacco; and other or unknown substances. While some major groupings of psychoactive substances are specifically identified, the use of other or unknown substances can also form the basis of a substance-related or addictive disorder.

The DSM-5 recognizes that people are not all automatically or equally vulnerable to developing substance-related disorders and that some people have lower levels of self-control that predispose them to develop problems if they're exposed to drugs.

There are two groups of substance-related disorders: *substance use disorders and substance-induced disorders.*

- Substance use disorders are patterns of symptoms resulting from the use of a substance that you continue to take, despite experiencing problems as a result.
- Substance-induced disorders, including intoxication, withdrawal, and other substance/medication-induced mental disorders, are detailed alongside substance use disorders.

CRITERIA FOR SUBSTANCE USE DISORDERS

Substance use disorders span a wide variety of problems arising from substance use, and cover 11 different criteria:

1. Taking the substance in larger amounts or for longer than you're meant to.
2. Wanting to cut down or stop using the substance but not managing to.
3. Spending a lot of time getting, using, or recovering from use of the substance.
4. Cravings and urges to use the substance.
5. Not managing to do what you should at work, home, or school because of substance use.
6. Continuing to use, even when it causes problems in relationships.

7. Giving up important social, occupational, or recreational activities because of substance use.
8. Using substances again and again, even when it puts you in danger.
9. Continuing to use, even when you know you have a physical or psychological problem that could have been caused or made worse by the substance.
10. Needing more of the substance to get the effect you want (tolerance).
11. Development of withdrawal symptoms, which can be relieved by taking more of the substance.

SEVERITY OF SUBSTANCE USE DISORDERS

The DSM-5 allows clinicians to specify how severe or how much of a problem the substance use disorder is, depending on how many symptoms are identified.

- *Two or three* symptoms indicate a **mild** substance use disorder.
- *Four or five* symptoms indicate a **moderate** substance use disorder.
- *Six or more* symptoms indicate a **severe** substance use disorder.

Clinicians can also add "in early remission," "in sustained remission," "on maintenance therapy," and "in a controlled environment."

PLACEMENT CRITERIA FOR SUD (ASAM)

ASAM's criteria, formerly known as the ASAM patient placement criteria, is the result of a collaboration that began in the 1980s to define one national set of criteria for providing outcome-oriented and results-based care in the treatment of addiction.[25] Today the criteria have become the most widely used and comprehensive set of guidelines for placement, continued stay, and transfer/discharge of patients with addiction and co-occurring conditions. ASAM's criteria are required in over 30 states.

ASAM (2015) definition of addiction:

> Addiction is a treatable, chronic medical disease involving complex interactions among brain circuits, genetics, the environment, and an individual's life experiences. People with addiction use substances or engage in behaviors that become compulsive and often continue despite harmful consequences. Prevention efforts and treatment approaches for addiction are generally as successful as those for other chronic diseases.

Addiction is characterized by the inability to consistently abstain, impairment in behavioral control, and craving, diminished recognition of significant problems with one's behaviors and interpersonal relationships, and a dysfunctional emotional response. Like other chronic diseases, addiction often involves cycles of relapse and remission. Without treatment or engagement in recovery activities, addiction is progressive and can result in disability or premature death.

Other factors that can contribute to the appearance of addiction, leading to its characteristic bio-psycho-socio-spiritual manifestations, include:

- The presence of an underlying biological deficit in the function of reward circuits, such that drugs and behaviors which enhance reward function are preferred and sought as reinforcers.
- The repeated engagement in drug use or other addictive behaviors, causing neuroadaptation in motivational circuitry, leading to impaired control over further drug use or engagement in addictive behaviors.

- Cognitive and affective distortions, which impair perceptions and compromise the ability to deal with feelings, resulting in significant self-deception.
- Disruption of healthy social supports and problems in interpersonal relationships which impact the development or impact of resiliencies.
- Exposure to trauma or stressors that overwhelm an individual's coping abilities.
- Distortion in meaning, purpose, and values that guide attitudes, thinking, and behavior.
- Distortions in a patient's connection with self, with others, and with the transcendent (referred to as God by many, the Higher Power by 12-steps groups, or higher consciousness by others).
- The presence of co-occurring psychiatric disorders in patients who engage in substance use or other addictive behaviors.

PATIENT INTERVENTION PROTOCOLS UNIQUE TO SUD

Current practices geared toward helping patients struggling with a substance use disorder still lack a clear understanding of some common protocols that can assist in planning for future considerations for care. Unfortunately it is still common for medical professionals to frequently "miss" opportunities to recognize and react appropriately to an SUD at their particular point of contact due to not knowing some of the experiences unique to an SUD patient. Knowledge of these experiences can improve decision-making and recommendations for follow-up care.

EARLY DETECTION

It is important to be able to detect when SUD has developed and symptomatology began during adolescence. When dealing with an adolescent, these patients will lack some of the overt medical symptoms associated with SUD and are often masked by other mental health-related concerns. Baler and Volkow[26] (2006) reported that patients with diagnosable SUD are known to have decreased executive functioning, low behavioral and emotional control, poor decision-making, and greater levels of deviant behavior and impulsivity. These symptoms are observably more pronounced when patients report initial use of substances in early adolescence. Knowledge of patient initiation of substance use is often associated with increased addiction severity when faced with an acute medical crisis. There is evidence of a relationship between accumulated adversity and addiction risk—the greater the number of stressors an individual is exposed to, the higher the risk of developing a greater addiction severity.

UNDERSTANDING A "MOMENT OF CLARITY"

When a patient's use gets interrupted, it is medical professionals that will often be the first person they come in contact with. Patients will often be in a state of despair, but within that despair many will experience something called a *moment of clarity—a period of mental and emotional reflection where they recognize the intersection of past and present and may be willing to take action.* This experience provides opportunity, albeit sometimes briefly, to "decide" rather than "react" to the pain, emotional dysregulation, and fear they will describe as overwhelming. There is a deep understanding and *power* surrounding the moment of clarity, and many might choose the path of recovery if treatment opportunities are immediately available. If treatment opportunities are not immediately available, it is likely they will return to active use once the acute episode is resolved.

This *power* to decide, rather than react, begins the process of healing. However, the fear of emotional and physical pain will return shortly after the healing process begins. The emotional consequences tied to extensive and frequent relapses instill little hope of initiating recovery. Remember that it will not take long for the patient to experience extreme depression where their feelings are more intense, their negative moods and emotions seem more severe, and their suicidal ideations more frequent. Survival during this period often depends on support from parents, siblings, and helping professionals. Lacking the skills of emotion regulation, they have to depend on others to help stabilize their lives.

Understanding Relapse Potential

Historically, this population has been documented as having a high risk and relapse potential. In many cases, medical professionals will have multiple experiences with the same patient related to overdose and withdrawal. Many patients who are addicted are looking to be understood and for medical professionals to understand what is motivating their use. Previous research has demonstrated that those addicted require additional support and attention to motivation to ensure improved outcomes.[27,28]

Understanding Patient "Reservations"

Reservation is a term universally used in the 12-step recovering community. Reservation refers to holding back a complete willingness to put full effort and internal and external energy into initiating and maintaining sobriety. Reservations are the belief that they should put some effort into getting sober but would still rather continue to use.

Most patients will come into an acute medical situation experiencing reservations, most frequently connected to feelings of fear or connected to feelings of anger/resentment, which result in previous failed attempts and a lack of full commitment to sobriety. The most common reservations can include serving jail time, losing a stable residence, needing to work, or the loss of a significant relationship. These reservations will be frustrating to the professionals attempting to triage the patient and assist them in finding treatment or recovery-oriented services. However, it is important to work with the patient in areas in which they are not showing reservations and connecting them to the treatment or services they require without gap or delay. Otherwise, emotional dysregulation will recur, and the patient may decide to not receive any assistance other than becoming medically stable.

Treatment Experience and Recovery Attempts

Previous Treatment Experiences

Many SUD patients will have experienced more than one treatment episode by the time you see them in a medical crisis. Many will have had near-death experiences and previous treatments during their lifetime. According to the Substance Abuse and Mental Health Services Administration (SAMHSA 2012) it is estimated that the number of adults who will need treatment for substance abuse has tripled since 2000.[29] Patients with diagnosable SUD typically will experience more than one treatment episode during their lifetime. Treatment experiences generally benefit patients with SUD even when the outcome isn't immediately successful. Current research does not support the relationship between treatment engagement and patient increases in motivation at this time. However, treatment experiences often can provide resources, support, and time away from active SUD which can extend a patient's life when properly diagnosed and placed.

Recovery Attempts

Previous recovery attempts can provide some benefit to patients as they will have some experience and knowledge. However, previous attempts at recovery can also be experienced as deflating or unattainable. Patients may describe their drive or motivation (often referred to as ambition) toward attempting recovery as lost once they become addicted and have experienced setbacks. Loss of motivation, to them, may instead look like a progressively deteriorating situation. Therefore, despite being in extreme crisis patients may appear unmotivated to accept help. Patients may recount decreased feelings of ambition to remain abstinent and decreased hope for the future. Motivation for change may appear as described as an external experience only, driven by fear of loss.

AVERSION

Patients will likely experience aversion to withdrawal (dope sickness). This can be viewed as potential internal motivation for abstinence. Spitsbergen[11] (2017) reported that the term withdrawal and the aversion to it was frequently associated with other terms or phrases like "depression," "wish I would die," and "I would do anything to make this stop," and patients acknowledged the psychological anxiety or fear of getting sick. Aversion is potent and impactful, even more than the thought of death when in an acute crisis. Aversion is helpful and attractive to a patient only when there are options to avoid withdrawal in lieu of recommencing the use of substances. This includes immediate detoxification services, residential SUD treatment, medically assisted treatments (MAT), and peer recovery coaches.

EXTERNAL MOTIVATION

For patients struggling with an SUD, increased motivation toward abstinence will more likely occur when external pressure is applied. Spitsbergen[11] (2017) found several indicators central to external motivation, including parental influence, worrying about disappointing their parents, losing the financial resources, loss of employment, jail or prison, or having nowhere to go once they ran out of money. In the same study participants most frequently reported attempting abstinence for the sake of their children, avoiding jail time, or losing a relationship with a significant other as the primary reason to attempt sobriety. Observable lack of motivation can be summarized by looking at fear of withdrawal (aversion), motivation likely influenced by consequence (external), and lack of full commitment to change (reservations).

IMPLICATIONS FOR MEDICAL PROFESSIONALS

Taken as a whole, further refinement of combined medical/clinical interventions when patients are at the peak of dysregulation and their mood is in its most vulnerable state is needed. The following recommendations are proposed:

1. Updating knowledge and intervention techniques aimed at improving immediate engagement when individuals are in their most vulnerable state. Without a strong connection, patients leave medical facilities before experiencing the benefits of abstinence. Focusing on techniques that assist in recognizing anxiety and improving emotional regulation even slightly could improve retention and recovery engagement.
2. SUD training on developing brief clinical competencies related to the role of emotional regulation during a patient's moment of clarity. Patients with SUD will experience a moment of clarity as one of extraordinary importance, but medical professionals must recognize this is also brief and fleeting. Symptom recognition and relief need to be combined with intervention techniques aimed at developing immediate rapport.
3. Medical professionals can improve outcomes when they recognize the patient's level of addiction severity. This will clarify itself further when professionals can identify early exposure and developmental readiness to receive assistance based on the age of first use.
4. Medical professionals can pay close attention to the role that the moment of clarity plays in increasing patient motivation. The moment of clarity is a key experience for most SUD persons with extended periods of sobriety. After several attempts at sobriety, some are able to return to their moment of clarity and come to believe that achieving and maintaining sobriety is attainable. The importance of breaking the isolation cycle becomes crucial

regardless of how uncomfortable socializing and problem solving with others make them feel. Reconnecting with others promotes value-driven decision-making which include a reliance on outside help to get through feelings of fear and pain.

5. Medical professionals should be prepared and equipped with immediate strategies to adequately deal with the associated depressed feelings and intense moods, especially when dealing with the trauma associated with detoxification and withdrawal. Detoxification appears to be the most likely time at which patients begin to experience a severe wave of emotions embedded in what many will later describe as trauma. Patients will likely have deficiencies in their emotional development and turn toward learned coping strategies. An example of this is social isolation, which might have helped them in the past to immediately cope with feelings of shame and of emotional inadequacy. But this pattern is pervasive and harmful and in the long term will move them further away from the emotional growth and development required to sustain sobriety.

SUMMARY

When patients experience a "miss" they are likely to become more frustrated and distrustful of medical professionals who do not "understand" or do not "really want to help." Patients with multiple admissions for acute SUD symptoms are more likely to be combative, non-compliant, and dishonest regarding the nature of their use.

It's probably not all that surprising that assisting patients with an SUD under current practices appears to the SUD patient as a set of fragmented services, and ineffective treatment recommendations resulting in repeat customers in emergency room settings.

Rather than implementing clear and regimented intervention protocols to stabilize patients and provide them with opportunities to recover, the current reactionary response to the SUD epidemic seems to be producing negative outcomes. There are significant consequences for the patient's emotional and physical health when they do not receive adequate care at their first point of contact. Increased relapse incidents will likely advance the severity of emotional and physical consequences associated with addiction and invariably destroy the individual piece by piece with each relapse while valuable time is lost for a patient to successfully recover.

When full integration occurs—when healthcare systems, academic institutions, and public safety and behavioral health specialists embrace and recognize the value of adopting a reliable educational base of knowledge about SUD and the option of supporting consistent protocols at all levels of care—we then might see significant progress.

REFERENCES

1. Volkow, N.D., Frieden, T.R., Hyde, P.S., & Cha, S.S. (2014). Medication-assisted therapies — tackling the opioid-overdose epidemic. *New England Journal of Medicine*, 370(22), 2063–2066.
2. Hawkins, J.D., Catalano, R.F., & Miller, J.Y. (1992). Risk and protective factors for alcohol and other drug problems in adolescence and early adulthood: implications for substance abuse prevention. *Psychological Bulletin*, 112(1), 64–105.
3. Stice, E., & Gonzales, N. (1998). Adolescent temperament moderates the relation of parenting to antisocial behavior and substance use. *Journal of Adolescent Research*, 13(1), 5–31.
4. Wills, T., McNamara, G., Vaccaro, D., & Hirky, A. (1996). Escalated substance use: a longitudinal grouping analysis from early to middle adolescence. *Journal of Abnormal Psychology*, 105(2), 166–180.
5. Wills, T.A., & Dishion, T.J. (2004). Temperament and adolescent substance use: a transactional analysis of emerging self-control. *Journal of Clinical Child and Adolescent Psychology*, 33(1), 69–81.
6. Rinaldi, R.C., Steindler, E.M., Wilford, B.B., & Goodwin, D. (1988). Clarification and standardization of substance abuse terminology. *JAMA*, 259(4), 555–557.
7. Baldacchino, A., Balfour, D.J., Passetti, F., Humphris, G., & Matthews, K. (2012). Neuropsychological consequences of chronic opioid use: a quantitative review and meta-analysis. *Neuroscience and Biobehavioral Reviews*, 36(9), 2056–2068.

8. McLellan, A.T., Luborsky, L., Woody, G.E., & O'Brien, C.P. (1980). An improved diagnostic evaluation instrument for substance abuse patients: the addiction severity index. *Journal of Nervous and Mental Disease*, 168(1), 26–33.

9. Tice, D., Bratslavsky, E., & Baumeister, R. (2001). Emotional distress regulation takes precedence over impulse control: if you feel bad, do it! *Journal of Personality and Social Psychology*, 80(1), 53–67.

10. Campbell, W.G. (2003). Addiction: a disease of volition caused by a cognitive impairment. *The Canadian Journal of Psychiatry*, 4, 669–674.

11. Spitsbergen, B. (2017). Drugs of choice and other explanatory factors in young adults understandings of adolescent addiction and recovery experiences. PhD Dissertation. Oakland University.

12. Davis, L., Uezato, A., Newell, J.M., & Frazier, E. (2008). Major depression and comorbid substance use disorders. *Current Opinion in Psychiatry*, 21(1), 14–18.

13. Driessen, M., Meier, S., Hill, A., Wetterling, T., Lange, W., & Junghanns, K. (2001). The course of anxiety, depression and drinking behaviours after completed detoxification in alcoholics with and without comorbid anxiety and depressive disorders. *Alcohol and Alcoholism*, 36(3), 249–255.

14. Anda, R.F., Whitfield, C.L., Felitti, V.J., Chapman, D., Edwards, V.J., Dube, S.R., & Williamson, D.F. (2002). Adverse childhood experiences, alcoholic parents, and later risk of alcoholism and depression. *Psychiatric Services*, 53(8), 1001–1009.

15. Blumenthal, H., Blanchard, L., Feldner, M.T., Babson, K.A., Leen-Feldner, E.W., & Dixon, L. (2008). Traumatic event exposure, posttraumatic stress, and substance use among youth: a critical review of the empirical literature. *Current Psychiatry Reviews*, 4(4), 228–254.

16. Chilcoat, H.D., & Breslau, N. (1998a). Investigations of causal pathways between PTSD and drug use disorders. *Addictive Behaviors*, 23(6), 827–840.

17. Chilcoat, H.D., & Breslau, N. (1998b). Posttraumatic stress disorder and drug disorders: testing causal pathways. *Archives of General Psychiatry*, 55(10), 913–917.

18. Dube, S.R., Anda, R.F., Felitti, V.J., Edwards, V.J., & Croft, J.B. (2002). Adverse childhood experiences and patiental alcohol abuse as an adult. *Addictive Behaviors*, 27(5), 713–725.

19. Dube, S.R., Felitti, V.J., Dong, M., Chapman, D.P., Giles, W.H., & Anda, R.F. (2003). Childhood abuse, neglect, and household dysfunction and the risk of illicit drug use: the adverse childhood experiences study. *Pediatrics*, 111(3), 564–572.

20. Bukstein, O.G., & Horner, M.S. (2010). Management of the adolescent with substance use disorders and comorbid psychopathology. *Child and Adolescent Psychiatric Clinics of North America*, 19(3), 609–623.

21. Anda, R.F., Dong, M., Brown, D.W., Felitti, V.J., Giles, W.H., Perry, G.S., et al. (2009). The relationship of adverse childhood experiences to history of premature death of family members. *BMC Public Health*, 9, 106.

22. Brown, D.W., Anda, R.F., Tiemeier, H., Felitti, V.J., Edwards, V.J., Croft, J.B., & Giles, W.H. (2009). Adverse childhood experiences and the risk of premature mortality. *American Journal of Preventive Medicine*, 37(5), 389–396.

23. Dube, S.R., Fairweather, D., Pearson, W.S., Felitti, V.J., Anda, R.F., & Croft, J.B. (2009). Cumulative childhood stress and autoimmune diseases in adults. *Psychosomatic Medicine*, 71(2), 243–250.

24. American Psychiatric Association. (2013). *Diagnostic and Statistical Manual of Mental Disorders* (5th ed.). Washington, DC: Author.

25. American Society of Addiction Medicine. (2018). American society of addiction medicine, ASAM placement criteria. Retrieved March 2019, from www.asam.org/.

26. Baler, R.D., & Volkow, N.D. (2006). Drug addiction: the neurobiology of disrupted self-control. *Trends in Molecular Medicine*, 12(12), 559–566.

27. Kollins, S.H., Barkley, R.A., & DuPaul, G.J. (2001). Use and management of medications for children diagnosed with attention deficit hyperactivity disorder (ADHD). *Focus on Exceptional Children*, 33(5), 1–24.

28. Poulin, C. (2001). Medical and nonmedical stimulant use among adolescents: from sanctioned to unsanctioned use. *Canadian Medical Association Journal*, 165(8), 1039–1044.

29. United States Department of Health and Human Services. (SAMHSA). (2012). Substance abuse and mental health services administration. *Center for Behavioral Health Statistics and Quality. Treatment Episode Data Set – Admissions (TEDS-A), ICPSR35037-v1.* Ann Arbor, MI: Inter-University Consortium for Political and Social Research [distributor] (2014-05-07).

23 Detoxification Strategies

Jennifer Kljajic and Ahmed Zaafran

CONTENTS

INTRODUCTION

The late 1990s marked a turning point in America's crisis with opioid consumption. With a surge in opioid production by pharmaceutical companies, the medical community received reassurances from pharmaceutical companies that patients would not become addicted to opioid pain relievers. As a result, an increased prescription rate of opioids and other habit-forming medications played a major factor in the current opioid epidemic. The incidence of prescribed and non-prescribed opioid misuse increased prior to a clear understanding of the highly addictive nature of these medications. Despite efforts to thwart the current opioid epidemic in the United States, drug overdose deaths continue to increase.

From 1999 to 2017, almost 400,000 people died from an overdose involving any opioid, including prescription and illicit opioids.[1] In October of 2017, the U.S. Department of Health and Human Services (HHS) declared a public health emergency regarding the opioid crisis and initiated strategies to help tackle the many issues surrounding the epidemic.

Alongside the opioid crisis, another crisis that is gaining momentum involves benzodiazepines. According to the National Institute of Drug Abuse, more than 30% of opioid overdoses included benzodiazepines. A study published in the U.S. National Library of Medicine National Institute of Health suggests that benzodiazepine prescriptions increased by 67% between 1996 and 2013 and likely contributed to an increase in accidental dependence.[2]

Benzodiazepines, a central nervous system depressant, are often sought out alongside opioids due to similar mechanisms of action on the brain and body.

The current landscape includes two groups of individuals affected by the opioid and benzodiazepine crisis: those who are traditionally addicted, and those who are accidentally dependent.

TRADITIONAL ADDICTION

Traditional addiction, or substance use disorder, is the result of changes in the brain that result in a loss of control, compulsive use, intensive cravings, and continued use despite consequences. Individuals struggling with addiction have a hijacked and/or disabled dopamine reward system.[3] Lastly, they continue to use the drug despite negative consequences, such as poor health, and loss of relationships and/or employment. Those individuals are more at risk for overdose due to the synergistic effects of opioids and benzodiazepines. Furthermore, there are questions now as to whether some of the overdoses are actually intentional, due to the side effect of risk of suicide with benzodiazepines.[4]

ACCIDENTAL DEPENDENCE

On the other side of the spectrum, there are those who are accidentally dependent. Habit-forming medications such as opioids or benzodiazepines prescribed by a physician may lead to dependency and, without a careful de-prescribing plan, may also lead to addiction.

Despite maintaining a therapeutic dose in many cases, tolerance to the medication is a risk, and patients may start to experience withdrawal symptoms. As a result, increasing doses become necessary in order to achieve a similar therapeutic effect. While physical dependence is one problem, medication withdrawal often leads to physiological as well as mental health symptomology. Those symptoms may include depersonalization, derealization, panic attacks, and anxiety, which may last long after withdrawal.[5]

In both addiction and accidental dependency, with the mechanisms of opiate (opioid) and GABA (benzodiazepine) receptors being downregulated, dependency can set in as early as under a week.[6] Access to executive functioning skills in the frontal cortex such as judgment, planning, prioritizing, emotional control, self-monitoring, understanding different points of view, and attention span may become impaired. Additionally, areas such as the cerebellum, which includes motor control, balance, attention, language, processing procedural memories, and regulating fear and pleasure responses, are impacted.

Cumulatively, this disequilibrium within the central nervous system leads to impaired functioning, particularly in quality of life measures. Simple tasks such as writing grocery lists or running errands can be overwhelming due to the cognitive impairments from the medication during and after withdrawal.[7,8]

GENETICS

Genetic predisposition is a contributing factor in addiction. In a recent publication looking at human endogenous retrovirus-K HML-2 integration within RASGRF2, the authors note that gene expression may be altered simply by dealing with a stressor such as loss of loved one or loss of a job.[9] The epigenetics of the dopamine reward center increase the chance for addiction or dependency to set in.[9] Until recently, patients were being prescribed opioids and benzodiazepines for an indefinite time. A multi-agency approach, that includes hospital systems and government entities, is being taken to solve this crisis.

There are many challenges in legislating change in regulations and guidelines for pain management while still addressing patient needs for adequate pain management. While it is imperative that the medical community works diligently to effectively taper patients off of habit-forming medications safely, it is equally important that patients needing complex pain management strategies are not left to suffer because of inadequate pain management regimes.

A lucid understanding of weaning and tapering strategies is crucial with this patient population. A mainstay methodology has been a cross over to a medication with a longer half-life. This allows for blood serum levels to stabilize. Further, the consensus has been to wean slowly to help mitigate the acute medication withdrawal process. Many primary care physicians and specialists do not have experience with the process and may do harm to the patient when attempting to remove these medications abruptly.

There are multiple strategies for tapering off of habit-forming medications, but only through a comprehensive approach, that includes behavioral health modalities with continuous support and empathy, will improved outcomes occur. The maintenance and containment of acute withdrawal symptoms that are seen alongside tapering strategies are of utmost importance, and the process may take months to years to successfully complete.

With the opioid and benzodiazepine epidemic garnering more national attention in the media, people are becoming more aware of the dangers of prescribing benzodiazepines and opioids concurrently. More education and mentoring of primary care physicians by specialists in addiction medicine are needed to help patients wean off their opioid and benzodiazepine slowly and safely. In addition, recovery centers are struggling with discharge planning when sending patients back to rural communities that lack resources to support their sobriety and/or healing from addiction or dependency.

Likewise, there is a gap in professional services outside of traditional hospital systems to tackle this epidemic. With the vast resources available on the Internet today, many patients are turning to informal online support groups where individuals seek to help each other come off of habit-forming medications. These informal groups include moderators and peers helping each other to manage 24/7 daily withdrawal symptoms, with positive results speaking to the utility and efficacy of group therapy. Limitations include incorrect advice and the lack of professional experience, in addition to the risk of inter- and intrapersonal issues, bullying, and/or risk of secondary trauma from being exposed to extreme symptomology. Learned helplessness is also a potential outcome of these groups that can't be easily identified if the moderator is ill-equipped to manage such group dynamics and incidents.

There is a great need to fill the gap in services and long-term recovery with professional support. Virtual medical teams that include recovery coaches that use cognitive behavioral therapy (CBT) and mindfulness, as well as wellness and health coaches supporting prescribing doctors and their patients, are helpful since withdrawal and healing are known to be a long process. Inpatient residential programs are not as effective as previously thought without long-term support and recovery plans. Addiction is a chronic relapsing and remitting disease that takes months to years of treatment. In addition, there is evidence that it takes that long for the brain to heal, even from taking a drug as prescribed.

In addition, evidence-based tapering protocols such as those outlined in the Asthon Manuel, which is currently being introduced into legislation in New Jersey, are a great tool that could be used as a guideline. Dr. Heather Ashton, creator of the Ashton Manual, ran a clinic in the United Kingdom from 1982 to 1994 for benzodiazepine withdrawal. Her research is centered on the effects of psychotropic drugs including nicotine, cannabis, benzodiazepines, antidepressants, and others. In the manual, the half-life of benzodiazepines and directions for cross over to longer-acting benzodiazepines with respect to dosing are outlined.[10] Physicians are in need of best practices in tapering benzodiazepines at a measured pace. Much work is needed to combat the stigma associated with this process.

The neurological system is the slowest healing system in the body. When a nerve is damaged, it takes 6–9 months to regenerate. Benzodiazepines work on GABA receptors, which are key in nerve functioning. When a benzodiazepine is ingested, it modulates the GABA receptors all over the body. GABA also works in balance with glutamate, an excitatory neurotransmitter. Therefore, when someone stops a benzodiazepine, glutamate becomes the dominant neurotransmitter in the brain, causing a whole host of very uncomfortable symptoms such as muscle twitches, spasms, and/or seizures.

What is needed is to follow a conservative protocol that facilitates a patient–physician relationship that is patient-centered. Empowering patients through education and planning is the crux of a successful tapering regimen. It is important to educate physicians and collaborate in a way that includes innovative methodologies such as digital health programs as well as the use of compounding pharmacies to measure accurate dosing and reductions. A common tapering strategy is based on the Ashton method and suggests no more than a 10% medication reduction every 2 to 4 weeks to help stave off severe withdrawal symptoms.[10] Compounding the medication into a liquid titration or capsules can simplify the process and allow for more accurate dosing. However, some individuals need slower tapering such as 2.5% every 7–10 days or 5% every 2 weeks. Some individuals need to cut 2.5% and hold until their symptoms stabilize so they can make their next cut/taper.

What is very important to note is that blood serum levels need to be stable throughout the day so that the individual tapering can maintain some manageable level of activities of daily living in between dose reduction. Practitioners in methadone clinics have known this for years, and benzodiazepines need the same amount of careful discernment in keeping individuals stable as they taper. Due to the half-life of the medication, it is important to factor that into the taper. If someone is taking alprazolam, they need to dose four times daily due to the approximate 6-hour half-life. Lorazepam in general is dosed three times daily due to the 8-hour half-life, and clonazepam is dosed twice daily due to the 12-hour half-life. Diazepam is dosed once daily due to 30-hour half-life. The half-life of all of these drugs is approximate due to inter-individual variability in metabolism and excretion rates. When tapering, a person would need to make even cuts across the doses. For example, if someone is taking 1 mg of Ativan a day (individual doses of 0.33 mg three times daily), a 5% dose decrease would be 0.316 mg three times daily for a total of 0.95 mg, and then the next step would be 0.3 mg three times daily for a total of 0.9 mg with a duration hold at each level anywhere from 7 to 14 days or holding until the withdrawal symptoms stabilize. The only accurate way of performing these dose tapers is to have the dose compounded at a compounding pharmacy or prescribing the liquid form of these medications for accurate measurement.

The need for daily support during this long process is crucial as indicated earlier with individuals looking to the informal groups on the Internet such as Benzo Buddies and closed Facebook groups for support and advice. Professional virtual support is much needed to provide privacy, confidentiality, and accessibility to those who may be homebound by temporary symptoms of agoraphobia, living in rural areas, or who are struggling to make it through the workday due to vestibular challenges, weakness, and/or stress-induced triggers to use again and/or panic attacks. Helping people understand their severe symptoms and identify the use of coping tools during withdrawal as well as the use of problem-solving skills to navigate the red tape around withdrawal will increase the chance of success. A person's radical acceptance of the severe symptoms is crucial to help manage daily challenges that present often for many months to sometimes years. Some are at risk of taking their own life due to the severity of the withdrawal symptoms. This process can only be done with sufficient support; sending someone home with a tapering plan and a follow-up check in 1–2 months is not sufficient.

The use of virtual recovery coaches, collaboration between doctors, and a virtual medical team are just some of the many ways to address this gap in services where behavioral health techniques to support emotional states in conjunction with patients' personalized tapering protocols can be taught and implemented. The introduction, practice, and tracking of coping tools such as affirmations, positive self-talk, and cognitive behavior therapy (CBT) techniques such as reality testing and journaling are also useful. Additional tools working with fears and feelings, such as Jin Shin Jyutsu, which include breathing techniques, grounding exercises, meditation, visualization, emotional freedom technique (tapping), and guided imagery, can be taught and modeled virtually to help in coping with some of the withdrawal symptoms.

Furthermore, assisting people in withdrawal with accessing community resources, such as community acupuncture and traditional acupuncture, along with the framework of Maslow's Hierarchy of Needs in mind, will help them to connect with others in the community and meet the need for the sense of belongingness. Likewise, daily reminders about the importance of keeping things simple by getting back to the basics in life such as eating nutrient-dense food and drinking clean purified water help to meet the physiological needs for feeling well. According to Maslow, one cannot connect with others unless one's physiological and security needs are met.[11]

Individuals in acute withdrawal are often weak, nauseous, and dizzy. Focusing on helping individual function by assessing their basic physiological needs, helping to simplify their life to meet their basic needs while in withdrawal, and accepting temporary limitations and setbacks are all very crucial to a successful healing journey. It can be a very long process, and living with the hundreds of symptoms in withdrawal 24/7 can be exhausting. Even during slow tapers, individuals experience a multitude of symptoms that affect activities of daily living.

Patience and support are central to sustaining the long-term healing of the central nervous system. Having access to family support systems fosters a sense of belongingness. According to the Rat Park Study by Bruce Aleksander, that sense of belonging has profound implications. Recovery was found to be more likely if individuals had connections with others and were involved in engaging activities in their environment.[12] Daily support keeps these areas in perspective through techniques such as motivational interviewing and can help keep those in recovery focused.

Services like Lucid Lane are helpful in long-term discharge planning from recovery centers for traditional addiction and partnering with those afflicted with accidental dependency, but they are only able to scratch the surface of the need at this point. The need is growing as we enter an epidemic emerging from the shadows of the opiate crisis. Clients facing arrested development, unhealed trauma, nutritional deficiencies, and/or genetic mutations, such as the MTHFR gene that has been indicated in mental health,[13] virtual ongoing support as well as daily on the ground support is much needed to fill the gap in services for long-term recovery. Through a holistic and comprehensive approach that includes personalized medication tapering strategies, and behavioral health techniques, along with innovative digital health programs, a cohesive effort needs to be made to combat the global epidemic caused by the uncontrolled misuse and overprescribing of habit-forming medications such as benzodiazepines and opioids and to support education in deprescribing practices.

REFERENCES

1. Bohnert A., Guy G., Losby J. Opioid Prescribing in the United States Before and After the Centers for Disease Control and Prevention's 2016 Opioid Guideline. *Ann Intern Med* 2018; 169(6): 367–375. doi:10.7326/M18-1243
2. Bachhuber M.A. Hennessy S. Cunningham C.O., Starrels J.L. Increasing Benzodiazepine Prescriptions and Overdose Mortality in the United States, 1996–2013. *Am J Public Health.* 2016 April; 106(4): 686–688. Published online April. doi:10.2105/AJPH.2016.303061
3. Hauser K.F., Knapp P.E. Opiate Drugs with Abuse Liability Hijack the Endogenous Opioid System to Disrupt Neuronal and Glial Maturation in the Central Nervous System. *Front Pediatr.* 2018; 23(5): 294. doi:10.3389/fped.2017.00294
4. Rocket I.R.H., Caine E.D., Connery H.S., et al. Mortality in the United Stated from Self-Injury Surpasses Diabetes: A Prevention Imperative Injury Prevention. Inj Prev 2019; 25(4): 331–333. Published online 27 August 2018. doi:10.1136/injuryprev-2018-042889
5. Busto U., Sellers E.M., Naranjo C.A., Cappell H., Sanchez-Craig M., Sykora K. Withdrawal Reaction after Long-Term Therapeutic Use of Benzodiazepines. *N Engl J Med* 1986; 315(14): 854–859. https://www.ncbi.nlm.nih.gov/pubmed/3092053
6. Shah A., Hayes C.J., Martin B.C. Characteristics of Initial Prescription Episodes and Likelihood of Long-Term Opioid Use — United States, 2006–2015. *MMWR Morb Mortal Wkly Rep* 2017; 66(10): 265–269. doi:10.15585/mmwr.mm6610a1
7. De Vries T.J., Shippenberg T.S. Neural Systems Underlying Opiate Addiction. *J Neurosci* 2002; 22(9): 3321–3325.
8. NIDA. Drugs, Brains, and Behavior: The Science of Addiction. 20 July 2018. Retrieved from https://www.drugabuse.gov/publications/drugs-brains-behavior-science-addiction. Accessed on 13 February 2019.
9. Karamitros, T., et al. Human Endogenous Retrovirus-K HML-2 Integration within RASGRF2 Is Associated with Intravenous Drug Abuse and Modulates Transcription in a Cell-Line Model. *Proc Nat Acad Sci* 2018; 115(41): 10434–10439.
10. Ashton H. Benzodiazepines: How They Work & How to Withdraw, the Ashton Manual. 2002. Benzo.org.uk. Retrieved from http://benzo.org.uk/manual/bzcha01.htm. Accessed on 3 March 2019.
11. McLeod S.A. Maslow's Hierarchy of Needs. 2017. Retrieved from www.simplypsychology.org/maslow.html
12. Peele S. *The Meaning of Addiction*. Lexington, MA: DC Heath; 1985: 77–96.
13. Wan L., Li Y., Zhang, Z. et al. Methylenetetrahydrofolate Reductase and Psychiatric Diseases. *Transl Psychiatry.* 2018; 8(1): 242. Published online 5 November 2018. doi:10.1038/s41398-018-0276-6

24 Naloxone Use in the Opioid Epidemic

Sahar Swidan and Ellen Klepack

CONTENTS

Drug overdose deaths continue to rise in the United States. Two out of three overdose deaths involve an opioid, which includes prescription opioids, heroin, and synthetic opioids such as fentanyl.[1] In 2017, opioid overdoses killed more than 47,000 people, with 36% involving prescription opioids.[2] Illicit opioids have now surpassed prescription opioids as the most common drug involved in overdose deaths in the United States.[3] Opioid overdose deaths have increased across all races and for both adult men and women of all ages.[1]

According to the U.S. Centers for Disease Control and Prevention,[4] the rise in opioid overdose deaths can be outlined in three distinct waves (Figure 24.1):

- The first wave began when opioid prescribing increased in the 1990s, with overdose deaths involving prescription opioids (natural and semi-synthetic opioids and methadone) increasing since at least 1999.
- The second wave began in 2010, with rapid increases in overdose deaths involving heroin.
- The third wave began in 2013, with significant increases in overdose deaths involving synthetic opioids—particularly those involving illicitly manufactured fentanyl. The illicit fentanyl market continues to change, and fentanyl can be found in combination with heroin, counterfeit pills, and cocaine. Carfentanil, a synthetic opioid used to tranquilize large animals, is also becoming more popular on the illicit market, used to "cut" heroin and increase profits for dealers. Carfentanil is estimated to be 100 times more potent than fentanyl and 10,000 times more potent than morphine. It has a quick onset and is short-acting.

Given current numbers, it is projected that 700,400 people in the United States will die of an opioid overdose between the years of 2016 and 2025, and 80% of these deaths will be attributed to illicit opioids.[5] The opioid crisis is now widely recognized as a complex problem that will require healthcare, legislative, and community support to effectively address. In 2017, the U.S. Department of Health and Human Services launched a comprehensive five-point strategy to combat the opioid crisis.[6] The five-point strategy consists of the following:

- Access: better prevention, treatment, and recovery services
- Data: better data on the epidemic
- Pain: better pain management
- Overdoses: better targeting of overdose-reversing drugs
- Research: better research on pain and addiction

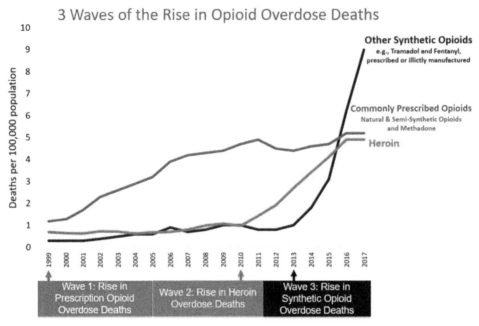

FIGURE 24.1   Three waves of the rise in opioid overdose deaths.

NALOXONE

Naloxone is thought to be a competitive antagonist of the mu- (highest affinity), kappa-, and delta-receptors, inhibiting both the toxic and clinical effects of opioids, making it an effective antidote for opioid overdoses.[7] An opioid overdose can be identified by a combination of three signs and symptoms known as the "opioid overdose triad":[8]

- Pinpoint pupils
- Unconsciousness
- Respiratory depression

Other symptoms of overdose can include chocking or gurgling sounds, limp body, and pale, blue, or cold skin.

When an overdose is suspected, naloxone should be used within 4–6 minutes to prevent major brain damage or death, making it a critical component in combating the opioid crisis. It generally takes effect within a few minutes and lasts for 30–90 minutes, depending on the individual's metabolism and the amount of opioid used. Because its antagonism is short-lived, repeat doses may be needed when long-acting opioids are involved, or if there is an insufficient response. Activating EMS 911 is critical and should be done immediately as medical management is necessary after overdose. Naloxone can precipitate opioid withdrawal if large doses are given. The person being revived may wake up combative and have other side effects due to withdrawal, which are generally not life-threatening. Additional signs of acute withdrawal include agitation, tachycardia, nausea, vomiting, piloerection, diarrhea, lacrimation, yawning, rhinorrhea, and hyperhidrosis. These symptoms tend to dissipate after 30–60 minutes due to the relatively short half-life of naloxone.[9] Naloxone cannot be abused and does not produce euphoria. In cases of maternal opioid overdose during pregnancy, naloxone use is safe and recommended as a life-saving measure; however, induced withdrawal may contribute to fetal distress.[10] Allergic reactions to naloxone are rare.

TABLE 24.1

Naloxone Product Comparison

	Injectable Generic (Atomizer Adapter)	Injectable Generic (Vial)	Intranasal	Auto-Injector
Brand name			Narcan	Evzio Auto-Injector
FDA-approved	X (Approved for IV, IM, SC, intranasal use off-label)	X	X	X
Assembly required	X	X		
Strength	1 mg/ml	0.4 mg/ml vial 4 mg/10 ml vial	4 mg/0.1 ml	2 mg/0.4 ml
Directions	Spray 1 ml (1/2 syringe) into each nostril. Repeat after 2–3 minutes if no or minimal response.	Inject 1 ml in shoulder or thigh. Repeat after 2–3 minutes if no or minimal response.	Spray 0.1 ml into one nostril. Repeat with second device into other nostril after 2–3 minutes if no or minimal response.	Inject into outer thigh as directed by English voice prompt system. Place black side firmly on outer thigh and depress and hold for 5 seconds. Repeat with second device in 2–3 minutes if no or minimal response.
Cost per kit	$$	$	$$	$$$
Storage (protect from light)	Store at 59–86° F.	Store at 68–77°F.	Store at 59–77°F. Excursions from 39 to 104°F.	Store at 59–77°F. Excursions from 39 to 104°F.

Source: Reference 11.

Naloxone is commercially available as a nasal spray and as an IV, SC, and IM injection (Table 24.1). Narcan® was the first U.S. Food and Drug Administration (FDA)-approved nasal spray in 2015. The first generic version of Narcan® nasal spray was approved in April 2019. A prefilled syringe of naloxone, administered with an atomizer for intranasal administration, can also be used as an off-label option in opioid overdose situations.

The most expensive option on the market is Evzio®. Approved in April 2014, Evzio® is a prefilled auto-injector that contains both voice and visual guidance for use during an overdose emergency. This product is intended for nonmedical persons. In December of 2018, the maker of Evzio® announced that a generic version of their product would be made available.

Larger doses of naloxone may be required to resuscitate individuals who have a suspected carfentanil overdose. A case study by Bardsley[12] looked at the use of high-dose naloxone in two patients who presented to a small community hospital with suspected carfentanil overdose. Both patients were successfully resuscitated with high doses of naloxone. Patient 1 required a total of 12 mg to be successfully resuscitated and patient 2 required a total of 10 mg for successful resuscitation. The authors of this study concluded that higher than standard doses of naloxone may be needed depending on the opioid overdose. Larger studies are needed to further explore naloxone dosing in cases where the overdose is due to an extremely high-potency opioid.

Overdoses can be the result of ingesting "cocktails" including opioids, alcohol, benzodiazepines, muscle relaxers, and sometimes stimulants. Naloxone will only reverse the opioid part of the overdose and does not work on alcohol, stimulant, or benzodiazepine overdoses. If first responders are unsure if opioids are in any way involved with an unresponsive person, it is recommended to give the person naloxone while waiting for EMS to arrive.

INCREASING ACCESS TO NALOXONE

Access to naloxone has been increasing in recent years. Between 2017 and 2018, naloxone prescriptions doubled from 270,000 prescriptions written in 2017 to 556,000 prescriptions written in 2018.[13] During this same time, prescriptions for high-dose opioids decreased from 48 million in 2017 to 38 million in 2018. Prescriptions for naloxone, while increasing, are still low compared to the number of patients who are prescribed high-dose opioids. To put these numbers into perspective, if each person prescribed a high-dose opioid in 2018 also received a prescription for naloxone, 9 million prescriptions for naloxone would have been written.[13] The CDC guidelines for prescribing opioids for chronic pain recommend that healthcare providers co-prescribe naloxone along with a high-dose opioid prescription in patients at risk for overdose including:[14]

- Patients with a history of overdose
- Patients with a history of substance use disorder
- Patients taking benzodiazepines with opioids
- Patients returning to a high dose to which they are no longer tolerant
- Patients taking opioids at a dose of ≥50 MME/day (Table 24.2)

Many states allow pharmacists to dispense naloxone without a prescription, otherwise known as "standing orders." In addition to providing greater access to naloxone, it is also necessary for

---

TABLE 24.2

Calculating Morphine Milligram Equivalents (MME)[a] for Commonly Prescribed Opioids

Opioid[b]	Conversion Factor[c]
Codeine	0.15
Fentanyl transdermal (mcg/hr)	2.4
Hydrocodone	1
Hydromorphone	4
Methadone: 1–20 mg/day	4
Methadone: 21–40 mg/day	8
Methadone: 41–60 mg/day	10
Methadone: ≥61–80 mg/day	12
Morphine	1
Oxycodone	1.5
Oxymorphone	3
Tapentadol[d]	0.4

[a] MME=dose of opioid multiplied by the conversion factor.

[b] All doses in mg/day, except fentanyl, which should be in mcg/hr before multiplying by conversion factor.

[c] Dose conversions are estimated and cannot account for all individual differences in genetics and pharmacokinetics.

[d] Tapentadol is a mu-receptor agonist and norepinephrine reuptake inhibitor. MMEs are based on degree of mu-receptor agonist activity, but it is unknown if this drug is associated with overdose in the same dose-dependent manner as observed with medications that are solely mu-receptor agonists.

Source: Reference 15.

healthcare providers to become actively involved in providing education on both opioid overdose and the proper use of naloxone during an emergency situation. Education is important not only for the patient, but also any household members and for the greater community.

The FDA has addressed better targeting of naloxone in the community through supporting the development of over-the-counter (OTC) forms of naloxone. In an effort to speed development of OTC versions, the FDA created labeling that can be used by sponsors to obtain approval of naloxone for OTC status.[16]

Cost can also be a barrier to naloxone access and use. In September of 2019, the FDA announced its commitment to prioritize and expedite the review of generic medications indicated for the emergency treatment of opioid overdoses.[17]

CONCLUSION

The opioid crisis was created by multiple factors, and it will take a concerted effort from multiple disciplines, including healthcare professionals, legislators, and the general public, to address it effectively. Wider access to naloxone is an important component to help fight opioid deaths and ensure that this crisis does not continue in the future.

REFERENCES

1. Hedegaard H., Miniño A.M., Warner M. Drug overdose deaths in the United States, 1999–2017. *NCHS Data Brief*. Hyattsville, MD: National Center for Health Statistics. 2018;329. Cited by: Center for disease control and prevention, national center for injury prevention and control. Overview of the drug overdose epidemic: behind the numbers. https://www.cdc.gov/drugoverdose/data/index.html. Accessed December 16, 2019.
2. Scholl L., Seth P., Kariisa M., Wilson N., Baldwin G. Drug and opioid-involved overdose deaths – United States. *Morb Mortal Wkly Rep*. ePub: December 21, 2018. 2013–2017. Cited by: center for disease control and prevention, national center for injury prevention and control. Overview of the drug overdose epidemic: behind the numbers. https://www.cdc.gov/drugoverdose/data/index.html. Accessed December 16, 2019.
3. Jones C.M., Einstein E.B., Compton W.M. Changes in synthetic opioid involvement in drug overdose deaths in the United States, 2010–2016. *JAMA* 2018;319(17):1819–1821. Cited by: National institute on drug abuse. Nearly half of opioid-related overdose deaths involve fentanyl. National institute on drug abuse website. May 1, 2018. https://www.drugabuse.gov/news-events/news-releases/2018/05/nearly-half-opioid-related-overdose-deaths-involve-fentanyl. Accessed December 16, 2019.
4. Center for Disease Control and Prevention, National Center for Injury Prevention and Control. Three waves of opioid overdose deaths. https://www.cdc.gov/drugoverdose/epidemic/index.html. Accessed December 16, 2019.
5. Chen Q., Larochelle M.R., Weaver D.T., Lietz A.P., Mueller P.P., Mercaldo S., et al. Prevention of prescription opioid misuse and projected overdose deaths in the United States. *JAMA Network Open* 2019;2(2):e187621.
6. U.S. Department of Health and Human Services. 5-point strategy to combat the opioid crisis. https://www.hhs.gov/opioids/about-the-epidemic/hhs-response/index.html. Accessed December 16, 2019.
7. Physicians' Desk Reference. Naloxone hydrochloride-drug summary. https://www.pdr.net/drug-summary/Narcan-naloxone-hydrochloride-3837.6202. Accessed December 16, 2019.
8. World Health Organization. Information sheet on opioid overdose. August 2018. https://www.who.int/substance_abuse/information-sheet/en/. Accessed December 16, 2019.
9. Wermeling D.P. Review of naloxone safety for opioid overdose: practical considerations for new technology and expanded public access. *Ther Adv Drug Saf* 2015;6(1):20–31.
10. Committee on Obstetric Practice. Committee opinion no.711: opioid use and opioid use disorder in pregnancy. *Obstet Gynecol* 2017;130(2):e81–e94.
11. Prescribe to Prevent. Naloxone Product Comparison. https://prescribetoprevent.org/wp2015/wp-content/uploads/Naloxone-product-chart.17_04_14.pdf. Accessed December 16, 2019.
12. Bardsley R. Higher dosing may be required for opioid overdose. *Am J Health Syst Pharm* 2019;76(22):1835–1837.

13. Center for Disease Control and Prevention, National Center for Injury Prevention and Control. Life-saving naloxone from pharmacies. More dispensing needed despite progress. https://www.cdc.gov/vital signs/naloxone/index.html. Accessed December 16, 2019.

14. Dowell D., Haegerich T.M., Chou R. CDC guideline for prescribing opioids for chronic pain — United States, 2016. *MMWR Recomm Rep* 2016;65(1):1–49.

15. Centers for Disease Control and Prevention, National Center for Injury Prevention. CDC guideline for prescribing opioids for chronic pain. https://www.cdc.gov/drugoverdose/prescribing/guideline.html. Accessed December 16, 2009.

16. Statement from FDA Commissioner Scott Gottlieb, M.D., on unprecedented new efforts to support development of over-the-counter naloxone to help reduce opioid overdose deaths [Press Announcement]. *U.S. Food and Drug Administration* January 17, 2019. https://www.fda.gov/news-events/press-announc ements/statement-fda-commissioner-scott-gottlieb-md-unprecedented-new-efforts-support-developme nt-over. Accessed December 16, 2019.

17. Statement on continued efforts to increase availability of all forms of naloxone to help reduce opioid over-dose deaths [Press Announcement]. *U.S. Food and Drug Administration*. September 20, 2019. https://www.fda.gov/news-events/press-announcements/statement-continued-efforts-increase-availability-all-forms-naloxone-help-reduce-opioid-overdose. Accessed December 16, 2019.

25 Psychological Intervention
Cognitive-Behavioral Therapy

Samantha Rafie, Sarah Rispinto, and Sarah Martin

CONTENTS

INTRODUCTION

The following chapter aims to introduce readers to the biopsychosocial model of managing chronic pain, with emphasis on the role of psychological intervention. To better understand the biopsychosocial model, the role of the brain in the pain experience will be expanded upon. A brief overview of cognitive-behavioral therapy will be presented, underscoring the importance of cognitive processes and behaviors in the management of chronic pain. Finally, the unique considerations in pediatric treatment will be presented and discussed including family and parent involvement and the role of school and social functioning.

Chronic pain is a pervasive public health problem associated with high costs for treatment and loss of productivity. Estimates according to the Centers for Disease Control and Prevention suggest up to 20.4% of U.S. adults experience chronic pain.[1] Approximately 5–38% of children and adolescents suffer from chronic pain,[2,3] and up to 73% of pediatric patients with chronic pain will continue to have pain into adulthood and are likely to later develop new pain conditions.[4,5]

The International Association for the Study of Pain defines pain as "an unpleasant sensory and emotional experience associated with, or resembling that associated with, actual or potential tissue damage."[6] Embedded within this global definition is not only the subjective experience of pain, but also the biological, psychological, and social aspects that contribute to a pain experience. This pain may be acute or chronic, each with distinct characteristics. Acute pain is typically associated with an injury or tissue damage, and the pain typically resolves itself within 3 months or less. This is in contrast to chronic pain, which may or may not be associated with an injury or tissue damage and tends to persist for 3 months or longer. Acute pain and chronic pain are treated within different frameworks; acute pain is best treated within a biomedical model, whereas chronic pain is best treated with a biopsychosocial model.

A biomedical approach to acute pain typically includes the expectation of "fixing" or "curing" the source of pain with the subsequent resolution of pain. For example, if a patient arrives at the physician's office with a laceration, the expectation is that a physician will either repair the injury through medical intervention, such as stitches, or provide analgesic medication. The period of discomfort or injury is expected to be time-limited. Biomedical approaches aim to cure or alleviate symptoms. Such an approach may be limited with chronic pain, which requires a comprehensive and holistic approach viewed through the biopsychosocial model of illness. This model, developed and introduced by George Engel in 1977, suggests that the biological, psychological, and social aspects of a person's functioning are to be considered as a whole and not in isolation.[7-9] The model was later applied to pain by Loeser (1982), who expanded on the model to include the multidimensional interaction of pain and disability.[10] The biopsychosocial approach has been touted as the optimal paradigm for the treatment of chronic pain. The biological factors are still addressed within this framework, and include, but are not limited to, physical health, genetic vulnerabilities, and nociception; however, psychosocial factors are critical considerations. These psychological experiences, for example, personality, coping skills, depression, fear, and catastrophizing, are important factors to address and treat as part of the pain experience. Socio-contextual factors including family, friends, and socioeconomic status also play a vital role in understanding a person's overall pain experience. When pain persists, psychosocial factors must be addressed and are known to be the strongest predictors of pain-related treatment outcomes.[11-13] While traditional biomedical approaches focus on curative treatments, the biopsychosocial model for treatment empowers patients to self-manage their pain through improved functioning and optimizing their overall quality of life. Biopsychosocial paradigms are best implemented as interdisciplinary approaches that integrate medicine, physical therapy, and psychology.

Psychology is embedded within the definition of pain. Not only can pain be a frustrating and depressing experience, but depression and other psychological experiences exacerbate the perception of pain. Chronic pain can affect mood, relationships, work, school, and overall ability to function. This can lead to feelings of anger, hopelessness, and depression. Psychologists and other psychotherapists specialized in chronic pain management help people living with chronic pain to better manage their reactions and improve their pain coping skills. A goal of treatment is to address the patient's overall pain experience by also exploring ways of thinking differently about their pain. Cognitive-behavioral therapy, considered the gold standard for the treatment of chronic pain, has the strongest evidence base for treatment and will be presented in greater detail later in this chapter. One of the main goals of psychological treatment is not to get rid of the pain, but for the patient to learn to accept the pain and improve their mood and functioning in spite of the pain using an adaptive set of behavioral pain management skills and techniques.

THE BRAIN

The first prominent theory of pain, proposed by Descartes, stated that pain was an injury or pathology-determined sensory process; however, it is now accepted that pain perception is a complex, biopsychosocial process that involves sensory, cognitive, and emotional processing. In 1965, Melzack and Wall proposed the Gate Control Theory of Pain, which revolutionized pain science. The Gate Control Theory of Pain emphasized the active role of central, neural mechanisms in pain perception and modulation.[14] Specifically, the Gate Control Theory proposed that a gating mechanism in the dorsal horn of the spine modulates nerve impulses from afferent fibers to spinal cord transmission cells, and small and large fibers can open and close the "Gate," respectively. Descending nerve impulses from the brain also act on the gating mechanism. Collectively, the Gate affects the output of spinal cord transmission cells in response to stimulation, and the level of central and sensory inputs affects brain activity. Ultimately, the experience of "pain" occurs when brain activity reaches a certain level.

The Gate Control Theory and the subsequent efforts to expand on this work highlighted the importance of central input modulation and biopsychosocial mechanisms in pain processing. With greater use of the spinal cordotomy procedure, phantom limb pain challenges led Melzack to expand on the Gate Control Theory and propose the *neuromatrix* concept. The development of the neuromatrix stemmed from the understanding that central neural processes and sensory perception can be modulated and experienced with or without peripheral inputs. The neuromatrix model postulates that the interaction of cognitive, sensory, and affective neural components determines pain perception and pain modulatory responses.[15] Thus, the brain interprets cognitive, sensory, and affective inputs to determine whether stimulation is dangerous (i.e., painful), how painful that stimulation is, and what descending modulatory or protective response is needed.

Advances in brain imaging methodologies have allowed for the identification of neural components implicated in pain processing and examination of chronic pain-related alterations in neural processes. Imaging data consistently indicate that brain areas associated with sensory, cognitive, emotional, social, and behavioral processes make up what is now often referred to as the *pain connectome*.[16] Specifically, key brain regions responsible for nociceptive and pain processing include the primary and secondary somatosensory cortices, primary motor and supplementary motor cortices, insular cortex, anterior cingulate cortex, prefrontal cortex, thalamus, and regions in the hippocampus, amygdala, and basal ganglia that process fear, emotion, and memory.[17,18] Although similar brain regions are implicated in chronic pain processing, extant data suggest that individuals with chronic pain exhibit dysfunction in endogenous pain modulatory systems, structural (i.e. grey matter density and volume) and functional (i.e., default mode network and regional connectivity) brain differences, and alterations in neurochemical systems (i.e., glutamatergic, GABAergic, opioidergic, and dopaminergic systems).[17–19]

Further, findings from imaging and experimental pain studies indicate that individuals with chronic pain may exhibit *central sensitization*. Central sensitization is a process by which the brain experiences pain in response to an innocuous stimulus and amplifies and/or prolongs this perception of pain. This amplified pain response may occur from both increased activation of nociceptive pathways and dysfunction in descending pain modulatory systems.

Given the evidence of neural dysfunction or alteration in regions or neurochemical processes associated with cognitive, and emotional functioning, it is not surprising that individuals with chronic pain exhibit impairment in these areas. Individuals with chronic pain demonstrate impairment in working memory tasks, emotional decision-making, awareness, and judgment.[20,21] More recent work highlights how the associated psychobiological stress associated with the progression of chronic pain may result in altered reward-aversion homeostatic function.[22] As chronic pain progresses, allostatic load increases, and surges in stress-related neurochemicals (e.g., norepinephrine, glutamate, vasopressin) result in reward deficiency and negative affective states, such as decreased motivation, anxiety, and depression.

Cognitive-behavioral and neuromodulatory (e.g., hypnosis and mindfulness) psychological treatment may help reduce the negative impact of chronic pain. Imaging studies show that these therapies have an effect on pain-related brain structure and function. Mindfulness meditation has been shown to increase activity in the anterior cingulate cortex and insula and induce analgesia through non-opioidergic mechanisms.[23,24] Imaging studies examining hypnosis report hypnotic analgesia activity in pain-processing supraspinal areas, including the thalamus, sensory cortices, insula, anterior cingulate cortex, and frontal attentional control systems.[25–27] Data also suggest that cognitive-behavioral-based therapies may affect cognitive control, or top-down processing of pain. Specifically, participation in cognitive-behavioral therapy has been shown to increase prefrontal cortex activation (ventrolateral prefrontal/lateral orbitofrontal cortex), increase gray matter in the posterior parietal and prefrontal cortices, and decrease the processing of painful input in somatosensory and midcingulate cortices.[17, 28–30]

Taken together, neuroimaging data provide important insights into the role of cognitive and emotional processing of pain and support a biopsychosocial approach to understanding and addressing chronic pain. Psychological factors affect how pain is experienced, and chronic pain is associated with altered neurological functioning and impaired functioning. Thus, the chronic pain state is likely to result in an unfortunate negative cycle if integrative treatment is not provided.

COGNITIVE-BEHAVIORAL THERAPY

Pain is complex and involves many factors including cognition, emotions, affect, mood, attention, and social factors.[31] Psychosocial approaches to pain management address the psychological, behavioral, social, and cultural domains in the pain experience. The goal of treatment is to empower people living with pain to better manage their pain and improve their overall functioning and well-being through applied skills and techniques acquired in a supportive treatment milieu. This care typically includes psychoeducation, cognitive-behavioral interventions, acceptance and commitment therapy, and mindfulness-based stress reduction. Cognitive behavioral therapy (CBT) is a first-line treatment for chronic pain, alone or in combination with interdisciplinary pain rehabilitation.[32,33] This treatment (CBT) aims to improve an individual's coping with chronic pain through a series of both cognitive (i.e., pertaining to thoughts) and behavioral (i.e., actions and choices) changes. Treatment often involves goal setting and problem solving to help individuals function better with an improvement in overall quality of life.

Numerous studies on behavioral and cognitive treatments for chronic pain demonstrate strong efficacy and establish its utility in stabilizing mood, restoring function, and decreasing pain and illness-focused behavior.[34] Futhermore, the use of CBT in treating chronic pain impacts the pain experience, the use of adaptive versus maladaptive coping, overall activity level, and social function.[35] Regardless of patient baseline characteristics, such as number of pain sites, rumination, stress before treatment, or the severity of the disability, the effects of CBT were consistently robust,[36] and outcomes were stable at 3, 6, and 12 months post-treatment.[37,38] Similar results as seen in adults were also found in pediatric populations.[39,40]

COGNITION

Cognitions play a vital role in the way a person experiences chronic pain. Cognitive distortions are negatively biased errors in thinking[41] that increase vulnerability to emotional and behavioral responses. There are common cognitive distortions, or thinking errors, that influence how an individual responds to pain, including the following: mindreading, catastrophizing, all-or-nothing thinking, emotional reasoning, labeling, mental filtering, overgeneralization, personalization, should statements, and minimizing.[42–44] Pain catastrophizing is commonly presented due to the high correlation between catastrophizing and adjustment to pain.[45]

Pain catastrophizing is the way in which an individual generates negative, worst-case scenarios regarding their pain and disability.[46] Sullivan defines catastrophizing as "an exaggerated negative mental set brought to bear during an actual or anticipated pain experience."[45] Pain catastrophizing is associated with poor pain-related outcomes and disability.[47,48] The impact on pain catastrophizing and pain-related outcomes has been well-documented in the literature, suggesting that patients with high pain catastrophizing have poor responses to pain treatment,[49,50] poor response following surgery,[51] and are more likely to misuse opioids.[52] In addition, pain catastrophizing is associated with heightened pain intensity, muscle tenderness,[48] and increased affective distress, including anxiety and depression.[49,53,54] Further, both child and parent catastrophizing is associated with poor child functioning and maladaptive pain behaviors.[55,56]

One's thoughts and beliefs about one's pain significantly affect one's pain experience. Ongoing catastrophization contributes to avoidance of activity and associated disability,[57] which perpetuates the chronic pain cycle. Cognitive restructuring, a core component of CBT,[58] is a technique that aims at challenging and changing one's unhealthy or maladaptive thoughts by identifying new alternatives to one's experiences.[44] Cognitive restructuring includes identifying the automatic thought or faulty thought, identifying the unpleasant or negative emotions, challenging the thought, and changing the thought.[59,60] The first step to changing maladaptive thought patterns is to bring awareness to the automatic thoughts we experience. Oftentimes, these thoughts happen outside of one's awareness and bringing them to the surface can aid in one's ability to modify them. Of importance is the ability to link how negative thoughts contribute to affective distress or negative emotional states including depression, anxiety, and anger.[45] As self-awareness grows and individuals are able to recognize how their thoughts influence their mood, and subsequently their pain, they are better able to challenge the validity of their distorted thoughts and incorporate more adaptive thoughts.[43]

BEHAVIOR

The purpose of modifying the individual's maladaptive thoughts regarding their pain is to achieve changes in emotion and behavior. Once the individual in pain learns a new relationship with their pain through psychoeducation, cognitive restructuring, and coping skills training, they are then prepared for behavior modification. This is an approach to behavior change that functions on the basic principles of operant and classical conditioning.[35,61,62] The primary target is behavioral activation, with the purpose of remedying muscle deterioration and depression associated with reduced activity.

Long-term goals are identified at the outset of treatment, and short-term goals are developed to gauge consistent progress. Setting weekly goals allows individuals with chronic pain to begin or increase recreational and social activities, work, school, and home duties, while working to decrease reliance on medications and rest as the primary tools for pain coping. Goal setting often includes consideration of medical and physical therapy recommendations, including adherence to a regimented home exercise program and medication changes. Activity pacing is an important part of the behavior plan to avoid over- and under-exertion.[63] Progress toward these goals should be reinforced by treating providers, and challenges problem-solved in order to develop more realistic goals and plans if needed.

Fear of re-injury is a significant contributor to reduced activity levels, in addition to catastrophization, which lead to avoidance behaviors.[64] Graded activity and graded exposure are commonly used to improve activity tolerance and to achieve functional goals.[65] Graded exposure allows for dosed confrontation to feared situations, gradually increasing through a defined hierarchy, and is effective in reducing pain-related fear and disability.[62,66] The focus with both interventions is on small, achievable goals, pacing activities, and inspiring self-reinforcement through objective feedback on progress.

PEDIATRIC CONSIDERATIONS

Studies estimate that up to 50% of children with pain report multiple pain sites, including back, abdominal, limb, and headache pain.[3,67,68] Overall, the prevalence of pediatric chronic pain tends to increase with age and is more common in females.[3] Studies of pain within clinical samples reveal that children with sickle cell disease, arthritis, and cancer often experience recurrent pain.[69–71] Furthermore, youth with chronic pain report significant impairment in physical, psychological, social, and academic functioning.[72–75]

Although some commonalities exist among adult and pediatric chronic pain prevalence and outcome data, children and adolescents should not be approached as "little adults." The assessment and treatment of pediatric chronic pain needs to account for important developmental and social considerations within a biopsychosocial perspective. The childhood and adolescent period is marked by significant changes in physical, neurological, cognitive, and social development, all of which need to be considered when treating youth with chronic pain. In addition, family, social, and school contexts all play an important role during this period and will likely affect treatment.[76] Although data on adults are more robust, research does support the use of cognitive-behavioral treatment for pediatric chronic pain.[39,77–80] This section will start with a general discussion of assessment of chronic pain in pediatric patients and then briefly discuss developmental, family, social, and academic considerations in the assessment and treatment of pediatric chronic pain.

The pediatric chronic pain prevalence data indicate that pediatric chronic pain exists and evidence-based assessment of pain is the first step to understanding how to best approach treatment. In general, expert consensus indicates that pediatric pain assessment should include the assessment of pain intensity, physical and emotional functioning, pain-related symptoms and adverse events, family economic factors, and sleep.[81–83] Depending on the age and cognitive capacity of the child, assessment methods may vary, but it is important to include both child self-report and caregiver-proxy reports. Although caregiver and child reports are often correlated, discrepancies exist, and it is important to understand the child's perception of pain and pain-related impairment.[83,84]

DEVELOPMENT

A child's age and developmental stage play an important role in pain assessment and treatment. For younger children, it may be more difficult for them to express their pain and/or describe how pain impairs their functioning so it is important to use developmentally appropriate assessment[85] and include caregivers. During the adolescent period, adolescents typically have an increased need for autonomy, are more peer-focused, and spend more time with peers than with their caregivers. The presence of chronic pain challenges this developmental process, as most adolescents with chronic pain have to rely on caregivers to help manage treatment, and pain may limit their social engagement. When assessing chronic pain, it is important to consider the adolescents' autonomy and developmental challenges. For example, it is important to (1) obtain the adolescent's self-reported perspective on his/her pain symptoms, physical and social impairment, and family interactions without the caregiver present, and (2) obtain the caregiver's perspective with the adolescent present. The childhood and adolescent period is marked by changes in neurobiological and social development and increased nervous system plasticity.[86,87] For example, because of increased prefrontal cortex maturity, adolescents may be better able to participate in more complex pain coping strategies that require cognitive control and planning. With younger children, treatment requires more caregiver involvement in pain management. Thus, developmental stage should also be considered in treatment planning.

RELATIONSHIPS

Pediatric chronic pain exists within a family and social context, which can affect a child's experience of pain and pain management. Caregivers' pain beliefs and responses have been shown to affect pain responses in children; thus, psychoeducation surrounding the biopsychosocial conceptualization of chronic pain is an important part of pediatric chronic pain treatment.[88–90] Caregiver protective responses (e.g., attending to pain, giving special privileges) and pain catastrophizing are associated with child pain behaviors and coping.[91–93] Biopsychosocial-based psychoeducation can help caregivers understand the importance of shifting from "emergency, pain-relief mode" to a "return to normal mode" regardless of the pain. Caregivers' distress surrounding their child's pain must also be acknowledged and addressed.[94,95] Socially, children and adolescents with chronic pain often experience social impairment and limited peer social support, which can be particularly problematic during adolescence.[90] Thus, cognitive-behavioral treatment addresses the social functioning of children and adolescents with chronic pain and encourages peer engagement.

ACADEMICS

Chronic pain often limits a child's ability to attend school and participate in school activities, and can negatively affect cognitive functioning.[96,97] Assessment of academic functioning and coordinating school reintegration and accommodations are important components of treatment. Specifically, treatment includes assessment of academic and cognitive functioning (e.g., school absences, grades, school stressors, and neuropsychological assessment). Ongoing assessment of these factors can inform treatment, which often includes the child, caregivers, and school personnel. In coordination with teachers and school personnel, cognitive-behavioral treatment may include developing behavioral plans to encourage school attendance and school-focused coping skills training.

Collectively, children and adolescents can experience chronic pain, and ineffective treatment may increase the likelihood of pediatric chronic pain continuing into adulthood. Evidence supports the use of cognitive and behaviorally based psychological therapies in the treatment of pediatric chronic pain. Given that childhood and adolescence represent unique developmental periods, psychological chronic pain treatment should include an appreciation for developmental, family, social, and academic factors.

REFERENCES

1. Dahlhamer, J., J. Lucas, C. Zelaya, R. Nahin, S. Mackey, L. DeBar, R. Kerns, M. Von Korff, L. Porter, and C. Helmick. "Prevalence of Chronic Pain and High-Impact Chronic Pain Among Adults—United States, 2016." *MMWR. Morbidity and Mortality Weekly Report* 67(36), 2018: 1001.
2. Huguet, A., and J. Miró. "The Severity of Chronic Pediatric Pain: An Epidemiological Study." *Journal of Pain* 9(3), 2008: 226–236. pii:S1526-5900(07)00903-0. doi:10.1016/j.jpain.2007.10.015.
3. King, S., C.T. Chambers, A. Huguet, R.C. MacNevin, P.J. McGrath, L. Parker, and A.J. MacDonald. "The Epidemiology of Chronic Pain in Children and Adolescents Revisited: A Systematic Review." *Pain* 152(12), 2011: 2729–2738.
4. Brna, P., J. Dooley, K. Gordon, and T. Dewan. "The Prognosis of Childhood Headache: A 20-Year Follow-Up." *Archives of Pediatrics and Adolescent Medicine* 159(12), 2005: 1157–1160.
5. Walker, L.S., C.M. Dengler-Crish, S. Rippel, and S. Bruehl. "Functional Abdominal Pain in Childhood and Adolescence Increases Risk for Chronic Pain in Adulthood." *Pain* 150(3), 2010: 568–572.
6. Raja, Srinivasa N., Daniel B. Carr, Milton Cohen, Nanna B. Finnerup, Herta Flor, Stephen Gibson, Francis J. Keefe et al. "The Revised International Association for the Study of Pain Definition of Pain: Concepts, Challenges, and Compromises." *Pain* 161(9), 2020: 1976–1982.
7. Engel, G.L. "The Need for a New Medical Model: A Challenge for Biomedicine." *Science* 196(4286), 1977: 129–136.
8. Gatchel, R.J., D.D. McGeary, C.A. McGeary, and B. Lippe. "Interdisciplinary Chronic Pain Management: Past, Present, and Future." *American Psychologist* 69(2), 2014: 119.
9. Papadimitriou, G. "The Biopsychosocial Model 40 Years of Application in Psychiatry." *Psychiatrike* 28(2), 2017: 107–110.
10. Loeser, J.D.. Concepts of pain. In: Stanton-Hicks M., Boas R., eds. *Chronic Low Back Pain*. New York: Raven Press, 1982: 145–148.
11. Edwards, R.R., R.H. Dworkin, M.D. Sullivan, D.C. Turk, and A.D. Wasan. "The Role of Psychosocial Processes in the Development and Maintenance of Chronic Pain." *The Journal of Pain* 17(9), 2016: T70–T92.
12. Davin, S., J. Scheman, and E. Covington. "Psychological Management of Pain." In: Cheng J., Rosenquist, R.W., eds. *Fundamentals of PAIN Medicine*. Cham: Springer, 2018: 43–52.
13. Hung, C.-I., C.-Y. Liu, and T.-S. Fu. "Depression: An Important Factor Associated with Disability Among Patients with Chronic Low Back Pain." *The International Journal of Psychiatry in Medicine* 49(3), 2015: 187–198.
14. Melzack, R., and P.D. Wall. "Pain Mechanisms: A New Theory." *Science* 150(699), 1965: 971–979.
15. Melzack, R.. "From the Gate to the Neuromatrix." *Pain* 82(6), 1999: S121–S126.
16. Kucyi, A., and K.D. Davis. "The Dynamic Pain Connectome." *Trends in Neurosciences* 38(2), 2015: 86–95.
17. Bushnell, M.C., M. Čeko, and L.A. Low. "Cognitive and Emotional Control of Pain and Its Disruption in Chronic Pain." *Nature Reviews. Neuroscience* 14(7), 2013: 502.
18. Martucci, K.T., and S.C. Mackey. "Neuroimaging of PainHuman Evidence and Clinical Relevance of Central Nervous System Processes and Modulation." *Anesthesiology* 128(6), 2018: 1241–1254.
19. Simons, L., I. Elman, and D. Borsook. "Psychological Processing in Chronic Pain: A Neural Systems Approach." *Neuroscience and Biobehavioral Reviews* 2014: 61–78. https://doi.org/10.1016/j.neubiorev.2013.12.006.
20. Eccleston, C., and G. Crombez. "Pain Demands Attention: A Cognitive-Affective Model of the Interruptive Function of Pain." *Psychological Bulletin* 125(3), 1999: 356–366.
21. Moriarty, O., B.E. McGuire, and D.P. Finn. "The Effect of Pain on Cognitive Function: A Review of Clinical and Preclinical Research." *Progress in Neurobiology* 93(3), 2011: 385–404.
22. Borsook, D., C. Linnman, V. Faria, A.M. Strassman, L. Becerra, and I. Elman. "Reward Deficiency and Anti-Reward in Pain Chronification." *Neuroscience and Biobehavioral Reviews* 68, 2016: 282–297.

23. Zeidan, F., N.M. Emerson, S.R. Farris, J.N. Ray, Y. Jung, J.G. McHaffie, and R.C. Coghill. "Mindfulness Meditation-Based Pain Relief Employs Different Neural Mechanisms than Placebo and Sham Mindfulness Meditation-Induced Analgesia." *Journal of Neuroscience: The Official Journal of the Society for Neuroscience* 35(46), 2015: 15307–15325.

24. Zeidan, F., K.T. Martucci, R.A. Kraft, N.S. Gordon, J.G. McHaffie, and R.C. Coghill. "Brain Mechanisms Supporting the Modulation of Pain by Mindfulness Meditation." *Journal of Neuroscience* 31(14), 2011: 5540–5548.

25. Vanhaudenhuyse, A., M. Boly, E. Balteau [et al.] "Pain and Non-Pain Processing During Hypnosis: A Thulium-YAG Event-Related fMRI Study." *Neuroimage* 47(3), 2009: 1047–1054.

26. Derbyshire, S.W.G., M.G. Whalley, and D.A. Oakley. "Fibromyalgia Pain and Its Modulation by Hypnotic and Non-Hypnotic Suggestion: An fMRI Analysis." *European Journal of Pain* 13(5), 2009: 542–550.

27. Jensen, M.P., G.A. Jamieson, A. Lutz [et al.] "New Directions in Hypnosis Research: Strategies for Advancing the Cognitive and Clinical Neuroscience of Hypnosis." *Neuroscience of Consciousness* 3(1), 2017: nix004.

28. Cole, L.J., K.L. Bennell, Y. Ahamed, C. Bryant, F. Keefe, G. Lorimer Moseley, P. Hodges, and M.J. Farrell. "Determining Brain Mechanisms that Underpin Analgesia Induced by the Use of Pain Coping Skills." *Pain Medicine* 19(11), 2018: 2177–2190. https://doi.org/10.1093/pm/pnx301.

29. Jensen, K.B., E. Kosek, R. Wicksell, M. Kemani, G. Olsson, J.V. Merle, D. Kadetoff, and M. Ingvar. "Cognitive Behavioral Therapy Increases Pain-Evoked Activation of the Prefrontal Cortex in Patients with Fibromyalgeia." *Pain* 153(7), 2012: 1495–1503.

30. Seminowicz, D.A., M. Shpaner, M.L. Keaser, G.M. Krauthamer, J. Mantegna, J.A. Dumas, P.A. Newhouse, C.G. Filippi, F.J. Keefe, and M.R. Naylor. "Cognitive-Behavioral Therapy Increases Prefrontal Cortex Gray Matter in Patients with Chronic Pain." *The Journal of Pain* 14(12), 2013: 1573–1584. https://doi.org/10.1016/j.jpain.2013.07.020.

31. Villemure, C., and M.C. Bushnell. "Cognitive Modulation of Pain: How Do Attention and Emotion Influence Pain Processing?" *Pain* 95(3), 2002: 195–199.

32. Ehde, D.M., T.M. Dillworth, and J.A. Turner. "Cognitive-Behavioral Therapy for Individuals with Chronic Pain: Efficacy, Innovations, and Directions for Research." *American Psychologist* 69(2), 2014: 153.

33. California Code of Regulations, Title 8, Section 9792.24.4. Medical Treatment Utilization Schedule, Chronic Pain Medical Treatment Guidelines; Effective. July 28, 2016.

34. Butler, A.C., J.E. Chapman, E.M. Forman, and A.T. Beck. "The Empirical Status of Cognitive-Behavioral Therapy: A Review of Meta-Analyses." *Clinical Psychology Review* 26(1), 2006: 17–31.

35. Morley, S., C. Eccleston, and A. Williams. "Systematic Review and Meta-Analysis of Randomized Controlled Trials of Cognitive Behaviour Therapy and Behaviour Therapy for Chronic Pain in Adults, Excluding Headache." *Pain* 80(1–2), 1999: 1–13.

36. Turner, J.A., S. Holtzman, and L. Mancl. "Mediators, Moderators, and Predictors of Therapeutic Change in Cognitive–Behavioral Therapy for Chronic Pain." *Pain* 127(3), 2007: 276–286.

37. McCracken, L.M., F. MacKichan, and C. Eccleston. "Contextual Cognitive-Behavioral Therapy for Severely Disabled Chronic Pain Sufferers: Effectiveness and Clinically Significant Change." *European Journal of Pain* 11(3), 2007: 314–322.

38. Dysvik, E., J.T. Kvaløy, and G.K. Natvig. "The Effectiveness of an Improved Multidisciplinary Pain Management Programme: A 6- and 12-Month Follow-Up Study." *Journal of Advanced Nursing* 68(5), 2012: 1061–1072.

39. Fisher, E., L. Heathcote, T.M. Palermo, A.C. de C Williams, J. Lau, and C. Eccleston. "Systematic Review and Meta-Analysis of Psychological Therapies for Children with Chronic Pain." *Journal of Pediatric Psychology* 39(8), 2014: 763–782.

40. Levy, R.L., S.L. Langer, L.S. Walker, [et al.] "Twelve-Month Follow-Up of Cognitive Behavioral Therapy for Children with Functional Abdominal Pain." *JAMA Pediatrics* 167(2), 2013: 178–184.

41. Dozois, D.J.A., and A.T. Beck. "Cognitive Schemas, Beliefs and Assumptions." *Risk Factors in Depression* 2008: 119–143.

42. Turk, D.C., and E.S. Monarch. "Biopsychosocial Perspective on Chronic Pain." Psychological Approaches to Pain Management: A Practitioner's Handbook 2, 2002: 3–29.

43. Beck, J.S. *Cognitive Therapy: Basics and Beyond*. New York: Guilford Press, 1995.

44. Burns, D.D. *Feeling Good: The New Mood Therapy*. New York: William Morrow and Company Inc., 1980.

45. Sullivan, M.J.L., B. Thorn, J.A. Haythornthwaite, F. Keefe, M. Martin, L.A. Bradley, and J.C. Lefebvre. "Theoretical Perspectives on the Relation Between Catastrophizing and Pain." *The Clinical Journal of Pain* 17(1), 2001: 52–64.

46. Chapman, C.R., and A. Okifuji. "Pain: Basic Mechanisms and Conscious Experience." *Progress in PAIN Research and Management* 27, 2004: 3–28.

47. Sullivan, M.J.L., W. Stanish, H. Waite, M. Sullivan, and D.A. Tripp. "Catastrophizing, Pain, and Disability in Patients with Soft-Tissue Injuries." *Pain* 77(3), 1998: 253–260.

48. Severeijns, R., J.W.S. Vlaeyen, M.A. van den Hout, and W.E.J. Weber. "Pain Catastrophizing Predicts Pain Intensity, Disability, and Psychological Distress Independent of the Level of Physical Impairment." *The Clinical Journal of Pain* 17(2), 2001: 165–172.

49. Spinhoven, P., M. Ter Kuile, A.M.J. Kole-Snijders, M.H. Mansfeld, D.-J. Den Ouden, and J.W.S. Vlaeyen. "Catastrophizing and Internal Pain Control as Mediators of Outcome in the Multidisciplinary Treatment of Chronic Low Back Pain." *European Journal of Pain* 8(3), 2004: 211–219.

50. Smeets, R.J.E.M., A.C. Van Geel, A.D. Kester, and J.A. Knottnerus. "Physical Capacity Tasks in Chronic Low Back Pain: What is the Contributing Role of Cardiovascular Capacity, Pain and Psychological Factors?" *Disability and Rehabilitation* 29(7), 2007: 577–586.

51. Papaioannou, M., P. Skapinakis, D. Damigos, V. Mavreas, G. Broumas, and A. Palgimesi. "The Role of Catastrophizing in the Prediction of Postoperative Pain." *Pain Medicine* 10(8), 2009: 1452–1459.

52. Martel, M.O., A.D. Wasan, R.N. Jamison, and R.R. Edwards. "Catastrophic Thinking and Increased Risk for Prescription Opioid Misuse in Patients with Chronic Pain." *Drug and Alcohol Dependence* 132(1–2), 2013: 335–341.

53. Spinhoven, P., M.M. Ter Kuile, A. Corry, G. Linssen, and B. Gazendam. "Pain Coping Strategies in a Dutch Population of Chronic Low Back Pain Patients." *Pain* 37(1), 1989: 77–83.

54. Sullivan, M.J.L., S.R. Bishop, and J. Pivik. "The Pain Catastrophizing Scale: Development and Validation." *Psychological Assessment* 7(4), 1995: 524.

55. Guite, J.W., R.L. McCue, J.L. Sherker, D.D. Sherry, and J.B. Rose. "Relationships Among Pain, Protective Parental Responses, and Disability for Adolescents with Chronic Musculoskeletal Pain: The Mediating Role of Pain Catastrophizing." *The Clinical Journal of Pain* 27(9), 2011: 775–781.

56. Lynch-Jordan, A.M., S. Kashikar-Zuck, A. Szabova, and K.R. Goldschneider. "The Interplay of Parent and Adolescent Catastrophizing and Its Impact on Adolescents' Pain, Functioning, and Pain Behavior." *The Clinical Journal of Pain* 29(8), 2013: 681–688. https://doi.org/10.1097/AJP.0b013e3182757720.

57. Picavet, H., J. Susan, J.W.S. Vlaeyen, and J.S. Schouten. "Pain Catastrophizing and Kinesiophobia: Predictors of Chronic Low Back Pain." *American Journal of Epidemiology* 156(11), 2002: 1028–1034.

58. Keefe, F.J. "Cognitive Behavioral Therapy for Managing Pain." *The Clinical Psychologist* 49(3), 1996: 4–5.

59. Gil, K.M., D.A. Williams, F.J. Keefe, and J.C. Beckham. "The Relationship of Negative Thoughts to Pain and Psychological Distress." *Behavior Therapy* 21(3), 1990: 349–362.

60. Waters, S.J., L.C. Campbell, F.J. Keefe, and J.W. Carson. "The Essence of Cognitive-Behavioral Pain Management." *Progress in PAIN Research and Management* 27, 2004: 261–284.

61. Fordyce, W.E., R.S. Fowler, J.F. Lehmann, B.J. Delateur, P.L. Sand, and R.B. Treischmann. "Operant Conditioning in the Treatment of Chronic Pain." *Archives of Physical Medicine and Rehabilitation* 54(9), 1973: 399–408.

62. Leeuw, M., M.E.J.B. Goossens, G.J.P. van Breukelen, J.R. de Jong, P.H.T.G. Heuts, R.J.E.M. Smeets, A.J.A. Köke, and J.W.S. Vlaeyen. "Exposure In Vivo Versus Operant Graded Activity in Chronic Low Back Pain Patients: Results of a Randomized Controlled Trial." *Pain* 138(1), 2008: 192–207.

63. Nicholas, M.K., P.H. Wilson, and J. Goyen. "Operant-Behavioural and Cognitive-Behavioural Treatment for Chronic Low Back Pain." *Behaviour Research and Therapy* 29(3), 1991: 225–238.

64. Lethem, J., P.D. Slade, J.D. Troup, and G. Bentley. "Outline of a Fear-Avoidance Model of Exaggerated Pain Perception–I." *Behaviour Research and Therapy* 21(4), 1983: 401–408.

65. Macedo, L.G., R.J.E.M. Smeets, C.G. Maher, J. Latimer, and J.H. McAuley. "Graded Activity and Graded Exposure for Persistent Nonspecific Low Back Pain: A Systematic Review." *Physical Therapy* 90(6), 2010: 860–879.

66. George, S.Z., V.T. Wittmer, R.B. Fillingim, and M.E. Robinson. "Comparison of Graded Exercise and Graded Exposure Clinical Outcomes for Patients with Chronic Low Back Pain." *Journal of Orthopaedic and Sports Physical Therapy* 40(11), 2010: 694–704.

67. Perquin, C.W., A.A.J.M. Hazebroek-Kampschreur, J.A.M. Hunfeld, A.M. Bohnen, L.W.A. van Suijlekom-Smit, J. Passchier, and J.C. van der Wouden. "Pain in Children and Adolescents: A Common Experience." *Pain* 87(1), 2000: 51–58.

68. Roth-Isigkeit, A., U. Thyen, H. Stoven, J. Schwarzenberger, and P. Schmucker. "Pain Among Children and Adolescents: Restrictions in Daily Living and Triggering Factors." *Pediatrics* 115(2), 2005: e152.

69. Sil, S., L.L. Cohen, and C. Dampier. "Psychosocial and Functional Outcomes in Youth with Chronic Sickle Cell Pain." *The Clinical Journal of Pain* 32(6), 2016: 527–533.

70. Twycross, A., R. Parker, A. Williams, and F. Gibson. "Cancer-Related Pain and Pain Management Sources, Prevalence, and the Experiences of Children and Parents." *Journal of Pediatric Oncology Nursing* 32(6), 2015: 369–384.

71. Fortier, M.A., A. Wahi, C. Bruce, E.L. Maurer, and R. Stevenson. "Pain Management at Home in Children with Cancer: A Daily Diary Study." *Pediatric Blood and Cancer* 61(6), 2014: 1029–1033.

72. Cunningham, N.R., S. Nelson, A. Jagpal, E. Moorman, M. Farrell, S. Pentiuk, and S. Kashikar-Zuck. "Development of the Aim to Decrease Anxiety and Pain Treatment for Pediatric Functional Abdominal Pain Disorders." *Journal of Pediatric Gastroenterology and Nutrition* 66(1), 2018: 16–20. https://doi.org/10.1097/MPG.0000000000001714.

73. Kashikar-Zuck, S., A.M. Lynch, S. Slater, T.B. Graham, N.F. Swain, and R.B. Noll. "Family Factors, Emotional Functioning, and Functional Impairment in Juvenile Fibromyalgia Syndrome." *Arthritis and Rheumatism* 59(10), 2008: 1392–1398. https://doi.org/10.1002/art.24099.

74. McKillop, H.N., and G.A. Banez. "A Broad Consideration of Risk Factors in Pediatric Chronic Pain: Where to Go from Here?" *Children* 3(4), 2016: 38.

75. Gauntlett-Gilbert, J., and C. Eccleston. "Disability in Adolescents with Chronic Pain: Patterns and Predictors Across Different Domains of Functioning." *Pain* 131(1–2), 2007: 132–141.

76. Palermo, T.M., and C.T. Chambers. "Parent and Family Factors in Pediatric Chronic Pain and Disability: An Integrative Approach." *Pain* 119(1–3), 2005: 1–4.

77. Palermo, T.M. *Cognitive-Behavioral Therapy for Chronic Pain in Children and Adolescents*. New York: Oxford University Press, 2012.

78. Simons, L.E., and M.C. Basch. "State of the Art in Biobehavioral Approaches to the Management of Chronic Pain in Childhood." *Pain Management* 6(1), 2016: 49–61.

79. Eccleston, C., T. Palermo, A.C.D.C. Williams, A. Lewandowski, S. Morley, E. Fisher, and E. Law. "Psychological Therapies for the Management of Chronic and Recurrent Pain in Children and Adolescents." *Cochrane Database of Systematic Reviews* 12, 2012. http://onlinelibrary.wiley.com/doi/10.1002/14651858.CD003968.pub3/pdf/standard.

80. Zeltzer, L., and P. Zeltzer *Pain in Children and Young Adults: The Journey Back to Normal*. Encino, CA: Shilysca Press, 2016.

81. McGrath, P.J., G.A. Walco, D.C. Turk [et al.] "Core Outcome Domains and Measures for Pediatric Acute and Chronic/Recurrent Pain Clinical Trials: PedIMMPACT Recommendations." *The Journal of Pain* 9(9), 2008: 771–783.

82. Walco, G.A., H. Rozelman, and D.A. Maroof. "The Assessment and Management of Chronic and Recurrent Pain in Adolescents." In: *Behavioral Approaches to Chronic Disease in Adolescence: A Guide to Integrative Care*, edited by W.T. O'Donohue. New York: Springer, 2009: 163–175. https://doi.org/10.1007/978-0-387-87687-0_14.

83. Cohen, L.L., K. Lemanek, R.L. Blount, L.M. Dahlquist, C.S. Lim, T.M. Palermo, K.D. McKenna, and K.E. Weiss. "Evidence-Based Assessment of Pediatric Pain." *Journal of Pediatric Psychology* 33(9), 2007: 939–955.

84. Varni, J.W., D. Thissen, B.D. Stucky, Y. Liu, B. Magnus, J. He, E.M. DeWitt, D.E. Irwin, J.-S. Lai, and D. Amtmann. "Item-Level Informant Discrepancies between Children and Their Parents on the PROMIS® Pediatric Scales." Quality of Life Research 24(8), 2015: 1921–1937.

85. Palermo, T.M., C.R. Valrie, and C.W. Karlson. "Family and Parent Influences on Pediatric Chronic Pain: A Developmental Perspective." *American Psychologist* 69(2), 2014: 142.

86. Kadosh, K.C., D.E.J. Linden, and J.Y.F. Lau. "Plasticity During Childhood and Adolescence: Innovative Approaches to Investigating Neurocognitive Development." *Developmental Science* 16(4), 2013: 574–583. https://doi.org/10.1111/desc.12054.

87. Jolles, D.D., and E.A. Crone. "Training the Developing Brain: A Neurocognitive Perspective." *Frontiers in Human Neuroscience* 6(76), 2012: 76. https://doi.org/10.3389/fnhum.2012.00076.

88. Lewandowski, A.S., T.M. Palermo, J. Stinson, S. Handley, and C.T. Chambers. "Systematic Review of Family Functioning in Families of Children and Adolescents with Chronic Pain." *The Journal of Pain* 11(11), 2010: 1027–1038.

89. Eccleston, C., G. Crombez, A. Scotford, J. Clinch, and H. Connell. "Adolescent Chronic Pain: Patterns and Predictors of Emotional Distress in Adolescents with Chronic Pain and Their Parents." *Pain* 108(3), 2004: 221–229.

90. Forgeron, P., S. King, J.N. Stinson, P.J. McGrath, A.J. MacDonald, and C.T. Chambers. "Social Functioning and Peer Relationships in Children and Adolescents with Chronic Pain: A Systematic Review." *Pain Research and Management* 15(1), 2010: 27.

91. Wilson, A.C., A.S. Lewandowski, and T.M. Palermo. "Fear-Avoidance Beliefs and Parental Responses to Pain in Adolescents with Chronic Pain." *Pain Research and Management* 16(3), 2011: 178–182.

92. Caes, L., T. Vervoort, Z. Trost, and L. Goubert. "Impact of Parental Catastrophizing and Contextual Threat on Parents' Emotional and Behavioral Responses to Their Child's Pain." *Pain* 153(3), 2012: 687–695. https://doi.org/10.1016/j.pain.2011.12.007.

93. Simons, L.E., L. Goubert, T. Vervoort, and D. Borsook. "Circles of Engagement: Childhood Pain and Parent Brain." *Neuroscience and Biobehavioral Reviews* 68(September), 2016: 537–546. https://doi.org/10.1016/j.neubiorev.2016.06.020.

94. Palermo, T.M. "Impact of Recurrent and Chronic Pain on Child and Family Daily Functioning: A Critical Review of the Literature." *Journal of Developmental and Behavioral Pediatrics: JDBP* 21(1), 2000: 58.

95. Palermo, T.M., and C. Eccleston. "Parents of Children and Adolescents with Chronic Pain." *Pain* 146(1–2), 2009: 15–17. https://doi.org/10.1016/j.pain.2009.05.009.

96. Logan, D.E., L.E. Simons, and K.J. Kaczynski. "School Functioning in Adolescents with Chronic Pain: The Role of Depressive Symptoms in School Impairment." *Journal of Pediatric Psychology* 2009. https://doi.org/10.1093/jpepsy/jsn143.

97. Logan, D.E., L.E. Simons, and E.A. Carpino. "Too Sick for School? Parent Influences on School Functioning Among Children with Chronic Pain." *Pain* 153(2), 2012: 437–443.

Index

A

Aβ-fibers, 2
Accidental dependence, 360
Acetyl L-carnitine, 123–124, 313–314
Acupuncture, 125, 336
Acute *vs.* chronic pain, 371
Adaptive pain, 280
Adaptogens, 124
Addiction Severity Index (ASI), 349
Aδ-fibers, 2
Adenomyosis, 138
Adipose-derived stem cells, 224–225, 231–232
Adrenal adaptogen, 93
Adverse events (AEs), 286
Allogeneic-derived stem cells, 232–233
Alpha-lipoic acid, 217
Alzheimer disease (AD), 326–327
Ambroxol, 119, 299
Aminosalicylates (ASAs), 278
Amitriptyline, 146, 293
Amygdala, 266
Androgens, 67
Anti-inflammatory therapy, 325
Antiviral/cyclooxygenase inhibitor combination (IMC-1), 120
ASAM patient placement criteria, 352–353
ASAs, *see* Aminosalicylates
ASC, *see* Autism spectrum conditions
ASI, *see* Addiction Severity Index
Aspartame, 339
Asthma, 285
Autism spectrum conditions (ASC), 283
Autoimmune disease (AD)
    biochemical and physiologic changes, 78
    diagnostic stool analysis, 94–97
    diagnostic testing, 81–92
    etiology, 78–79
    food sensitivity test, 99–102
    immune system set point, 79–81, 104–106
    polyautoimmunity, 77
    potential testing limitations, 106
    provocative heavy metal test, 97–99
    salivary cortisol, 92–93
    traditional setting, 103
    treatment, 102–103
Autologous bone marrow mononuclear cells, 228
Autonomic nervous system, 11–13
Axons, 2–3

B

Baclofen, 148, 294
Basic fibroblast growth factor (b-FGF), 224
Bayesian model, 212
BBB, *see* Blood-brain barrier

BDNF, *see* Brain-derived neurotropic factor
Benzodiazepines, 260, 359–361, 363
Best corrected visual acuity (BCVA), 328
Beta glucuronidase, 96
6-Beta-naltrexol, 275
Bilstrom's nuclearitis, 104
Biocidin, 92
Biofeedback, 125, 208
Biomechanics, 183
Biopsychosocial model, 371–373
Biotensegrity
    anatomy and biomechanics, 183
    bodybuilder with degenerative arthrosis
        apprehension test, posterior pain and limited PROM, 179, 180
        glenohumeral arthrosis and limited AROM, 179
        MRI, 179, 181
        speed's test, pronated/internally rotated position, 179, 180
        speed's test, supinated/externally rotated position, 179, 180
    dynamic ultrasonography, 179–181
    fascia, body-wide signaling mechanism, 183
    history, 184
    ligaments, 186–187
    myofascial pain, 178
    neurologic control, 178
    orthopedic injury and neuromuscular dysfunction, 177
    physical exam, 184–186
    principles, 184
    restoration of tensional integrity, 188–190
    tensegrity theory, 181–183
    treatment, 187–188
Biotin, 315
Biotoxin illness, 214
Bladder dysfunction, 145
Blood–brain barrier (BBB), 12, 276–277
Bloodwork
    interpretation, 84–85
    men and women (fasting), 81, 82
    nutrients, 81–82
    treatment, 86–92
Bone marrow aspirate concentration (BMAC), 223–225, 228, 232
Bone marrow-derived stem cells, 224, 230–231
Bone marrow *vs.* adipose tissue, 227
Bone morphogenetic protein-2 (BMP-2), 224
Botulinum toxin type A, 157
Brain
    chronic neuropathic pain, 16
    ischemia, 326–327
    limbic system dysfunction, 17
    psychological intervention, 372–373
    thermal stimulation, 16
Brain-derived neurotropic factor (BDNF), 27, 28, 234–235
Brain–gut connection, 51

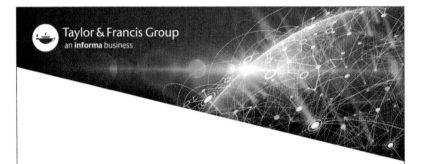

Printed and bound by CPI Group (UK) Ltd, Croydon, CR0 4YY

24/10/2024

01778286-0015